Handbook of binding and memory: perspectives from cognitive neuroscience

Handbook of binding and memory: perspectives from cognitive neuroscience

Edited by

Hubert D. Zimmer,

Department of Psychology, Brain and Cognition Unit,

Saarland University, Germany

Axel Mecklinger,

Department of Psychology, Experimental Psychology Unit,

Saarland University, Germany

and

Ulman Lindenberger,

Director, Center for Lifespan Psychology,

Max Planck Institute for Human Development, Germany

OXFORD

UNIVERSITY PRESS

OXFORD
UNIVERSITY PRESS

Great Clarendon Street, Oxford OX2 6DP

Oxford University Press is a department of the University of Oxford.
It furthers the University's objective of excellence in research, scholarship,
and education by publishing worldwide in

Oxford New York

Auckland Cape Town Dar es Salaam Hong Kong Karachi
Kuala Lumpur Madrid Melbourne Mexico City Nairobi
New Delhi Shanghai Taipei Toronto

With offices in

Argentina Austria Brazil Chile Czech Republic France Greece
Guatemala Hungary Italy Japan Poland Portugal Singapore
South Korea Switzerland Thailand Turkey Ukraine Vietnam

Oxford is a registered trade mark of Oxford University Press
in the UK and in certain other countries

Published in the United States
by Oxford University Press Inc., New York

First published 2006

British Library Cataloguing in Publication Data
Data available

Library of Congress Cataloging in Publication Data
Data available

Typeset by Newgen Imaging Systems (P) Ltd., Chennai, India
Printed in Great Britain
on acid-free paper by
Biddles Ltd., King's Lynn, UK

ISBN 0–19–852967–8 978–0–19–852967–5

10 9 8 7 6 5 4 3 2 1

Preface

The idea for this book originated at the conference *Binding in Human Memory: A Neurocognitive Approach,* which took place in 2002 at Saarland University in honour of Johannes Engelkamp and his contribution to memory psychology. The conference was also the opening event for Research Unit 448, 'Binding: Functional Architecture, Neural Correlates, and Ontogeny' funded by Deutsche Forschungsgemeinschaft (German Research Foundation). The aim of the conference was to establish the theoretical and empirical basis of a neurocognitive model of memory. For that purpose, the editors brought together two groups of researchers: those investigating memory processes mainly with experimental methods, and those using ERP/EEG and functional imaging techniques. The specific focus on binding was chosen because we consider this process a core operation in human cognitive and neural processing.

The conference strengthened our view that feature binding is a fundamental process in perception and memory, and that the exploration of binding mechanisms may help to extend our understanding of key memory processes such as encoding, consolidation, and retrieval. We asked the conference participants as well as a number of other researchers for contributions to a book on this topic. As the feedback from the authors and from the external reviewer was very positive, Oxford University Press decided that the book should be published.

The result is the present book comprising 28 chapters on aspects of binding in different domains of memory research. The main focus is the contribution of different medial temporal lobe structures to the retrieval of episodic information, and the role of familiarity and recollection in remembering. Another focus is the neural mechanisms of binding. In these chapters the authors discuss how binding might emerge from neural processing. A core concept in this regard is the synchronization of neural activity which may support different functions depending on synchronization frequency.

The contributions to this book provide an exhaustive survey of recent views on binding and its importance for remembering. In addition, they provide a promising approach offering an integrative view of the functions of binding in memory, as well as insights into the neural mechanisms which enable these processes. We hope that the book will enhance our understanding of binding and instigate new ideas in research.

Saarbrücken, 2006

Hubert D. Zimmer, Axel Mecklinger, and Ulman Lindenberger

Contents

Contributors

Lars Bäckman
Aging Research Center,
Department of Geriatric Epidemiology,
Neurotec, Karolinska Institute,
Stockholm, Sweden

Karl-Heinz Bäuml
Department of Experimental
Psychology, Regensburg University,
93040 Regensburg, Germany

Moshe Naveh-Benjamin
Department of Psychological Sciences,
University of Missouri,
106 McAlester Hall,
Columbia, MO 65211, USA

Jochen Brandstädter
Department of Psychology,
University of Trier,
D-54286 Trier, Germany

Gordon D. A. Brown
Department of Psychology,
University of Warwick, UK

M. W. Brown
MRC Centre for Synaptic Plasticity,
Department of Anatomy, School of
Medical Sciences,
University of Bristol,
Bristol, BS8 1TD, UK

Neil Burgess
Institute of Cognitive Neuroscience,
and Department of Anatomy and
Developmental Biology,
University College London,
17 Queen Square,
London WC1N 3AR, UK

Karin M. Butler
Department of Psychology,
University of New Mexico,
Albuquerque, NM 87131, USA

Roberto Cabeza
Center for Cognitive Neuroscience,
Duke University,
Durham, NC 27708, USA

Daniel M. Cer
Department of Psychology,
University of Colorado Boulder,
345 UCB, Boulder,
CO 80309, USA

Fergus I. M. Craik
Rotman Research Institute,
Baycrest Centre,
3560 Bathurst Street,
Toronto, M6A 2E1, Canada

Tim Curran
Department of Psychology,
University of Colorado,
HUCB 345,
Boulder, CO 80309–0345, USA

Courtney C. Dornburg
Sandia Natiónal Laboratories,
PO Box 5800, Mail Stop 0830,
Albuquerque, NM 87185, USA

Emrah Düzel
Department of Neurology II,
Otto-von-Guericke University,

Leipziger Straße 44, 39120
Magdeburg, Germany

Howard Eichenbaum
Center for Memory and Brain,
Boston University,
Boston, MA 02215, USA

Laura L. Eldridge
Department of Psychology,
University of California
at Los Angeles, Los Angeles,
CA, USA

Jürgen Fell
Department of Epileptology,
University of Bonn,
Sigmund-Freud Straße 25, D-53105
Bonn, Germany

Guillén Fernández
F.C. Donders Centre for Cognitive
Neuroimaging,
PO Box 9101, 6500 HB Nijmegen,
The Netherlands

David Friedman
Cognitive Electrophysiology
Laboratory, 1051 Riverside Drive,
Unit 6, New York,
NY 10032, USA

Esther Fujiwara
Department of Physiological
Psychology, University of Bielefeld,
University of Bielefeld,
PO Box 100131, D-33501 Bielefeld,
Germany

Sebastian Guderian
Department of Neurology II,
Otto-von-Guericke University,
Leipziger Straße 44, 39120
Magdeburg, Germany

Kerstin Jost
Experimental and Biological Psychology,
Philipps University, 35032 Marburg,
Germany

John A. King
Institute of Cognitive Neuroscience,
and Department of Anatomy and
Developmental Biology,
University College London,
17 Queen Square,
London WC1N 3AR, UK

Wolfgang Klimesch
Department of Physiological
Psychology,
University of Salzburg,
Institute of Psychology,
Hellbrunnerstraße 34, A-5020
Salzburg, Austria

Barbara J. Knowlton
Department of Psychology,
University of California
at Los Angeles, Los Angeles, CA, USA

Neal E. A. Kroll
Department of Psychology,
University of California Davis,
One Shields Avenue,
Davis, CA 95616, USA

Shu-Chen Li
Center for Lifespan Psychology,
Max Planck Institute for Human
Development,
Lentzeallee 94, D-14195 Berlin,
Germany

Ulman Lindenberger
Centre for Lifespan Psychology,
Max Planck Institute for Human
Development, D-14195 Berlin, and

School of Psychology, Saarland University, D-66041 Saarbrücken, Germany

Phan Luu
Electrical Geodesics Inc., University of Oregon, Eugene, OR, USA

Hans J. Markowitsch
Department of Physiological Psychology, University of Bielefeld, PO Box 100131, D-33501 Bielefeld, Germany

Teresa McCormack
Department of Psychology, Queen's University, Belfast, UK

Mark A. McDaniel
Department of Psychology, Washington University in St Louis, One Brookings Drive, St Louis, MO 63130, USA

Axel Mecklinger
Experimental Neuropsychology Unit, Saarland University, D-66041 Saarbrücken, Germany

Jaap M. J. Murre
Department of Psychology, University of Amsterdam, Roetersstraat 15, 1018 WB Amsterdam, The Netherlands

Markus Neufang
Department of Neurology II, Otto-von-Guericke University, Leipziger Straße 44, 39120 Magdeburg, Germany

Michael Niedeggen
Experimental Psychology, Heinrich Heine University, 40225 Düsseldorf, Germany

Lars Nyberg
Department of Radiation Sciences and Integrative Medical Biology, Umeå University, Sweden

Randall C. O'Reilly
Department of Psychology, University of Colorado Boulder, 345 UCB, Boulder, CO 80309, USA

Ken A. Paller
Institute for Neuroscience and Department of Psychology, 2029 Sheridan Road, Northwestern University, Evanston, IL 60208-2710, USA

Carley Piatt
Department of Psychology, University of Victoria, Victoria, BCV8W3P5 Canada

Joel R. Quamme
Department of Psychology, Green Hall, Princeton University, Princeton, NJ 08540, USA

Antonino Raffone
Business School, University of Sunderland, Reg Vardy Centre, St Peter's Way, Sunderland, SR6 ODD, UK

Frank Rösler
Experimental and Biological Psychology,
Philipps University,
35032 Marburg, Germany

Klaus Rothermund
Department of Psychology,
University of Trier, D-54286 Trier,
Germany

Brent J. Small
School of Aging Studies,
MHC1346,
University of South Florida,
4202 East Fowler Ave.,
Tampa, FL 33620, USA

Hugo J. Spiers
Functional Imaging Laboratory,
Wellcome Department of Imaging
Neuroscience,
University College London,
12 Queen Square,
London WC1N 3BG, UK

Katharine L. Tepe
Department of Psychology,
University of Colorado,
HUCB 345,
Boulder, CO 80309–0345, USA

Anne Treisman
Department of Psychology,
Green Hall,
Princeton University,
Princeton, NJ 08544, USA

Iris Trinkler
Institute of Cognitive Neuroscience,
and Department of Anatomy and
Developmental Biology,
University College London,
17 Queen Square,
London WC1N 3AR, UK

Don M. Tucker
Electrical Geodesics Inc.,
University of Oregon,
Eugene, OR, USA

Andreas Voss
Department of Psychology,
Albert-Ludwigs-Universität
Freiburg, Social Psychology
and Statistics,
79085 Freiburg, Germany

E. C. Warburton
MRC Centre for Synaptic Plasticity,
Department of Anatomy,
School of Medical Sciences,
University of Bristol,
Bristol, BS8 1TD, UK

Gezinus Wolters
Department of Cognetive Psychology,
University of Leiden,
Po Box 9500, 2300 RA Leiden,
The Netherlands

Andrew P. Yonelinas
Department of Psychology,
University of California Davis,
One Shields Avenue,
Davis, CA 95616, USA

Hubert D. Zimmer
Cognitive Psychology: Brain and
Cognition Unit,
Saarland University, D-66041
Saarbrücken, Germany

Abbreviations

ACC	anterior cingulate cortex
ADH	associative deficit hypothesis
ANOVA	analysis of variance
BOLD signal	blood oxygenation-dependent signal
CCDR	coarse-coded distributed representation
CLS	complementary learning systems model
CRT	choice reaction time
CSD	current source density
DA	divided attention
Dm	difference in subsequent memory
DRM	Deese–Roediger–McDermott
DTI	diffusion tensor imaging
efMRI	event-related functional MRI
EM	episodic memory
ERBP	event-related band power
ERD	event-related desynchronization
ERN	error-related negativity
ERP	event-related potential
ERS	event-related synchronization
FA	full attention
FF	frontal function
Fmq	frontal midline theta
HERA	hemispheric encoding–retrieval asymmetry
IM	item memory
ISI	inter-stimulus interval
ITC	inferotemporal cortex
LFP	local field potential
LIPC	left inferior prefrontal cortex
LPC	late positive component
LPN	late posterior negativity
LTD	long-term depotentiation
LTM	long-term memory
LTP	long-term potentiation
MFN	medial frontal negativity
MS/DBv	medial septum/vertical limb
MTL	medial temporal lobe
MTLH	medial temporal–hippocampal
NMDA	*N*-methyl-D-aspartate
PET	positron-emission tomography
PFC	prefrontal cortex
PLS	partial least-squares
RA	retrograde amnesia
RM	relational memory
ROC	receiver operating characteristic
RPO	pontis oralis nucleus
RT	response time, reaction time
SAM model	search of associative memory model
SIMPLE model	scale-invariant memory, perception, and learning model
SMA	supplementary motor area
SME	subsequent memory effect
SNRGE	specialized neural regions for global efficiency
STDP	spike-timing-dependent Hebbian plasticity
SUM	supramammillary nucleus

TODAM	theory of distributed associative memory
VCM	virtual context-dependent memory
VR	virtual reality
VTA	ventral tegmental area
WAIS-R	Wechsler Adult Intelligence Scale Revised
WM	working memory
WMH	white matter hyperintensity
WMS-III	Wechsler Memory Scale III

Introduction

Chapter 1

Levels of binding: types, mechanisms, and functions of binding in remembering

Hubert D. Zimmer, Axel Mecklinger, and Ulman Lindenberger

Introduction

When considering binding one might first think of perception and not memory, because the problem of binding is most frequently discussed at lower perceptual processing levels in which elementary stimulus features are encoded (Kanwisher and Driver 1992). If it is assumed that different features are separately represented in a distributed neural structure, a problem arises if more than one object is in view, namely, how to represent the fact that a set of specific features belongs to object A, and others, although active at the same time, belong to object B (Treisman 1996). This problem of analysing and representing relations among features is not restricted to perception, but is a general problem of cognitive processing. In thinking, remembering, and knowledge representation, features are processed within distributed systems as sets of separate units in a highly parallel way. As a consequence, elements belonging to the same cognitive 'event' have to be bound and separated from other features belonging to a different 'event'. Similarly, during enactment, binding is necessary in the form of attachment of task-relevant features to the intended action (see Chapter 13). Finally, memories are traces of processes performed during encoding, and therefore binding mechanisms strongly specify the input to memory. Moreover, binding may even be highly relevant for consolidation of distinctive memory traces and for retrieval because features have to be re-bound at the time of remembering (Nader 2003). Hence, the binding problem is a ubiquitous one that has to be solved in perception and in action; it is also a problem in memory because binding of features is necessary during encoding, consolidation, and retrieval.

Therefore we consider binding mechanisms to be basic operations of cognitive systems, performing different functions at various processing levels, with their efficiencies being a limiting factor for a number of mental processes. If this is correct, factors that either enhance or impair the efficacy of binding may explain much of the variance in performance between different situations, between different individuals, and over the lifespan. Therefore changes in binding processes may explain changes in a wide range of behaviour, and knowing how the neural system enables binding at various levels would enable us to closely relate cognitive performances to neural mechanisms. Hence, in our view, an adequate conception of binding is a cornerstone of a neurocognitive model of memory. This book should contribute to the grounding of such a model.

A selective view of the history of binding

Assuming that memory entries are made up of bound features is not a new idea. In many theories, memory entries are treated as sets of attributes which must be grouped in some way in order to constitute distinctive episodes. An early example is the suggestion of associative memory (Underwood 1969); other examples are formal models of memory, such as the search of associative memory (SAM) model (Raaijmakers and Shiffrin 1980) and the various types of 'vector' models (e.g. the theory of distributed associative memory (TODAM) (Murdock 1993)) which represent an event as a vector of features.

Similarly, the idea of conjoining attributes to units is not new in memory research (Ceraso 1985). For instance, the concept of 'chunking' (Miller 1956) refers to a binding effect. Entities are grouped by some mechanism to form larger entities, which can be used as units in further processing (if binding is successful). Grouping also has an important role in SAM theory (Raaijmakers and Shiffrin 1980); units are formed by association of concepts in working memory, and they strongly influence retrieval. Similarly, the problem of binding is explicitly addressed in vector models (Humphreys *et al.* 1994). Empirically, binding in mental processes has been investigated in a number of different experimental paradigms. Garner's research on integrated and separable dimensions is a good example of the investigation of binding in perception (e.g. Garner 1974). The work of Asch *et al.* (1960) on memory for unitary versus separate stimuli and the work of Jones (1976) on feature binding in memory retrieval are examples of behavioural studies on binding in memory. The best known research is probably that on feature integration (Treisman and Gelade 1980); for a summary and an extension, see Chapter12.

Obviously, considering memory entries not as holistic units but as sets of separate features is a relatively common assumption in psychology, and as a consequence some kind of binding mechanism must often be assumed. What is new in recent research is the attempt to search for neurophysiological correlates of these mechanisms and to disclose binding processes at the neural level. When representing entities in distributed neural nets, one has to solve the problem of indicating which elements belong to each other. Since the 1980s this topic has been explicitly addressed in neuropsychological and computational models as 'the binding problem' (e.g. Damasio 1989).

Several suggestions as to how the brain solves this problem have been made (e.g. von der Malsburg 1995). The most popular explanation currently is **temporal synchronization** of the discharges of individual and feature-specific neurons which form dynamic cell assemblies (Singer *et al.* 1997). Synchronization within cell assemblies was first used to model the perception of objects (Hummel and Biederman 1992), and physiological evidence for the synchronization of oscillating neural patterns has been reported for both animals (Engel *et al.* 1991, 1992) and humans (reviewed by Tallon-Baudry and Bertrand 1999). Synchronization has also been suggested as a mechanism for other kinds of binding, including task sets in actions (von Stein *et al.* 2000), binding before and during voluntary movements (Tallon-Baudry and Bertrand 1999), and binding in memory, as discussed in several contributions to this book (e.g. Chapter 9). Dynamic binding by synchronized cell assemblies may even play an important role in consciousness (Singer 2001).

Whereas with synchronization a fundamental mechanism for binding is in focus, other equally important aspects concern the neural structures that mediate binding and their relations with different types of binding. From this perspective, it is of interest to establish whether qualitatively different forms of binding exist, and whether they are provided by different neural structures. For example, it has been proposed that the frequency of the oscillatory patterns in which synchronization is observed decreases as one proceeds from low to higher processing levels (Singer *et al.* 1997). It follows that injuries to specific brain structures should lead to impairments in performing specific tasks, depending upon the forms of binding that are affected. From the viewpoint of memory, an interesting distinction in this respect is that between **recollection** and **familiarity** in remembering (reviewed by Yonelinas 2002), and their neural implementation. The importance of these processes for the understanding of remembering is reflected by the fact that this distinction is a central topic of many chapters in this book.

As early as 1980, Mandler had suggested that recognition can be based on either a feeling of familiarity, caused by integration of item-specific information without any context association, or recollection, which includes retrieving the context of an item, giving the individual a strong impression of when and where it was previously encountered. Stimulated by this proposal, several experimental paradigms were suggested to distinguish these subcomponents of recognition memory. According to Tulving (1985) and Gardiner (reviewed by Gardiner and

Richardson-Klavehn 2000), different types of subjective awareness are associated with both types of recognition, i.e. **remembering** and **knowing.** Because this classification is based on self-reports in recognition memory tasks, it is called the first-person view of memory. Subjects label a memory 'remembered' when they consciously retrieve specific contextual details of a study episode, and 'known' when they feel familiar with the event but are not able to retrieve any contextual details of its prior occurrence. Because the remember–know procedure is easy to use, it has become quite popular in experimental memory research. Another procedure is estimating familiarity and recollection from **receiver operating characteristics** (ROC), sometimes called memory operating curves, which are constructed by plotting memory performance as a function of response confidence that participants assign to their recognition judgements (Yonelinas 1994; see also Chapter 17).

Jacoby (1991) had less confidence in individuals' introspective abilities. He developed the **process-dissociation procedure** for estimating the contribution of familiarity (automatic retrieval) and recollection. Participants study two lists and are then assigned to one of two test conditions. In the inclusion condition, they have to accept all old items and reject new ones. In the exclusion condition, they have to discriminate between lists and accept only items from one list, while rejecting those from the second list together with new items. In the inclusion condition, familiarity and recollection work in concert. In the exclusion condition, particularly when considering the items from the to-be-rejected list, the two processes work in opposition. Performance in both tasks is used to estimate the contribution of both components to recognition judgements. Erroneously accepted old items from the to-be-rejected list indicate that the item evokes familiarity but no recollection. Stimulated by Jacoby's proposal, multinomial approaches to modelling participants' decisions have been developed which give better estimations of familiarity and recollection, and which also take guessing into account (Buchner *et al.* 1997).

Finally, research on **source memory** needs to be discussed in this context. Studies on source memory distinguish between item memory and memory for the context in which the item was presented (i.e. its source). Research on source memory has isolated many factors that differently influence item and source memory, and thus has demonstrated that these are two separable aspects of remembering (reviewed by Johnson *et al.* 1993). Ageing, for example, exerts differential influences on item and source memory. In childhood and old age, source memory is more strongly impaired than item memory (Czernochowski *et al.* 2005; reviewed by Zacks *et al.* 2000). The association-deficit hypothesis of memory in the elderly (Naveh-Benjamin 2000) generalizes this aspect of binding between items in general (see Chapter 25) and binding of features within items (Chalfonte and Johnson 1996; see also Chapter 11). Based on such results, Johnson and Chalfonte (1994) postulated that for the conscious binding of information, as in source memory, specific higher mental processes are necessary. The concept of levels of binding described by Craik (Chapter 23) develops this idea further.

Item and source memory also differ with respect to **retrieval requirements**. Successful memory performance requires the initiation and maintenance of task-specific retrieval strategies, for which prefrontal brain areas are relevant. Several recent studies that examined neural activity in the test phase of item and source memory tasks found pronounced differences in event-related potentials (ERPs) over frontal scalp regions (Senkfor and Van Petten 1998; reviewed by Rugg and Wilding 2000). Similarly, the requirement to retrieve item-context bindings (as in source memory tasks) gives rise to a pronounced negative ERP slow wave over posterior parietal regions, which is known as the late posterior negativity (LPN). It starts around the time of the subject's response and is absent when items rather than attribute conjunctions have to be retrieved. It has been proposed that the LPN may reflect the search for or retrieval of attribute conjunctions from long-term memory (reviewed by Johansson and Mecklinger 2003).

In addition to experimental memory research, progress in **cognitive neuroscience** and new methodological developments in functional brain imaging have promoted research on familiarity, recollection, and binding mechanisms. Cognitive brain research quickly expanded and obtained increasing evidence that different states of remembering are mediated by different brain systems and binding mechanisms. Early indications of the relevance of specific brain structures for memory came from patient HM, who suffered anterograde amnesia after resection of medio-temporal brain areas for treatment of epilepsy (Milner 1958). Later, more differentiated analyses of the effects of selective impairments of memory revealed that specific brain areas are relevant for different memory processes and binding mechanisms. Mayes *et al.* (2004) described patient YR, who had suffered a selective bilateral hippocampus atrophy which left adjacent temporal lobe structures unaffected. She showed a selective deficit in a subgroup of association memory tests requiring the binding of items of different kinds, whereas her memory for items and intra-item associations was largely unaffected. This suggests that, while the hippocampus is engaged in the encoding and retrieval of memory records composed of arbitrary features, adjacent medial temporal lobe structures may mediate binding of features within an item and representations of unitized associations. This form of binding is preserved after hippocampal damage and may give rise to a familiarity signal in the respective brain structures.

In this view, the hippocampus appears to be specifically relevant for recollection, whereas perirhinal structures provide the familiarity signal (Aggleton and Brown 1999; for an updated review see Chapter 16). However, alternative positions have also been put forward, as demonstrated in Chapter 19. Two main controversies can be noted. The first refers to the relevance of the hippocampus for non-episodic declarative memory, i.e. semantic memory (see Chapter 2). The second addresses the issue of whether familiarity and recollection are qualitatively different memory states in the sense that they are mediated by different brain structures and binding mechanisms, or whether they are quantitatively different expressions of one and the same declarative memory system. Proponents of the latter position quote in support of their view that hippocampal impairment influences not only recall, i.e. recollection, but also recognition, i.e. familiarity (Wixted and Squire 2004).

While these ideas about the brain systems mediating memory processes were originally derived from neuropsychological case studies and animal research, this situation was strongly changed by the development of functional brain imaging techniques. Currently, we have excellent techniques for observing neural processes correlated with memory function, with sufficiently high spatial and temporal resolution in healthy participants. ERPs allow resolution of the temporal dynamics of encoding and retrieval processes (Friedman and Johnson 2000; Mecklinger 2000), and event-related fMRI enables identification of the neural structures involved in these processes during encoding (Wagner *et al.* 1999) and retrieval (see Chapter20). Many examples of both methodological approaches can be found in the contributions to Parts 4 and 5.

Types of binding

Before giving an overview of the book's central topics, we will examine more closely the differences between types of binding. Although we are interested in binding mechanisms in memory, we will start with encoding and hence with perception. The simplest case is perception of an isolated object presented on an unstructured background, but even here binding is necessary. It is assumed that in perception different features, such as colour, shape, location, etc., are processed in parallel in distributed networks. The relations between these features have to be processed by means of synchronized activity within a cell assembly, giving rise to a coherent percept. Treisman postulated that these features are collected in an object file (e.g. Kahneman *et al.* 1992). She suggests that these files, called object tokens when representing specific objects, are the units of both working memory and long-term memory (see Chapter 12). Therefore **'binding of features within object tokens'** is the first type of binding relevant for memory. Presumably, it operates automatically during perception if objects are attended to and separated as figures from the ground (O'Craven *et al.* 1999).

When more than one object is in view, binding between objects is required. This can be considered a higher type of binding because object tokens, the units of elementary binding processes, are themselves bound into assemblies. Context can be treated like an object; therefore between-item and item-context binding might be provided by the same process. However, one might even go one step further and classify any binding operation between explicitly encoded units, thus having the status of declarative knowledge, as between-item binding. Cabeza (Chapter 24) calls tasks in which one asks for the existence of specific information 'relational memory tasks', in order to distinguish them from item memory tasks in which relational information is not task relevant. Following his suggestion, we will call these forms of binding **'relational binding'**. Cabeza also shows that the distinction between item and relational memory is highly relevant for memory performances. However, he also demonstrates that, within relational binding, different types of relations show different effects (see also Chapter 3). Examples of features that have specific relational qualities are information on an item's perceptual characteristics, the perceptual elaboration of an item, the generation of cross-modal information, the processing of spatial relational information, the item context, and temporal relational information. According to this analysis, it is not justified to consider all types of relational binding as equivalent, although they are frequently treated as homogeneous. One consequence of this shortcoming is that in experimental research, the features which are critical for relational binding are often selected by chance and are rarely systematically compared because differences are not considered.

A further relevant dimension for the analysis of binding arises from the fact that objects and items are usually embedded in larger units. This may be a scene or an event. Therefore it is all but clear what the actual item is (see also Chapter 10). Hence, it is important to know the characteristics which define an item and the border between item and context. Depending on the task characteristics, either the item alone or the item together with spatial, temporal, or any other contextual features may constitute the object. If indeed within-item and between-item binding effects differ, and thus the outcome depends on whether elementary features are processed as part of the same or of different items, then this border is critical (see also Chapter 26). The following example illustrates this point: Yonelinas *et al.* (1999) presented upright or upside-down faces and changed the combination of inner and outer features of faces from study to test.

At test, old faces were to be discriminated either from completely new faces or from faces constructed by rearranging features from different old faces. As participants had to discriminate between the same and recombined features, the test was classified as an associative memory test and thus was based on relational binding. There was a contribution of familiarity to recognition, estimated from ROC curves, when the faces were presented upright but not when they were presented upside down. Yonelinas *et al.* suggested that an influence of familiarity on associative recognition can be found for unitized associations, i.e. if 'items' (the features of a face in this experiment) can be treated as coherent wholes. Putting it differently, in an upright orientation faces are items, whereas when they are presented upside down, features are items. The former characteristic causes within-item binding that supports familiarity-based recognition, whereas the latter causes between-item binding and recollection-based recognition.

Thus in order to predict memory effects as a function of binding, we should know the relevant factors that constitute an item. Perceptual characteristics are one defining factor, as was shown in the experiment of Yonelinas *et al.* From this perspective, object tokens (see Chapter 12) are a good starting point for the definition of within-item binding. However, any features even across processing modalities can be constituent elements of an item, and when their relations allow grouping into a unitized association they are subject of within-item binding processes (Mayes *et al.* 2004).

Thus object tokens can be bound by relational binding into larger units, which can be called episodic tokens. Object tokens generated within a perceptual modality may influence familiarity via perirhinal structures, whereas episodic tokens need relational binding via hippocampal structures and influence recollection (Ecker *et al.* 2004). However, because objects are partially defined by interacting bottom-up and top-down processes, not only perceptual factors, but also **subject's task** and **pre-existing knowledge** contribute to the definition of an item (see also the discussion of levels of binding in Chapter 23). Therefore semantic knowledge can influence whether features are processed as within-item or between-item information. Consistent with this view, Czernochowski *et al.* (2005) recently reported an ERP correlate of familiarity for learned materials that had to be rejected in the test phase of an exclusion task, even though study and test materials were presented in different modalities (see also Nessler *et al.* (2005) for an evaluation of the putative ERP correlates of familiarity and semantic knowledge).

A third factor that plays a critical role in binding is **attention**. Because attention is often considered the glue that binds features to object tokens, one may even consider it a precondition for binding. However, attention is not a homogeneous construct either, and it also influences memory in different ways. An effect of attention on binding at the object level was demonstrated by Reinitz and Hannigan (2001). In a sequential presentation, they found enhanced false conjunctions in face recognition when the two faces from which the rearranged features were taken were presented in an interleaved fashion so that attention switched back and forth between them during encoding. Another example is the effect of attention on relational binding in a divided attention task. It has been shown that dividing attention during encoding influences the putative ERP correlates of recollection but not familiarity (Curran 2004). In addition, the selective association deficit shown by elderly people is sometimes attributed to a selective impairment of relational binding caused by an attentional deficit. However, inconsistent with this position, young adults show equal impairment in the learning of item versus relational information under divided attention (see Chapter 25). Finally, during retrieval, attentional processes are necessary for setting up retrieval strategies and adapting retrieval to the current task demands. Therefore attention may influence memory in many ways.

The brain not only has to solve the task of binding the episodic features to items and separating different items within an episode, but also has to maintain the distinction between **episodic** and **semantic representations**, the type-token problem. Seeing a deviant exemplar, for example a blue banana, should set up a specific episodic entry, but it should not instantly change the type representation so that from this time on it is assumed bananas were blue. One solution to this problem is postulating different learning mechanisms for episodic and semantic networks (McClelland and Rumelhart 1985; see also Chapter 8). This also has consequences for the question of binding in memory. Binding of sensory features in episodic tasks should be distinguished from changes of binding in semantic representations, which are probably the basis of repetition priming (Groh-Bordin *et al.* 2005). These differences may also explain why amnesics show repetition priming effects and why they can acquire semantic knowledge (see Chapter 19).

Finally, types of binding should be differentiated in the **temporal domain**, and this should be done in at least two ways. Thus the temporal domain should be considered both as a dimension of encoding and referring to the duration of retention. The temporal encoding dimension is discussed by Brown and McCormack in Chapter 10. They suggest that time, similar to space, plays a privileged role in memory binding. Time stamps may define memory events. The temporal duration refers to the difference between temporary and long-term binding (see Chapter 9). An example of a transient process is the binding of features of seen objects during perception. Other examples are the binding of stimulus-response codes when actions are performed (Hommel 1998; Hommel *et al.* 2001) and the separation of different streams of parallel processes in a multitasking system, which also makes it necessary to bind same-goal processes. In the latter case, the prefrontal cortex probably plays a critical role (see Chapter 26). Binding for long-term remembering is a different issue. One aspect is that the neural synchronization suggested for temporary binding has to be transformed into a more durable form of representation because otherwise, when synchronization is gone, the brain is left without a trace (Wagner 2001). For this purpose, some form of consolidation must occur. Long-range cross-cortical coordination has been discussed as a relevant factor for consolidation (Paller 2000; see also Chapter 21). Synchronization may also play an important role in this process, but it may operate at other frequency ranges than synchronization in local binding (see Chapter 5). Another aspect is that consolidation may not be achieved immediately, but in a sequence of processing steps.

Considering these different aspects of binding, it is obvious that binding in human memory is a multifaceted research topic. Several different forms of binding exist, associated with different processes. Craik (see Chapter 23) coined the term 'levels of binding' to illustrate the hierarchical organization of these processes, starting with low-level perceptual binding mechanisms, continuing with the encoding of events requiring the binding of more complex constellations of features and making necessary between-item binding, and ending at a relatively context-free semantic encoding. The levels of this hierarchy may be associated with several trade-offs. Low-level encoding is rather automatic and presumably determined by the discharges of feature-selective neurons. Thereby, the response properties of the neurons provide much direct support for grouping, so that no additional cues are necessary during encoding. In contrast, high-level encoding is more effortful and context dependent, and therefore is in need of environmental support. Ageing effects are also rank-ordered along this dimension. In good agreement with the idea of such a hierarchy, Cabeza (Chapter 24) demonstrates that a well-functioning prefrontal cortex determines higher forms of between-item binding, whereas the efficiency of these brain structures is less important for within-item binding.

We can go one step further. At the computational level, Li and Lindenberger (Chapter 11) show that between-item binding (association) can be selectively impaired while leaving within-item binding intact. One critical variable in their model is the gain parameter, i.e. the adjustment of connections between units according to the feedback during learning. If they are correct and gain is related to the availability of specific neurotransmitters, the efficiency of between-item binding would finally be limited by a neurochemical factor.

In summary, differences between types of binding seem to exist at all levels of analysis. At the behavioural level, we find differences according to the types of binding that are task relevant, and from a first-person viewpoint these different types of binding are associated with different states of experience. Correlates of these processes can be found in electrophysiological signals of familiarity and recollection. Different neural structures (the perirhinal structures and the hippocampus, respectively) are suggested as sources of these electrophysiological changes. Results from brain imaging as well as neuropsychological case studies are in good agreement with these assumptions. Additionally, prefrontal brain areas seem to be relevant for active volitional binding during encoding and for an adjustment of retrieval orientation. These processes modulate the mediotemporal binding mechanisms. Analogous differences may exist in computational modelling, with more or less straightforward relations to neurochemical mechanisms. The latter differences would explain why binding processes can be selectively and gradually impaired without specific damage to the hippocampus. The contributions to this book develop these different views and demonstrate that we have made a real step forward in grounding a neurocognitive model of binding in memory.

The contributions: mechanisms of bindings and their variations

The book is organized into five thematic parts focusing on specific aspects of binding. Parts 1 and 2 deal with the neural mechanisms of binding and related computational models. On the basis of recent neurocognitive evidence, Part 1 provides a comprehensive overview of the neural mechanisms of binding. In Part 2, binding mechanisms are discussed from a computational point of view. Part 3 addresses binding in different cognitive domains, as well as the passage from transient to permanent binding states. Part 4 provides in-depth analyses of binding during episodic retrieval. Finally, Part 5 describes normal and pathological changes of memory in ageing and Alzheimer's disease, and their relation to various binding mechanisms.

The chapters in Part 1 address various mechanisms of feature binding. Eichenbaum (Chapter 2) presents evidence that the hippocampus is involved in different forms of relational binding including non-episodic declarative (semantic) knowledge. In contrast, Trinkler *et al.* (Chapter 3) see this brain structure as mainly involved in episodic but not semantic binding. Tucker and Luu (Chapter 4) discuss different forms of binding from the perspective of their adaptive utility, including the modulatory aspects of limbic networks which may serve a gating function. The next three chapters relate the mechanisms of binding to synchronizations in specific frequency bands and/or brain structures. Klimesch (Chapter 5) presents evidence for a contribution of theta frequencies to memory formation, and for the nesting of higher frequencies in lower ones during memory encoding. Düzel *et al.* (Chapter 6) discuss theta, delta, and gamma oscillations and their covariance in relation to binding and the different electrophysiological correlates of memory. Finally, Fernandez and Fell (Chapter 7) present data from depth electrodes, demonstrating that rhinal–hippocampal synchronization contributes to memory formation. In these contributions it becomes apparent that different neural structures and different mechanisms mediate different types of binding.

Part 2 presents various computational approaches to binding mechanisms. A variety of computational models that formalize binding processes are presented. Cer and O'Reilly (Chapter 8) present a complementary learning model that allows gradual adaptation of low-level conjunctions during generalization in semantic learning tasks, but also fast learning of higher-order bindings in an episodic task. A transient binding in working memory is suggested as a third form. Similarly, Murre *et al.* (Chapter 9) discuss different mechanisms for binding in long-term and working memory. Brown and McCormack (Chapter 10) consider the role of time in these binding processes. Finally, simulating ageing effects in a computational network, Li and Lindenberger (Chapter 11) demonstrate a selective impairment of relational binding and spared within-item binding mechanisms, and discuss how these effects are related to dopaminergic neuromodulation. In sum, the approaches covered in this part support the view that human memory needs multiple and interactive binding mechanisms to function effectively.

The contributions in Part 3 deal with binding processes in perception and knowledge representation. As an integral part of encoding operations, these processes partially determine the input of memory processes. Treisman (Chapter 12) gives an overview of her research on feature integration and also demonstrates how these processes may define object tokens as entries in working memory. Rösler *et al.* (Chapter 13) use the N400, an ERP component associated with semantic processing, to examine binding processes during fact retrieval in arithmetic tasks. Using an individual differences approach, Voss *et al.* (Chapter 14) show that top-down influences can modulate binding processes. Similarly, Fujiwara and Markowitsch (Chapter 15) discuss the binding of episodes to the self and show influences of negative emotions on autobiographical memory and autonoetic awareness. Taken together, the chapters indicate that binding not only plays an important role in perception, but also contributes to the formation of durable memory traces that can be modulated by emotions.

Part 4 addresses binding processes during episodic retrieval. Retrieval, the process by which memory information is made available for behavioural responses, can be triggered automatically by appropriate retrieval cues. In other instances, control processes responsible for the specification of retrieval task parameters and/or the verification of retrieved information are required for successful task performance. Brown and Warburton (Chapter 16) show how the perirhinal cortex and the hippocampus may contribute to familiarity and conscious recollection, respectively, suggesting that different binding mechanisms are influenced by different neural processes and parameters. The same differentiation is suggested by Quamme *et al.* (Chapter 17) on the basis of behavioural data. Curran *et al.* (Chapter 18) review work on the putative ERP correlates of familiarity and recollection, and discuss the role of binding for both processes. Knowlton and Eldridge (Chapter 19) review the role of the medial temporal lobe in declarative memory, including neuropsychological case studies and brain imaging data, and also giving some credit to controversial topics. In contrast, Nyberg's focus (Chapter 20) is not the binding process itself, but the content that is bound, i.e. the modality of the stimulus. He shows that the same modality- specific structures that encode information are also active during retrieval. Next, Paller (Chapter 21) discusses various forms of binding fragments represented in multiple neocortical zones in different memory tasks and their ERP correlates. Declarative memory binding and cross-cortical storage are discussed as critical components of episodic memory. Finally, Bäuml (Chapter 22) shows that retrieval is not only the reactivation of old traces, but rather can be considered a constructive process during which memories are changed by new binding processes which may cause other information to be forgotten. Overall, the contributions of this part give an exhaustive picture of binding processes during episodic retrieval, and they sketch the neural structures mediating these binding mechanisms.

Part 5 extends these discussions to binding mechanisms in the ageing brain. Episodic memory deficits are present in normal ageing and in Alzheimer's disease. It is shown that in normal ageing strategic and associative components of episodic memory are more impaired than non-strategic components. Specifically, item-context or, more generally, associative binding appears to lose efficiency in old age. In Alzheimer's disease, episodic memory decline is less selective and more pronounced. Craik (Chapter 23) demonstrates that reduced processing efficiency may impair memory and binding in various ways. These and other results lead to his concept of 'levels of binding'. Similarly, Cabeza (Chapter 24) identifies a relational binding deficit as the main memory impairment of elderly people, and he relates this to a reduced processing efficiency of the prefrontal cortex. In Chapter 25, Naveh-Benjamin presents a series of data showing that this impairment leads to an association deficit which is specific to the elderly and difficult to simulate by dividing attention in younger adults. McDaniel *et al.* (Chapter 26) also focus on prefrontal processes and show that the type of relation that is processed is also relevant. Friedman (Chapter 27) makes the same point concerning relational processing. He reviews a series of data that support the view of a specific deficit of conscious recollection in the elderly. In the closing chapter, Small and Bäckman relate binding to preclinical symptoms of Alzheimer's disease (AD). The results are still ambiguous, but suggest that memory impairments in preclinical AD may be less specific than previously assumed. Therefore normal ageing may be associated with a specific impairment of relational binding (associative deficit), whereas AD appears to cause a global binding impairment.

A short summary and some unresolved issues

The contributions to this book demonstrate that we already know a great deal about the relationship between binding and memory. However, many details of binding processes are not yet fully understood.

We can distinguish different types of binding. A main distinction is the one of within- and between-item or relational binding. The former type of binding is associated with familiarity and the latter with recollection. It is conceivable that the latter type of binding may even be associated with declarative knowledge in general, and not specifically tied to episodic knowledge. On the neural level, the former type of binding, and the familiarity signal associated with it, is mediated by perirhinal structures, whereas hippocampal processing is involved in the latter type of binding. However, these mediotemporal structures are not stores of memory traces; they only provide the mechanisms which bind contents represented in modality-specific processing areas. Correlates of these components can be found in electrophysiological and brain imaging data. Additionally, prefrontal areas play a critical role in memory formation and retrieval. They exert a top-down influence on binding mechanisms by specification of retrieval cues, initiation of memory search, and selection of task-appropriate ensembles of bound features. Another factor that influences the efficiency of binding may be the energetic level, for example the availability of neurotransmitters. They may influence binding by modulating the synchronization between different brain areas. For example, stress hormones and the amygdala have been shown to be important modulators of memory consolidation for emotional events (Cahill and McGaugh 1998). These synchronizations are possible mechanisms for transient binding, and oscillations in different EEG frequency bands may support grouping operations at different levels of the processing hierarchy. These levels may also differ in the distances between neural structures across which information is bound—local versus long range. These temporary forms of binding have to be consolidated for long-term memory.

The different chapters in the book provide excellent overviews of the details of these processes, and so it is not necessary to reiterate all of them here. We only want to highlight some topics that can be found in several papers, and we also want to mention a few issues which in our view have not yet attracted the necessary attention. In the following, we briefly discuss some of these topics, hoping to instigate further research in these areas.

The first issue is the **different types of relational binding**. In this book, there are several allusions to the suggestion that relational binding is not homogeneous (e.g. Chapters 3, 10, 20, and 23–26). Bindings of locations/spatial context, temporal context, and different items seem to be different. Similarly, within- and cross-modal features differ, and modality also plays a role. Considering these differences, we argue for a more systematic analysis of different types of binding within the same experiment, across different memory tasks. This would not only result in a better understanding of binding differences, but would also add to the understanding of association memory deficits in elderly people (see Chapters 25 and 26). Additionally, we suggest multi-method studies. If the same task is investigated by means of behavioural, electrophysiological, and brain imaging techniques in parallel, we may be able to disclose the brain–behaviour relationship with respect to binding mechanisms.

A second issue is the **definition of an item**. We need an independent definition of an item if we want to explain differences in behaviour by the difference between bindings of within-item and between-item features. This definition probably cannot be given on the basis of the input structure alone, although considering results from perceptual psychology is a first step in that direction (see Chapter 12). The examination of structural and functional connectivities between selected brain areas may be a promising next step in this quest. Top-down processes, pre-semantic knowledge, task demands, etc. are modulating factors that play an important role in the flexible adaptation of bound representations to changing task and environmental demands (see Chapters 3, 14, 25, and 26). It follows from this that the analysis of binding mechanisms must be extended to other domains of memory (see Chapter13), in particular working memory (see Chapters 8 and 9).

A third issue is the distinction between **familiarity** and **recollection**, or more generally the question of the relationship between **states of memory** and **awareness**. It is still not clear what these mechanisms are and what types of processes their correlates reflect (see Chapters 17, 18, 21, and 27). A relevant aspect here is the definition of the mental processes and their computational basis that generates these signals (e.g. O'Reilly and Norman 2002). Another aspect is the relationship between episodic and semantic tasks. We need to explicate in what respect episodic declarative knowledge is different from semantic declarative knowledge (see Chapters 2, 3, and 19).

It is assumed that familiarity is based on a global match that may be associated with cognitive impenetrability (Fodor 1983) and hence the absence of declarative knowledge. Familiarity seems to be sensitive to intra-item binding mechanisms that lead to memory representations of unitized associations. However, the circumstances under which unitization of features into a coherent representation occurs are poorly understood. Familiarity reflects a quantitatively graded memory signal, while recollection reflects the retrieval of qualitative information from a study episode, i.e. declarative knowledge. Therefore the availability of declarative and context-rich knowledge seems to be critical for recollection but not for familiarity.

A final issue we want to mention is the distinction between **transient bindings** and more **durable bindings**. The existence of these two forms of binding has at least two consequences. First, different mechanisms probably bind features for different ranges of time (Chapters 5, 8, and 9). Further, as yet undiscovered physiological mechanisms may pertain to more extended time intervals (Arshavsky 2003). Having identified different binding mechanisms necessitates an additional process of **consolidation** that transforms transient into durable bindings (Chapter 21). We are only at the beginning of understanding these processes at the systems level, even though at a cellular level the importance of long-term potentiation for trace consolidation is undisputed (Zalutsky and Nicoll 1990). We partially understand correlates of encoding that cause successful remembering in long-term memory, at least for intervals used in the laboratory (Chapters 6, 7, and 24). However, these are only correlates. We do not really understand the neural states triggering those neural processes that enable effective and long lasting bindings. In other words, we need to understand the gating mechanisms that facilitate and enable binding to occur in the first place. Emotional qualities, personal relevance of an event, and its relatedness to the observer's self may be relevant variables in this regard (see Chapters 4 and 15). In order to learn more about this pivotal issue, experiments with enhanced personal relevance of the material and extended retention intervals seem desirable.

Therefore we expect that more veridical and ecologically valid theories of memory will emerge in the future. These theories will allow suggestions to be made for a more efficient memory encoding based on a neurocognitive model. They will also account for memory impairments, individual differences in memory performance, and ontogenetic changes in memory functioning, and they will provide clues about ways to enhance memory functioning. Whatever form these theories take, binding mechanisms will occupy a central place. Hence, we are confident that some of the key elements of such future theories can and will be found in the contributions to this book.

Acknowledgements

This work was supported by grants from German Science Foundation (Deutsche Forschungsgemeinschaft) within the Research Unit 448, 'Binding: Functional Architecture, Neural Correlates, and Ontogeny'.

References

Aggleton, J.P. and Brown, M.W. (1999). Episodic memory, amnesia, and the hippocampal–anterior thalamic axis. *Behavioral and Brain Sciences*, **22**, 425–489.

Arshavsky Y.I. (2003). Long-term memory: does it have a structural or chemical basis? *Trends in Neurosciences*, **26**, 465–466.

Asch, S.E., Ceraso, F., and Heimer, W. (1960). Perceptional conditions of association. *Psychological Monographs*, **74.**

Buchner, A., Erdfelder, E., Steffens, M.C., and Martensen, H. (1997). The nature of memory processes underlying recognition judgments in the process dissociation procedure. *Memory and Cognition*, **25**, 508–518.

Cahill, L and McGaugh, J.L. (1998). Mechanisms of emotional arousal and lasting declarative memory. Trends in Cognitive Sciences, **21**, 294–298.

Chalfonte, B.L. and Johnson, M.K. (1996). Feature memory and binding in young and older adults. *Memory and Cognition*, **24**, 403–416.

Ceraso, F. (1985). Unit formation in perception and memory. *The Psychology of Learning and Motivation*, **19**, 179–210.

Curran, T. (2004). Effects of attention and confidence on the hypothesized ERP correlates of recollection and familiarity. *Neuropsychologia*, **42**, 1088–1106.

Czernochowski, D., Mecklinger, A., Johansson, M., and Brinkmann, M. (2005). Age-related differences in familiarity and recollection: ERP evidence from a recognition memory study in children and young adults. *Cognitive, Affective and Behavioral Neuroscience*, in press.

Damasio, A.R. (1989). The brain binds entities and events by multiregional activation from convergence zones. *Neural Computation*, **1**, 123–132.

Ecker, U.K.H., Groh-Bordin, C., and Zimmer, H.D. (2004). Electrophysiological correlates of specific feature binding in remembering: introducing a neurocognitive model of human memory. In *Bound in Memory: Insights from Behavioral and Neuropsychological Studies* (ed A. Mecklinger, H.D. Zimmer and U. Lindenberger). Aachen: Shaker.

Engel A.K., Kreiter A.K., König P., and Singer, W. (1991). Synchronization of oscillatory neural responses between striate and extrastriate visual cortical areas of the cat. *Proceedings of the National Academy of Sciences of the United States of America*, **88**, 6048–6052.

Engel A.K., König P., Kreiter A.K., Schillen T.B., and Singer W. (1992).Temporal coding in the visual cortex: new vistas on integration in the nervous system. *Trends in Neurosciences*, **15**, 218–226.

Fodor, A. (1983). *The Modularity of Mind.* Cambridge, MA: MIT Press.

Friedman, D. and Johnson, R. (2000). Event-related potential (ERP) studies of memory encoding and retrieval: a selective review. *Microscopy Research and Technique*, **51**, 6–28.

Gardiner, J.M. and Richardson-Klavehn, A. (2000). Remembering and knowing. In *Oxford Handbook of Memory* (ed E. Tulving and F.I.M. Craik). Oxford: Oxford University Press, pp. 229–244.

Garner, W.R. (1974). *The Processing of Information and Structure.* **Hillsdale, NJ: Erlbaum.**

Groh-Bordin, C., Zimmer, H.D. and Mecklinger, A. (2005). Feature binding in perceptual priming and in episodic object recognition: evidence from event-related brain potentials. *Brain Research: Cognitive Brain Research*, **24**, 556–567.

Hommel, B. (1998). Event files: evidence for automatic integration of stimulus-response episodes. *Visual Cognition*, **5**, 183–216.

Hommel, B., Müsseler, J., Aschersleben, G., and Prinz, W. (2001). The theory of event coding (TEC): A framework for perception and action planning. *Behavioral and Brain Research*, **24**, 849–937.

Hummel, J.E. and Biederman, I. (1992). Dynamic binding in a neural network for shape recognition. *Psychological Review*, **99**, 480–517.

Humphreys, M.S., Wiles, J. and Dennis, S. (1994). Toward a theory of human memory: data structures and access processes. *Behavioral and Brain Sciences*, **17**, 655–692.

Jacoby, L.L. (1991). A process dissociation framework: Separating automatic from intentional uses of memory. *Journal of Memory and Language*, **30**, 513–541.0

Johansson, M. and Mecklinger, A. (2003). Action monitoring and episodic memory retrieval: An ERP evaluation. *Biological Psychology*, **64**, 99–125.

Johnson, M.K., and Chalfonte, B.L. (1994). Binding complex memories: the role of reactivation and the hippocampus. In *Memory Systems 1994* (ed D.L. Schacter and E. Tulving). Cambridge, MA: MIT Press, pp. 311–350.

Johnson, M.K., Hashtroudi, S. and Lindsay, D.S. (1993). Source monitoring. *Psychological Bulletin*, **114**, 3–28.

Jones, G.V. (1976). A fragmentation hypothesis of memory: cued recall of pictures and of sequential position. *Journal of Experimental Psychology: General*, **105**, 277–293.

Kahneman, D., Treisman, A., and Gibbs, B. (1992). The reviewing of object files: object-specific integration of information. *Cognitive Psychology*, **24**, 175–219.

Kanwisher, N. and Driver, J. (1992). Objects, attributes, and visual attention: which, what, and where. *Current Directions in Psychological Science*, **1**, 26–31.

McClelland, J.L. and Rumelhart, D.E. (1985). Distributed memory and the representation of general and specific information. *Journal of Experimental Psychology: General*, **114**, 159–197.

Mandler, G. (1980). Recognizing: the judgement of previous occurrence. *Psychological Review*, **87**, 252–271.

Mayes, A.R., Holdstock, J.S., Isaac, C.L., *et al.* (2004). Associative recognition in a patient with selective hippocampal lesions and relatively normal item recognition. *Hippocampus*, **14**, 763–784.

Mecklinger, A. (2000). Interfacing mind and brain: a neurocognitive model of recognition memory. *Psychophysiology*, **37**, 565–582.

Miller, G.A. (1956). The magical number seven plus or minus two: some limits on our capacity for processing information. *Psychological Review*, **63**, 81–97.

Milner, B. (1958). Psychological defects produced by temporal lobe excision. *Research Publications of the Association for Research in Nervous and Mental Disease*, **36**, 244–257.

Murdock, B.B. (1993). TODAM2: A model for the storage and retrieval of item, associative, and serial-order information. *Psychological Review*, **100**, 183–203.

Nader. K. (2003). Memory traces unbound. *Trends in Neurosciences*, **26**, 65–72.

Naveh-Benjamin, M. (2000). Adult age differences in memory performance: tests of an associative deficit hypothesis. *Journal of Experimental Psychology: Learning, Memory, and Cognition*, **26**, 1170–1187.

Nessler, D., Mecklinger, A., and Penney, T.B. (2005). Perceptual fluency, semantic familiarity, and recognition-related familiarity: An electrophysiological exploration. *Brain Research: Cognitive Brain Research*, **22**, 265–288

O'Reilly, R. and Norman, K. (2002). Hippocampal and neocortical contributions to memory: advances in the complementary learning systems framework. *Trends in Cognitive Sciences*, **6**, 505–510.

O'Craven, K.M., Downing, P.E., and Kanwisher, N. (1999). fMRI evidence for objects as the units of attentional selection. *Nature*, **401**, 584–587.

Paller, K.A. (2000). Neurocognitive foundations of human memory. In *The Psychology of Learning and Motivation*, **40** (ed. D.L. Medin). San Diego, CA: Academic Press, pp. 121–145.

Raaijmakers, J.G.W. and Shiffrin, R.M. (1980). SAM: A theory of probabilistic search of associative memory. *The Psychology of Learning and Motivation*, Vol. 14 (ed G.H. Bower). New York: Academic Press, pp. 207–262.

Reinitz, M.T. and Hannigan, S.L. (2001). Effects of simultaneous stimulus presentation and attention switching on memory conjunction errors. *Journal of Memory and Language*, **44**, 206–219.

Rugg, M.D. and Wilding, E.L. (2000). Retrieval processing and episodic memory. *Trends in Cognitive Sciences*, **4**, 108–115.

Senkfor, A. and Van Petten, C. (1998). Who said what? An event-related potential investigation of source and item memory. *Journal of Experimental Psychology: Learning, Memory, and Cognition*, **24**, 1005–1025.

Singer, W. (1993). Synchronization of cortical activity and its putative role in information processing and learning. *Annual Review of Physiology*, **55**, 349–374.

Singer W. (2001). Consciousness and the binding problem. *Annals of the New York Academy of Sciences*, **929**, 123–146.

Singer, W., Engel, A.K., Kreiter, A.K., Munk, M.H.J., Neuenschwander, S., and Roelfsema, P.R. (1997). Neural assemblies: necessity, signature and detectability. *Trends in Cognitive Sciences*, **1**, 252–261.

Tallon-Baudry, C. and Bertrand O. (1999). Oscillatory gamma activity in humans and its role in object representation. *Trends in Cognitive Sciences*, **3**, 151–162.

Treisman, A. (1996). The binding problem. *Current Opinion in Neurobiology*, **6**, 171–178.

Treisman, A. and Gelade, G.A. (1980). A feature integration theory of attention. *Cognitive Psychology*, **12**, 97–130.

Tulving, E. (1985). How many memory systems are there? *American Psychologist*, **40**, 385–398.

Underwood, B.J. (1969). Attributes of memory. *Psychological Review*, **76**, 559–573.

von der Malsburg, C. (1995). Binding in models of perception and brain function. *Current Opinion in Neurobiology*, **5**, 520–526.

von Stein, A., Chiang, C., and König, P. (2000). Top-down processing mediated by interareal synchronization. *Proceedings of the National Academy of Sciences of the United States of America*, **97**, 14748–14753.

Wagner, A.D. (2001). Synchronicity: when you're gone I'm lost without a trace? *Nature Neuroscience*, **4**, 1159–1160.

Wagner, A.D., Koutstaal, W., and Schacter, D.L. (1999). When encoding yields remembering: insights from event-related neuroimaging. *Philosophical Transactions of the Royal Society of London, Series B, Biological Sciences*, **354**, 1307–1324.

Wixted, J.T. and Squire, L.R. (2004). Recall and recognition are equally impaired in patients with selective hippocampal damage. *Cognitive, Affective and Behavioral Neuroscience*, **4**, 58–66.

Yonelinas, A.P. (1994). Receiver-operating characteristics in recognition memory: evidence for a dual-process model. *Journal of Experimental Psychology: Learning, Memory, and Cognition*, **20**, 1341–1354.

Yonelinas, A.P. (2002). The nature of recollection and familiarity: A review of 30 years of research. *Journal of Memory and Language*, **46**, 441–517.

Yonelinas, A.P., Kroll, N.E.A., Dobbins, I.G., and Soltani, M. (1999). Recognition memory of faces: when familiarity supports associative recognition judgments. *Psychonomic Bulletin and Review*, **6**, 654–661

Zacks, R.T., Hasher, L., and Li, K.Z.H. (2000). Human memory. In *Handbook of Aging and Cognition* (ed F.I.M. Craik and T.A. Salthouse. Mahwah, NJ: Erlbaum, pp. 293–357.

Zalutsky, R.A. and Nicoll, R.A. (1990). Comparison of two forms of long-term potentiation in single hippocampal neurons. *Science*, **248**, 1619–1624.

Section 1

Neural mechanisms of binding

Chapter 2

Memory binding in hippocampal relational networks

Howard Eichenbaum

Introduction

A decade ago my colleagues and I offered a proposal that sought common ground among competing theories of hippocampal function (Eichenbaum *et al.* 1992a,b, 1994; Cohen and Eichenbaum 1993; Eichenbaum 1994). Here I will update the relational memory theory and outline an information processing syntax that contributes to a broad range of phenomena in declarative memory, including episodic and semantic memory, flexibility in memory expression, and cognitive mapping. I will outline a set of specific biologically realistic 'binding' mechanisms performed within the hippocampus in support of these phenomena in declarative memory processing. It is proposed that the hippocampus (1) binds together information about stimuli, actions, and places to compose representations of events, (2) binds these events in the order in which they were experienced to compose representations of unique episodes, and (3) binds together representations of distinct episodes, thereby abstracting common 'semantic' information and linking overlapping representations to construct a relational memory network. Relational networks retrieve multiple, related, episodic, and semantic memories and support cortical processing that identifies relationships among those memories. In addition, the same relational processing of memories for journeys through space could support the development and utilization of cognitive maps.

Mechanisms of relational memory representation

The present extensions of the relational memory hypothesis are aimed at providing a mechanistic framework of hippocampal functional circuitry that contributes to the phenomenology of episodic memory and semantic memory, the broad domain of relationships represented by the hippocampal system, and the important place of spatial mapping within a general declarative memory function. The model offered here is cognitively robust, in that it incorporates high-level psychological phenomena attributed to declarative memory. It is also biologically plausible, in that well-established features of hippocampal circuitry and plasticity could implement the proposed relational processing. Thus the account is derived from a top-down analysis of declarative memory that characterizes basic cognitive properties attributed to this form of memory. At the same time, the hypothesis is bottom-up in that it is formulated as a qualitative model of hippocampal neural representation that could emerge from the known properties of the circuitry and plasticity of the hippocampus.

There is a growing body of evidence that the hippocampus binds together representations of stimuli, actions, and places that compose discrete events. Several functional imaging studies have examined whether the hippocampus is more activated during the encoding or retrieval of associations among many elements of a memory, a characteristic of context-rich episodic memories. Henke *et al.* (1997) observed greater hippocampal activation when subjects associated a person with a house than when they made independent judgements about the person and house. Giovanello *et al.* (2003a) reported greater hippocampal activation when subjects recognized previously presented word pairings compared with rearranged word pairs or words studied separately. Davachi and Wagner (2002) found that the hippocampus is activated during encoding of multiple items, and is more activated when subjects are required to link the items to one another by systematic comparisons, compared with rote rehearsal of individual items. Furthermore, the magnitude of hippocampal activation during the comparison and linkage of the items predicted later success in recognition. Other recent studies have revealed activation within subfields of the hippocampus during the encoding of face–name associations (Small *et al.* 2001; Sperling *et al.* 2003; Zeineh *et al.* 2003). Correspondingly, recent neuropsychological studies have found that recognition of associations is impaired in amnesic patients even when recognition for single items is spared (Giovanello *et al.* 2003b; Turriziani *et al.* 2004). These studies reported impairment in recognition memory for associations between words or between faces or face–occupation pairs compared with normal performance in recognition of single items. At the same time, other functional imaging studies on characterizations of amnesia have suggested that the hippocampus is sometimes involved in both associative and single-item recognition, highlighting the need to clarify the nature of associative information that composes an 'event' (Squire *et al.* 2004). Nevertheless, these findings are generally consistent with the notion that the hippocampus plays a distinct role in binding features of items and their context to represent salient events.

We live our lives through personal experience, and our initial construction of reality within consciousness is a form of episodic buffer that contains a representation of the stream of events as they just occurred (Baddeley 2000). For example, a vivid episodic memory of your morning experience might include a series of salient events, including going to the kitchen, examining several choices of breakfast foods, then selecting and then eating Cheerios cereal. Of the many characteristics of episodic memory that have been highlighted in different accounts, the most striking is that vivid episodic memories capture the flow of events in experience (Fig. 2.1A). In an early construal, Tulving (1983) distinguished episodic memory as organized in the temporal dimension, and contrasted this scheme with a conceptual organization of semantic memory. Tulving argued that the central organizing feature of episodic memory is that 'one event precedes, co-occurs, or follows another'. This is reminiscent of Aristotle's (350 BC) characterization of vivid remembering: 'Acts of recollection, as they occur in experience, are due to the fact that one thought has by nature another that succeeds it in regular order'. The current account emphasizes the temporal organization of episodic memories, and suggests that the hippocampus encodes sequences of events that compose any attended experience (Morris and Frey 1997). It is proposed here that the hippocampus represents each event as the associations between the salient stimuli and actions and the background context in which they occur, and the hippocampal network represents the orderliness of events within episodes (Fig. 2.1A).

In addition, further consideration of the cognitive properties of episodic memory suggests how related episodic representations might be integrated with one

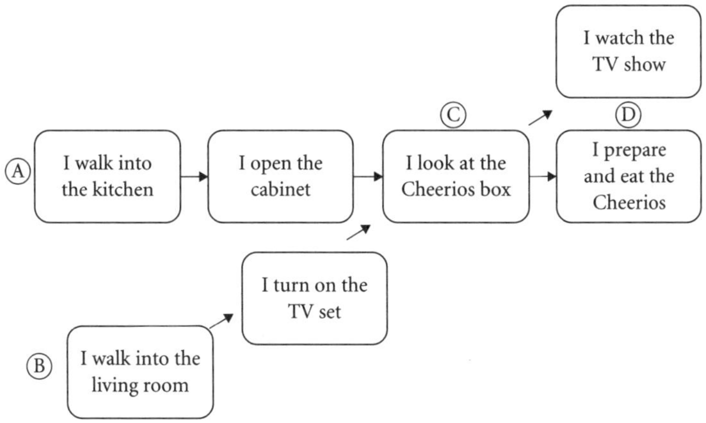

Figure 2.1 A schematic diagram of a simple relational network composed of two episodic memories (A and B). Each is construed as a sequence of elements (1–6) that represent a salient event as the conjunction of stimuli, actions, and the place where these occurred. C is an element that contains the same features in both episodes. D lies between two elements from distinct experiences that can be related via the common element C.

another to support additional aspects of declarative memory, specifically semantic memory and the flexibility of recollection. Referring to how different memories are integrated with one another, William James (1890) emphasized that

> . . . in mental terms, the more other facts a fact is associated with in the mind, the better possession of it our memory retains. Each of its associates becomes a hook to which it hangs, a means by which to fish it up by when sunk beneath the surface. Together they form a network of attachments by which it is woven into the entire tissue of our thought.

James saw semantic memory as a systematic organization of information wherein the usefulness of memories was determined by how well they are linked together. In the example, the breakfast episode may be linked to other episodes with Cheerios, such as seeing a television commercial for Cheerios (Fig. 2.1B), by the common element of the Cheerios box in both experiences (Fig. 2.1C).

There are two main outcomes of the linking of representations of specific experiences. One is a common base of associations that are not dependent on the episodic context in which the information was acquired. Thus when several experiences share considerable common information, the overlapping elements and common links among them will be reinforced such that those items and associations become general regularities. The representation of these general regularities constitutes semantic 'knowledge' that is not bound to the particular episode or context in which the information was encoded. In the example, multiple experiences with Cheerios may be linked to provide to the general knowledge about Cheerios and other breakfast foods. The proposed networking of episodic memories by common elements provides a mechanism for the commonly, albeit not universally (Tulving 2002), held view that semantic knowledge is derived from information repeated within and abstracted from episodic memories.

The second proposed outcome from a network of linked memories is a capacity to use the common elements to retrieve multiple memories that include that element. Thus, when one is asked about Cheerios, one can employ that cue to recall the last occasion on which one ate Cheerios for breakfast or what a Cheerios box looks like. Furthermore, hippocampal representations could support a capacity to 'surf' the network of linked memories and identify relationships and associations among items that were experienced in distinct memories and therefore are only indirectly related. A single cue could generate the retrieval of multiple episodic and semantic memories, and cortical areas can access these multiple memories to analyse the consequential, logical, spatial, and other abstract relationships among items that appeared separately in distinct memories. These logical operations on indirectly related memories can support inferences from memory. In the example, the cue of a Cheerios box could evoke memories about pictures on the Cheerios cereal box where you found your breakfast with those seen on the Cheerios box in a television commercial. You could then compare these memories and conclude that the Cheerios you had seen during the television show was the cereal you ate that morning (Fig. 2.1D). The activity of searching and surfing networks of memories, and then comparing and contrasting memories, could underlie our awareness of memories and the experience of conscious recollection. The organization of linked experience-specific and experience-general memories with the capacity for association and inference among memories is called a 'relational memory network'.

Neural circuit and plasticity mechanisms that underlie relational memory networks

Are relational memory networks biologically plausible? Three well-known features of hippocampal circuitry, particularly that of area CA3, can work in combination to support all the properties of relational memory networks described above (Fig. 2.2).

1. The hippocampus receives convergent afferents from virtually all cortical association areas, and these inputs are widely distributed onto the cell population in multiple subdivisions of the hippocampus including CA3 (Amaral and Witter 1995). Thus CA3 principle cells have as their main afferents considerable high-level perceptual information about attended stimuli and spatial cues, as well as signals about emotions, actions, motivations, and virtually all forms of attended personal information.

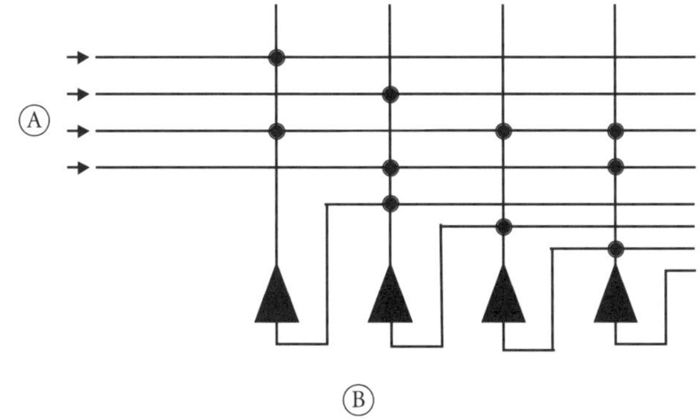

Figure 2.2 A schematic diagram of some of the principal neurons and their key connections in hippocampal area CA3 that might represent an episodic sequence. The large dots represent connections enhanced by LTP. A represents the flow of convergent multisensory information from the parahippocampal region. B indicates the recurrent connections by which outputs of the principal cells project diffusely to one another.

2. The principal neurons of area CA3 send considerable projections to other CA3 principal cells. These recurrent connections are broad across the CA3 population, sparse in that each cell connects with 5–20 per cent of the other cells, and involve mainly excitatory glutamatergic synapses.
3. The hippocampus is noted for the prevalence of rapid synaptic plasticity, known as long-term potentiation (LTP) (Bliss and Collingridge, 1993). In particular, a form of LTP that is dependent on *N*-methyl-D-aspartate (NMDA) receptors has been strongly linked to memory (Martin *et al.* 2000) and to the memory-associated firing properties of hippocampal neurons (Shapiro and Eichenbaum 1999).

These properties can work in combination to support key features of relational memory networks, specifically the development of associative representations of events, the sequential organization of event codings, and the linking of related memories. With regard to associative representations, simultaneous activation of multiple high-level afferents to CA3 principal cells could support rapid induction of associative LTP such that the synapses of each of the inputs are all enhanced for an extended duration (Fig. 2.2A). This associative LTP would support pattern completion, such that subsequent presentation of any part of the conjunctive coding would fire the cell, constituting retrieval of the pattern initially occurring during binding of all the high-level features.

With regard to sequential organization, several recent computational models have emphasized temporal coding as a main organizing feature of the memory representations supported by the hippocampus, and in particular area CA3. Levy (1989, 1996) proposed that unique characteristics of hippocampal area CA3, specifically the sparseness and largely excitatory nature of its recurrent connectivity, combined with rapid synaptic plasticity inherently produces asymmetric connections that can represent sequences of information from a single patterned input, and can spontaneously reproduce these sequences (Fig. 2.2B). Thus, according to these models, when temporally patterned inputs reach the hippocampus, a rapid LTP mechanism enhances connections between cells that fire in sequence. The likelihood of a reciprocal (backward) connection of forward connected cells is very low because of the overall sparse connectivity. Therefore the enhancement of recurrent connections is mostly unidirectional, leading to an asymmetry of the enhanced connectivity. When partial inputs are reproduced, the network is more likely to complete the sequence of the full initial input pattern. In addition, when sequences are repeated (practised) just a few times, cells representing neighbouring sequential events converge on background cells that enhance sustained activity, providing a context that bridges the firings of neurons representing salient sequential events (Levy 1989, 1996; Wallenstein *et al.* 1998). Although sequence storage and recall was initially proposed as characteristic of CA3, subsequent models (Lisman 1999) have shown how more complex and reciprocally connected recurrent networks in the dentate gyrus and CA3 can coordinate to provide more faithful recall of sequences, leaving CA1 to decode the sequence signals back to the cortex and to compare predictions of the network for the next sequential item with actual information as it arrives.

With regard to linking memories, the same computational models that emphasize temporal organization in episodic memory representations provide a mechanism for binding distinct memory representations and for extracting the common information among them that is independent of their episodic context. Thus the proposed networks include cells that receive no external inputs but develop firing patterns that are regularly associated with a particular sequence or with overlapping sequences (Levy 1996; Sohal and Hasselmo 1998; Wallenstein *et al.* 1998). In the situation where episodes are repeated, these cells provide a local temporal context in which items within a particular sequence are linked together. When these links incorporate events that are unique to a particular episode, they can assist the network in disambiguating successive patterns in overlapping but distinct sequences. At the same time, when the links are activated similarly by separate episodes that share a series of overlapping features, they can allow the association of discontiguous episodes that share those features. Thus the same network properties that support encoding episodes as sequences of events also contain means to link and disambiguate related episodes (see Agster *et al.* (2002) for an experimental test).

Validation of the theoretical framework described above rests on evidence that (1) the hippocampus is critical to the representation of the order of events that compose unique experiences, (2) the hippocampus is critical to linking overlapping memories and the consequent flexibility of memory expression, (3) the hippocampal network encodes sequences of events and these codings include both conjunctions of events and places that are unique to particular episodes and common features of events that could link overlapping experiences, and (4) the properties of relational memory networks apply equally well to both spatial and non-spatial memory. The following sections discuss evidence supporting each of these points.

The hippocampus is critical to memory for the flow of events in unique experiences

To investigate the specific role of the hippocampus in remembering the order of events in unique experiences, recent studies have employed a behavioural protocol that assesses memory for episodes composed of a unique sequence of olfactory stimuli (Fortin *et al.* 2002; Kesner *et al.* 2002). In our study, memory for the sequential order of odour events was directly compared with recognition of the odours in the list independent of memory for their order. On each trial rats were presented with a unique series of five odours, selected randomly from a large pool of common household scents. Memory for each series was subsequently probed using a choice test where the animal was reinforced for selecting the earlier of two of the odours that had appeared in the series. For example, the rat was initially presented with odours A, B, C, D, and E sequentially. Following a delay, two non-adjacent odours (e.g. B and D) were presented and the animal was rewarded for selecting odour that appeared earlier (in this case B). Animals were tested with six different types of probes that assessed memory for different separations (lags) between odour presentations in the series. In each trial, any pair of non-adjacent odours might be presented as the probe, so that the animal had to remember the entire sequence in order to perform well throughout the testing session.

Normal rats performed sequential order judgements across all lags, and performance on probes was dependent on the lag, indicating that order judgements were easier for more widely separated items. In contrast, rats with hippocampal lesions performed the sequential order task at near-chance levels and were impaired at all lags. The same rats were then tested on their ability to recognize the recent occurrence of odours presented in the series. in each trial, a unique series of five odours was presented in a format identical to that used in the sequential order task. Then recognition was probed using a choice test in which the animal was presented with one of the odours from the series and another odour from the pool that was not in the series. Reinforcement was given for selecting the odour not presented in the series. For example, the rat might instead be presented with the series K to O and then, following a delay, an odour selected randomly from those initially sampled and an odour not presented in the sequence (e.g. N or X). In this case, the rat would be rewarded for choosing X. Five types of probes that differed in the recency of the initially presented odour were used.

Both control rats and rats with selective hippocampal damage acquired the task rapidly and there was no overall performance difference between the groups in acquisition rate. Subsequent analyses of performance on the different types of probes showed that rats with hippocampal lesions performed as well as normal rats in recognition throughout the series. Furthermore, in both groups, recognition scores were consistently superior on probes involving odours that appeared later in the series, suggesting some forgetting of items that had to be remembered for a longer period and through more intervening items. Rats with hippocampal damage showed normal differences in the strengths of memories for items that were experienced at different times, strongly suggesting that the relative strengths of memories could not support order judgements. Therefore we concluded that normal rats based their sequential order judgements directly on remembering the odour sequence. Contrary to the argument that animals lack episodic memory because they are 'stuck in time' (Roberts 2002; Tulving 2002), these observations suggest that animals have the capacity to recollect the flow of events in unique experiences.

These findings suggest that humans should also depend on the hippocampus in memory for the order of events. In a study using a design similar to that described above, Hopkins *et al.* (1995) found that patients with hypoxic brain injury involving shrinkage of the hippocampus were impaired in memory for the order of a series of six words, pictures, or spatial locations. However, these patients were also impaired in recognition of the items, undermining an unambiguous interpretation of a deficit in the order of the events independent of memory for the events. More recently, Spiers *et al.* (2001) reported a selective deficit in order memory independent of item memory in a patient with selective hippocampal damage due to perinatal transient anoxia (Vargha-Khadem *et al.* 1997). In this study the patient explored a virtual reality town in which he received objects from virtual characters. His recognition of the familiar objects was intact, but he was severely impaired in memory for the order in which he received objects, as well as for where he received them. Downes *et al.* (2002) reported that patients with medial temporal lobe damage that included bilateral hippocampal damage (as well as some parahippocampal cortical damage) were impaired in memory for the order of presentation of words for which recognition of the items was equivalent. Thus, as in rats with selective hippocampal damage, humans with hippocampal damage are impaired in memory for the order of events in unique episodes even in cases where recognition memory is intact.

The hippocampus is critical to the networking of memories, supporting the flexibility of declarative memory expression

Previous conceptions of hippocampal function have focused on the notion that the hippocampus mediates a binding of disparate cortical representations of stimuli and contextual backgrounds (e.g. Squire *et al.* 1984), and this characteristic has also been attributed to relational memory (Cohen *et al.* 1997, 1999; Reed and Squire 1997; Spiers *et al.* 2001; Davachi and Wagner 2002). The current proposal incorporates this feature of hippocampal binding as well, and attributes this processing to the coding of associations among elements of events and the sequential coding of serial events within episodes, as described above. In addition, with the current proposal, the hippocampal relational network also mediates the linking of distinct episodes that may contain items that have not been experienced in the same episode or the same context. In doing so, the hippocampus plays a role not only in simply binding items within memories, but also in mediating associations between distinct memories.

As desscribed above, the hippocampus supports a capacity to generate multiple memories that share a common element, and the information contained within these memories can be used by many brain systems to make judgements about causal, logical, temporal, and spatial relations among the items in those memories (Cohen and Eichenbaum 1993). Iterations of association, retrieval, and recoding memories according to deduced relationships among the items would lead to the development of a systematic organization of items and episodes in memory wherein facts and events are linked to one another by a broad range of causal, logical, temporal, spatial, and other relevant relationships among the items. This organization supports flexibility in the expression of memory, specifically involving inferences between items that are only indirectly related.

In a series of studies we have used a model system of rodent olfactory memory to explore the importance of the hippocampus in the linking memories and using the resulting relational networks to make associational and logical inferences from memory. One study examined the role of the hippocampus in making indirect associations between stimuli that were each directly associated with a common stimulus. Initially, we trained normal rats and rats with hippocampal lesions on a series of overlapping 'paired associates' (Bunsey and Eichenbaum 1996). On each trial, the rat was initially presented with one of two initial items in a pairing and then had to select the arbitrarily assigned associate. For example, for training on the pairs A–B and X–Y, if A was the initial item, the rat had to select B and not Y; conversely, if X was the initial item, the rat had to select Y and not B. Then the rats were trained on a second paired associated list where the initial items were the second items in the first list and new items were the associates (B–C and Y–Z). Thus, when B was presented initially, the rat was required to select C and not Z, and when Y was presented initially, the rat was required to select Z and not C.

After training on all four paired associates, the rats were tested on their knowledge of the indirect relations among the pairings. These tests involved presentations of an initial item from the first learned paired associates (A or X) followed by a choice between the second items of the later learned associates (C or Z). Normal rats demonstrated their ability to express these indirect relations by selecting C when A was presented and Z when X was presented, whereas rats with selective hippocampal damage showed no capacity for this inference from memory. These findings, combined with observations on another transitive inference task (Dusek and Eichenbaum 1997), indicate that the hippocampus is critical to binding distinct memories into a relational network that supports flexible memory expression.

Hippocampal neuronal networks encode sequences of events that define distinct experiences as well as events that are common across experiences

We have also studied the content of information captured by populations of hippocampal neurons in animals performing a variety of learning and memory tasks. Based on the model presented in Figure 2.1, three general hypotheses were explored. First, we expected that elements of the hippocampal neuronal network would be activated serially during sequential events that compose an episode in any behavioural protocol. Secondly, with regard to the contents of the events encoded, we expected that many cells would fire associated with complex conjunctions of the salient stimuli, behavioural actions, and spatial context (location) that define each event. Thirdly, we expected that other cells would fire associated with common features of overlapping experiences. These codings could link representations of related experiences and, in doing so, mediate the establishment of semantic representations and the retrieval of related episodic memories.

How well do the observations of the firing properties of hippocampal neurons conform to these expectations? With regard to the expectation that hippocampal cells should fire associated with sequential events, in many studies we have observed that different hippocampal neurons were activated during virtually every moment of task performance, including during the approach and stimulus sampling behaviours, discriminative responses, and consummatory behaviours (Eichenbaum *et al.* 1999). In addition, many other studies using classical conditioning, discrimination learning, and matching to sample paradigms also found that hippocampal neurons fire associated with each sequential task-relevant event (Berger *et al.* 1983; Eichenbaum *et al.* 1987; Deadwyler *et al.* 1996; McEchron and Disterhoft 1997; Wiebe and Staubli, 1999). In each of these paradigms, animals are repeatedly presented with specific stimuli and reinforcers, and execute appropriate cognitive judgements and conditioned behaviours. Corresponding to each of these regular events, many hippocampal cells show time-locked activations associated with each sequential stimulus and behavioural action.

A criticism raised about these studies is that the firing associated with various events occurred consistently in a particular location, leaving open the possibility that the firing patterns reflected largely spatial information. We addressed this issue by training animals to perform the same behavioural judgements at many locations in the same environment (Wood *et al.* 1999). Rats were trained to perform a recognition memory task in which cups with scented sand were the relevant cues. In each trial the cup was placed in any of nine locations and the place was not predictive. The rats approached the cup and sniffed the odour, and then dug for a reward if the odour was a non-match with the odour presented on the preceding trial, or turned away if it was a match. Because the location of the discriminative stimuli was varied systematically, cellular activity related to the stimuli and behaviour could be dissociated from that related to the animal's location.

As observed in the previous studies, hippocampal cells were active during all aspects of task performance, consistent with the view that the hippocampus encoded the continuous flow of events. Regarding the contents of the codings, some cells fired only if the animal began the approach from a particular location, or fired only if the odour was a particular conjunction of the odour, the place where it was sampled, and the match–non-match status of the odour. These firing patterns are consistent with the representation of events unique to a particular rarely repeated episode. Other cells fired associated with a feature of the task independent of other features. Thus some cells fired during a particular phase of the approach towards any stimulus cup. Others fired differentially as the rat sampled a particular odour, regardless of its location or match–non-match status. Other cells fired only when the rat sampled the odour at a particular place, regardless of the odour or its status. Yet other cells fired differentially associated with the match and non-match status of the odour, regardless of the odour or where it was sampled.

Very similar findings have been obtained in a study where hippocampal neuronal activity was recorded from humans performing a navigational task in a virtual town (Ekstrom *et al.* 2003). As subjects drove a 'taxi' round the town, different neurons fired throughout task performance. Some cells fired associated with specific conjunctions of viewing a particular building, being at a particular place, and having a particular goal that characterized specific trial episodes. Other cells fired associated with features of events that overlapped across episodes, including viewing a particular building, or being in a particular place, or having a specific goal.

Other studies confirm and extend these general findings within different behavioural paradigms. In one study rats were trained on an auditory fear- conditioning task (Moita *et al.* 2003). Prior to fear conditioning, few hippocampal cells were activated by an auditory stimulus. Following pairings of tone presentations and shocks, many cells fired briskly to the tone when the animal was in a particular place where the cell fired above baseline (the place field), although some fired associated with the tone across locations in the environment. These findings support the view that hippocampal cells rapidly encode conjunctions of specific salient stimuli and the places where they occur associated with a particular training experience, and some cells encode cues that are common across similar experiences. Another study characterized hippocampal firing patterns in humans during presentations of a variety of visual stimuli (Kreiman *et al.* 2000). They reported a substantial number of hippocampal neurons that fired when the subject viewed specific categories of material, (e.g. faces, famous people, animals, scenes, houses) across many exemplars of each. This observation is consistent with the notion that some hippocampal cells represent common features among the various episodes that could serve to link memories obtained in separate experiences. In addition, in studies that have examined the spatial firing properties of the same hippocampal neurons as animals explore different environments that share common features, some of the neurons fired differentially in each of the environments whereas other cells fired associated with features that are common across environments (Shapiro *et al.* 1997; Tanila *et al.* 1997; Skaggs and McNaughton 1998).

These observations are consistent with the proposal that the organization of hippocampal neuronal representations is structured to represent behavioural sequences across a broad range of behavioural protocols and species. A subset of hippocampal neurons are selectively activated at every moment throughout task performance across a broad range of behavioural protocols. Furthermore, the contents of hippocampal neuronal representations can be characterized as each and every regularity of the events that is salient during the performance of any task (Eichenbaum *et al.* 1999, Eichenbaum and Cohen 2001). These include both regularities of places where events occur and a broad range of non-spatial stimulus and behavioural events and contingencies that characterize the task in hand. The full scope of information encoded by the hippocampal population is precisely as broad as the set of attended and regular events that compose the behavioural protocol. Thus hippocampal population activity can be viewed as a continuous and automatic recording of attended experiences (Morris and Frey 1997). This characterization is consistent with the view that hippocampal ensembles encode experiences as sequences of events that define both rare experiences and common stimuli, places, and events that are shared across episodes, providing a framework for linking related memories (Eichenbaum *et al.* 1999).

The properties of relational memory account for findings on the role of the hippocampus in spatial memory

The hippocampus is critical to spatial memory in animals and humans, leading to the view that it mediates the creation and operation of cognitive maps

(O'Keefe and Nadel 1978; Burgess *et al.* 2002). Here, through a consideration of the findings on spatial memory and the spatial firing properties of hippocampal neurons, I propose that the cognitive mapping view can be reconciled with the relational memory hypothesis.

Recent studies on the spatial firing patterns of hippocampal neurons provide compelling data consistent with the present framework and inconsistent with the notion that the hippocampus creates spatial maps of the environment. In a study designed to contrast these theories, rats were trained on the classic spatial alternation task in a modified T-maze (Wood *et al.* 2000). Performance on this task requires that the animal distinguishes left-turn and right-turn episodes, and that it remembers the immediately preceding episode to guide its choice on the current trial. Thus, Olton (1984, 1986) considered this class of task similar in demand to that of episodic memory. The analysis of firing patterns in animals performing this task directly contrasted predictions of the cognitive mapping hypothesis and the relational memory hypothesis. The key comparison focused on the central 'stem' of the maze, i.e. the portion that the rat traversed on both trial types before making a left or right choice. According to the cognitive mapping hypothesis (O'Keefe and Nadel 1978), the activity of each cell should identify the locus of the rat within its map of the room in which the maze is situated, regardless of the demands of the ongoing alternation task. Therefore, according to this view, each place cell that fired when the rat was on the stem should fire similarly on left-turn and right-turn trials. Alternatively, according to the relational memory hypothesis, each hippocampal neuron encodes an event and its locus within one type of episode, leading to the prediction that most cells should fire when the rat was on the stem during either the left-turn or right-turn episode, but not both. Notably, the activity of some cells was expected to reflect the common features of the two types of episodes, in this case the common locations traversed on both trial types.

The findings strongly supported the relational memory hypothesis. Virtually all cells that fired when the rat was on the maze stem, and whose differential activity could not be accounted for by differences in head direction, running speed, or location on the two trial types, fired differentially on left-turn versus right-turn trials. The majority of cells showed striking selectivity, firing at over 10 times the rate on one trial type, suggesting that they were part of the representations of only one type of episode. Other cells fired substantially on both trial types, potentially providing a link between left-turn and right-turn representations by the common places traversed on both trial types. Similar results have been observed in other versions of this task (Frank *et al.* 2000; Ferbinteanu and Shapiro 2003; but see Lenck-Santini *et al.* 2002).

A consideration of these findings from the perspective of the literature on human spatial cognition suggests a framework for reconciliation of the cognitive mapping and relational memory hypotheses. Studies of human spatial cognition have revealed that there are multiple forms of representation of large-scale spatial environments, and these are differentially emphasized in numerous theories about the nature of cognitive maps (reviewed by Kitchin and Blades 2002). The most prominent among these forms of spatial representation are 'route' and 'survey' knowledge (McNamara 2002). Survey knowledge refers to the construction and use of a map-like representation of the overall layout of the environment. This strategy predominates when people have the aid of a map or if the goal is to create a map-like representation. Alternatively, when a map is not available and the goal is to learn a particular path, the initial knowledge is usually constituted as a representation of a route. With sufficient experience on routes within the same environment, people may learn global spatial dimensions, including distances and directions, and may subsequently construct a map-like representation. Whether or not a survey representation exists, it is easier for people to retrieve information from some perspectives than from others, suggesting that memory of space from egocentric views is the primary means of representation, and the ability to make judgements from novel views involves manipulation and integration of these representations (Wang and Spelke 2000; McNamara 2002).

Imagine that you have arrived at a hotel in a city that you have not previously visited and for which you have not obtained a map. As you go out for dinner on the first evening, you travel along a route, taking in several views and making several turns along the way to the restaurant. At this point, it is very unlikely you have a map-like representation of the environment, but it is likely that you can recall much of the route you have followed. The next day you go out again to a meeting in a different direction. A similar route representation is formed for that journey. However, imagine that today's journey intersects with the route followed yesterday. You may recognize the scene at the locus of intersection of the two journeys and recall the routes back to the hotel and to the restaurant along the previous journey. As you make additional journeys through the city, these also intersect, allowing you to construct a large-scale representation wherein route representations are linked by their intersections. Eventually, as more and more of the journeys share common locations and the particular routes are less important to remember, you develop a representation of the common loci and their spatial relations independent of particular routes, i.e. a map-like 'semantic' representation of the environment constrained and organized by the spatial regularities. At this point, you can probably draw a reasonable map of those parts of the city you have visited and can navigate along new routes deduced from the map-like representation.

This example suggests a common role for the hippocampus in spatial and non-spatial memory, consistent with the relational memory hypothesis. Just as in non-spatial learning, in spatial learning the hippocampus initially forms a representation of each spatially extended episode. In this case, a spatial episode consists of a series of views from places and your own movements through space, as well as any events witnessed along the way, that constitute a route for each journey. As multiple routes intersect, the common places are represented by some of the same hippocampal neurons, such that the route representations become linked, just as in the examples of learning overlapping non-spatial problems described above. Eventually, as more intersections are shared among journeys, some of those neurons represent only the common places, and those cells constitute true 'place cells'. In addition, when you arrive at a common location, the hippocampus may be able to generate many of the routes that included that location, mediating a capacity for navigation in novel directions.

The evidence on hippocampal neuronal firing patterns described above supports this accounting of spatial representations. Thus, in the study by Wood *et al.* (2000), separate subpopulations of hippocampal neurons can be described as representing the series of successive places that compose each type of episode, and some cells in each population represent the common places that link the different types of episodes. In addition, recent evidence from functional brain imaging suggests that the human hippocampus is also specifically involved in the representation of routes. Several functional imaging studies have now been performed on humans performing spatial tasks, and these reveal a common network of cortical areas activated during different aspects of spatial performance (Flitman *et al.* 1997; Mellet *et al.* 2000). Furthermore, when humans simply view complex spatial scenes, both the parahippocampal region and parts of the hippocampus can be activated (Epstein and Kanwisher 1998; Kohler *et al.* 2002). Other studies have directly investigated hippocampal activation during recall or encoding of large-scale environments. In one study humans initially explored an imaginary town using virtual reality technology (Maguire *et al.* 1997). Strong activation was observed in the right hippocampus during successful recall of routes compared with following arrows through a route or unsuccessful navigational attempts. Similarly, in London taxi drivers, the hippocampus is strongly activated when they recall specific routes through the city (Maguire *et al.* 1998).

These studies demonstrate hippocampal activation during route retrieval, but they do not distinguish whether the activations reflect recollection of specific routes or generation of a route from a map-like representation. Indeed, following initial study of either routes or maps, the hippocampus is activated during subsequent navigation of an environment (Mellet *et al.* 2000). A recent study that examined hippocampal activation specifically during the encoding of a novel environment speaks more directly to the nature of initial spatial representation (Shelton and Gabrieli 2002). In this study, subjects were scanned as they explored a large-scale virtual reality environment in one of two ways. Under one condition, they explored the environment from a 'bird's eye' view, encouraging a survey representation. Under the other condition, they explored the environment from a 'ground' perspective by entering through a doorway and traversing corridors and rooms, encouraging the representation of routes. As in previous imaging studies, a common network of cortical areas was activated in both conditions, but there were differences as well. In particular, survey encoding recruited greater activation in the inferior temporal and posterior parietal cortex, suggesting that survey representations are mainly encoded as complex visual scenes. In contrast, route encoding recruited regions not activated by survey encoding, including other cortical areas, the parahippocampal region, and the hippocampus.

These findings suggest a concept that contrasts with the view of Burgess *et al.* (2002), who suggested that the hippocampus encodes episodic memory by adding a temporal dimension to a fundamentally map-like survey representation. Instead, Shelton and Gabrieli's findings support the view that the hippocampus initially encodes a large-scale space as a representation of routes. These episodic representations can then be recalled and used to develop survey representations and in the navigation of well-known environments. The strong consistency in data on route encoding from studies on hippocampal neuronal firing patterns in rats and hippocampal activation in human functional imaging support the notion that hippocampal representations of space, like those for non-spatial memory, are fundamentally organized as sequences of events and places where they occur.

The hippocampal memory system

The present review has focused on the role of the hippocampus. However, surely a comprehensive understanding will require consideration of the large system of cortical (and other) areas with which the hippocampus is connected. Among these are some of neocortical association areas that play specific roles in episodic and semantic memory, and the parahippocampal cortical region surrounding the hippocampus. Brief considerations of the contributions of those cortical areas will precede a final summary of the present proposal about the mechanisms of relational memory representation.

Widespread neocortical areas play important roles in episodic and semantic memory (reviewed by Fuster 1995; Eichenbaum 2000; Buckner and Wheeler,

2001). Evidence from both neuropsychological studies and functional brain imaging indicate that the prefrontal cortex plays a complex but specific role in the retrieval of episodic memories. For example, patients with prefrontal damage are impaired in the organization of their search strategies for the order or grouping of words in a list they are attempting to recall (Milner *et al.* 1985; Gershberg and Shimamura 1995; Wheeler *et al.* 1995). Accordingly, areas of the prefrontal cortex are activated in normal human subjects during episodic retrieval in a variety of tasks. While the specific functional nature and localization of the activations is still an evolving story, the domain of activations includes semantic analysis, recollective monitoring, and rehearsal (Dobbins *et al.* 2002). Activation of the prefrontal cortex may reflect aspects of retrieval effort, rather than success in retrieval, consistent with the role of the prefrontal areas in working memory and rule learning (Miller 2000).

Recent studies have contrasted the differences in the role of cortical and hippocampal contributions to episodic memory. In one comparison, amnesic subjects maintained a capacity for immediate recall of episodes but were impaired if retrieval was delayed, consistent with the findings described above (Baddeley and Wilson 2002). In contrast, Alzheimer's patients, who have widespread cortical as well as hippocampal damage, are impaired with and without the delay, suggesting that cortical areas support an 'episodic buffer' that mediates temporary storage and rehearsal of episodic memories independent of involvement of the hippocampus. Conversely, posterior cortical areas are activated more in association with with success in retrieval. For example, activity in lateral temporal and parietal regions predicts whether a subject will successfully identify familiar items in recall tests (Kirchhoff *et al.* 2000; reviewed by Buckner and Wheeler, 2001). Also, the same sensory-specific cortical areas that are involved in processing of perceptual information are vigorously reactivated during vivid remembering in a recall test (Wheeler *et al.* 2000). This phenomenon probably reflects the activation of perceptual processing elements for stimuli associated with memory cues (Sakai and Miyashita 1991) and combinations of elements that compose configural cues (Baker *et al.* 2002).

In addition, the parahippocampal region plays a critical role in the convergence of multisensory information (Bussey *et al.*, 2002) and in mediating memory based on familiarity of stimuli (Eichenbaum, 2002). Thus animals with parahippocampal damage are impaired in discrimination tasks involving configurations of sensory cues, and indeed animals without a hippocampus may be more prone to configure stimuli than normal animals (Eichenbaum and Cohen 2001). Also, in some simple recognition tasks, in particular the delayed non-match to sample task, monkeys and rats with damage to the hippocampus are minimally impaired, whereas damage to the parahippocampal region results in severe loss of memory over brief periods (Murray 1996; Eichenbaum and Cohen 2001), consistent with some form of representation that can support recognition independent of the hippocampus.

Accordingly, recording studies in monkeys and rats have reported that neurons in the parahippocampal region can be active during memory delays in simple recognition tasks, and they show striking stimulus-selective differential responses to familiar and unfamiliar stimuli (Eichenbaum 2002). Furthermore, whereas neurons in the parahippocampal region respond differentially to the familiarity of a single stimulus, hippocampal neurons respond to alterations in relationships among familiar stimuli (Wan *et al.* 1999). Correspondingly, functional brain imaging studies in humans have revealed activations specifically in the parahippocampal region and not in the hippocampus associated with stimulus familiarity (Stern *et al.* 1996; Henson *et al.* 2003). The parahippocampal region is activated more during successful coding of independent items than in memory for relations among items, whereas the hippocampus is activated more during encoding of relations among items (Davachi and Wagner 2002; see also Duzel *et al.* 2003). Similarly, a recent study reported that hippocampal activation predicted later recollection of specific contextual details about learned materials, whereas perirhinal cortex activation predicted recognition of the learned items (Davachi *et al.* 2003). Furthermore, parahippocampal activation associated with familiarity can be dissociated from activation of the hippocampus during cued recall (Gabrieli *et al.* 1997). These studies strongly suggest that processing of neurons in the parahippocampal region is different from the kind of processing performed by hippocampal neurons. These findings, combined with the characterization of hippocampal neurons provided above, are consistent with the view that neurons in parahippocampal regions construct and maintain representations of single simple or configural items, whereas hippocampal neurons encode conjunctions or relations among independent items.

The combination of observations from all these studies suggests that multiple neocortical areas, the parahippocampal region, and the hippocampus work in concert to mediate relational memory (Eichenbaum 2000; Eichenbaum and Cohen 2001). According to this view, neocortical areas mediate the representation of stimulus details. These converge within the parahippocampal region as configural representations that compose distinct items in memory that can be recognized as familiar. The hippocampus binds complex perceptual representations as associations between items within an event, supporting conscious recall of events. Also, the hippocampus binds these events in order to record their flow in the memory of an experience. In addition, by iterative interactions between the hippocampal and parahippocampal region, the hippocampus can employ the persistent stimulus representations of the parahippocampal region to identify common features along episodes (Fell *et al.* 2001). The output of hippocampal representation is called up by strategic processing in the prefrontal cortex, which directs the contents and timing of recovery of the detailed cortical representations and can mediate in working memory other types of cognitive processing on the retrieved memories. Such a scheme could account for the phenomenology of declarative memory in both the non-spatial and spatial domains.

Conclusions

The present theoretical considerations and experimental evidence support the proposal that the hippocampus is involved in three types of 'binding' fundamental to declarative memory. First, the activity of hippocampal neurons reflects the binding of multiple stimuli, behavioural actions, and the context in which these occur, composing representations of complex unique events. The observations on single neurons reviewed above are consistent with recent evidence from studies on humans indicating that the hippocampus is more activated during the encoding and retrieval of associations among stimuli and their context (Gabrieli *et al.* 1997; Davachi and Wagner 2002; Davachi *et al.* 2003) and that amnesic patients with hippocampal damage are selectively impaired in memory for associations among stimuli compared with intact memory for single items (Giovanello *et al.* 2003b). However, there is evidence that cortical areas surrounding the hippocampus are also more activated during associative processing (Kirwan and Stark 2004), highlighting the need to distinguish the roles of the hippocampus and cortical components of the hippocampal system in the binding of elements that compose an event (Bussey *et al.* 2002). In addition, there is evidence that amnesic patients can be impaired in simple as well as associative memory (Stark *et al.* 2002), highlighting the need to distinguish how events might be differentially constituted as associations among distinct items (e.g. an object carried by a person) or configured as elements of a single item (e.g. the features of an object). The particular kind of associative binding supported by the hippocampus may be essential to recollection of events as contrasted with familiarity with the same items (Yonelinas 2002; Fortin *et al.* 2004).

Secondly, the hippocampus plays a central role in binding sequential events composing unique episodes. The requisite role for the hippocampus in this kind of binding is evident in a selective deficit in memory for the orderliness of events in unique episodes as contrasted with intact recognition of individual events (Fortin *et al.* 2002). In addition, the activity of hippocampal neurons distinguishes events by the unique episodes in which they occur (Frank *et al.* 2000; Wood *et al.* 2000; Ferbinteanu and Shapiro 2003). Additional evidence indicates that the binding of sequential events into distinct episodes plays a critical role in our ability to disambiguate experiences that share common elements (Levy 1989). A recent examination of this hypothesis showed that whereas normal rats can distinguish overlapping sequences of odours, rats with selective hippocampal damage are severely impaired (Agster *et al.* 2002). Considerable further research on humans and animals is required to elaborate the role of the hippocampus in the representation of order and to integrate that function with its role in disambiguation of overlapping experiences.

Thirdly, the hippocampus plays a critical role in binding distinct experiences into a network of memories that supports the flexibility of declarative memory. Animals with selective hippocampal damage can acquire a set of complex and conflicting discrimination problems but are severely impaired in making transitive inferences between items that are only indirectly related by common elements between problems (Bunsey and Eichenbaum 1996; Dusek and Eichenbaum 1997). The involvement of the hippocampus in binding indirectly related items was recently confirmed in studies showing activation of the hippocampus in humans performing similar transitive inference judgements (Heckers *et al.* 2004; Preston *et al.* 2004). Also, these findings are consistent with recent evidence concerning the role of the hippocampus in semantic memory. Several recent studies have emphasized the preservation of semantic memory compared with severe impairment in episodic memory in humans with hippocampal damage (Vargha-Khadem *et al.* 1997; Verfaellie *et al.* 2000; O'Kane *et al.* 2004). In contrast, Manns *et al.* (2003) reported severe impairment for semantic as well as episodic information in patients with damage limited to the hippocampal formation. A resolution of this issue was suggested in the findings of Bayley and Squire (2002) who successfully trained amnesic patients to recall and recognize word sequences, but these patients were severely impaired in the flexibility with which they could employ their memories. Within the present framework, the details of semantic memory are considered the province of cortical representation, providing a basis for sparing of semantic memory capacities in amnesia. However, the binding of distinct experiences that share common (semantic) elements contributes critically to the flexibility with which those semantic memories can be expressed.

Acknowledgements

This work was supported by grants from the national Institute of Mental Health (NIMH) and the national Institute on Aging (NIA). The author is indebted to

Yadin Dudai, Joseph Manns, and Neal Cohen for their comments on a preliminary version of this chapter.

References

Agster, K.L., Fortin, N.J., and Eichenbaum, H. (2002). The hippocampus and disambiguation of overlapping sequences. *Journal of Neuroscience*, **22**, 5760–5768.

Amaral, D.G., and Witter, M.P. (1995). Hippocampal formation. In *The Rat Nervous System* (2nd edn) (ed G. Pacinos). San Diego, CA: Academic Press, pp. 443–493.

Aristotle (350 BC). *On Memory and Reminiscence* (trans J.I. Beare). Available online at: http://www.knuten.liu.se/~bjoch509/works/aristotle/memory.txt (accessed 3 February 2003).

Baddeley, A. (2000). The episodic buffer: a new component of working memory? *Trends in Cognitive Sciences*, **4**, 417–423.

Baddeley, A. and Wilson, B.A. (2002). Prose recall and amnesia: implications for the structure of working memory. *Neuropsychologia*, **40**, 1737–1743.

Baker, C.I., Behrmann, M., and Olson, C.R. (2002). Impact of learning on representation of parts and wholes in the monkey inferotemporal cortex. *Nature Neuroscience*, **5**, 1210–1216.

Bayley, P.J. and Squire, L.R. (2002). Medial temporal lobe amnesia: gradual acquisition of factual information by nondeclarative memory. *Journal of Neuroscience*, **22**, 5741–5748.

Berger, T.W., Rinaldi, P.C., Weisz, D.J., and Thompson, R.F. (1983). Single-unit analysis of different hippocampal cell types during classical conditioning of rabbit nictitating membrane response. *Journal of Neurophysiology*, **50**, 1197–1219.

Bliss, T.V.P. and Collinridge, G.L. (1993). A synaptic model of memory: long-term potentiation in the hippocampus. *Nature*, **361**, 31–39.

Buckner, R.L. and Wheeler, M.E. (2001). The cognitive neuroscience of remembering. *Nature Reviews Neuroscience*, **2**, 624–634.

Bunsey, M. and Eichenbaum, H. (1996). Conservation of hippocampal memory function in rats and humans. *Nature*, **379**, 255–257.

Burgess, N., Maguire, E.A., and O'Keefe, J. (2002). The human hippocampus and spatial and episodic memory. *Neuron*, **35**, 625–641.

Bussey, T.J., Saksida, L.M., and Murray, E.A. (2002). The role of perirhinal cortex in memory and perception: conjunctive representations for object identification. In *The Parahippocampal Region: Organization and Role in Cognitive Function* (ed M.P. Witter and F. Wouterlood). Oxford: Oxford University Press, pp. 239–254.

Cohen, N.J. and Eichenbaum, H. (1993). *Memory, Amnesia, and the Hippocampal System.* Cambridge, MA: MIT Press.

Cohen, N.J., Poldrack, R.A., and Eichenbaum, H. (1997). Memory for items and memory for relations in the procedural/declarative memory framework. *Memory*, **5**, 131–178.

Cohen, N.J., Ryan, J., Hunt, C., Romine, L., Wszalek, T., and Nash, C. (1999). Hippocampal system and declarative (relational) memory: summarizing the data from functional neuroimaging studies. *Hippocampus*, **9**, 83–98.

Davachi, L. and Wagner, A.G. (2002). Hippocampal contributions to episodic encoding: insights from relational and item-based learning. *Journal of Neurophysiology*, **88**, 982–990.

Davachi, L., Mitchell, J.P. and Wagner, A.D. (2003). Multiple routes to memory: distinct medial temporal lobe processes build item and source memories. *Proceedings of the National Academy of Sciences of the United States of America*, **100**, 2157–2162.

Deadwyler, S.A., Bunn, T., and Hampson, R.E. (1996). Hippocampal ensemble activity during spatial delayed-nonmatch-to-sample performance in rats. *Journal of Neuroscience*, **16**, 354–372.

Dobbins, I.G., Foley, H., Schacter, D.L., and Wagner, A.D. (2002). Executive control during episodic retrieval: multiple prefrontal processes subserve source memory. *Neuron*, **35**, 989–996.

Downes, J.J., Mayes, A.R., MacDonald, C., and Humkin, N.M. (2002). Temporal order memory in patients with Korsakoff's syndrome and medial temporal amnesia. *Neuropsychologia*, **40**, 853–861.

Dusek, J.A., Eichenbaum, H. (1997). The hippocampus and memory for orderly stimulus relations. *Proceedings of the National Academy of Sciences of the United States of America*, **94**, 7109–7114.

Duzel, E., Habib, R., Rotte, M., Guderian, S., Tulving, E., and Heinze, H.-J. (2003). Human hippocampal and parahippocampal activity during visual associative recognition memory for spatial and nonspatial stimulus configurations. *Journal of Neuroscience* **23**, 9439–9444.

Eichenbaum, H. (2000). A cortical-hippocampal system for declarative memory. *Nature Reviews Neuroscience*, **1**, 41–50.

Eichenbaum, H. (2002). Memory representations in the parahippocampal region. In *The Parahippocampal Region, Organization and Role in Cognitive Function* (ed M. Witter and F. Wouterlood). Oxford: Oxford University Press, pp. 165–184.

Eichenbaum, H. (1994). The hippocampal system and declarative memory in humans and animals: experimental analysis and historical origins. In *Memory Systems* (ed D.L. Schacter and E. Tulving). Cambridge, MA: MIT Press.

Eichenbaum, H. and Cohen, N.J. (2001). *From Conditioning to Conscious Recollection: Memory Systems of the Brain*. New York: Oxford University Press.

Eichenbaum, H., Kuperstein, M., Fagan, A., and Nagode, J. (1987). Cue-sampling and goal-approach correlates of hippocampal unit activity in rats performing an odor discrimination task. *Journal of Neuroscience*, **7**, 716–732.

Eichenbaum, H., Cohen, N.J., Otto, T. and Wible, C. (1992a). Memory representation in the hippocampus: functional domain and functional organization. In *Memory: Organization and Locus of Change* (ed L.R. Squire, G. Lynch, N.M. Weinberger and J.L. McGaugh). New York: Oxford University Press, pp. 163–204.

Eichenbaum, H., Otto, T., and Cohen, N.J. (1992b). The hippocampus. What does it do? *Behavioral and Neural Biology*, **57**, 2–36.

Eichenbaum, H., Otto, T., and Cohen, N.J. (1994). Two functional components of the hippocampal memory system. *Brain and Behavioral Sciences*, **17**, 449–518.

Eichenbaum, H., Dudchencko, P., Wood, E., Shapiro, M., and Tanila, H. (1999). The hippocampus, memory, and place cells, Is it spatial memory or a memory space? *Neuron*, **23**, 209–226.

Ekstrom, A.D., Kahana, M.J., Caplan, J.B., *et al.* (2003). Cellular networks underlying human spatial navigation. *Nature*, **425**, 184–188.

Epstein, R. and Kanwisher, N. (1998). A cortical representation of the local visual environment. *Nature*, **392**, 598–601.

Fell, J., Klaver, P., Lehnertz, K., Grunwald, T., Schaller, C., Elger, C.E., and Fernandez, G. (2001). Human memory formation is accompanied by rhinal-hippocampal coupling and decoupling. *Nature Neuroscience*, **4**, 1259–1264.

Ferbinteanu, J. and Shapiro, M.L. (2003). Prospective and retrospective memory coding in the hippocampus. *Neuron*, **40**, 1227–1239.

Flitman, S., O'Grady, J., Cooper, V., and Grafman, J. (1997). Pet imaging of maze processing. *Neuropsychologia*, **35**, 409–420.

Fortin, N.J., Agster, K.L., and Eichenbaum, H. (2002). Critical role of the hippocampus in memory for sequences of events. *Nature Neuroscience*, **5**, 458–462.

Fortin, N.J., Wright, S.P., and Eichenbaum, H. (2004). Recollection-like memory retrieval in rats is dependent on the hippocampus. *Nature*, **431**, 188–191.

Frank, L.M., Brown, E.N., and Wilson, M. (2000). Trajectory encoding in the hippocampus and entorhinal cortex. *Neuron*, **27**, 169–178.

Fuster, J.M. (1995). *Memory in the Cerebral Cortex*. Cambridge, MA: MIT Press.

Gabrieli, J.D.E., Brewer, J.B., Desmond, J.E., and Glover G.H. (1997). Separate neural bases of two fundamental memory processes in the human medial temporal lobe. *Science*, **276**, 264–266.

Gershberg, F.B. and Shimamura, A.P. (1995). Impaired use of organizational strategies in free recall following frontal lobe damage. *Neuropsychologia*, **33**, 1305–1333.

Giovanello, K.S., Schnyer, D.M., and Verfaellie, M. (2003a). A critical role for the anterior hippocampus in relational memory: evidence from an fMRI study comparing associative and item recognition. *Hippocampus*, **14**, 5–8.

Giovanello, K.S., Verfaellie, M., and Keane, M.M. (2003b). Disproportionate deficit in associative recognition relative to item recognition in global amnesia. *Cognitive, Affective, and Behavioral Neuroscience* **3**, 186–194.

Heckers, S., Zalezak, M., Weiss, A.P., Ditman, T., and Titone, D. (2004). Hippocampal activation during transitive inference in humans. *Hippocampus*, **14**, 153–162.

Henke, K., Buck, A., Weber, B., and Wieser, H.G. (1997). Human hippocampus establishes associations in memory. *Hippocampus*, **7**, 249–256.

Henson, R.N.A., Cansino, S., Herron, J.E., Robb, W.G.K., and Rugg, M.D. (2003). A familiarity signal in human anterior medial temporal cortex? *Hippocampus*, **13**, 301–304.

Hopkins, R.O., Kesner, R.P., and Goldstein, M. (1995). Item and order recognition memory in subjects with hypoxic brain injury. *Brain and Cognition*, **27**, 180–201.

James, W. (1890). *The Principles of Psychology* (1918 edn). New York: Holt.

Kesner, R.P., Gilbert, P.E., and Barua, L.A. (2002). The role of the hippocampus in memory for the temporal order of a sequence of odors. *Behavioral Neuroscience*, **116**, 286–290.

Kirchhoff, B.A., Wagner, A.D., Maril, A., and Stern, C.E. (2000). Prefrontal-temporal circuitry for novel stimulus encoding and subsequent memory. *Journal of Neuroscience*, **20**, 6173–6180.

Kirwan, C.B. and Stark, C.E.L. (2004). Medial temporal lobe activation during encoding and retrieval of novel face–name pairs. *Hippocampus*, **14**, 919–930.

Kitchin, R. and Blades, M. (2002). *The Cognition of Geographic Space*. London: IB Tauris.

Kohler, S., Crane, J., and Milner, B. (2002). Differential contributions of the parahippocampal place area and anterior hippocampus to human memory for scenes. *Hippocampus*, **12**, 718–723.

Kreiman, K., Kock, C., and Fried, I. (2000). Catgegory specific visual responses of single neurons in the human medial temporal lobe. *Nature Neuroscience*, **3**, 946–953.

Lenck-Santini, P.P., Muller, R.U., Save, E., and Poucet, B. (2002). Relationships between place cell firing fields and navigational decisions by rats. *Journal of Neuroscience*, **22**, 9035–9047.

Levy, W.B. (1989). A computational approach to hippocampal function. In *Computational Models of Learning in Simple Systems* (ed R.D. Hawkins and G.H. Bower). New York: Academic Press, pp. 243–305.

Levy, W.B. (1996). A sequence predicting CA3 is a flexible associator that learns and uses context to solve hippocampal-like tasks. *Hippocampus*, **6**, 579–590.

Lisman, J.E. (1999). Relating hippocampal circuitry to function: recall of memory sequences by reciprocal dentate–CA3 interactions. *Neuron*, **22**, 233–242.

McEchron, M.D. and Disterhoft, J.F. (1997). Sequence of single neuron changes in CA1 hippocampus of rabbits during acquisition of trace eyeblink conditioned responses. *Journal of Neurophysiology*, **78**, 1030–1044.

McNamara, T.P. (2002). Spatial memory. In *Learning and Memory* (2nd edn) (ed J. R. Byrne). New York: Macmillan, pp. 633–636.

Maguire, E.A., Frackowiak, R.S.J., and Frith, C.D. (1997). Recalling routes around London, activation of the right hippocampus in taxi drivers. *Journal of Neuroscience*, **17**, 7103–7110.

Maguire, E.A., Burgess, N., Donnett, J.G., Frackowiak, R.S.J., Frith, C.D., and O'Keefe, J. (1998). Knowing where and getting there: a human navigational network. *Science*, **280**, 921–924.

Manns, J.R., Hopkins, R.O., and Squire, L.R. (2003). Semantic memory and the human hippocampus. *Neuron* **38**, 127–133.

Martin, S.J., Grimwood, P.D., and Morris, R.G.M. (2000). Synaptic plasticity and memory, an evaluation of the hypothesis. *Annual Review of Neuroscience*, **23**, 649–711.

Mellet, E., Bricogne, S., Tzourio-Mazoyer, N., *et al.* (2000). Neural correlates of topographic mental exploration: The impact of route versus survey perspective encoding. *NeuroImage*, **12**, 588–600.

Miller, E.K. (2000). The prefrontal cortex and cognitive control. *Nature Reviews Neuroscience*, **1**, 59–65.

Milner, B., Petrides, M., and Smith, M.L. (1985). Frontal lobes and the temporal organization of memory. *Human Neurobiology*, **4**, 137–142.

Moita, M.A.P., Moisis, S., Zhou, Y., LeDoux, J.E., and Blair, H.T. (2003). Hippocampal place cells acquire location specific location specific responses to the conditioned stimulus during auditory fear conditioning. *Neuron*, **37**, 485–497.

Morris, R.G.M. and Frey, U. (1997). Hippocampal synaptic plasticity, role in spatial learning or the automatic recording of attended experience? *Philosophical Transactions of the Royal Society of London, Series B, Biological Sciences*, **352**, 1489–1503.

Murray, E.A. (1996). What have ablation studies told us about the neural substrates of stimulus memory? *Seminars in the Neurosciences*, **8**, 13–22.

O'Kane, G., Kensinger, E.A., and Corkin, S. (2004). Evidence for semantic learning in profound amnesia: an investigation with patient HM. *Hippocampus* **14**, 417–425.

O'Keefe, J. and Nadel, L. (1978). *The Hippocampus as a Cognitive Map*. New York: Oxford University Press.

Olton, D.S. (1984). Comparative analyses of episodic memory. *Brain and Behavioral Sciences*, **7**, 250–251.

Olton, D.S. (1986). Hippocampal function and memory for temporal context. In *The Hippocampus* (ed R.L. Isaacson and K.H. Pribram), Vol. **4**. New York: Plenum Press.

Preston, A., Shrager, Y., Dudukovic, N.M., and Gabrieli, J.D.E. (2004). Hippocampal contribution to the novel use of relational information in declarative memory. *Hippocampus* **14**, 148–152.

Reed, J.M. and Squire, L.R. (1997). Impaired recognition memory in patients with lesions limited to the hippocampal formation. *Behavioral Neuroscience*, **111**, 667–675.

Roberts, W. (2002). Are animals stuck in time? *Psychological Bulletin*, **128**, 473–489.

Sakai, K. and Miyashita, Y. (1991). Neural organization for the long-term memory of paired associates. *Nature*, **354**, 152–155.

Shapiro, M.L. and Eichenbaum, H. (1999). Hippocampus as a memory map, synaptic plasticity and memory encoding by hippocampal neurons. *Hippocampus*, **9**, 365–384.

Shapiro, M.L., Tanila, H., and Eichenbaum, H. (1997). The cues that hippocampal place cells encode, Dynamic and hierarchical representation of local and distal stimuli. *Hippocampus*, **7**, 624–642.

Shelton, A.L. and Gabrieli, J.D.E. (2002). Neural correlates of encoding space from route and survey perspectives. *Journal of Neuroscience*, **22**, 2711–2717.

Skaggs, W.E. and McNaughton, B.L. (1998). Spatial firing properties of hippocampal CA1 populations in an environment containing two visually identical regions. *Journal of Neuroscience*, **18**, 8455–8466.

Small, S.A., Nava, A.S., Perera, G.M., DeLaPaz, R., Mayeux, R., and Stern, Y. (2001). Circuit mechanisms underlying memory encoding and retrieval in the long axis of the hippocampal formation. *Nature Neuroscience*, **4**, 442–449.

Sohal, V.S. and Hasselmo, M.E. (1998). Changes in $GABA_B$ modulation during a theta cycle may be analogous to the fall of temperature during annealing. *Neural Computation*, **10**, 889–902.

Sperling, R., Chua, E., Cocchiarella, A., *et al.* (2003). Putting names to faces: successful encoding of associative memories activates the anterior hippocampal formation. *NeuroImage*, **20**, 1400–1410.

Spiers, H.J., Burgess, N., Hartley, T., Vargha-Khadem, F., and O'Keefe, J. (2001). Bilateral hippocampal pathology impairs topographical and episodic memory but not visual pattern matching. *Hippocampus*, **11**, 715–725.

Squire, L.R., Cohen, N.J., and Nadel, L. (1984). The medial temporal region and memory consolidation: a new hypothesis. In *Memory Consolidation* (ed H. Weingartner and E. Parker). Hillsdale, NJ: Erlbaum.

Squire, L.R., Stark, C.E.L., and Clark, R.E. (2004). The medial temporal lobe. *Annual Review of Neuroscience*, **27**, 279–306.

Stark, C.E.L., Bayley, P.J., and Squire, L.R. (2002). Recognition memory for single items and for associations is similarly impaired following damage to the hippocampal region. *Learning and Memory*, **9**, 238–242.

Stern, C.E., Corkin, S., Gonzalez, R.G., *et al.* (1996). The hippocampal formation participates in novel picture encoding: evidence from functional MRI. *Proceedings of the National Academy of Sciences of the United States of America*, **93**, 8660–8665.

Tanila, H., Sipila, P., Shapiro, M., and Eichenbaum, H. (1997). Brain aging, changes in the nature of information coding by the hippocampus. *Journal of Neuroscience*, **17**, 5155–5166.

Tulving, E. (1983). *Elements of Episodic Memory*. New York: Oxford University Press.

Tulving, E. (2002). Episodic memory: from mind to brain. *Annual Review of Psychology*, **53**, 1–25.

Turriziani, P., Fadda, L., Caltagirone, C., and Carlesimo, G.A. (2004). Recognition memory for single items and associations in amnesia patients. *Neuropsychologia* **42**: 426–433.

Vargha-Khadem, F., Gadin, D.G., Watkins, K.E., Connelly, A., Van Paesschen, W. and Mishkin, M. (1997). Differential effects of early hippocampal pathology on episodic and semantic memory. *Science*, **277**, 376–380.

Verfaellie, M., Koseff, P., and Alexander, M.P. (2000). Acquisition of novel semantic information in amnesia: effects of lesion location. *Neuropsychologia* **38**, 484–492.

Wallenstein, G.V., Eichenbaum, H., and Hasselmo, M.E. (1998). The hippocampus as an associator of discontiguous events. *Trends in Neurosciences*, **21**, 315–365.

Wan, H., Aggleton, J.P., and Brown, M.W. (1999). Different contributions of the hippocampus and perirhinal cortex to recognition memory. *Journal of Neuroscience* **19**, 1142–1148.

Wang, R.F. and Spelke, E.S. (2000). Updating egocentric representations in human navigation. *Cognition*, **77**, 215–250.

Wheeler, M.A., Stuss, D.T. and Tulving, E. (1995). Frontal lobe damage produces episodic memory impairment. *Journal of the International Neuropsychological Society*, **1**, 525–536.

Wheeler, M.E., Petersen, S.E. and Buckner, R.L. (2000). Memory's echo: vivid remembering reactivates sensory-specific cortex. *Proceedings of the National Academy of Sciences of the United States of America*, **97**, 11125–11129.

Wiebe, S.P. and Staubli, U.V. (1999). Dynamic filtering of recognition memory codes in the hippocampus. *Journal of Neuroscience*, **19**, 10562–10574.

Wood, E., Dudchenko, P.A., and Eichenbaum, H. (1999). The global record of memory in hippocampal neuronal activity. *Nature*, **397**, 613–616.

Wood, E., Dudchenko, P., Robitsek, J.R., and Eichenbaum, H. (2000). Hippocampal neurons encode information about different types of memory episodes occurring in the same location. *Neuron*, **27**, 623–633.

Yonelinas, A.P. (2002). The nature of recollection and familiarity: a review of 30 years of research. *Journal of Memory and Language* **46**, 441–517.

Zeineh, M.M., Engel, S.A., Thompson, P.M., and Brookheimer, S.Y. (2003). Dynamics of the hippocampus during encoding and retrieval of face–name pairs. *Science*, **299**, 577–580.

Chapter 3

Part or parcel? Contextual binding of events in episodic memory

Iris Trinkler, John A. King, Hugo J. Spiers, and Neil Burgess

Introduction

In our daily life we experience a vast number of events involving objects, people, and places. Memory for personally experienced events is often referred to as episodic memory and has been distinguished from semantic memory, memory for factual information, by the fact that episodic memories contain both information about what happened and a specific spatial and temporal context (Tulving 1972). Tulving (1983, p. 223) hassuggested that the 'prototypical unit of an episodic memory is an event', and the different elements of an event are believed to be strongly tied together to provide a single encapsulated unit, allowing 're-experience' of all aspects of the event at retrieval (Tulving 2002, 1983, 1972).

In this chapter we examine whether events are the units of episodic memory. Taken at face value this would imply that episodic memory is holistic: when an event is remembered, *all* of its elements including the spatiotemporal context are remembered together. In contrast, if this viewpoint were completely untrue, memory for different elements of an event might be remembered or forgotten *independently*. Between these theoretical extremes, we might characterize the argument that episodic memory for events is holistic in terms of the size of the correlation between performance when an event is retrieved via one cue and performance when the same event is retrieved via another cue. A fully holistic view would predict maximal correlation. A fully fragmented view or 'independent model' of memory for the many types of association comprising an event would predict no such correlation.

Support for the different interpretations (holistic or fragmentary) can be found in previous research. The holistic view is strongly implied by the theoretical stand point of Tulving and his co-authors. For example, episodic remembering is 'the kind of awareness that characterizes "mental re-living" of happenings from one's personal past. It is phemenologically known to all healthy people who can "travel back in time in their own minds"." (Duzel *et al.* 1997, p. 5973). Tulving and his colleagues are not alone in their suggestion that events might be the units of episodic memory. Fisher and Chandler remark that the episodic memory system 'treats information in a close temporal-spatial proximity as an event that is represented in an *isolated* trace. Later activation of that trace produces recollection of that specific event' (Fisher and Chandler 1991, p. 722, emphasis added), based on observed interdependence between the recall of different event sets. A study by Brewer and Dupree (1983) suggests that, for at least some types of events, recall appears to be all or none. In their experiments participants were shown films in which actors performed goal-directed actions. In some cases there was a causal link between elements in the event and in others the link was solely temporal. Recall of the causally related events tended to be all or none, while the recall of the non-causally related events tended to be less well correlated.

Jones (1976) examined the recall of different elements of an event using one or several elements as retrieval cues. Participants observed sequences of pictures of coloured objects, each in a specific location within the scene. They were then cued with the colour, shape, spatial position, or sequential position, or with combinations of these cues, and their ability to retrieve the remaining elements was tested. Jones noticed several patterns in these data. First, the nature of sequential position as a memory cue was different from the other elements in being asymmetrical. Retrieval of sequential position was poor compared with its usefulness as a retrieval cue (in addition, retrieval of serial position decreased with serial position, while retrieval of other information from serial position followed a U-shaped curve, being best near to the start or end of a sequence). In contrast, other elements were used symmetrically: retrieval of element A by element B was as good as retrieval of element B by element A. This symmetrical use of cues was also proposed by Asch and Ebenholz (1962). Secondly, recall performance was not found to increase dramatically with additional cues, ruling out a fully independent model in which each pairwise association contributes independently to the probability of success. Jones suggested that memories of the visual characteristics of his events (object, colour, and location, i.e. ignoring sequential position) were stored as independent but holistic fragments. Thus those elements represented within the same fragment would act holistically (all being equally effective and used symmetrically and non-additively), while cueing with multiple elements would increase the chance of accessing a fragment containing a given element required for recall.

In a long-term study of his own memory, Wagenaar (1986) attempted to recall different autobiographical events recorded over 4 years by probing himself with different elements of each event (who, what, when, and where). Consistent with

Jones's (1976) study, he found that temporal information (when) was a very poor cue even though it could be retrieved reasonably well. However, unlike Jones, he also found marked differences in the usefulness of the remaining elements as cues and asymmetry in their processing: He found 'what' to be the best cue, while 'where' was slightly better than 'who'. Correspondingly, 'what' was also used asymmetrically in being less well retrieved via other elements than they were retrieved by it. The observation that not all elements of an event will serve as equally effective retrieval cues is also stressed in the 'headed records' model of memory (Morton *et al.* 1985; Morton and Bekerian 1986). Finally, also unlike Jones, Wagenaar found that the advantage of retrieving an element by cueing with multiple other elements slightly exceeded that predicted by a fully independent model in many cases.

Wagenaar interpreted the differences between his study and that of Jones in terms of differences in cue specificity. In Jones's study, within each list of nine events, each cue was specific to only one event, whereas Wagenaar's cues varied in specificity, with 'what' being the most specific, and who and where varying in specificity. Thus more specific cues might be more efficient in prompting retrieval, and many less specific cues might, in Jones's terms, be contained in very many fragments. This latter consideration raises the possibility that multiple cues are combined into configural cues that could overcome the lack of specificity, as has also been suggested by Foss and Harwood's (1975) model of sentence recall. An alternative interpretation would simply be that the elements of Wagenaar's events were stored independently, perhaps differing from Jones's stimuli in being truly multimodal. The slight increase in the advantage found for multiple cueing might result from the multiple-cue retrieval attempts occurring after the single-cue attempts.

Here we investigate the binding of the context of an event with the event's content in episodic memory using a computer-based virtual reality (VR) paradigm involving pseudo-realistic simulated events. We hope to combine some of the contextual richness of autobiography with some of the control of stimuli across participants of traditional laboratory-based memory experiments. In this virtual context-dependent memory (VCM) paradigm, participants move through the virtual environment and encounter virtual characters within it. The events for which memory will be tested consist of the presentation of an object to the participant by a virtual character (see Fig. 3.2 below). We distinguish between the 'content' of the event, i.e. the change in the world that marks the event (in this case the presentation of an object), from the ongoing 'context' of the event, including the surrounding spatial environment, time, and the person giving the object (Burgess *et al.* 2001).

Participants experience a series of such events as they move about the virtual town. After this learning phase, participants are tested on their memory for the events using a context-dependent two-alternative forced-choice paradigm: pairs of objects are presented in a particular place, with a particular character present. Different types of questions probe memories for different elements of the context of the events experienced in the learning phase (e.g. 'which object did you receive in this place?'). In addition, one question type tests the memory for the content of the events alone (i.e. the object given), in which the familiar object that was present in the learning phase must be recognized compared wth a similar-looking novel foil. In one variation of this paradigm, we added odour as an additional contextual element. Our scope was to explicitly look for any relationships between the probability of retrieving one element of an event and the probability of retrieving another element of that same event.

The categorization of memory into subtypes, such as 'episodic memory', goes hand-in-hand with consideration of its neural bases. Indeed, the aim of much of the neuroscience research into memory is to match structure to function. As we discuss below, the hippocampus has been strongly implicated in supporting episodic memory. Here, we note that discussion concerns the specific role in memory played by the hippocampus as often as it concerns the specification of the psychological process of 'episodic memory', exemplified by the term 'hippocampal-dependent memory'. Before we present the methods and results of our experiments in detail, we discuss the neuropsychological and neuroimaging findings relating to the neural bases of episodic memory, and of our VCM task in particular (reviewed by Burgess *et al.* 2002).

Neural bases of episodic memory

There is a consensus that context-dependent memory for personally experienced events (i.e. 'episodic' memory) is supported by the hippocampus (Kinsbourne and Wood 1975; O'Keefe and Nadel 1978; Squire and Zola-Morgan 1991; Vargha-Khadem *et al.* 1997; Eichenbaum and Cohen 2001; reviewed by Spiers *et al.* 2001c, Burgess *et al.* 2002), although opinion remains divided about what possible other roles the human hippocampus might perform and over the role of other brain regions in episodic memory. This controversy includes debate concerning the possible hippocampal contribution to acontextual forms of memory such as memory for factual knowledge ('semantic memory'). Declarative memory theory (e.g. Squire and Zola-Morgan 1991) sees the medial temporal lobe (including the amygdala and surrounding neocortex as well as the hippocampus) as supporting all forms of explicit memory in an undifferentiated manner.

A further dissociation has been postulated between different types of retrieval: psychological studies (Mandler 1980, 1991, Jacoby *et al.* 1993, reviewed by Yonelinas 2002) suggest that two distinct processes are involved in recognition memory, one based on a general sense that the stimulus has been encountered before ('familiarity-based recognition') and the other entailing specific retrieval of an event and its context ('episodic recollection'). It has been suggested that these processes are dissociated in the brain, with a circuit including the mamillary bodies, anterior thalamus, and hippocampus supporting episodic recollection, while a distinct parallel system, including the medial thalamus and perirhinal cortex, supports familiarity-based recognition (Delay and Brion 1969; Gaffan and Parker 1996; Vargha-Khadem *et al.* 1997; Aggleton and Brown 1999; Wan *et al.* 1999; Bogacz *et al.* 2001; Tulving 2001; Holdstock *et al.* 2002; Yonelinas 2002). In a recent review, Rugg and Yonelinas (2003) concluded that clinical data support the dual-process model, suggesting that, while familiarity is commonly impaired in amnesia, recollection is disrupted to a greater degree.

We have used the VCM paradigm introduced above in some recent neuropsychological investigations to address the issue of the neural bases of familiarity-based recognition and episodic recollection (Spiers *et al.* 2001a, b; King *et al.* 2004). First, we discuss our experiments with Jon, a young man with focal bilateral hippocampal pathology (Vargha-Khadem *et al.* 1997). He was between 5 and 6 years old when it was discovered that he was experiencing spatial, temporal, and episodic memory problems. Further investigation revealed selective bilateral hippocampal pathology apparently caused by perinatal anoxia. His hippocampal volumes are approximately half those of control participants (Gadian *et al.* 2000). There is also evidence that the remaining hippocampal tissue is compromised, but that extra-hippocampal regions are largely preserved. Jon's educational record suggests few problems with semantic memory; for instance, he passed a UK General Certificate of Secondary Education (GCSE) examination in history. His verbal IQ was assessed to be 108 and his performance IQ 120 when tested at the age of 19.

We tested Jon using the VCM paradigm (for details see Experiment 1 and Spiers *et al.* (2001a)) and found that his ability to recognize the objects used in the events was spared but his context-dependent recognition memory was impaired. However, there were two potential problems with this study. First, control participants also showed lower scores for the context-dependent task than the object-recognition task in this experiment, so that we could not exclude the possibility that a non-linear effect of difficulty compromised Jon's performance. Secondly, we were concerned that a high degree of similarity between the contexts of different events might have reduced their distinctiveness, possibly

Table 3.1 Hippocampal patient Jon's performance shows a comparable score for a purely familiarity-based recognition task (context-free Object condition) as control participants, as opposed to impaired performance in two context-dependent episodic-memory recognition tasks (Person and Place conditions)

Participant(s)	Question type		
	Context-free	Context-dependent	
	Object	Person	Place
Jon (%)	85	60	55
Control group average (%)	86	83	84
Control group SD (%)	6	12	9

See King *et al.* (2004) for details.

introducing a lack of specificity in the contextual retrieval cues. These concerns were addressed in a second experiment (see Experiment 2 and King *et al.* (2004)) in which performance was matched across all conditions and each event occurred in a unique context. This experiment replicated the earlier findings in that Jon was impaired in the context-dependent recognition tasks but not impaired when asked to recognize objects on the basis of their familiarity (Table 3.1).

The pattern of performance shown by patient Jon conflicts with the declarative memory theory (Squire and Zola-Morgan 1991) since both the spared item recognition and the impaired context-dependent recognition are 'declarative' tasks. Note, however, that other patients with hippocampal damage have been described with impaired item recognition memory (Manns and Squire 1999; reviewed by Spiers *et al.* 2001c). In contrast, the above findings do conform to the idea that the hippocampus and related structures along Papez's circuit (Papez 1937) support episodic recollection, while a separate circuit including the perirhinal cortex supports familiarity-based recognition (Gaffan and Parker 1996; Aggleton and Brown 1999; Baxter and Murray 2001). Interestingly, the pattern of performance of patients who had had unilateral anterior temporal lobectomies (removing tissue from both hippocampus and perirhinal cortex) in the VCM paradigm was also consistent with the assumption of separate processes: Patients with left anterior temporal lobectomies were found to be significantly impaired on the context-dependent questions, while those with right anterior temporal lobectomies were found to be impaired on the object recognition question (Spiers *et al.* 2001b). The pattern shown by both these patients and Jon is consistent with hippocampal involvement in context-dependent memory (and more so on the left consistent with functional neuroimaging data) and perirhinal involvement in object recognition (and more so on the right). See Burgess *et al.* (2002) for further discussion.

With regard to the nature of the episodic information stored by the medial temporal lobes, Marr's (1971) seminal hippocampo-cortical model of memory saw the hippocampus as providing a mechanism for the rapid storage of a simple representation of an event, from which semantic information could later be abstracted and stored in the neocortex. Importantly, these simple representations were thought to be formed of only those elements through which an event is later addressed, consistent with the ideas of cue specificity discussed with respect to Wagenaar's data. On the other hand, O'Keefe and Nadel's (1978, Chapter 14, p. 380 ff.) extension of the cognitive map theory to humans has more similarities with the holistic viewpoint of equal and symmetric cue processing. O'Keefe and Nadel take up Tulving's semantic-epsiodic memory distinction, opposing 'memory for items independent of time or place of their occurrence' in the 'taxon system' with 'memory for items within *a spatio-temporal context*' in the hippocampal 'locale system'. Specifically, the locale system provides multiple channels of access for the retrieval of any of the relationships embodied in the map, such that any relationship in the map can be retrieved by activating any other portion of the map, whether or not these relationships were noticed at the time of input (O'Keefe and Nadel, 1978, p. 384). Eichenbaum and Cohen's (1988; 2001) characterization of the hippocampus as supporting flexible-relational memory maintains the idea of flexibility from the cognitive map (e.g. information should be retrievable via a variety of cues), but puts more stress on pairwise associations, and so need not necessarily imply holistic representation.

Another idea related to binding in episodic memory is that of the hippocampus as a 'convergence zone' (Damasio 1989; Alvarez and Squire 1994; Murre 1996; Moll and Miikkulainen 1997), linking information from different sensory modalities that are represented in disparate cortical areas. In Experiment 3, we added an olfactory component to our (visual) VR events in order to compare unimodal and cross-modal binding. Olfactory cues have further been seen as particularly potent reminders of past experiences, which is sometimes referred to as the 'Proust phenomenon' after Proust's (1922) description of such an event (Chu and Downes 2000). Such a role might reflect the direct connections between primary olfactory regions and the hippocampus (Dade *et al.* 2002). However, scientific evidence rather undermined this notion (Bolger and Titchener 1907; Davis 1975; Rubin *et al.* 1984; Herz 1998). The only evidence for privileged olfactory cueing of memory comes from Chu and Downes (2002) who found that solely odour cues enhance autobiographical memory retrieval in a second retrieval attempt (following a first memory search cued by a label) compared with other cues. Alternatively, Rubin *et al.* (1984) argue that long-term retention in olfactory memory is due to odour cues to memory suffering from less interference than verbal cues during the retention interval, a hypothesis that is supported by evidence for reduced retroactive interference in olfactory memory (Lawless and Engen 1977).

For completeness, we should also mention that many areas outside the medial temporal lobes also play important roles in episodic memory. For example, the frontal lobes are vital for the strategic organization of retrieval, editing, selecting, categorizing, and inhibiting memories as appropriate (Burgess and Shallice 1996). How the frontal lobes interact with the medial temporal lobes to provide a full episodic memory system is an area of increasing interest (reviewed by Wheeler *et al.* 1997; Simons and Spiers 2003). The VCM paradigm described in this chapter has also been used in functional imaging studies to investigate the wider neural systems supporting context-dependent memory. Memory for the spatial context ('where') of an event was associated with hippocampal, parahippocampal, retrosplenial, and medial and posterior parietal activations in two studies (Burgess *et al.* 2001; King *et al.* 2005). Moreover, these studies relate to the dual-process argument above, in that they did not find activation of the medial temporal structures for familiarity-based object recognition, consistent with our neuropsychological findings on the same tasks (Spiers *et al.* 2001a; King *et al.* 2004). They also relate to the role of the frontal lobes in episodic memory. In the first study (Burgess *et al.* 2001), the 16 events in a trial shared only two people and two places as their contexts (see Experiment 1 for details). The widespread lateral and anterior prefrontal activation found in this study, but not seen in previous studies of autobiographical memory (Maguire and Mummery 1999; Maguire *et al.* 2000) was interpreted as reflecting the interference resulting from such overlapping contextual cues. This interpretation is consistent with neuropsychological studies (Incisa della Rocchetta and Milner 1993) and with our more recent functional neuroimaging study involving 20 events with distinct people and places (see Experiment 2) in which the prefrontal activations from the earlier study were much reduced (King *et al.* 2005).

Experiment 1

In the first version of the VCM experiment, participants experienced a series of 16 events that took place in two different places within a VR environment, and with two different 'people' (VR characters) from whom participants 'received' a different object at each encounter. This encoding phase was followed by a forced-choice test of recognition memory probing each event four times addressing memory for different aspects. The whole sequence was then repeated with 16 new objects in two new places with two new characters. In total, participants answered 128 memory questions on the VR events experienced. For further details see Spiers 2002.

Methods

Participants

Thirty-five participants (nine female, 26 male), with an age range of 18–33 years (mean 25 years), took part in the study. Their mean IQ was 105 (inferred from a mean score of 9.5 (SD 1.7) on Raven's Progressive Matrices, Set 1).

Encoding task

Participants followed a marked route through a VR town designed using Duke Nukem 3D (see Burgess *et al.* 2001). They repeatedly encountered one of two characters in one of two rooms along the route (not always in the same part of the room). When they encountered a character, they pressed a key, causing the virtual character to present an object (e.g. a light bulb). Participants were told that they would subsequently be tested on which of two objects they had received, who gave them each object, where they received each object, and in which order they received them.

Recognition test

Immediately after each encoding phase, participants performed 4 × 16 forced-choice recognition trials. For each they re-entered one of the two rooms (in a counterbalanced sequence), encountered one of the two characters, and saw two objects that appeared on the nearest wall along with a word indicating the type of memory question. There were four different memory questions.

- Object: 'Which of the two objects displayed were you given?'
- Person: 'Which of the two objects did you receive from the present character?'
- Place: 'Which of the two objects did you receive in this location?'
- First: 'Which of the two objects did you collect first?'

The foil for the Object question was a similar looking version of the original, while foil objects in the other conditions were from other events in the encoding task and thus were equally familiar.

Practice trial

Participants were given a practice trial during which they followed each of the two routes and encountered two characters who presented them with four objects in different places. They were then given one of each type of question concerning memory for these objects and asked whether they had used any particular encoding strategies. If they did, they were asked to refrain from using these strategies in the test and simply to pay attention to the various elements of each event.

Results

There was a significant effect of question type on performance (Fig. 3.1). Post hoc single comparisons revealed significant differences for each pair ($t(34) > 3.5$; $P < 0.01$) except for the Person versus First comparison. In particular, object recognition (the Object task) was most successful. Of interest regarding the question of binding is the comparison between the context-dependent question types (Person versus Place versus First). Overall, retrieval was more successful via the Person cue and the temporal cue First than via the Place cue.

We then wished to find out whether retrieving the object associated with one element of an event was correlated with retrieving that object via another element of the *same* event. We present theoretical contingency tables for a pair of question types under a Fully Dependent Model (where retrieving one element of an event is maximally correlated to retrieving another element of the same event) in Table 3.2, and under a Fully Independent Model (where retrieving one element of an event is independent of retrieving another element of that event) in Table 3.3. In the Fully Dependent Model, if one retrieval cue is more successful than another, then both cues should be successful every time the least successful is, hence cell *a* (proportion correct for both questions) represents the proportion correct of the least successful ($a = p$). Also, there should be no cases where the

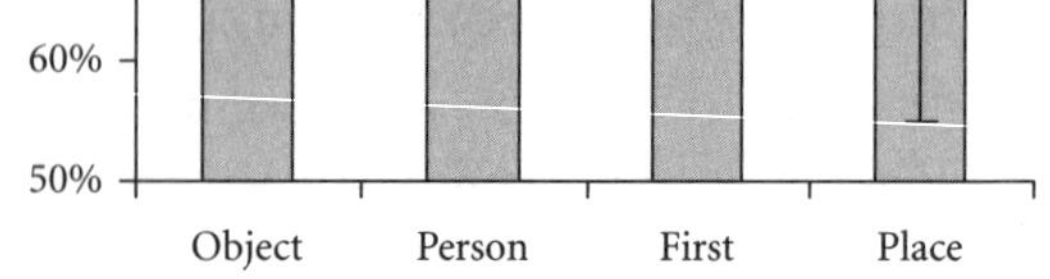

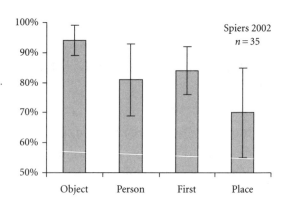

Figure 3.1 Average performance over all participants per question type in Experiment 1. Error bars show one standard deviation. Object refers to a question solvable by familiarity-based recognition; Person, Place, and First refer to questions requiring context-dependent memory.

Table 3.2 Contingency table for a Fully Dependent Model

Retrieval with another cue	Retrieval with one cue (more successful)	
	Proportion correct (f)	**Proportion incorrect ($1 - f$)**
Proportion correct (p)	$a = p$	$b = 0$
Proportion incorrect ($1 - p$)	$c = f - p$	$d = (1 - f)$

See text for explanation.

least successful is correct and the more successful incorrect; hence cell $b = 0$. Further, all incorrect cases of the more successful cue $(1 - f)$ must occur in the case where neither cue is successful, (cell $d = 1 - f$) and finally, cell c expresses the case where only the more successful cue retrieves the correct answer $(c = f - p)$. In the Fully Independent Model, the proportions of a, b, c, and d can be estimated by combining the assumed probabilities of correct and incorrect cases of two cues (see Table 3.3).

Observed responses and predicted values from the Fully Dependent and Fully Independent Models were subjected to a χ^2 analysis. Table 3.4 shows the corresponding statistics and P-values. Four out of the six contingency tables (i.e. question pairs) showed statistically significant differences between the Dependent Model and the observed data, whereas there was a close fit between the data and the Independent Model in all cases, suggesting that the associations formed between objects and context are encoded independently in memory.

In addition, each individual participant's data were analysed using a corrected correlation statistic, as suggested by Hayman and Tulving (1989), in order to avoid Simpson's paradox when interpreting contingency tables from group data. Results at the single-participant level corroborate the above findings on group data (for details see Spiers 2002).

Table 3.3 Contingency table for the Independent Model

Retrieval with another cue	**Retrieval with one cue (more successful)**	
	Proportion correct (f)	**Proportion incorrect ($1 - f$)**
Proportion correct (p)	$a = p \times f$	$b = p \times (1 - f)$
Proportion incorrect ($1 - p$)	$c = f \times (1 - p)$	$d = (1 - p) \times (1 - f)$

See text for explanation.

Table 3.4 χ^2 analysis for comparison of empirical data from Experiment 1 with both the Dependent and the Independent Models (see Tables 3.2 and 3.3)

Comparison	***P*-value (χ^2 statistic)**	
	Difference from Independent Model	**Difference from Dependent Model**
Object vs Person	0.09 (0.99)	0.06 (7.38)
Object vs First	0.99 (0.07)	0.02 (9.66)
Object vs Place	0.99 (0.01)	<0.001 (30.79)
Person vs Place	0.99 (0.09)	0.001 (20.34)
First vs Person	0.95 (0.34)	0.07 (7.18)
First vs Place	0.99 (0.09)	<0.001 (37.18)

Discussion

Evidence from Experiment 1 casts doubt on the suggestion that events are encoded holistically in our hippocampal-dependent episodic memory test. A very good fit of the data is provided by a model assuming an independent probability of success in retrieving the same event from different contextual elements. The independence between performance in the Object question and the context-dependent questions might be specifically related to use of an additional process of familiarity-based recognition that does not depend on the hippocampus (King *et al.* 2004). Further, performance in the First question might also be influenced by an additional factor as this question requires retrieving and comparing the place in temporal sequence of both objects (with the exception of the first and last objects received). However, a holistic encoding theory would at the very least predict some dependence between performance on the Place and Person questions, and no such dependence was observed.

The generally low performance in the context-dependent questions is of concern because it might imply a high degree of guessing. Therefore random answers could be obscuring some possible dependencies in the data. Furthermore, the high degree of interference between 16 events involving only two characters and two places may have resulted in recollection being less 'truly episodic' in Tulving's sense of fully re-experiencing distinct events. Similarly, the re-use of contextual cues in different events might prevent simple use of a fragmentation model such as that of Jones (1976), as discussed by Wagenaar (1986). Finally, performance differed between the various question types which in itself rules out complete dependence between performance in different questions relating to a given event. These issues were addressed in Experiment 2.

Experiment 2

In this experiment we used a VCM paradigm involving 20 events with unique contexts, each involving a distinct virtual character and location. We again attempted to look at whether the probability to retrieve an event via one contextual cue was dependent or independent of the probability of retrieving the same event via another contextual cue. In addition, we attempted to equalize performance across the question types. For further details see King *et al.* (2004).

Methods

Participants

Twelve male participants, who were age and IQ matched for comparisons of performance with patient Jon (see above), took part in this experiment. Their age range was 21–28 years (mean age 23.4) and their mean IQ was 114 (inferred from a mean score of 10.43 (SD 1.22) on Raven's Advanced Matrices, Set I).

Encoding task

A VR town, built on the commercially available Computer Game Deus Ex, provided the environment for the test. It was presented on an AMD Athlon XP2200 computer with a standard 19-inch monitor at a resolution of 800 × 600 pixels and a vertical refresh rate of 60 Hz. To manoeuvre within the town, participants used the cursor keys of the keyboard and followed a trail of green icons (Fig. 3.2(a)). In distinct places along the route, participants encountered virtual characters who presented them with an image of an object (display size 7 × 7 cm) (Fig. 3.2(b)). Subsequently, a new trail of icons would appear for the

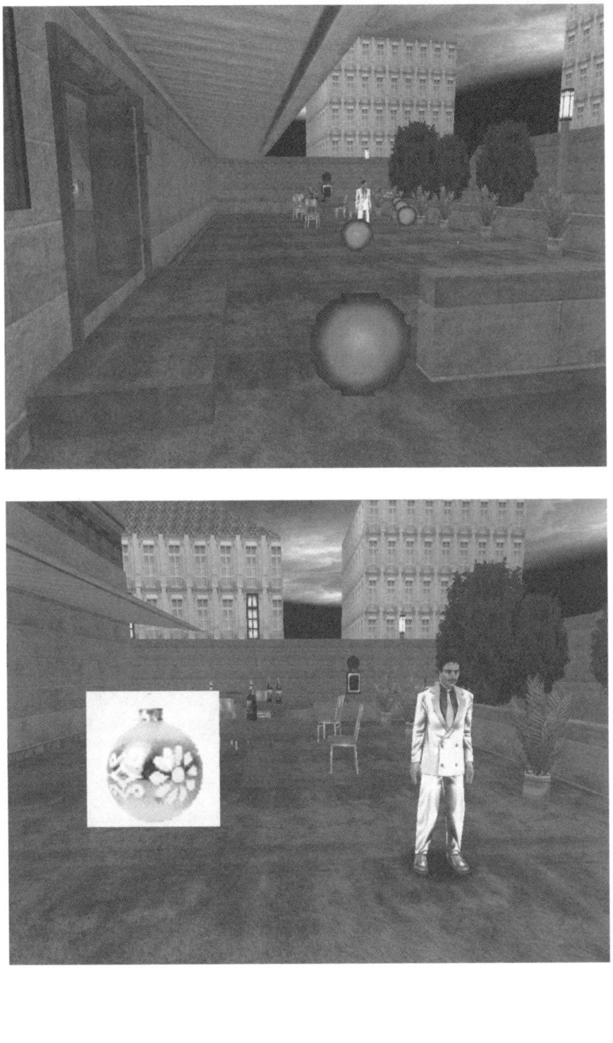

Figure 3.2 Snapshot of the encoding phase of Experiment 2. (a) The participant follows a trail of green dots (the next dot to move over is coloured red), and (b) encounters a distinct person in a distinct location and is presented with the image of a distinct object. See colour plate section.

participant to follow to the next encounter. Participants were told that they would be tested on these events afterwards and instructed to try and remember the person, object, and place of each event. All participants experienced the same sequence of 20 events (rather than counterbalancing order, objects, etc.) as the data were also used to assess the memory performance of patient Jon. The encoding phase took about 15 min on average.

Recognition task

Immediately after the encoding task, participants were given paired forced-choice recognition tests on all aspects of all events (3 × 20 tests): they were presented with two objects, on the left and right of the screen, a virtual character in the foreground, and a snapshot of one of the locations in the background. A word appearing on the top of the screen indicated what type of event information was being probed (Fig. 3.3).

Two questions probed context-dependent memory (Place and Person) and one question (Object) probed recognition of the content of the events, as in Experiment 1. Participants responded by button press, indicating whether the left or the right object was associated with the cue in question. In the Object condition, the foil object was a similar looking version of the original image that had been presented in the encoding task.

Practice trial

Before testing, participants were given a trial run of both the encoding task (consisting of three events presented in an alternative VR town) and the recognition memory test.

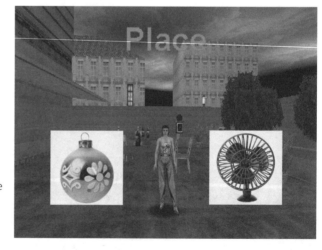

Figure 3.3 An example of a context-dependent paired forced choice question from Experiment 2, showing a Place question: 'Which object did you see in this place?' See colour plate section.

Results

The average performance over all participants is shown in Table 3.1. Note that average performance does not differ between the different question types. As before, our main focus of interest was whether performance on the different question types was correlated across events or not. As in Experiment 1, we constructed contingency tables for each pair of questions (e.g. Person and Place) for each participant. This time we analysed the contingency table for each participant individually using Fisher's exact test. There was a good match between the observed results in that the Independent Model assumed by Fisher's exact test was far from being rejected (Table 3.5).

We also explicitly created the contingency tables expected under an Independent Model (as explained in Experiment 1; see Table 3.3) on the basis of the frequencies of each type of paired response (e.g. correct–correct, correct–incorrect, etc.) for the 20 events. Because performance was approximately equal across conditions in Experiment 2 we were also able to create a Fully Dependent model that included guessing (Table 3.6).

Table 3.5 *P*-values (Fisher's exact test) for h_0 = rejection of Independent Model per participant and event-element-pairing in Experiment 2

Participant no.	***P*-value**		
	Object vs Person	**Object vs Place**	**Person vs Place**
1	1.00	1.00	1.00
2	0.85	0.72	0.90
3	0.49	0.40	0.25
4	0.63	0.40	0.60
5	0.63	0.38	0.63
6	1.00	0.81	1.00
7	0.63	0.80	0.90
8	0.08	0.63	0.34
9	0.02	0.28	0.52
10	0.21	0.34	0.61
11	0.80	0.75	0.72
12	0.75	0.80	0.72

There is no sign of similarity in performance on different questions about the same event. Note that, for our performance levels (e.g. 0.85), a Fully Dependent Model With Guessing (see Table 3.6) would score $P = 0.15$, i.e. we do not have the power to reject the Independent Model at $P < 0.05$. However, the average *P*-values are clearly >0.15, consistent with an Independent Model.

Table 3.6 Contingency table for a Fully Dependent Model With Guessing in the case of equally good retrieval via either cue (as for Experiment 2)

Retrieval with another cue	**Retrieval with one cue** **Proportion correct** **($p = p' + g/2$)**	**Proportion incorrect** **($1 - p$)**
Proportion correct ($p = p' + g/2$)	$a = p' + g/4$	$b = g/4$
Proportion incorrect ($1 - p$)	$c = g/4$	$d = 1 - p' - 3g/4 = g/4$

The proportion correct is p in both cases.The proportion of events in which both cues are correctly retrieved from memory is p' and the proportion of guessed answers is g. All responses are due to either correct retrieval of both aspects or random guessing, i.e. $p' + g = 1$.

Table 3.7 *P*-values and χ^2 statistics for comparison of data with the expectation according to both the Independent Model and the Dependent Model With Guessing over all participants (n = 240)

Comparison	***P*-value (χ^2, 1 degree of freedom)**	
	Independent Model	**Dependent Model With Guessing**
Object vs Person	0.92 (0.009)	< 0.0001 (28.2)
Object vs Place	0.23 (1.461)	< 0.0001 (39.2)
Person vs Place	0.099 (2.717)	< 0.0001 (15.2)

The Dependent Model can clearly be rejected whereas the Independent Model provides a reasonable fit.

Table 3.8 Direct comparison of model and data

Comparison	**Mean squared difference[a] between data and**		***P*-value (*t*-test of mean squared differences)**
	Independent Model	**Dependent Model With Guessing**	
Object vs Person	0.0018 (0.0003)	0.0065 (0.0003)	< 0.005
Object vs Place	0.0007 (5.6×10^{-5})	0.0062 (0.0003)	< 0.001
Person vs Place	0.0004 (6.6×10^{-5})	0.0031 (0.0002)	< 0.005

For all three comparisons the mean squared difference $[(a - a')^2 + (b - b')^2 + (c - c')^2 + (d - d')^2)]/4$ between model and data for the Independent Model is significantly smaller than that for the Dependent Model With Guessing.

[a] Average over participants; SD in parentheses

The χ^2test applied to a contingency table over all participants corroborates data from the analysis of single participants (Table 3.7), fitting the Independent Model and rejecting the Dependent Model With Guessing.

Furthermore, we sought to compare the two models directly, evaluating the difference between both models and the data (Table 3.8). For all three pairs of questions compared, the sum of squared differences between model and data was significantly smaller for the Independent Model than for the Dependent Model With Guessing.

In summary, as in Experiment 1, we found no evidence in favour of events being encoded holistically.

Discussion

The results of Experiment 2 further support a model where all elements of an event are encoded and retrieved as independent pairwise associations. In this experiment some of the concerns regarding the interpretation of Experiment 1 could be eliminated. Performance was reasonably high, suggesting a reduced role for guessing, and also well-matched across conditions, removing one potential obstacle to finding evidence in favour of a fully dependent model.

There is one remaining difficulty in interpreting the results from Experiment 1 and Experiment 2 in terms of whether or not retrieval is holistic i.e. all-or-none. Even if participants answer the Person question correctly, but not the Place question regarding the same event, there remains the possibility that in the instant of retrieving the Person information, they successfully retrieve the whole event, but that at the instant of retrieving the Place information, they fail to recall any elements of the event. Thus, our simple cued-recognition paradigm only allows us to conclude that events are not encoded holistically, in which case variations in the strength of encoding of different events would produce some dependencies among the performance of the different questions concerning the same event. However, it is still possible that events are retrieved holistically, because a separate retrieval process is required for each question regarding a given event. To address this issue, in Experiment 3 we added a cued-recall test to our paradigm, in which memory for different elements of an event could be probed simultaneously.

Experiment 3

In this experiment we made a further modification to the VCM paradigm to test cued recall in addition to forced-choice recognition of context–object pairs and familiar objects. After the encoding phase, we additionally presented participants with the individual components of all events and asked them to reconstruct the events they had experienced. This also allowed us to look at possible 'retrieval hierarchies', i.e. whether some contextual cues may be preferred over others to retrieve information about an event. Furthermore, in this experiment, each VR event included a distinct olfactory cue in addition to distinct people and places. This allowed us to begin to investigate retrieval of events via truly cross-modal contextual cues.

Methods

Participants

Twelve participants (five females and seven males) with an average age of 28 years (range 22–39 years), took part in the experiment. Their mean IQ was 108 (inferred from a mean score of 9.75 (SD 2.0) on Raven's Advanced Matrices,

Set 1). Only people who rated their sense of smell 5 or above were included (self-rating on a scale from 1 to 7).

Practice trial

Before testing, participants wee given the same trial run as in Experiment 2 with the addition of an odour cue for each event.

Pre-experimental exposure to olfactory stimuli

After participants had conducted the practice trial, they were presented with the 10 phials used in the experiment and asked to sample all smells, one after another, and to describe them verbally. If participants failed to come up with a label, they were given a hint (e.g. 'Is it a flower?') and further prompted until they had a specific label for each of the 10 odour stimuli.

Encoding task

The virtual town, computer, and manner of navigating and responding were identical to Experiment 2. At distinct places along the route, participants would meet virtual characters who would present them with an object. Simultaneously with the occurrence of the object, the experimenter would also present an odorous stimulus from a phial (about 1 cm from the participant's nose) for the duration of one sniff. Participants then continued their journey through the virtual town along a new trail of green icons. They were told that they would be tested on these events subsequently and instructed to try to remember the person, object, place, and odour of each event.

Each participant experienced a unique composition of 10 events, i.e. assignment of objects, people, places, and odours was randomly varied between participants. There were five different possible first places that were always reached from the same start location within the town and the sequence of locations was the same for all participants. The whole 'encoding-walk' took about 15 min on average.

Odour stimuli

Odours were presented in medicine bottles labelled with numbers visible to the experimenter only. Through extensive pilot experiments we sought out odorous liquids that were rated neutral in hedonic quality, were matched in perceived intensity, and were easily distinguished from one another. They were rated 'familiar' and could be described verbally, e.g. 'rose', 'peanut butter', 'white spirit', 'spearmint', etc.

Recognition test

After the encoding task, participants were given paired forced-choice recognition tests: A question word on the screen preceded the presentation of two objects on the left and right of the screen, together with one contextual cue corresponding to the question word: in the Place condition, the two objects appeared in front of a snapshot of one of the 10 event locations; in the Person condition, one of the 10 characters appeared between the two objects in front of a plain brown background; in the Odour condition, the participants were presented with one of the 10 odours from a phial together with the visual presentation of two objects in front of a plain brown background. Participants indicated by button press whether they had received the left or the right object in the presence of the respective cue. For the Object condition, an object from the encoding phase was presented together with a similar looking new lure in front of a plain brown background.

Cued-recall test

After the recognition memory task, participants were shown randomly arranged laminated paper copies of all elements of the events they had experienced in the encoding task: virtual characters, images of objects, and snapshots of locations. The odour stimuli were presented on commercially used test-strips on pegs. Participants were instructed to try and reconstruct as well as possible 'what they could remember'. They were further told that their reconstruction process would be recorded online by the experimenter. We recorded which card–odour clip was put together with which other card–clip and in what sequence. Participants were allowed to finish before they had recombined all single elements, when they felt they 'could not remember anything more'. Finally, participants were asked what strategies they had used to encode the events.

Results

Recognition test

Table 3.9 shows the results of the recognition memory test in Experiment 3. Performance on the Object question was significantly better than performance on any other question type (repeated measures analysis of variance: overall

Table 3.9 Overall performance in the paired forced-choice test of Experiment 3 by question type

	Question type			
	Object	**Odour**	**Person**	**Place**
Average performance (%)	100	64	80	71
SD (%)	0	17	14	22

See text for details.

$F = 15.7$, df $= 9$, $P < 0.001$; simple contrasts between Object and any other condition: F values of 51.5, 24, and 20.4 respectively, df $= 1$, all $P < 0.001$) and better than in Experiments 1 and 2, probably because of the smaller number of events used. Within the context-dependent question types, we found significantly better performance for Person questions than for either Place or Odour questions (paired t-tests, one-tailed, $P < 0.01$ for Person versus Odour, $P < 0.05$ for Person versus Place), but no significant difference between performance on Place and Odour questions.

Regarding the Odour cue, we assessed a possible relation between recognition memory score and odour identification ability: Odour identification as assessed pre-experimentally was estimated 1 for a correct label, 0.5 for an approximate description, and 0 for no description There was no correlation between individual participants' identification scores and their memory scores for odour-cued recognition ($R^2 = 0.0048$); however, there was a high correlation between an odour's identification score and how well it elicited odour-cued recognition ($R^2 = 0.80$).

Cued recall

Data from participants' reconstruction processes were scored as follows. As participants were allowed to continue reconstructing one event after having attempted to reconstruct another event in the meantime, and made frequent use of this possibility, all participants' reconstructions of all 10 events were scored in two ways. Firsty, we counted how many elements of an event a participant correctly put together in the first attempt before going on to reconstructing another event. We refer to this as the 'initially remembered' score. Secondly, we counted how many elements of an event participants had correctly put together at the end of their reconstruction process. We refer to this as the 'eventually remembered' score.

Overall, for 'initially remembered' items, 66 per cent of all events (total $= 10$ events $\times$ 12 participants) were at least partially correctly reconstructed as opposed to 34 per cent of events for which no two elements were correctly matched. For 'eventually remembered' items, these percentages amounted to 81 per cent at least partially correctly reconstructed events versus 19 per cent entirely forgotten (Table 3.10).

The percentage of events for which all four elements were remembered together correctly does not exceed 19 per cent. Thus the full retrieval of a complete event is rare compared with the retrieval of the object via a single cue in the recognition test (which was 64 per cent for the worst case, Odour). Table 3.11 shows which elements were not recombined with the others correctly when the other three elements were correctly matched, revealing that the association with odour was the weakest overall; it could not be reattributed to the other elements

Table 3.10 Proportions of correctly remembered elements over all events and all participants in the cued-recall task of Experiment 3

No. of combined elements remembered	Initially remembered		Eventually remembered	
4	7%		19%	
3	18%	Combined 66%	29%	Combined 81%
2	41%		33%	
<2 (i.e. forgotten)	34%		19%	

Table 3.11 Percentage of events in which all elements but one are reconstructed correctly, by omitted element

Three elements remembered	Missing element				
	Object	Odour	Person	Place	Total
Initially	0%	16.4%	0%	1.6%	18%
Eventually	1.7%	23.2%	3.2%	0.9%	29%

Odour is most frequently omitted.

of an event in 91 per cent of all cases that missed one element. Note that initial and eventual reconstruction cannot be compared directly, as some events may have become fully reconstructed in the meantime and are thus no longer counted in the three-elements category, or participants may have taken the element combinations apart again and recombined them differently.

Events were retrieved via the following cues first: Person, 38 per cent; Object, 18 per cent; Odour, 7 per cent; Place, 5 per cent (note that these percentages do not sum to the total number of 66 per cent 'initially remembered' because some events were retrieved by two cues simultaneously). Participants thus show an overall cue preference in favour of the Person cue over the Place and Odour cues in our cued-recall setting, where the cues themselves do not have to be recalled from memory but are already present and merely have to be combined correctly.

Strategies

Participants did not seem to employ distinct strategies throughout. However, they often gave examples of well-remembered associations, which hinted at a facilitation for associations with a common semantic theme that was either inherent, e.g. 'chef' and 'kitchen', or easy enough to be thought of, e.g. '*cream*-coloured glove and smell of *coffee* liquor'. Note that all aspect combinations per event, and thus their semantic coherence, varied between participants.

Discussion

The cued-recall experiment revealed clearly that participants did not successfully retrieve complete events consisting of all four testable elements either at an initial retrieval attempt or after the final retrieval attempt. However, the percentage of events for which more than two elements are correctly associated together increases from 25 per cent initially remembered to 48 per cent eventually remembered. Thus participants are often successful at re-attempting retrieval after a first attempt, and mostly add a third (and eventually fourth) element. This could reflect the use of (independent) pairwise associations with either of the elements of the first pair.

In contrast with Experiment 2, which shared the VR setting of Experiment 3 (but not the odour element), performance in the Object condition was much higher than in the other (context-dependent) conditions of the recognition test. Possible explanations are as follows: first, the total number of events was only 10 rather thn 20; second, the number of repeated exposures to objects in the recognition test was increased because of an additional Odour condition; thirdly, presentation of the odour distracted participants from the other elements of context. These last two factors may also have contributed to the worse performance in the context-dependent question types in this experiment. However, we note that we previously found that retrieval of different elements of an event was independent of whether difficulty was matched (Experiment 2) or not (Experiment 1).

Retrieval independence is complemented by retrieval asymmetry: The Person cue featured predominantly as the element by which other elements of an event were retrieved. In contrast, Odour was most noticeably forgotten and hardly served as a primary cue for the reconstruction of the event. Similarly, performance of the Odour cue in the forced-choice recognition test was worst. The success of a particular Odour cue stimulus was correlated with how nameable it was considered to be overall, thus indicating odour memory facilitation through available semantic information, as also shown by Rabin and Cain (1984). However, this correlation was not found within participants, suggesting that performance was not necessarily influenced by a participant's (momentary) ability in naming, which could in turn be due to a 'tip-of-the-nose-state' (Lawless and Engen 1977), but rather the relative nameability of the stimuli in general.

General discussion

We used a VR paradigm to study memory for the context and content of a series of pseudo-realistic events in which the participant encounters a person in a place and receives an object from them. Memory for context was tested via paired forced choice of which of two objects were received in a given place or from a given person (context-dependent memory). Memory for the content of an event took the form of a paired forced choice of which of two similar looking objects had been received before (object recognition). In neuropsychological and functional neuroimaging experiments we found the hippocampus to be implicated in the context-dependent memory questions, but not in the object-recognition questions. We also correlated memory performance for each contextual aspect and for the content per event in order to test whether encoding of these events was holistic or fragmented.

Events are not encoded as holistic units

We found that participants' retrieval success when cued with one element of an event does not correlate with retrieval success when cued with another element of that same event (Experiment 1). Moreover, this finding holds when the overall retrieval performance is the same on average for retrieval cued by the different elements, and when each event occurs in a distinct context (Experiment 2). We thus conclude that, in our experiments, events are not encoded holistically since this would predict dependencies between the retrieval of the same event by different cues. In contrast, a model based on independent pairwise associations between elements provides a good fit to the data.

Whether or not each retrieval of an event might be holistic (i.e. all-or-none) was investigated by using an additional cued-recall test in which the participants had to recombine all the individual elements into the events that they had experienced (Experiment 3). We found that at the initial retrieval attempt only 7 per cent of all events were retrieved fully, with 59 per cent remembered partially and 33 per cent not remembered at all. Importantly, this performance increases to 19 per cent entirely remembered in the end, as opposed to 62 per cent partially remembered and 19 per cent forgotten completely. This suggests that recollection of events is also not holistic, but rather is partial and iterative in nature: more and more information is added in subsequent retrieval attempts.

Relation to previous work

Our results are inconsistent with the idea that episodic recollection corresponds to 're-experiencing' an event complete with its multimodal context in such a realistic way that a mechanism of autonoetic awareness (Tulving 2002) is required to disambiguate it from current perception. They are also inconsistent with the spirit of the 'locale system' proposed by O'Keefe and Nadel (1978) in which an event is stored in a map-like set of relations such that it can be equally well retrieved via different relationships.

Is it possible that our stimuli somehow fail to capture the essence of autobiographical episodic information? For example, even though we took care to use distinct contextual elements for each event in Experiment 2, all the events involved the same action: walking up to a person and 'receiving' the object that appears as a result of that encounter. In Brewer and Dupree's (1983) study, different goal-directed actions, viewed on film, were remembered holistically. It may be that the similarity of the actions in our events caused interference between them that disrupts the holistic and distinct recollection of each one. However, this interpretation is undermined by the similarity between our results and those in Wagenaar's (1986) study of his own autobiographical memory. Wagenaar found that some elements of an event formed better cues than others and also found that multiple cueing by different elements of an event increased the probability of retrieval in line with (and sometimes exceeding) the prediction of independent pairwise associations. In addition, he reports many events that were only partially remembered, and a failure to retrieve around 20 per cent of events (consistent with the final result in the cued recall of our Experiment 3).

Our results also contrast with Jones's (1976) finding of independent but holistically encoded fragments. Or, put another way, we only found evidence for fragments including pairs of elements but not triples. As argued by Wagenaar (1986), some differences might be due to Jones's paradigm, using nine lists of each of nine objects in nine different colours and nine different locations. In this paradigm, participants might quickly learn that, within a list, each element of an event is unique and thus any fragment containing a given element will be specific to the single event containing that element. In autobiographical studies, and in our VCM paradigm, the participant will not in general be able to make that assumption (even though it would have been correct in Experiments 2 and 3, the participants would not have had time to learn it as they performed only one full trial). In the case of multiple fragments potentially containing the same single elements, a simple fragment model may not be sufficient to describe performance and other processes may become the performance-limiting factor. For instance, as Wichawut and Martin (1971) found, retrieval independence is related to the strength of a formed association. They found that, after learning A–B and A–C associations, the responses B and C are retrieved independently as long as at least one of the pairs is well stored in memory, but that retrieval dependencies arise if both are weakly stored.

Retrieval cue hierarchy

We found that different levels of access to the memory of the content of the event (the object) are afforded by different contextual cues. This is consistent with

Wagenaar's findings. It is also consistent with Marr's (1971) model, the 'filing cabinet' model referred to by Wagenaar (1986), and the model of headed records (Morton *et al.* 1985; Morton and Bekerian 1986) in which some elements of a memory are seen to be efficient retrieval cues (e.g. the name of a person) but are much less easily retrieved themselves.

In our cued-recall experiment, the Person cue was most frequently chosen to start retrieval of episodic information. At first sight, this contrasts with Jones's (1976) findings that cued recall was symmetric in that the probability for either of two (perceptual) components of an event to promptly recall the other was the same. There are several potential explanations to account for this. As well as the chances for participants to evaluate cue specificity over several trials (discussed above), the elements of context in Jones's experiments perhaps had more similar, and reduced, semantic complexity than the elements of context in our experiment. In Jones's experiment, one element ('location') was one of nine grid positions on a backdrop and was thus similar to the other element ('colour') in its (lack of) semantic complexity. Asch and Ebenholtz (1962) similarly demonstrated approximate symmetry in the recall of two-component visual patterns but argued that asymmetry in other circumstances could be due to differential availability of the components, perhaps differential levels of semantic association.

Clayton *et al.* (2001), in their investigation of episodic-like memory in scrub jays, suggested that 'where' is the predominant element binding an episode together compared with 'what' and 'when'. This clearly contrasts with our findings from Experiment 1 where recognition performance was equal for Person and First (the temporal order question) and better than for the Place question. However, we hypothesize that retrieval cue success (and preference) depends on the circumstances; the crucial cue of retrieval might well shift away from Place to People, depending on the nature of information to be remembered. Whereas for scrub jays caching food, for example, the most successful memory cues might well be places (triggering additional episodic information), for human participants wandering around in (VR) towns, the most relevant cues would be the people who provide them with objects. The Person might be given preference because she could hypothetically walk away and disrupt the 'where' whilst taking the 'what' away with her. The original paradigm used by Clayton and colleagues (Clayton and Dickinson 1998; Clayton *et al.* 2001) did not test memory for 'who' was involved in a caching event (but see Emery and Clayton 2001). An alternative explanation would be that cue preference is dependent on the distinctiveness of cues of the same category across events. For example, if the places are very similar, other cues will contribute more to the distinctiveness of the event.

Role of semantics in episodic memory

In our experiment, where we had created episodes of random semantic consistency, there were only a few combinations of places, people, objects, and smells, created by chance, that were inherently consistent (e.g. imagine 'kitchen', 'chef', 'cup and saucer', and 'smell of peanut-butter' in Experiment 3). Notably, participants happily made use of any semantic consistency (which they reported in the post-experimental assessment of strategies used). Furthermore, we found that those odorants which were more easily given a label (in a perceptual test before the VCM experiment), and thus a meaning, proved to be better cues to episodic memory. Thus semantic relations may play a role in binding of episodic memory, as emphasized by Tulving and Markowitsch (1998), and as shown in earlier experimental investigations of human memory (Jenkins and Russell 1952; Deese 1959) and recently in people with dementia (Rusted *et al.* 2000). However, at the same time, our example also highlights the problem of knowing which of several semantically consistent alternatives to use. For example, how does one succeed in recalling that the 'chef' was paired with the 'cup and saucer' and not the 'teapot'? In a future experiment, we could test whether semantically related items tend to be confounded (see also 'false-memory phenomena' (Roediger and McDermott (1995) and, most interestingly, whether this would affect single pairings within an event as would be predicted by an independent model of encoding and retrieval, or whether its affect would be more holistic.

Olfactory cues are not especially evocative

Despite the use of familiar, distinct, and identifiable odours, the success of olfactory cues in retrieving episodes was relatively small compared with the other cues (place and person). Taking into account that perceptual features might account for this, and admitting that there is no information available about the extent to which the cues were matched semantically and perceptually across modality, we would nonetheless like to add another potential explanation. Olfactory stimuli are generally not easily tagged with a label, despite their perceived familiarity and the fact that the very same stimuli had just been labelled some minutes ago (Engen and Ross 1973, Cain and Potts 1996), with participants sometimes becoming trapped in a 'tip-of-the-nose-state' (Lawless and Engen 1977). The binding of label and olfactory percept is volatile. Therefore, on the one hand, semantic integration of an odour enhances its success as a retrieval cue, as reported above and shown previously (Lawless and Engen 1977; Rabin and Cain 1984; Lyman and McDaniel 1990). On the other hand, an olfactory cue's frequent temporary failure to elicit a label might result in it being preserved in memory as a rather isolated and inaccessible trace. As such it might be a poor contextual cue, although by being recalled relatively rarely it might also remain a highly distinctive cue. Corroborating this 'rarity argument', there is indeed experimental evidence showing reduced retroactive interference in olfactory memory compared with other modalities (Lawless and Engen 1977; Rubin *et al.* 1984).

Conclusion

In a chain of pseudo-realistic events which consist of the same element categories throughout, each event appears to be encoded in terms of independent pairwise associations between its elements. We found no evidence of a more holistic encoding in which all elements are associated together. On the contrary, performance on remembering the content of an event via one element of its context appeared to be independent of performance in remembering it via a second element. This finding argues against the idea that whole events are the units of episodic memory and are necessarily re-experienced in all their detail at retrieval.

The context-dependent memory task was shown to be hippocampal dependent, in accordance with the idea that episodic memory is supported by the hippocampus (Kinsbourne and Wood 1975; Mishkin *et al.* 1997; O'Keefe and Nadel 1978; Squire and Zola-Morgan 1991; Eichenbaum and Cohen 2001). Thus our results also argue that the hippocampal contribution to episodic memory is not specifically to encode events in a 'map' of associations in which all elements can contribute equally. Elements of an event can be retrieved individually and in various combinations and, in our experiment of cued recollection, most favourably via the Person cue as opposed to the Place, Object, or Odour cues. Finally, in our experiment including olfactory stimuli, we found that olfactory information is less closely tied to the event and serves as a less potent retrieval cue than the other elements of our events. This might be linked to poor semantic representation of olfactory information.

Acknowledgements

This research was supported by an MRC senior research fellowship to NB, UCL Graduate School and ORS studentships to IT, and an MRC studentship to HS. We thank Rebecca Dukeson for help with collecting data, and Tom Hartley and John Morton for many useful discussions and for commenting on an early version of this manuscript. We also thank the editors and an anonymous referee for helpful comments.

References

Aggleton, J.P. and Brown, M.W. (1999). Episodic memory, amnesia, and the hippocampal–anterior thalamic axis. *Behavioral and Brain Sciences*, **22**, 425–490.

Alvarez, P. and Squire, L.R. (1994). Memory consolidation and the medial temporal lobe: a simple network model. *Proceedings of the National Academy of Sciences of the United States of America*, **91**, 7041–7045.

Asch, S.E. and Ebenholtz, S.M. (1962). The principle of associative symmetry. *Proceedings of the American Philosophical Society*, **106**, 135–163.

Baxter, M.G. and Murray, E.A. (2001). Opposite relationship of hippocampal and rhinal cortex damage to delayed nonmatching-to-sample deficits in monkeys. *Hippocampus*, **11**, 61–71.

Bogacz, R., Brown, M.W., and Giraud-Carrier, C. (2001). Model of familiarity discrimination in the perirhinal cortex. *Journal of Computational Neuroscience*, **10**, 5–23.

Bolger, E.M. and Titchener, E.B. (1907). Some experiments on the association power of smells. *American Journal of Psychology*, **18**, 326–327.

Brewer, W.F. and Dupree, D.A. (1983). Use of plan schemata in the recall and recognition of goal-directed actions. *Journal of Experimental Psychology: Learning, Memory, and Cognition*, **9**, 117–129.

Burgess, N., Maguire, E.A., Spiers, H.J. and O'Keefe, J. (2001). A temporoparietal and prefrontal network for retrieving the spatial context of lifelike events. *NeuroImage*, **14**, 439–453.

Burgess, N., Maguire, E., and O'Keefe, J. (2002). The human hippocampus and spatial and episodic memory. *Neuron*, **35**, 625–641.

Burgess, P.W. and Shallice, T. (1996). Confabulation and the control of recollection. *Memory*, **4**, 359–411.

Cain, W.S. and Potts, B.C. (1996). Switch and bait: probing the discriminative basis of odor identification via recognition memory. *Chemical Senses*, **21**, 35–44.

Chu, S. and Downes, J.J. (2000). Odor-evoked autobiographical memories: psychological investigations of Proustian phenomena. *Chemical Senses*, **25**, 111–116.

Chu, S. and Downes, J.J. (2002). Proust nose best: odors are better cues of autobiographical memory. *Memory and Cognition*, **30**, 511–518.

Clayton, N.S. and Dickinson, A. (1998). Episodic-like memory during cache recovery by scrub jays. *Nature*, **395**, 272–274.

Clayton, N.S., Griffiths, D.P., Emery, N.J., and Dickinson, A. (2001). Elements of episodic-like memory in animals. *Philosophical Transactions of the Royal Society of London, Series B, Biological Sciences*, **356**, 1483–1491.

Dade, L.A., Zatorre, R.J., and Gotman, M. (2002). Olfactory learning: convergent findings from lesion and brain imaging studies in humans. *Brain*, **125**, 86–101.

Damasio, A.R. (1989). The brain binds entities and events by multiregional activation from convergence zones. *Neural Computation*, **1**, 123–132.

Davis, R.G. (1975). Acquisition of verbal associations to olfactory stimuli of varying familiarity and to abstract visual stimuli. *Journal of Experimental Psychology: Learning, Memory, and Cognition*, **1**, 134–142.

Deese, J. (1959). Influence of inter-item associative strength upon immediate free recall. *Psychological Reports*, **5**, 305–312.

Delay, J. and Brion, S. (1969). *Le syndrome de Korsakoff*. Paris: Masson.

Duzel, E., Yonelinas, A.P., Mangun, G.R., Heinze, H.J., and Tulving, E. (1997). Event-related brain potential correlates of two states of conscious awareness in memory. *Proceedings of the National Academy of Sciences of the United States of America*, **94**, 5973–5978.

Eichenbaum, H. and Cohen, N.J. (1988). Representation in the hippocampus. What do hippocampal neurons code? *Trends in Neurosciences*, **11**, 244–248.

Eichenbaum, H. and Cohen, N.J. (2001). *From Conditioning to Conscious Recollection: Memory Systems of the Brain*. Oxford: Oxford University Press.

Emery, N.J. and Clayton, N.S. (2001). Effects of experience and social context on prospective caching strategies by scrub jays. *Nature*, **414**, 443–446.

Engen, T. and Ross, B.M. (1973). Long-term memory of odors with and without verbal description. *Journal of Environmental Psychology*, **100**, 221–227.

Fisher, R.P. and Chandler, C.C. (1991). Independence between recalling interevent relations and specific events. *Journal of Experimental Psychology: Learning, Memory, and Cognition*, **17**, 722–733.

Foss, D.J. and Harwood, D.A. (1975). Memory for sentences: implications for human associative memory. *Journal of Verbal Learning and Verbal Behavior*, **14**, 1–16.

Gadian, D.G., Aicardi, J., Watkins, K.E., Porter, D.A., Mishkin, M., and Vargha-Khadem, F. (2000). Developmental amnesia associated with early hypoxic-ischaemic injury. *Brain*, **123**, 499–507.

Gaffan, D. and Parker, A. (1996). Interaction of perirhinal cortex with the fornix-fimbria: memory for objects and 'object-in-place' memory. *Journal of Neuroscience*, **16**, 5864–5869.

Hayman, C.A. and Tulving, E. (1989). Contingent dissociation between recognition and fragment completion: the method of triangulation. *Journal of Experimental Psychology: Learning, Memory, and Cognition*, **15**, 228–240.

Herz, R.S. (1998). Are odors the best cues to memory? *Annals of the New York Academy of Sciences*, **855**, 670–674.

Holdstock, J.S., Mayes, A.R., Roberts, N., *et al.* (2002). Under what conditions is recognition spared relative to recall after selective hippocampal damage in humans? *Hippocampus*, **12**, 341–351.

Incisa della Rocchetta, A. and Milner, B. (1993). Strategic search and retrieval inhibition: the role of the frontal lobes. *Neuropsychologia*, **31**, 503–524.

Jacoby, L.L., Toth, J.P., and Yonelinas, A.P. (1993). Separating conscious and unconscious influences of memory: measuring recollection. *Journal of Experimental Psychology: General*, **122**, 139–154.

Jenkins, J.J. and Russell, W.A. (1952). Associative clustering during recall. *Journal of Abnormal and Social Psychology*, **47**, 818–821.

Jones, G.V. (1976). A fragmentation hypothesis of memory: cued recall of pictures and of sequential position. *Journal of Experimental Psychology: General*, **105**, 277–293.

King, J.A., Trinkler, I., Hartley, T., Vargha-Khadem, F., and Burgess, N. (2004). The hippocampal role in spatial memory and the familiarity-recollection distinction: a single case study. *Neuropsychology*, ***18***, 405–417.

King, J.A., Hartley, T., Spiers, H.J., Maguire, E.A, and Burgess, N. (2005) Anterior prefrontal involvement in episodic retrieval reflects contextual interference. *NeuroImage*, **28**, 256–267.

Kinsbourne, M. and Wood, F. (1975). In *Short-Term Memory* (ed D. Deutsch and J.A. Deutsch). New York: Academic Press, pp 257–291.

Lawless, H.T. and Engen, T. (1977). Associations to odors: interference, memories, and verbal labelling. *Journal of Experimental Psychology: Human Learning and Memory*, **3**, 52–59.

Lyman, B.J. and McDaniel, M.A. (1990). Memory for odors and odor names: modalities of elaboration and imagery. *Journal of Experimental Psychology: Learning, Memory, and Cognition*, **16**, 656–664.

Maguire, E.A. and Mummery, C.J. (1999). Differential modulation of a common memory retrieval network revealed by positron emission tomography. *Hippocampus*, **9**, 54–61.

Maguire, E.A., Mummery, C.J., and Büchel, C. (2000). Patterns of hippocampal-cortical interaction dissociate temporal lobe memory subsystems. *Hippocampus*, **10**, 475–482.

Mandler, G. (1980). Recognizing: The judgment of previous occurence. *Psychological Review*, **87**, 252–271.

Mandler, G. (1991). Your face looks familiar but I can't remember your name: a review of dual process theory. In *RelatingTtheory and Data: Essays on Human Memory in Honor of Bennet B. Murdock* (ed E. William, E. Hockley, and E. S. Lewandowsky). Hillsdale, NJ: Erlbaum, pp. 207–225.

Manns, J.R. and Squire, L.R. (1999). Impaired recognition memory on the Doors and People Test after damage limited to the hippocampal region. *Hippocampus*, **9**, 495–499.

Marr, D. (1971). Simple memory: a theory for archicortex. *Philosophical Transactions of the Royal Society of London, Series B, Biological Sciences*, **262**, 23–81.

Mishkin *et al.* (1997).

Moll, M. and Miikkulainen, R. (1997). Convergence-zone episodic memory: analysis and simulations. *Neural Networks*, **10**, 1017–1036.

Morton, J. and Bekerian, D.A. (1986). Three ways of looking at memory. In *Advances in Cognitive Science 1* (ed N.E. Sharkey). Ellis Horwood, pp. 43–71.

Morton, J., Hammersley, R.H., and Bekerian, D.A. (1985). Headed records: a model for memory and its failure. *Cognition*, **20**, 1–23.

Murre, J.M. (1996). Trace link: a model of amnesia and consolidation of memory. *Hippocampus*, **6**, 675–684.

O'Keefe, J. and Nadel, L. (1978). *The Hippocampus as a Cognitive Map*. Oxford: Oxford University Press.

Papez, J.W. (1937). A proposed mechanism of emotion. *Archives of Neurology and Psychiatry*, **38**, 724–744.

Proust, M. (1922). *Swann's Way* (trans C.K. Scott Moncrieff). London: Chatto and Windus, 1960.

Rabin, M.D. and Cain, W.S. (1984). Odor recognition: familiarity, identifiability, and encoding consistency. *Journal of Experimental Psychology: Learning, Memory, and Cognition*, **10**, 316–325.

Roediger, H.L. and McDermott, K.B. (1995). Creating false memories: remembering words not presented in lists. *Journal of Experimental Psychology: Learning, Memory, and Cognition*, **21**, 803–814.

Rubin, D.C., Groth, E., and Goldsmith, D.J. (1984). Olfactory cueing of autobiographical memory. *American Journal of Psychology*, **97**, 493–507.

Rugg, M.D. and Yonelinas, A.P. (2003). Human recognition memory: a cognitive neuroscience perspective. *Trends in Cognitive Sciences*, **7**, 313–319.

Rusted, J., Gaskell, M., Watts, S., and Sheppard, L. (2000). People with dementia use schemata to support episodic memory. *Dementia and Geriatric Cognitive Disorders*, **11**, 350–356.

Simons, J.S. and Spiers, H.J. (2003). Prefrontal and medial temporal lobe interactions in long-term memory. *Nature Reviews Neuroscience*, **4**, 637–648.

Spiers, H.J. (2002). Temporal lobe contributions to topographical and episodic memory. Doctoral Thesis. University College London.

Spiers, H.J., Burgess, N., Hartley, T., Vargha-Khadem, F., and O'Keefe, J. (2001a). Bilateral hippocampal pathology impairs topographical and episodic memory but not visual pattern matching. *Hippocampus*, **11**, 715–725.

Spiers, H.J., Burgess, N., Maguire, E.A., *et al.* (2001b). Unilateral temporal lobectomy patients show lateralised topographical and episodic memory deficits in a virtual town. *Brain*, **124**, 2476–2489.

Spiers, H.J., Maguire, E.A., and Burgess, N. (2001c). Hippocampal amnesia. *Neurocase*, **7**, 357–382.

Squire, L.R. and Zola-Morgan, S. (1991). The medial temporal lobe memory system. *Science*, *253*, 1380–1386.

Tulving, E. (1972). Episodic and semantic memory. In *Organization of Memory* (ed E.Tulving and W. Donaldson). New York: Academic Press, pp. 381–403.

Tulving, E. (1983). *Elements of Episodic Memory*. Oxford: Clarendon Press.

Tulving, E. (2001). Episodic memory and common sense: how far apart? *Philosophical Transactions of the Royal Society of London, Series B, Biological Sciences*, **356**, 1505–1515.

Tulving, E. (2002). Episodic memory: from mind to brain. *Annual Review of Psychology*, **53**, 1–25.

Tulving, E. and Markowitsch, H.J. (1998). Encoding of information into the episodic system depends critically on the semantic system, p.200.

Vargha-Khadem, F., Gadian, D.G., Watkins, K.E., Connelly, A., Van Paesschen, W., and Mishkin, M. (1997). Differential effects of early hippocampal pathology on episodic and semantic memory. *Science*, **277**, 376–380.

Wagenaar, W.A. (1986). My memory: a study of autobiographical memory over six years. *Cognitive Psychology*, **18**, 225–252.

Wan, H., Aggleton, J.P. and Brown, M.W. (1999). Different contributions of the hippocampus and perirhinal cortex to recognition memory. *Journal of Neuroscience*, **19**, 1142–1148.

Wheeler, M.A., Stuss, D.T., and Tulving, E. (1997). Toward a theory of episodic memory: the frontal lobes and autonoetic consciousness. *Psychological Bulletin*, **121**, 331–354.

Wichawut, C. and Martin, E. (1971). Independence of A–B and A–C associations in retroaction. *Journal of Verbal Learning and Verbal Behavior*, **10**, 316–321.

Yonelinas, A.P. (2002). The nature of recollection and familiarity: a review of 30 years of research. *Journal of Memory and Language*, **46**, 441–517.

Chapter 4

Adaptive binding

Don M. Tucker and Phan Luu

Introduction

Current research is providing the opportunity for new insights into the binding of mental representations from informational elements. Neurophysiological mechanisms, such as gamma band oscillatory coupling of perceptual features across the sensory neocortex, may explain how dynamic processes bind enduring synaptic patterns within corticolimbic networks (Singer 1993; Menon *et al.* 1996). At larger scales of network integration, growing evidence suggests that synaptic coordination in memory consolidation is achieved through oscillatory coupling across limbic regions in the theta band (Freeman 1998; Buzsáki 2002). The intriguing implication is that if only we could read these oscillatory codes, we could examine directly how mental representations take neural form.

In this chapter, we first outline a theoretical model for understanding the adaptive neural systems underlying human memory. This model begins with the specific circuits mediating corticolimbic interactions, including the amygdala and hippocampus, their thalamic and hypothalamic projections, and the regions of limbic cortex and neocortex that are engaged by each circuit. These circuits appear to support dual corticolimbic memory systems, one centred on the hippocampus and the dorsal networks derived from the archicortex and the other centred on the amygdala and the ventral networks derived from the palaeocortex (Mesulam 2000). A key question is how these systems support the re-entrant interactions between limbic networks and neocortical networks that are required for memory consolidation (Ungerleider and Mishkin 1982; Squire 1986; Tucker 2001). Important controls on the memory process are provided not only by the primary limbic circuits through diencephalic structures (thalamus and hypothalamus), but also by the arousal mechanisms of the mesencephalic reticular activating system. In this brief outline, we attempt to illustrate how adaptive motivational control of memory is achieved through vertical integration, coordinating essential contributions from multiple levels of the neuraxis.

We then review recent findings in current human research on the self-control of memory and performance. These findings suggest that vertical integration may be critical not only to elementary motivational controls on arousal and effort, but also to the executive control of human memory systems. Research with both dense-array EEG and BOLD functional MRI (fMRI) points to activity in cingulate and insular cortices that supports not only the emotional evaluation of goals and outcomes, but also the monitoring and control of cognitions and actions. We focus on preliminary but intriguing clues to the neurophysiological mechanism of these corticolimbic circuits, specifically the limbic theta rhythm of the EEG.

Neurophysiological studies in animals have suggested that limbic theta may provide a method for coordinating the binding of significant representations across large-scale corticolimbic networks. We speculate from our EEG studies that cognitive representations can compete for control of the theta synchronizing signal by re-entrant interactions among networks. This competition may be evidenced by theta phase shifting, observable with human EEG and magnetoencephalographic (MEG) measures. In attempting to understand the possible mechanisms of these effects, we review the neurophysiological mechanisms in the control of limbic theta, considering both local modulations of synaptic synchronization and the global synchronization of limbic circuits by rhythmic oscillatory coupling. Although the evidence crosses widely different species and widely divergent levels of experimental analysis, there are important clues in this research to the adaptive controls that regulate the binding of large-scale network patterns in the human brain.

Vertical integration of memory systems

Research into the neural substrates of memory is delineating specific forms of memory related to specific neural mechanisms. Perceptual priming, for example, appears to engage neocortical networks of the sensory modality. In procedural memory, motor skills may be supported by elementary circuits within the neostriatum (Squire 1987). Even for the general processes of memory mediated by corticolimbic mechanisms, there appear to be two unique forms, each with a specialized corticolimbic circuit for its formation and maintenance (Mishkin 1982). Perceptual objects, achieved as differentiated packages of sensory-informational features, are organized within the ventral palaeocortical pathway, including perirhinal and extended amygdalar and orbital frontal corticolimbic networks (Aggleton and Brown 1999; Tucker *et al.* 2000; Luu and Tucker 2003). Spatial and relational contexts, achieved through inclusion of multiple elements and their configural relations, are organized within the dorsal archicortical pathway, including the hippocampal, cingulate, and diencephalic targets of the classical Papez circuit (Aggleton and Brown 1999; Tucker *et al.* 2000; Luu and Tucker 2003). The delineation of these memory systems has provided a possible neural substrate for the classical dual process models of memory functions in cognitive research, distinguishing between a familiarity process (ventral limbic) and a recollection process (dorsal limbic). Findings with both electrophysiological (EEG/ERP) and haemodynamic measures (fMRI) have provided consistent evidence in human studies (Rugg 1987; Rugg *et al.* 1998; Curran 2000; Wagner 2002). The possibility of reasoning from animal neurophysiological studies to human cognition presents important opportunities for a theoretical analysis of memory mechanisms. In the dorsal archicortical pathway, relational encoding appears to allow a rich elaboration of experiential elements, such that with an appropriate single cue we can readily recall a fully concrete episode of memory (Tucker 2001; Luu and Tucker 2003). In contrast, in the ventral palaeocortical pathway, although routinized and stereotyped operations on objects may play critical roles in cognitive representations such as language, the mnemonic information appears to be apprehended more vaguely, with a remembered item failing to engender its place in an episode of experience as it presents only the impression of isolated familiarity (Tucker 2001; Luu and Tucker 2003).

Mechanisms of adaptive synchronization

A key issue for both neurophysiological and psychological accounts is temporal binding, the formation of representations that span behavioural time. Binding often refers to a structure at one point in time: features bound into an object, or locations bound into an environment. However, because consolidation must extend in time before memories are encoded, the control of the temporal extent of consolidation is a critical parameter. Therefore classical questions of behavioural learning theory, including the relation of expectancy to associational learning (Rescorla and Wagner 1972), become critical to understanding adaptive binding. Because of the stability–plasticity dilemma, in which new input to a distributed representation invariably threatens the integrity of the existing memory store (Grossberg 1982; McClelland *et al.* 1995), the control of consolidation appears to be a balancing act between failure to learn and catastrophic decline of the existing representations.

The mammalian learning circuits seem to have adapted to the reality of both motivational and representational problems, applying strategic control systems to tune the stability–plasticity balance to meet adaptive demands. In this process, there appears to be extensive vertical integration, through which not only telencephalic regulatory circuits, but also mesencephalic and diencephalic projections provide essential modulatory controls to the corticolimbic interaction that achieves memory consolidation.

At the telencephalic level, the cholinergic projections from the nucleus basalis provide widespread innervation of the cortical mantle to regulate the activity level of the cortex in relation to adaptive demands. Importantly, this basal forebrain cholinergic control increases in density as cortical networks approach the limbic regions, providing a mechanism for motivational tuning of sensory processing (Mesulam *et al.* 1983). An even steeper gradient towards limbic networks is found for afferent inputs into the basal forebrain cholinergic system. The inputs to the nucleus basalis are not gathered from the entire cortex, but originate specifically in the limbic cortex, suggesting a mechanism through which the motivational reactivity of the limbic cortex may engage a fundamental mechanism of memory consolidation which then controls broader regions of the neocortex as well (Mesulam and Mufson 1984; Mesulam 1988).

Biasing towards the visceral core or the somatic shell

The regulation of the interactions between limbic cortex and neocortex may also engage diencephalic controls differentially, with hypothalamic and thalamic influences regulating what could be described as a core–shell dimension (Tucker 2001). At the internal limbic core of each hemisphere, network representations appear to be modulated by hypothalamic motivational constraints (Swanson 2000). At the external neocortical shell of each hemisphere, the primary sensory and motor cortices integrate the thalamic traffic mediating the interface with the environment (Steriade *et al.* 1990). Memory consolidation appears to require not only re-entrant interaction but a kind of negotiation between the core and the shell, linking both hypothalamic and thalamic roots of corticolimbic systems (Tucker 2001).

Several lines of evidence suggest that, at least in rodents, corticolimbic mechanisms shift the balance between the core and the shell adaptively as experiences are bound in memory. At certain times, marked in rodents by exploratory behaviour and the appearance of oscillations of the EEG at the theta frequency, the intake of new information is facilitated by dominance of input from the sensorimotor shell (Chrobak and Buzsáki 1998). At other times, marked in rodents by consummatory behaviour or resting, and hippocampal sharp waves, consolidation appears to be dominated by the integrative motivational constraints from the limbic core (Buzsáki 1996, 2002). Although these shifts in core–shell balance, and the associated changes in modulation by limbic theta, appear to be more flexible and transient in humans than in rodents, the necessity of coordinating both sensorimotor and motivational constraints on learning may remain an integral challenge for adaptive binding in human cognition.

Habituation and redundancy biases in regulating corticolimbic binding

In addition to engaging basal forebrain cholinergic mechanisms and hypothalamic controls, the limbic networks may recruit specific forms of arousal control from the mesencephalic reticular activating system (Pribram and McGuinness 1975). Following the analysis of limbic learning circuits by Gabriel and associates (Gabriel, Taylor, and Burhans 2003), we hypothesize that the process of core–shell arbitration may be achieved differently within the archicortical (dorsal) and palaeocortical (ventral) corticolimbic pathways (Tucker 2001; Luu and Tucker 2003). Each form of control, by biasing the operation of consolidation in time, may offer a different way of negotiating the stability–plasticity dilemma.

The stability–plasticity dilemma may be solved by segregating control of learning and memory into two functionally distinct yet interrelated systems with unique cybernetic control biases, each system expressing the opposite pole of the control dilemma. We hypothesize that in the dorsal archicortical pathway, the fundamental control appears to be a habituation bias, driven by internal representations of past experiences (Goldberg 1987). Because experience builds internal representations, the inherent bias is to habituate rapidly to external stimuli, preserving internal representations and thus the history of the organism. Rapid habituation permits a brief temporal window into internal representations, only allowing gradual learning to occur through updating of contexts (Tucker and Williamson 1984). The resulting contextual model, with strong representation in episodic memory, forms an ongoing expectancy for what will happen. The implicit expectancy of the contextual model of the dorsal memory circuit may be an essential mechanism supporting the continuity of episodic experience. Because of the inherently inward bias for representations and action generation, this mode of temporal binding facilitates a global scope of working memory. The habituation bias appears to be supported by mesencephalic noradrenergic projections, which are dense in the posterior cingulate and other regions of the archicortex but sparse in ventral limbic sites (Descarries and Lapierre 1973; Morrison *et al.* 1979; Foote and Morrison 1987).

In contrast, we hypothesize that, within the ventral palaeocortical pathway, another form of learning is engaged when implicit expectancies are violated by significant events and rapid adjustments must be made. This learning and memory system is externally driven, adjusting action to meet the demands of the external world (Goldberg 1987, 1996). The bias inherent in this learning and memory system is for redundancy. This is because, under external control, information is transient, changing with the environment. To counter this, the system has a built-in redundancy bias which sustains the information in working memory. The focused attention of this redundancy bias is an opposite mode of temporal binding from that of the habituation bias, maintaining a limited scope of the current stores of working memory over time. When the ventral memory circuit and its redundancy bias become dominant, the effect is to sacrifice the stability of the contextual model to support plasticity of control by the immediate focused contents of working memory (Tucker and Williamson 1984). The result is switching from the prior configural context to engage rapid learning of new behavioural contingencies. By focusing the contents of working memory in this way, the redundancy bias may be integral to its own structure of cognitive representation, allowing not only rapid acquisition of new contingencies, but also the separation of figure from ground which allows the object-encoding skills of the ventral corticolimbic pathways. This learning may be supported by mesencephalic dopamine projections which apply a redundancy bias on working memory. These projections are particularly dense not only in the supragenual anterior cingulate, but also in the perirhinal and other ventral limbic cortices (Morrison *et al.* 1979; Descarries *et al.* 1987; Foote and Morrison, 1987).

Strategies of action regulation

Thus the organization of memory appears to be a strategic process, regulated by unique limbic circuits which recruit vertically integrated systems with differing biases on working memory. If our theorizing is correct, these biases provide different strategies of adaptive control, which in combination allow memory formation to be motivated effectively, while at the same time being sensitive to the integrity of existing knowledge. Although they appear to support cognitive representations in memory in higher animals, these strategic learning biases appear to have evolved to support elementary mechanisms of action regulation.

Redundancy and viscerosensory feedback control

The ventral corticolimbic pathway may be suited to parse groups of elements from their embedding contexts, thus achieving strong representations of discrete objects. These skills may result from the focused attention and rapid switching of learning resources supported by the amygdala and ventral limbic circuitry. From the unique cybernetics of this ventral limbic circuit (Tucker and Williamson 1984; Tucker and Derryberry 1992), in which attention is restricted to maintain continuity of working memory, there appears to emerge a feedback form of action regulation that extends to the ventral (ventrolateral) frontal lobe.

Consistent with the viscerosensory functions of the insular perirhinal cortex of the ventral limbic networks (Neafsey *et al.* 1993), feedback from somatic as well as visceral afferents appears to provide ongoing guidance of actions within the orbital frontal (palaeocortical) cortex (Goldberg 1985; Passingham 1987; Tanji and Shima 1994; Shima and Tanji 1998; Luu and Tucker 2003). The redundancy bias appears to be required for holding the sensory criteria constant in working memory so that they can apply goal-oriented feedback control to ongoing actions.

Habituation and visceromotor feedforward control

In a similar vertical integration of matched control systems across mesencephalic, diencephalic, and telencephalic systems, the dorsal corticolimbic pathway may be suited to relational encoding of both spatial and non-spatial cognitive contexts through engaging the gradual incremental updating of contextual representations by the posterior cingulate cortex (Gabriel *et al.* 2002). The essential attentional operation for this process appears to be the phasic orienting response, through which changes in the environment are processed in a way that updates the ongoing contextual representation (Tucker and Williamson 1984). We propose that this context-updating process evolved as one strategy for mediating the stability–plasticity dilemma, such that the current representational store is altered incrementally, by the habituation bias, so as to minimize its disruption by the inclusion of new information. In the learning process, the unique cybernetics of this dorsal limbic circuit appear to produce a feedforward form of action regulation, in which mediodorsal frontal cortex integrates internal motives and goals for projectional feedforward launching of actions (Goldberg 1985; Passingham 1987; Tanji and Shima 1994; Shima and Tanji 1998; Luu and Tucker 2003). The phasic modulation of working memory by the habituation bias provides an impulsive form of action control (Tucker and Williamson 1984) generated by an internal urge from the archicortical visceromotor networks of the anterior cingulate cortex (Neafsey *et al.* 1993). The inherently phasic control of the dorsal pathway provides a unique temporal bias on binding that is well suited to a projectional feedforward form of action regulation.

Arousal, time, and consolidation

Thus action, and we propose cognition, emerges from two major representational forms, each supported by a unique mode of strategic memory consolidation. These consolidation modes are in turn supported by specific learning and behaviour control systems whose cybernetics result in distinct ways of structuring the temporal binding of information: habituation or redundancy. In the next section, we review electrophysiological evidence from our laboratory suggesting that activity in limbic cortices (anterior cingulate cortex and insula) is integral to the executive control of actions and cognitions. Although many of the findings are preliminary and the studies are often directed by methodology as much as theory, this research is beginning to provide clues to the differential role of dorsal and ventral limbic circuits in action regulation. Then, in the final section, we review neurophysiological mechanisms of memory consolidation that may explain the synchronization, and thus binding, of cognitive representations by vertically integrated motivational control systems.

Limbic mechanisms of executive control

Examining the anatomy of a human cerebral hemisphere shows that the neocortical networks are interconnected, and must be integrated, by the limbic networks at the hemispheric core. Since the early studies of neural mechanisms of executive control in humans (Pribram 1950), it has been apparent that the limbic base of the frontal and temporal lobes is critical to effective self-regulation in relation to adaptive goals. Modern studies of both cognition and emotion by neuroimaging methods have been consistent with the need for frontal networks to negotiate regulatory influences from limbic circuits (Tucker *et al.* 1995). In emotional self-regulation, for example, it has long been apparent that a hemispheric lesion may disinhibit subcortical emotional responses, such that the patient shows exaggerated emotional reactivity or crude and poorly modulated motive impulsivity (Monrad-Krohn 1924; Brodal 1969). In models of hemispheric contributions to emotion and psychopathology, the issue of disinhibition of subcortical influences has been a continuing question (Tucker 1981; Sackeim *et al.* 1982; Davidson 2001). Recent neuroimaging observations with psychiatric patients have suggested that emotional disorder may be associated with exaggerated limbic activation, whereas clinical improvement may be associated with a shift towards decreased limbic and greater neocortical activity (Drevets *et al.* 1998; Mayberg *et al.* 1999; Liotti and Mayberg 2001).

Evaluating events

In attempting to understand such corticolimbic interactions, we designed research to examine the neural mechanisms that motivate working memory. We asked subjects to memorize locations of doors that randomly appear in a video game and recorded dense-array EEGs (Tucker *et al.* 1994). Some doors were those of benefactors, who bestow points, and others were those of demons, who take points away. In addition to electrical activity in the posterior cortex that tracked the visual field of the stimulus, we observed electrical activity over the medial frontal cortex between 400 and 500 ms that discriminated between good (benefactor) and bad (demon) locations. The demons were associated with relatively negative medial frontal electrical activity, and dipole source analysis suggested the anterior cingulate cortex (ACC) as the proable neural source of this effect (Tucker *et al.* 1999).

Evaluating errors

At about the time that we first observed this good–bad evaluative discrimination effect, other researchers (Falkenstein *et al.* 1991; Gehring *et al.* 1993) reported a negative deflection over frontal regions as subjects made errors in simple motor conflict tasks. Replicating this effect with a dense-array EEG recording, Dehaene *et al.* (1994) found that this effect, called the Ne or error-related negativity (ERN), also seemed to emanate from the ACC.

Thus monitoring errors and detecting bad locations appeared to engage similar networks at the limbic base of the frontal lobe, suggesting that these networks may be integral to the binding of elements in working memory by motivational and evaluative processes. Interestingly, at the time these observations were made, ACC activation was being observed in many positron-emission tomography (PET) studies that demanded effortful control of attention, leading to the notion that the anterior cingulate cortex is integral to the 'anterior attention system' (Posner and Petersen 1990).

Self-evaluation and the executive functions

Thus several findings converged to suggest that the ACC is a fundamental neural mechanism of the executive functions in humans. However, surgical remove of the ACC in patients who suffered excessive anxiety or chronic pain was fairly common practice in the USA in the middle of the twentieth century (Pribram 1950; Tow and Whitty 1953; Foltz and White 1962). Perhaps one explanation is that the ACC is only one network in an extensive cortex in humans that has sufficient parallelism to function more or less normally in the absence of the ACC. However, among the important personality deficits in patients with ACC lesions (Rylander 1948; Tow and Whitty 1953), a critical deficit may be the effortful motivation of action. In fact, a review of psychosurgery with ACC and frontal targets concluded that psychiatric symptoms were never eliminated. The consistent effect was that patients showed a remarkable decrease in concern over their conditions (Flor-Henry 1977).

Consistent with the lesion evidence, recent neuroimaging studies have observed ACC activation when pain is administered as an experimental manipulation (Talbot *et al.* 1991; Vogt *et al.* 1993; Derbyshire *et al.* 1994; Zubieta *et al.* 2001). Psychologically, it has long been observed that intolerance of pain, as well as decreased stamina, are observed in persons who are anxious (Luu 1998). If ACC activity reflects affective or motivational impetus to effort and arousal, then the various findings on ACC activation in executive control may suggest the importance of anxiety in regulating working memory (Luu *et al.* 1998). To examine this issue specifically, Luu *et al.* (2000a) measured dense-array EEG during error monitoring in subjects varying in negative affect (a summary psychometric dimension reflecting anxiety and hostility). In the initial phase of the experiment, when subjects remained engaged in the task, greater negative affect was associated with stronger ERN responses from ACC in response to errors.

Thus error monitoring appears to engage frontolimbic circuits in relation to both affective and attentional functions. To examine the role of medial frontal regions in evaluative decisions, we asked normal subjects to read trait words as dense-array EEG was recorded, and to make a decision within one second as to whether the trait word was an accurate description of them (Tucker *et al.* 2003a). Within 300 ms, a focal negativity appeared over the medial frontal cortex that discriminated between good and bad words. Greater medial frontal (ACC) negativity was observed for the bad words, similar to the effect seen in discriminating benefactors from demons in the video game study (Tucker *et al.* 1999).

Corticolimbic circuits of action regulation

ACC activity in neuroimaging studies is common not only in effortful tasks (Posner and Petersen 1990; Paus *et al.* 1998;), but also in studies that involve conflict in response selection (Carter *et al.* 1998; Botvinick *et al.* 1999). To examine the time course of executive control of responses, we measured both medial frontal and motor cortex EEG activity as subjects completed a task with a reaction time deadline. In this procedure, subjects understand that late responses as well as incorrect responses are errors (Luu *et al.* 2000b). For incorrect responses, analysis of motor cortical activity suggested no response conflict before the error (i.e. only the incorrect hand was activated), yet there was a large ERN. For late responses, the ERN was found to increase in amplitude in proportion to the lateness of the response as if the ACC activity reflected the subject's monitoring of the status of the response continuously in time (Luu *et al.* 2000b).

Evaluating events in the context of the self

Although many of the tasks used in error-monitoring experiments are simple, the psychological processes are not easily separated. When subjects receive negative feedback on performance, for example, there is a negative wave over the medial frontal cortex that appears similar to the ERN (Miltner *et al.* 1997).

Although this may reflect an emotional or evaluative response to the feedback, it is not clear whether response-correction mechanisms are also engaged. In experimental studies of motivational control of action, Derryberry and associates have developed a method to separate the emotional response to feedback from ongoing response control, specifically by delaying feedback until it is no longer relevant for response correction (Derryberry 1991). We applied these methods in a dense-array EEG study of a reaction time deadline response compatibility task, using letter grades (A, C, and F) as feedback on whether responses were speedy, acceptable, or tardy (Luu *et al.* 2003). Even when the feedback was irrelevant to response correction, subjects evidenced a marked negativity over the medial frontal cortex in response to a poor letter grade (Luu *et al.* 2003). By similar reasoning to that used in the studies of negative affect (Luu 1998), we hypothesized that clinically depressed subjects may be biased to respond aversively to negative feedback. Examining the dense-array EEG in the speeded response feedback task in a range of normal and clinically depressed subjects, we found partial support for this hypothesis. As predicted, the depressed subjects as a group showed large ERNs, particularly to the F grade. For subjects that were moderately depressed, greater depression was associated with a larger ERN in response to the F grade. Importantly, this study used 256-channel EEG recording for the first time, and the improved measurement allowed source modelling that showed activity in insular cortex as well as the ACC in the response to negative grades.

Action regulation in learned helplessness

Unexpectedly, however, the more severely depressed subjects in this sample showed a reduction of the ERN rather than a continued increase in response to the negative feedback (Tucker *et al.* 2003b). Given the importance of the ACC in motivational control of the dorsal motor pathway (linked to the supplemental motor area, the premotor area, and the primary motor cortex), it may be important to note that severe depression is associated not only with impairment of working memory, but also with anhedonia and psychomotor retardation. Although these findings require replication, one implication may be that the dorsal limbic base of the frontal lobe (the ACC) is integral not only to hedonic tone but also to the initiation of cognitive as well as motor actions.

Deficits in action regulation in depression may thus be integral to the classical model of learned helplessness. In attempting to understand these effects, we reviewed the neurophysiological evidence on frontolimbic circuits in motivational control of actions (Luu and Tucker 2003). Drawing on experiments and theoretical analysis of corticothalamic and corticolimbic mechanisms in animal learning (Gabriel 1990), and on the theory and observations of limbic theta in binding the representations of behavioural contexts (Miller 1991), we interpreted the neuroimaging and electrophysiological findings in the medial frontal cortex within the model of action regulation outlined above. The ACC appears to form a pivotal control network for action control. Although it is part of archicortex and is responsible for visceromotor controls, it also appears to receive substantial control from the amygdala and ventral limbic memory circuit (Luu and Tucker 2003). Whereas the dorsal learning circuit is capable of gradual shaping and maintenance of projectional control of actions in line with the current contextual model and visceromotor state, it is not capable of rapid focused adjustment in response to changing environmental contingencies, such as are required when the animal's expectancies are violated (Rescorla and Wagner 1972). Under such conditions, the ventral perirhinal limbic circuit involving the amygdala, mediodorsal thalamus, and anterior cingulate cortex is required (Gabriel *et al.* 1991). This palaeocortical network and circuit appears to be integral not only to viscerosensory motivational mechanisms (Luu and Tucker, in press), but also to the feedback mode of action control of the orbital and ventrolateral motor pathway of the frontal lobe. Under conditions in which events violate the implicit expectancy of the configural contextual model, the ACC and ventral memory circuit are essential for the redundancy of current information stores to direct rapid adjustment of learning and resetting of priority to cues relevant to the new contingencies, a process Gabriel *et al.* (1991) term 'salience compensation.'

Electrophysiological signs of activity in limbic learning circuits

Increasingly, researchers examining executive processes are providing evidence of motivational and evaluative influences on ACC contributions to judgements and actions (Gehring and Willoughby 2002). We have attempted to understand how such electrophysiological measures may reflect the specific memory strategies engaged by limbic control systems. Could the sensitivity of late positive ERP responses over parietal regions to manipulations of recognition memory (Rugg *et al.* 1998; Curran 2000) reflect dorsal limbic circuit contributions to context updating (Gabriel *et al.* 1983; Donchin and Coles 1988)? Could the medial frontal negativity (MFN) reviewed in the studies above reflect the unique influence of the ventral limbic circuit, both to familiarization and to prediction discrepancies (Rugg *et al.* 1998; Wagner 1999; Curran 2000)? Could some of the ACC discriminations related to erroneous or affectively negative events in our research reflect not only affective evaluation but also context discrepancies when the subject's intrinsic contextual expectancy for a good outcome is violated by an unexpected bad event (Luu and Pedersen, in press)?

As we attempted to understand these questions of motivational and memory processes in limbic networks, we were surprised to observe that in individual trials the ACC showed oscillatory electrical waves in the theta band (4–7 Hz). Breaking down the EEG time series using Independent Components Analysis showed certain components with clear theta oscillations, and these were enhanced in amplitude for error trials (Makeig *et al.*, in preparation). When examined carefully, the theta bursts following error trials appeared to sum to create the ERN component in the averaged ERP (Luu and Tucker 2001; Luu *et al.* 2004).

Studying response-locked potentials over the motor cortex, we also observed brief oscillatory perturbations of the ongoing EEG with an approximate period in the theta band. These appeared to be particularly strong for the error trials. In many cases, the motor oscillations seemed to alternate with the theta oscillations over medial frontal (ACC) networks. Statistical analysis of the correlation of ACC theta with motor cortex theta across subjects showed that this limbic–neocortical correlation was significant for error, but not correct, trials (Luu and Tucker 2001). The implication appears to be that coordination of the large-scale networks of motor control may require synchronization with the limbic theta rhythm.

More recently, we found that when correct and error responses are compared with respect to EEG activity within the theta band, error responses are associated with greater theta band amplitude and that this increase starts at the time of the response and is sustained for approximately 400 ms post-response (Luu *et al.* 2004). We then analysed the phase-locked and non-phase-locked theta components of the EEG on error trials and found that the ERN is that part of the theta rhythm that is phase locked to the erroneous response. Approximately 100 ms before the erroneous button press, the ongoing theta rhythm of the EEG became phase locked to the action and lasted for approximately 200 ms post-response. However, the non-phase-locked component of the theta rhythm showed sustained amplitude, compared with correct responses, for approximately 400 ms post-response. These results suggest that the ERN may be generated through similar mechanisms to those of the EEG theta rhythm.

Control of limbic theta and binding in cortical networks

In rats, theta is observed as a rhythmic slow (4–12 Hz) activity recorded in the hippocampus under conditions in which the animal is exploring the environment (i.e. acquiring information). Cells within the hippocampal complex are easily activated at the theta frequency because they have intrinsic resonant properties tuned to this frequency (Bland and Oddie 1998). The anatomical circuit involved in the generation of the hippocampal EEG theta rhythm begins in the brainstem (reviewed by Vertes and Kocis 1997). The pedunculopontine tegmental nucleus of the brainstem projects to the pontis oralis nucleus (RPO) of the reticular formation. This input releases the RPO from inhibition, whose activity in turn is sent to the supramammillary nucleus (SUM). The SUM converts tonic RPO activity into a phasic theta-bursting pattern of discharge. This activity is then relayed to the medial septum/vertical limb of the diagonal band (MS/DBv). The MS/DBv contains two major classes of rhythmically bursting hippocampal projecting neurons, cholinergic and GABAergic. Within this circuit, it is believed the SUM controls the frequency of the EEG theta rhythm and that the MS/DBv controls the amplitude (Bland and Oddie 1998).

Overall, the majority of pyramidal cells are virtually silent during the theta state. Those that are active appear to code the currently relevant stimuli (Buzsáki 1996). For example, place-responsive cells that are active in one environment will be silent in other environments, at which time their lack of response is similar to silent cells which make up a majority of hippocampal cells (Thompson and Best 1989). This selective enhancement of cellular response to relevant stimuli may be specific to motivationally significant events. A model of this form of motivationally adaptive response may be provided by observations of hippocampal theta in response to nociceptive stimuli.

Cells in the medial septum are especially responsive to noxious stimulation, whether mechanical or thermal (Dutar *et al.* 1985). The receptive fields of these cells are broad, a characteristic feature of cells found in the medial pain system coding the affective, rather than locating, response to pain (Vogt *et al.* 1993). The pain-responsive cells of the medial septum project to the hippocampus to produce changes in the activity of pyramidal neurons. In the hippocampus, these changes produce a depression of population spikes together with an increase in theta activity and a selective activation of a small number of pain-responsive cells (Khanna 1997).

The inhibition of a majority of hippocampal cells, simultaneous with selective enhancement of stimulus-specific cell responses, appears to result specifically from MS/DBv projections. Lesion to the MS/DBv or application of a cholinergic antagonist will eliminate this effect (Zheng and Khanna 1999). It is possible that this selective suppression/enhancement of stimulus-responsive hippocampal cells is a consequence of active inhibition by the theta cells (pyramidal, granular, and interneuron) of the hippocampus (Thompson and Best 1989). It may also be possible, because of massive hippocampal efferents, that the theta rhythm also achieves active suppression of currently irrelevant neocortical sensory areas (Sainsbury 1998). Such an effect would allow stimulus-relevant cells within the sensory cortex and thalamus to become synchronized with the theta rhythm (Gambini *et al.* 2002). Thus the EEG theta rhythm may not only enhance the signal-to-noise ratio within the hippocampal circuit, but may also achieve a similar effect within more extensive corticlimbic networks. Of course, this implies the existence of very specific hippocampal circuitry that would allow for selective inhibition and excitation. The topographically specific nature of hippocampal architecture still remains to be clarified.

It will be important to characterize the neuroanatomical circuits responsible for control of the hippocampal EEG theta rhythm, and to understand how memory for stimulus information is regulated by this rhythm. More specifically, we need to understand how the multiple mesencephalic reticular activating systems can influence the properties and functions of limbic theta. We can now see that brainstem cholinergic mechanisms directly impinge upon limbic functions via the SUM and MS/DBv, which translate the brainstem inputs into physiological rhythms that have direct consequences for stimulus processing and representation. We have interesting clues to the differential limbic circuits modulated by the targeted projection zones of the noradrenergic (dorsal) and dopaminergic (ventral) neuromodulator systems. The control exerted by these brainstem systems appears to involve strategic biases applied to the synchronizing mechanisms of corticolimbic consolidation, and thus the binding of neuronal assemblies.

Theta rhythm and binding of short-term memory representations

The effects of the EEG theta rhythm, such as increased signal-to-noise ratio, may be integral to the binding of relevant stimuli. The result of selective suppression and enhancement appears to be that specific neuronal ensembles within the hippocampus are isolated and coherent in their activities. The components of a particular ensemble may be spatially distant, but through the binding influence of the hippocampal EEG theta rhythm a coherent representation of a particular stimulus can be achieved in short-term memory. In addition to this form of binding, the fact that place cells shift their firing to different phases of the hippocampal EEG theta rhythm as an animal moves through their spatial field (O'Keefe and Burgess 1999) implies that events can be segregated into temporal episodes, and, together with the configural information of the events within that particular episode, binding can now result in discrete representations necessary for episodic memory.

Exactly how limbic theta is related to neocortical binding such as may be achieved by gamma oscillations (40–100 Hz) remains a mystery. However, it is clear that both types of oscillation occur within the hippocampus, and that the gamma oscillations are modulated by the hippocampal EEG theta rhythm (Bragin *et al.* 1995). Perhaps the gamma oscillations reflect binding mechanisms related to percepts formed from sensory information, whereas the hippocampal EEG theta rhythm reflects a broader binding of configurations of events on the basis of motivational significance. Motivational significance would be gathered not only from brainstem and diencephalic inputs, but perhaps from corticolimbic structures as well, providing for adaptive control of memory representation.

It is now well known that long-term potentiation (LTP) is readily established within the hippocampal complex, and that the hippocampal EEG theta rhythm plays a central role in this establishment (Buzsáki 1996; Vertes and Kocis 1997). Initially, the large-amplitude antidromic stimulation required for experimentally inducing LTP was not physiologically plausible. However, it was then discovered that more physiological stimulation could be effective if it were delivered at the theta rhythm (Diamond and Rose 1994). Theta-patterned stimuli not only permit rapid formation of LTP, but a stimulus delivered in the presence of the hippocampal EEG theta rhythm also facilitates the establishment of LTP (Huerta and Lisman 1993). Furthermore, many studies have shown that the phase of the theta rhythm at which stimulus delivery is applied will determine whether the effect is LTP or long-term depotentiation (LTD) (Plavides *et al.* 1988; Huerta and Lisman 1993; Hyman *et al.* 2003; Yaniv *et al.* 2003). The mechanisms of theta regulation of LTP and LTD remain to be elucidated, but it appears clear that the EEG theta rhythm is likely to play a role in short-term memory representation within the hippocampus.

Theta rhythm and binding of large-scale networks involved in memory

Establishing long-term memory appears to require consolidation of traces within neocortical areas, achieved through some form of interaction with limbic regions (Squire 1987). One candidate for this consolidation of neocortical networks may be the sharp waves and high-frequency ripples that emanate from the hippocampus when the animal is quiet (Buzsáki 1996). In addition, however, several findings have suggested that the theta rhythm may also support binding on a larger inter-region scale (Miller 1991). The EEG theta rhythm is recorded not only in the hippocampus but also in corticolimbic regions with connections to the hippocampus, such as the cingulate cortex (Leung and Borst 1987). An obvious network in which the EEG theta rhythm may play an integral role in inter-region binding is the Papez or dorsal limbic circuit made up of the hippocampus, the mammillary body, th anterior nucleus of the thalamus, and the posterior cingulate cortex. Classical experimental evidence shows that a bilateral lesion to either the anterior nucleus of the thalamus or the cingulate gyrus reduces the duration of hippocampal theta induced by electrical stimulation (Azzaroni and Parmeggiani 1967). Such effects suggest that the EEG theta rhythm is maintained as it propagates through the network. Similarly, stimulation to either the cingulate cortex or the anterior thalamus induces theta activity in the ipsilateral hippocampus (Azzaroni and Parmeggiani 1967).

Intracranial as well as scalp recordings in humans show increased EEG power at the theta frequency in tasks that require working memory (Gevins *et al.* 1997; Tesche and Karhu 2000). Importantly, the location of the theta increase in these studies was observed in regions outside the hippocampus, such as the ACC and the frontal cortex, suggesting that an extended network is involved in the theta modulation of working memory. Evidence from both animal and human studies shows inter-regional coherence of the EEG theta rhythm during the performance of learning and memory tasks. When an animal learns the association between a conditioned stimulus and the delivery of a shock, the amygdalar and hippocampal EEG theta rhythms become synchronized (Seidenbecher *et al.* 2003). In humans, the requirement to hold information in working memory is associated with intercortical EEG coherence in the theta frequency band (Sarnthein *et al.* 1998). These findings are consistent with the proposal that limbic theta engages long-range binding of distant brain structures to support short-term memory (Miller 1991).

So far we have emphasized the EEG theta rhythm in the dorsal limbic circuit, which we have implicated in the feedforward control of learning and memory. However, as mentioned above (Seidenbecher *et al.* 2003), EEG theta rhythms are also present in the ventral limbic learning and memory circuit, operating through feedback control and centred on the amygdala (Paré *et al.* 2002). It is believed that the theta rhythm recorded within the amygdala does not simply reflect processes controlled by the hippocampal EEG theta rhythm. Rather, it reflects learning and memory processes inherent to the functions of the amygdala and, we would argue, to the ventral limbic circuit that recruits not only the perirhinal cortex but also the orbital frontal lobe and the anterior cingulate gyrus.

Paralleling the apparent binding functions of hippocampal theta, the amygdalar theta rhythm appears to be involved in processes associated with fear learning (Paré 2003). The EEG theta rhythm recorded in the basolateral complex of the amygdala is readily elicited by emotional arousal, such as when the animal is expecting delivery of a painful stimulus. Interestingly, the firing rate of cells in the basolateral complex does not increase in the emotional state. Rather, the activity of these cells becomes synchronized in this state through the modulating influence of the EEG theta rhythm (Paré 2003). This suggests that the amygdalar EEG theta rhythm acts to bind the activity of the cells of the basolateral complex into a coherent ensemble, paralleling the action of the hippocampal EEG theta rhythm on the activity of hippocampal cells.

In addition, the amygdalar EEG theta rhythm is important to memory functions, as illustrated by the facilitation of LTP. Theta-patterned stimulation of the entorhinal cortex, which has connections to both the basolateral complex and the hippocampus, readily establishes LTP in both the amygdala and hippocampus (Yaniv *et al* 2003). However, Yaniv *et al.* observed that the mechanisms underlying LTP in the two structures are different, consistent with the notion that the ventral and dorsal limbic circuits are indeed functionally distinct. Although there has been less research on the mechanisms underlying amygdalar theta than hippocampal theta, it is possible that the cells within the basolateral complex have membrane potentials tuned to the theta frequency that can be driven by the theta rhythm of the hippocampus (Paré 2003).

Phase reset of the theta rhythm and dynamics of network control

If the relation of neural activity to the phase of theta is important to binding, there must be a mechanism for aligning incoming information to the theta rhythm. Indeed, the evidence for phase alignment of EEG theta with task-relevant stimuli has existed for several decades. In the early stages of learning, when an animal is still trying to learn the association between the condition auditory stimulus and reward, the theta rhythm is prominent and is phased-locked to the auditory cue (Adey 1967; Buzsáki *et al.* 1979). When the animal's performance indicates that it has learned the task, the EEG theta amplitude decreases because of either a loss of phase-locked activity or a loss of synchronization of the rhythm generally. However, if the cue is reversed, the EEG theta rhythm re-emerges, again phase locked to the stimulus. Similarly, in tasks in which the animal is required to remember whether the current stimulus is the same or different from a previous stimulus in order to determine which response to make, Givens (1996) found that the hippocampal EEG theta rhythm became phase locked to the stimulus. However, when performing a much simpler, well-learned task of stimulus-response mapping, the hippocampal EEG theta rhythm was not phase locked to the stimulus (Givens 1996). The implication may be that greater demands for binding information in short-term memory lead to increased theta synchronization.

More recently, Williams and Givens (2003) demonstrated that reset of the hippocampal EEG theta rhythm to an incoming stimulus may occur through a phase-resetting signal delivered to either the perforant path or the fornix. Ultimately, these authors acknowledged, the resetting signal must reach the MS/DBv. Brazhnik *et al.* (1985) recorded the theta rhythm from the medial septum and found that stimulating the lateral septum resulted in phase locking of the theta rhythm to the stimulation. According to Brazhnik *et al.*, the resetting of the theta rhythm could be produced by either a temporary pause of cell activity, which lasts for 40–90 ms, or a cellular 'burst' which is time-locked to the stimulus.

Phase resetting and binding in executive control

These mechanisms of theta phase shifting in the septum are quite interesting to us, given our efforts to understand the apparent phase shifting of theta that we have recorded in humans over the medial frontal lobe (Luu and Tucker 2001, 2003). We have proposed that similar phase-resetting mechanisms underlie the phase alignment of the scalp-recorded EEG theta rhythm, an effect that creates an average ERN wave in the trials average (Luu and Tucker 2001; Makeig *et al.*, in preparation). We have also speculated that resetting the phase of the theta rhythm, such as through error signals or switching signals under dopaminergic or striatal control, may coordinate the response of multiple networks to important events (Luu and Tucker 2003). According to the Holroyd–Coles model of the ERN (Holroyd and Coles 2002), when an error occurs, dopaminergic activity is decreased. This dopaminergic decrement results in a disinhibition of neurons in the ACC; the ERN is observed as a consequence of this disinhibition. However, as we have observed, the ERN appears to arise not as a discrete negative transient, but rather as a phase shifting of mediofrontal sources that are modulated at the theta rhythm (Luu *et al.* 2004). Nonetheless, it could still be that the mechanism for the phase reset is the dopaminergic signal from the ventral tegmental area, possibly under control from the ventral limbic or striatal networks.

Although Luu and Tucker (2003) and Holroyd and Coles (2002) have proposed a direct effect of dopaminergic projections on the ACC, it is also possible that theta phase shifting results from a dopamine influence on the medial septum–diagonal band complex. Cells from the ventral tegmental area (VTA) and substantia nigra have been shown to project to cholinergic cells of the MS/DBv (Gaykema and Zaborszky 1996). Miura *et al.* (1987) injected dopamine into the medial septum and found an increase in hippocampal EEG theta activity. Therefore it is possible that, during an error response, an abrupt decrement of dopaminergic input into the medial septum or diagonal band results in a pause (or reduction) in cholinergic activity. This pause results in a phase resetting of the theta rhythm to the error event. Such an effect would involve a dopamine influence at the basal forebrain rather than in the ACC.

However, it is entirely possible that phase resetting can be initiated intrinsically within the cortical network, such as within the ACC itself. Of relevance to this proposal is the finding by Gabriel and Taylor (1998) of salience compensation functions carried out by the ACC. As described above, salience compensation appears to be a mechanism engaged during violation of contextual expectancies to allow non-salient, yet significant, stimuli to receive processing. When presented with motivationally significant but non-salient stimuli, cells within the ACC demonstrate a brief pause (40–80 ms) in their activity followed by enhanced firing. Gabriel and Taylor proposed that this pause is a resetting mechanism which recruits neurons that would otherwise not have been available for the processing of the low salience stimulus. Perhaps mechanisms such as this permit phase resetting of the EEG theta rhythm. Signals from multiple brain regions may be able to reset the phase of the theta rhythm based on error information. Such effects may be achieved by modulating the passage of the theta wave through the local network, or by competition for the binding and pacemaking functions of the MS/DBv.

Although most of the research on theta synchronization has focused on specific limbic structures, such as the amygdala or hippocampus, or the dominant memory circuits linking these structures to the thalamus, the process of memory consolidation also engages re-entrant connections of the major pathways of the cortex between paralimbic networks, association cortices, and finally primary sensory and motor neocortices (Tucker 2001). It is highly likely that the coordination of binding activities across these linked networks is accomplished through utilization of the EEG theta rhythm.

We have observed multiple cortical regions involved in the generation of the ERN, and these regions show phase relations that may be consistent with synchronized integration. Initially, localization of MEG recordings suggested that specific regions of the ACC and midline frontal cortex oscillate at theta, at phase relations that would be observed for a theta wave travelling through a corticolimbic circuit (Asada *et al.* 1999). In examining dense-array EEG with similar source-localization methods, we found similar ACC or supplementary motor area (SMA) sources for the EEG ERN, and these sources showed the same (60° out of phase) wave propagation as the MEG sources (Luu *et al.* 2003, 2004). In a separate study, we found that the midline oscillations making up the ERN alternated with motor potentials recorded at scalp sites, also with phase relations that suggested that the midline and motor regions may share a common theta wave propagation. Interestingly, the midline (ACC) and lateral (motor) theta waves were significantly correlated only when an error was made (Luu and Tucker 2001). The implication may be that the error-monitoring process of the ACC engages, and possibly resets, the limbic theta rhythm as a mechanism for coordinating the binding of action plans across multiple limbic and neocortical networks.

Conclusions: adaptive binding in space and time

We began this chapter with an analysis of the anatomical mechanisms of memory, including the vertical integration of brainstem and diencephalic homeostatic mechanisms that are essential for adaptive control. Even though the framework began with anatomical spatial organization, the temporal component of binding became the primary functional question. The functional spatial organization of the cortex appears to have been determined by the orthogonal elaboration of somatic systems (specializing for somatic sensory networks in the posterior cortex and somatic motor networks in the anterior cortex) and visceral systems (specializing for visceral sensory networks in the ventral limbic cortex and visceral motor networks in the dorsal limbic cortex). Although they are thus identified by their anatomical separation, we find that the functional roles of the dorsal and ventral limbic networks may best be described by differing biases in the temporal modulation of adaptive binding. The dorsal archicortical limbic network appears to operate through a habituation bias, allowing new information to be taken in rapidly, but maintaining the balance of control by the existing internal representation. The ventral palaeocortical limbic network appears to operate through a redundancy bias, providing extended representation of new information such that it dominates over existing memory, thus favouring plasticity over stability under conditions in which the internal neuronal model is not adaptive.

We reviewed several findings suggesting that the functional differentiation of dorsal and ventral memory systems can be observed in human studies, with both haemodynamic (fMRI) and electrophysiological (EEG) measures. The adaptive control of limbic networks has become a central question, whether in relation to conflict management in the anterior cingulate or the evaluation of pain and negative feedback in insular cortex. In the electrophysiological evidence, spatial localization is obviously important for differentiating the function of specific circuits, but it has also become clear in this research that the temporal resolution of binding operations is a critical factor. Functional changes in the limbic theta rhythm appear to reflect 100 ms phase shifts in response to arbitration among multiple networks in processes such as error monitoring, evaluating feedback, and self-evaluation. Thus adequate resolution in space and time will be required not only for measurement methodology but also for theoretical analysis of adaptive binding in relation to multiple issues of human psychological function.

References

Adey, W.R. (1967). Intrinisic organization of cerebral tissue in alterting, orienting, and discriminative reponses. In *The Neurosciences* (ed G.C. Quarton, T. Melnechuck, and F.O. Schmitt). New York: Rockefeller University Press, pp. 615–633.

Aggleton, J.R., and Brown, M.W. (1999). Episodic memory, amnesia, and the hippocampal-anterior thalamic axis. *Behavioral and Brain Sciences*, **22**, 425–489.

Asada, H., Fukuda, Y., Tsunoda, S., Yamaguchi, M., and Tonoike, M. (1999). Frontal midline theta rhythms reflect alternative activation of prefrontal cortex and anterior cingulate cortex in humans. *Neuroscience Letters*, **274**, 29–32.

Azzaroni, A., and Parmeggiani, P.L. (1967). Feedback regulation of the hippocampal theta-rhythm. *Helvetica Physiologica et Pharmacologica Acta*, **25**, 309–321.

Bland, B.H., and Oddie, S.D. (1998). Anatomical, electrophysiological and pharmacological studies of ascending brainstem hippocampal synchronizing pathways. *Neuroscience and Biobehavioral Reviews*, **22**, 259–273.

Botvinick, M., Nystrom, L.E., Fissell, K., Carter, C.S., and Cohen, J.D. (1999). Conflict monitoring versus selection-for-action in anterior cingulate cortex. *Nature*, **402**, 179–181.

Bragin, A., Jando, G., Nadasdy, Z., Hetke, J., Wise, K., and Buzsáki, G. (1995). Gamma (40–100 Hz) oscillations in the hippocampus of the behaving rat. *Journal of Neuroscience*, **15**, 47–60.

Brazhnik, E.S., Vinogradova, O.S., and Karanov, A.M. (1985). Frequency modulation of neuronal theta-bursts in rabbit's septum by low-frequency repetitive stimulation of the afferent pathways. *Neuroscience*, **14**, 501–508.

Brodal, A. (1969). *Neurological Anatomy in Relation to Clinical Medicine.* New York: Oxford University Press.

Buzsáki, G. (1996). The hippocampal–neocortical dialogue. *Cerebral Cortex*, **6**, 81–92.

Buzsáki, G. (2002). Theta oscillations in the hippocampus. *Neuron*, **33**, 325–340.

Buzsáki, G., Grastyán, E., Tveritskaya, I.N., and Czopf, J. (1979). Hippocampal evoked potentials and EEG changes during classical conditioning in the rat. *Electroencephalography and Clinical Neurophysiology*, **47**, 64–74.

Carter, C.S., Braver, T.S., Barch, D.M., Botvinick, M.M., Noll, D., and Cohen, J.D. (1998). Anterior cingulate cortex, error detection, and the online monitoring of performance. *Science*, **280**, 747–749.

Chrobak, J.J., and Buzsáki, G. (1998). Operational dynamics in the hippocampal-entorhinal axis. *Neuroscience and Biobehavioral Reviews*, **22**, 303–310.

Curran, T. (2000). Brain potentials of recollection and familiarity. *Memory and Cognition*, **28**, 923–938.

Davachi, L., Mitchell, J. P., and Wagner, A. D. (2003). Multiple routes to memory: distinct medial temporal lobe processes build item and source memories. *Proceedings of the National Academy of Sciences*, **100**, 2157–2162.

Davidson, R. J. (2001). Toward a biology of personality and emotion. *Annals of the New York Academy of Sciences*, **935**, 191–207.

Dehaene, S., Posner, M.I., and Tucker, D.M. (1994). Localization of a neural system for error detection and compensation. *Psychological Science*, **5**, 303–305.

Derbyshire, S.W.G., Jones, A.K.P., Devani, P., *et al.* (1994). Cerebral responses to pain in patients with atypical facial pain measured by positron emission tomography. *Journal of Neurology, Neurosurgery, and Psychiatry*, **57**, 1166–1172.

Derryberry, D. (1991). The immediate effects of positive and negative feedback signals. *Journal of Personality and Social Psychology*, **61**, 267–278.

Descarries, L., and Lapierre, Y. (1973). Norepinephrine and axon terminals in the cerebral cortex of the rat. *Brain Research*, **51**, 141–160.

Descarries, L., Lemay, B., Doucet, G., and Berger, B. (1987). Regional and laminar density of the dopamine innervation in adult rat cerebral cortex. *Neuroscience*, **21**, 807–824.

Diamond, D.M., and Rose, G. M. (1994). Does associative LTP underlie classical conditioning? *Psychobiology*, **22**, 263–269.

Donchin, E., and Coles, M.G.H. (1988). Is the P300 component a manifestation of context updating? *Behavioral and Brain Sciences*, **11**, 357–374.

Drevets, W.C., Ongur, D., and Price, J.L. (1998). Neuroimaging abnormalities in the subgenual prefrontal cortex: implications for the pathophysiology of familial mood disorders. *Molecular Psychiatry*, **3**, 220–226, 190–221.

Dutar, P., Lamour, Y., and Jobert, A. (1985). Activation of identified septo-hippocampal neurons by noxious peripheral stimulation. *Brain Research*, **328**, 15–21.

Falkenstein, M., Hohnsbein, J., Hoormann, J., and Blanke, L. (1991). Effects of crossmodal divided attention on late ERP components. II: Error processing in choice reaction tasks. *Electroencephalography and Clinical Neurophysiology*, **78**, 447–455.

Flor-Henry, P. (1977). Progress and problems in psychosurgery. In *Current Psychiatric Therapies* (ed J.H. Masserman). New York: Grune and Stratton, pp. 283–298.

Foltz, E., and White, L.E. (1962). Pain 'relief' by frontal cingulotomy. *Journal of Neurosurgery*, **19**, 89–100.

Foote, S.L., and Morrison, J.H. (1987). Extrathalamic modulation of cortical function. *Annual Review of Neuroscience*, **10**, 67–95.

Freeman, W.J. (1998). The neurobiology of multimodal sensory integration. *Integrative Physiological and Behavioral Science*, **33**, 124–129.

Gabriel, M. (1990). Functions of anterior and posterior cingulate cortex during avoidance learning in rabbits. *Progress in Brain Research*, **85**, 467–483.

Gabriel, M., and Taylor, C. (1998). Prenatal exposure to cocaine impairs neuronal coding of attention and discriminative learning. *Annals of the New York Academy of Sciences*, **846**, 194–212.

Gabriel, M., Lambert, R.W., Foster, K., Orona, E., Sparenborg, S., and Maiorca, R R. (1983). Anterior thalamic lesions and neuronal activity in the cingulate and retrosplenial cortices during discriminative avoidance behavior in rabbits. *Behavioral Neuroscience*, **97**, 675–696.

Gabriel, M., Taylor, C., and Burhans, L. (2003). In utero cocaine, discriminative avoidance learning with low-salient stimuli and learning-related neuronal activity in rabbits (*oryctolagus cuniculus*). *Behavioral Neuroscience*, **117**, 912–926.

Gabriel, M., Vogt, B.A., Kubota, Y., Poremba, A., and Kang, E. (1991). Training-stage related neuronal plasticity in limbic thalamus and cingulate cortex during learning: a possible key to mnemonic retrieval. *Behavioral and Brain Research*, **46**, 175–185.

Gambini, J.P., Velluti, R.A., and Pedemonte, M. (2002). Hippocampal theta rhythm synchronizes visual neurons in sleep and waking. *Brain Research*, **926**, 137–141.

Gaykema, R.P., and Zaborszky, L. (1996). Direct catecolaminergic-cholinergic interactions in the basal forebrain. II: Substantia nigra–ventral tegmental area projections. *Journal of Comparative Neurology*, **374**, 555–577.

Gehring, W.J., and Willoughby, A.R. (2002). The medial frontal cortex and the rapid processing of monetary gains and losses. *Science*, **295**, 2279–2282.

Gehring, W.J., Goss, B., Coles, M.G.H., Meyer, D.E., and Donchin, E. (1993). A neural system for error detection and compensation. *Psychological Science*, **4**, 385–390.

Gevins, A., Smith, M.E., McEvoy, L., and Yu, D. (1997). High-resolution EEG mapping of cortical activation related to working memory: effects of task difficulty, type of processing, and practice. *Cerebral Cortex*, **7**, 374–385.

Givens, B. (1996). Stimulus-evoked resetting of the dentate theta rhythm: relation to working memory. *Neuroreport*, **8**, 159–163.

Goldberg, G. (1985). Supplementary motor area structure and function: review and hypotheses. *Behavioral and Brain Sciences*, **8**, 567–616.

Goldberg, G. (1987). From intent to action: evolution and function of the premotor systems of the frontal lobe. In *The frontal lobes revisited* (ed E. Perceman). New York: The IRBN Press, pp. 273–306.

Grossberg, S. (1982). Processing of expected and unexpected events during conditioning and attention: a psychophysiological theory. *Psychological Review*, **89**, 529–572.

Holroyd, C.B., and Coles, M.G.H. (2002). The basis of human error processing: reinforcement learning, dopamine, and the error-related negativity. *Psychological Review*, **109**, 679–709.

Huerta, P.T., and Lisman, J.E. (1993). Heightened synaptic plasticity of hippocampal CA1 neurons during a cholinergically induced rhythmic state. *Nature*, **364**, 723–725.

Hyman, J.M., Wyble, B.P., Goyal, V., Rossi, C.A., and Hasselmo, M.E. (2003). Stimulation in hippocampal region CA1 in behaving rats yields long-term potentiation when delivered to the peak of theta and long-term depression when delivered to the trough. *Journal of Neuroscience*, **23**, 11725–11731.

Khanna, S. (1997). Dorsal hippocampus field CA1 pyramidal cell responses to a persistent versus an acute nociceptive stimulus and their septal modulation. *Neuroscience*, **77**, 713–721.

Leung, L.W.S., and Borst, J. G. G. (1987). Electrical activity of the cingulate cortex. I: Generating mechanisms and relations to behavior. *Brain Research*, **407**, 68–80.

Liotti, M., and Mayberg, H. S. (2001). The role of functional neuroimaging in the neuropsychology of depression. *Journal of Clinical and Experimental Neuropsychology*, **23**, 121–136.

Luu, P. (1998). Negative effect/emotionality and evaluation. *Dissertation Abstracts International: Section B: Sciences and Engineering*, **58**, 3928.

Luu, P. and Pedersen, S. M. (in press). The anterior cingulate cortext: regulating actions in context. New York: Guildford Publication Inc.

Luu, P., and Tucker, D.M. (2001). Regulating action: Alternating activation of midline frontal and motor cortical networks. *Clinical Neurophysiology, **112***, 1295–1306.

Luu, P., and Tucker, D.M. (2003). Self-regulation and the executive functions: electrophysiological clues. In *The Cognitive Electrophysiology of Mind and Brain* (ed A. Zani and A.M. Preverbio). San Diego, CA: Academic Press, pp. 199–223.

Luu, P., and Tucker, D.M. (in press). Action regulation by the medial frontal cortex: the representation of set-points and self-regulation. In *Consciousness, Emotional Self-Regulation and the Brain* (ed M. Beauregard). Amsterdam: John Benjamin.

Luu, P., Tucker, D.M., and Derryberry, D. (1998). Anxiety and the motivational basis of working memory. *Cognitive Therapy and Research*, **22**, 577–594.

Luu, P., Collins, P., and Tucker, D.M. (2000a). Mood, personality, and self-monitoring: negative affect and emotionality in relation to frontal lobe mechanisms of error monitoring. *Journal of Experimental Psychology: General*, **129**, 43–60.

Luu, P., Flaisch, T., and Tucker, D.M. (2000b). Medial frontal cortex in action monitoring. *Journal of Neuroscience*, **20**, 464–469.

Luu, P., Tucker, D.M., Derryberry, D., Reed, M., and Poulsen, C. (2003). Electrophysiological responses to errors and feedback in the process of action regulation. *Psychological Science*, **14**, 47–53.

Luu, P., Tucker, D.M., and Makeig, S. (2004). Frontal midline theta and the error-related negativity: neurophysiological mechanisms of action regulation. *Clinical Neurophysiology*, **115**, 1821–1835.

McClelland, J.L., McNaughton, B.L., and O'Reilly, R.C. (1995). Why there are complementary learning systems in the hippocampus and neocortex: Insights from the successes and failures of connectionist models of learning and memory. *Psychological Review*, **102**, 419–457.

Makeig, S., Luu, P., Briggman, K., Visser, E., Sejnowski, T. J., and Tucker, D.M. (in preparation). Error-related dynamics in distributed brain networks.

Mayberg, H.S., Liotti, M., Brannan, S.K., *et al.* (1999). Reciprocal limbic-cortical function and negative mood: converging PET findings in depression and normal sadness. *American Journal of Psychiatry*, **156**, 675–682.

Menon, V., Freeman, W.J., Cutillo, B.A., *et al.* (1996). Spatio-temporal correlations in human gamma band electrocorticograms. *Electroencephalography and Clinical Neurophysiology*, **98**, 89–102.

Mesulam, M. (1988). Central cholinergic pathways: neuroanatomy and some behavioral implications. In *Neurotransmitters and Cortical Function: From Molecules to Mind* (ed M. Avoli, T.A. Reader, R.W. Dykes, and P. Gloor). New York: Plenum Press, pp. 237–260.

Mesulam, M.M. (2000). Behavioral neuroanatomy: large-scale networks, association, cortex, frontal syndromes, the limbic system, and hemispheric specializations. In *Principles of Behavioral and Cognitive Neurology* (ed M.M. Mesulam). Oxford: Oxford University Press, pp. 1–120.

Mesulam, M.M., and Mufson, E.J. (1984). Neural inputs into the nucleus basalis of the substantia innominata (Ch4) in the rhesus monkey. *Brain*, **107**, 253–274.

Mesulam, M.M., Mufson, E.J., Levey, A.I., and Wainer, B.H. (1983). Cholinergic innervation of cortex by the basal forebrain: cytochemistry and cortical connections of the septal area, diagonal band nuclei, nucleus basalis (substantia innominata), and hypothalamus in the rhesus monkey. *Journal of Comparative Neurology*, **214**, 170–197.

Miller, R. (1991). *Cortico-Hippocampal Interplay and the Representation of Contexts in the Brain*. New York: Springer-Verlag.

Miltner, W.H.R., Braun, C.H., and Coles, M.G.H. (1997). Event-related brain potentials following incorrect feedback in a time-estimation task: evidence for a 'generic' neural system for error detection. *Journal of Cognitive Neuroscience*, **9**, 787–797.

Mishkin, M. (1982). A memory system in the monkey. *Philosophical Transactions of the Royal Societyof London, Series B, Biological Sciences*, **298**, 83–95.

Miura, Y., Ito, T., and Kadokawa, T. (1987). Effects of intraseptally injected dopamine and noradrenaline on hippocampal synchronized theta wave activity in rats. *Japanese Journal of Pharmacology*, **44**, 471–479.

Monrad-Krohn, G.H. (1924). On the dissociation of voluntary and emotional innervation in facial paresis of central origin. *Brain*, **47**, 22–35.

Morrison, J.H., Molliver, M.E., Grzanna, R., and Coyle, J.T. (1979). Noradrenergic innervation patterns in three regions of medial cortex: an immunofluorescence characterization. *Brain Research Bulletin*, **4**, 849–857.

Neafsey, E.J., Terreberry, R.R., Hurley, K.M., Ruit, K.G., and Frysztak, R.J. (1993). Anterior cingulate cortex in rodents: connections, visceral control functions, and implications for emotion. In *Neurobiology of the Cingulate Cortex and Limbic Thalamus* (ed B.A. Vogt and M. Gabriel). Boston, MA: Birkhauser, pp. 206–223.

O'Keefe, J. and Burgess, N. (1999). Theta activity, virtual navigation and the human hippocampus. *Trends in Cognitive Sciences*, **3**, 403–406.

Paré, D. (2003). Role of the basolateral amygdala in memory consolidation. *Progress in Neurobiology*, **70**, 409–420.

Paré, D., Collins, D.R., and Pelletier, J.G. (2002). Amygdala oscillations and the consolidation of emotional memories. *Trends in Cognitive Sciences*, **6**, 306–314.

Passingham, R.E. (1987). Two cortical systems for directing movement. *Ciba Foundation Symposium*, **132**, 151–164.

Paus, T., Koski, L., Caramanos, Z., and Westbury, C. (1998). Regional differences in the effects of task difficulty and motor output on blood flow response in the human anterior cingulate cortex: a review of 107 PET activation studies. *Neuroreport*, **9**, R37–R47.

Plavides, C., Greenstein, Y.J., Grudman, M., and Winson, J. (1988). Long-term potentiation in the dentate gyrus is unduced preferentially on the positive phase of theta rhythm. *Brain Research*, **439**, 383–387.

Posner, M.I., and Petersen, S. E. (1990). The attention system of the human brain. *Annual Review of Neuroscience*, **13**, 25–42.

Pribram, K.H. (1950). Psychosurgery in midcentury. *Surgery, Gynecology, and Obstetrics*, **91**, 364–367.

Pribram, K.H., and McGuinness, D. (1975). Arousal, activation, and effort in the control of attention. *Psychological Review*, **82**, 6–149.

Rescorla, R.A., and Wagner, A.R. (1972). A theory of Pavlovian conditioning: variations in the effectiveness of reinforcement and nonreinforcement. In *Classical Conditioning*. II: *Current Research and Theory*, Vol. 65–99 (ed A.H. Black and W.F. Prokasy). New York: Appleton-Century-Crofts.

Rugg, M.D. (1987). Dissociation of semantic priming, word and non-word repetition effects by event-related potentials. *Quarterly Journal of Experimental Psychology*, 123–148.

Rugg, M.D., Mark, R.E., Walla, P., Schloerscheidt, A.M., Birch, C.S., and Allan, K. (1998). Dissociation of the neural correlates of implicit and explicit memory. *Nature*, **392**, 595–598.

Rylander, G. (1948). Personality analysis before and after frontal lobotomy. In *The Frontal Lobes: Proceedings of the Association for Research in Nervous and Mental Disease*, Vol. XXVII (ed J.F. Fulton, C.D. Aring and S.B. Wortis). Baltimore, MD: Williams & Wilkins.

Sackeim, H.A., Greenberg, M.S., Weiman, A.L., Gur, R.C., Hungerbuhler, J.P., and Geschwind, M. (1982). Hemispheric asymmetry in the expression of positive and negative emotions: neurologic evidence. *Archives of Neurology*, **39**, 210–218.

Sainsbury, R.S. (1998). Hippocampal theta: a sensory-inhibition theory of function. *Neuroscience Biobehavioral Review*, **22**, 237–241.

Sarnthein, J., Petsche, H., Rappelsberger, P., Shaw, G.L., and von Stein, A. (1998). Synchronization between prefrontal and posterior association cortex during human working memory. *Proceedings of the National Academy of Sciences of the United States of America*, **95**, 7092–7096.

Seidenbecher, T., Laxmi, T.R., Stork, O., and Pape, H.-C. (2003). Amygdalar and hippocampal theta rhythm synchronization during fear memory retrieval. *Science*, **301**, 846–850.

Shima, K., and Tanji, J. (1998). Role for cingulate motor area cells in voluntary movement selection based on reward. *Science*, **282**, 1335–1338.

Singer, W. (1993). Synchronization of cortical activity and its putative role in information processing and learning. *Annual Review of Physiology*, **55**, 349–374.

Squire, L.R. (1986). Mechanisms of memory. *Science*, **232**, 1612–1619.

Squire, L.R. (1987). *Memory and Brain*. New York: Oxford University Press.

Steriade, M., Jones, E.G., and Llinas, R.R. (1990). *Thalamic Oscillations and Signaling*. New York: John Wiley.

Swanson, L.W. (2000). Cerebral hemisphere regulation of motivated behavior. *Brain Research*, **886**, 113–164.

Talbot, J.D., Marrett, S., Evans, A.C., Meyer, E., Bushnell, C.M., and Duncan, G.H. (1991). Multiple representations of pain in human cerebral cortex. *Science*, **251**, 1355–1358.

Tanji, J., and Shima, K. (1994). Role for supplementary motor area cells in planning several movements ahead. *Nature*, **371**, 413–416.

Tesche, C.D., and Karhu, J. (2000). Theta oscillations index human hippocampal activation during a working memory task. *Proceedings of the National Academy of Sciences of the United States of America*, **97**, 919–924.

Thompson, L.T., and Best, P.J. (1989). Place cells and silent cells in the hippocampus of freely-behaving rats. *Journal of Neuroscience*, **9**, 2382–2390.

Tow, P.M. and Whitty, C.W. (1953). Personality changes after operations on the cingulate gyrus in man. *Journal of Neurology, Neurosurgery, and Psychiatry*, **16**, 186–193.

Tucker, D.M. (1981). Lateral brain function, emotion, and conceptualization. *Psychological Bulletin*, **89**, 19–46.

Tucker, D.M. (2001). Motivated anatomy: a core-and-shell model of corticolimbic architecture. In *Handbook of Neuropsychology* (2nd edn). Vol. 5: *Emotional Behavior and its Disorders* (ed G. Gainotti). Amsterdam: Elsevier, pp. 125–160.

Tucker, D.M. and Derryberry, D. (1992). Motivated attention: anxiety and the frontal executive functions. *Neuropsychiatry, Neuropsychology, and Behavioral Neurology*, **5**, 233–252.

Tucker, D.M. and Williamson, P.A. (1984). Asymmetric neural control systems in human self-regulation. *Psychological Review*, **91**, 185–215.

Tucker, D.M., Liotti, M., Potts, G.F., Russell, G.S., and Posner, M.I. (1994). Spatiotemporal analysis of brain electrical fields. *Human Brain Mapping*, **1**, 134–152.

Tucker, D.M., Luu, P., and Pribram, K.H. (1995). Social and emotional self-regulation. *Annals of the New York Academy of Sciences*, **769**, 213–239.

Tucker, D.M., Hartry-Speiser, A., McDougal, L., Luu, P., and deGrandpre, D. (1999). Mood and spatial memory: emotion and right hemisphere contribution to spatial cognition. *Biological Psychology*, **50**, 103–125.

Tucker, D.M., Derryberry, D., and Luu, P. (2000). Anatomy and physiology of human emotion: vertical integration of brainstem, limbic, and cortical systems. In *Handbook of the Neuropsychology of Emotion* (ed J. Borod). New York: Oxford University Press, pp. 56–79.

Tucker, D.M., Luu, P., Richard, E., *et al.* (2003a). Corticolimbic mechanisms in emotional decisions. *Emotion*, **3**, 127–149.

Tucker, D.M., Luu, P., Frishkoff, G., Quiring, J., and Poulsen, C. (2003b). Frontolimbic response to negative feedback in clinical depression. *Journal of Abnormal Psychology*, **112**, 667–678.

Ungerleider, L.G. and Mishkin, M. (1982). Two cortical visual systems. In *The Analysis of Visual Behavior* (ed D.J. Ingle, R.J.W. Mansfield, and M.A. Goodale). Cambridge, MA: MIT Press, pp. 549–586.

Vertes, R.P. and Kocis, B. (1997). Brainstem-diencephalo-septohippocampal systems controlling the theta rhythm of the hippocampus. *Neuroscience*, **81**, 893–926.

Vogt, B.A., Sikes, R.W., and Vogt, L.J. (1993). Anterior cingulate cortex and the medial pain system. In *Neurobiology of the Cingulate Cortex and Limbic Thalamus* (ed B.A. Vogt and M. Gabriel). Boston, MA: Birkhäuser, pp. 314–344.

Wagner, A.D. (1999). Working memory contributions to human learning and remembering. *Neuron*, **22**, 19–22.

Williams, J.M. and Givens, B. (2003). Stimulation-induced reset of hippocampal theta in the freely moving rat. *Hippocampus*, **13**, 109–116.

Yaniv, D., Vouimba, R.M., Diamond, D.M., and Richter-Levin, G. (2003). Simultaneous induction of long-term potentiation in the hippocampus and the amygdala by enthorhinal cortex activation: mechanistic and temporal profiles. *Neuroscience*, **120**, 1125–1135.

Zheng, F. and Khanna, S. (1999). Hippocampal field CA1 interneuronal nociceptive responses: modulation by medial septal region and morphine. *Neuroscience*, **93**, 45–55.

Zubieta, J.K., Smith, Y.R., Bueller, J.A., *et al.* (2001). Regional mu opioid receptor regulation of sensory and affective dimensions of pain. *Science*, **293**, 311–315.

Chapter 5

Binding principles in the theta frequency range

Wolfgang Klimesch

Working memory and the functional meaning of theta

Converging evidence suggests that EEG theta is particularly 'responsive' to working memory (WM) demands. However, the question is whether theta reflects global WM processes or more specific subprocesses such as central executive and/or episodic encoding processes.

WM represents a limited capacity store both for retaining information over a period of seconds to minutes and for performing mental operations on the contents of this store (Baddeley 1992). Thus WM comprises two different aspects, short-term storage and the representation of those processes operating on the contents of this store (also termed central control, executive, and attentional control processes). Recently, an episodic buffer has been included in addition to the phonological loop (auditory–verbal short-term memory) and the visuospatial sketchpad (visual short-term memory) (Baddeley 2000).

A crucial function of WM is to encode information that is integrated in space and time (Baddeley 2000, p. 421). It should be noted that encoding has at least three different meanings: sensory, semantic, and episodic. The type of process that is primarily related to WM is episodic (or multidimensional) encoding. As an example, let us consider a recognition task in which a series of 'old' words which have already been presented during a study session (e.g. wheel, sun, car) are shown again during recognition, together with 'new' words (e.g. river, wheel). Because all the words are familiar, sensory and semantic codes already exist. Thus, the question is what type of information will allow a subject to decide that 'wheel' is 'old' and 'river' new? This type of information is termed 'episodic' because it refers to the context in which the word appeared. Context is defined by time, space, and personal experience (Tulving 1984). Thus episodic information is not provided by the stimulus *per se* but by subjective experience within the framework of WM processes, and is represented as a multidimensional code.

Thus any information represented and maintained in WM by central control processes is episodic.

The basic assumption is that theta serves to establish a multidimensional episodic code and thus provides the basis for storage in declarative memory. Although it is now generally believed that neuronal synchronicity plays a key role in the establishment of episodic codes (Baddeley 2000; Wagner 2001; Otten and Rugg 2002), what type of synchronization processes are involved remains an open question.

In this chapter the most important findings about different types of theta synchronization processes in WM and episodic tasks and their possible meaning for binding are critically reviewed. With respect to the frequency range of theta (usually defined as a frequency between 4 and 7 Hz), it is important to emphasize that in recent studies theta is used for an extended frequency range of about 3–9 Hz, including fast delta and slow alpha activity.

Different types of synchronization processes and their potential meaning for binding

For theta, as for any other EEG frequency, several different measures of synchronization can be considered. We distinguish between measures of amplitude and phase that are used to analyse event-related and ongoing EEG.

The findings reported below suggest that two different types of theta synchronization, event-related (or phasic) and task-related (or tonic), can be distinguished. Whereas the event-related theta increase is short lasting and occurs over a period of several hundred milliseconds after a relevant stimulus over brain regions involved in encoding and retrieval processes, tonic theta synchronization occurs over time periods of several seconds to minutes primarily over frontal sites. Thus there are reasons to assume that at least two different types of theta oscillation might be distinguished.

Event-related theta synchronization (theta ERS)

Three different parameters can be analysed for event-related EEG,: amplitude, phase angle, and phase alignment (synchronization) with other frequencies. A popular method of analysing amplitude changes is the event-related desynchronization/synchronization (ERD/ERS) method developed by Pfurtscheller and colleagues (Pfurtscheller and Aranibar 1977; reviewed by Pfurtscheller and Lopes da Silva 1999). In using this method, it was shown consistently that, with respect to a prestimulus reference interval, band power increases in response to stimulus presentation and/or task demands. Theta phase resetting was reported for both human EEG (Rahn and Basar 1993a,b; Tesche and Karhu 2000; Rizzuto *et al.* 2003) and animal studies (Givens 1996). Resetting, which has also been demonstrated for alpha oscillations (Brandt,1997; Makeig *et al.* 2002) means that, in a statistical sense, the phase angle (within a narrow time window around stimulus presentation) becomes redistributed and centred within a preferred range. Finally, during theta phase resetting, other oscillations (e.g. in the alpha or gamma band) may also undergo phase resetting and may become transiently aligned in absolute phase with the absolute phase angle of theta. This type of an evoked phase synchronization between frequencies leads to the superposition of evoked oscillations and is probably the mechanism underlying the generation of event-related potentials (reviewed by Basar 1999a,b).

Task-related theta synchronization in the ongoing EEG

During task performance tonic longer-lasting EEG changes (compared with the short-lasting event-related response) can be observed. Several studies indicate that prolonged and increased WM task requirements lead to increased theta power (Gevins *et al.* 1997, 1998; Gevins and Smith 2000), particularly at frontal midline sites.

In the ongoing EEG phase-sensitive measures can be used to determine the degree of a stable phase relationship between different brain regions. Two measures should be distinguished: (pure) phase synchronization and coherence. The latter is a type of correlation reflecting the combined influence of phase and amplitude. Both measures are used to detect networks of coactivated brain regions.

Finally, phase synchronization (in the ongoing EEG) between two frequencies can also be studied. This method is called m:n synchronization and has been used in only a few studies (e.g. Schack *et al.* 2001).

Binding processes within and between networks

Basically, binding may have two different meanings, one referring to the synchronous activation of a neural assembly (consisting of different distributed elements of one network) or the other to the activation of different assemblies (consisting of distributed elements of different networks). The logic of this approach is nicely outlined by Varela *et al.* (2001). The idea is that cognitive processes are related to the activation of neural assemblies, defined as distributed networks that are transiently linked by reciprocal dynamic connections. The activation of an assembly is reflected by an oscillatory process within a certain frequency range. The frequency is determined at least in part by geometric properties of the assembly, particularly by the length of reciprocal connections or feedback loops. For example, large networks connecting cortical and subcortical areas will operate at a low frequency, possibly in the delta, theta, or alpha range, whereas cortico-cortical networks will oscillate at higher frequencies, possibly in the beta or gamma range (von Stein *et al.* 1999, 2000; von Stein and Sarnthein 2000).

Neurons within a given assembly will fire synchronously in phase within the same frequency range. The power of that frequency range might be considered a functional correlate of the number of neurons or functional elements (e.g. clusters of dendrites) that are active within the same time interval. Phase synchronization or coherence may be used to investigate the topography of the activated assembly. If different assemblies (e.g. differing in size and dominant frequency) are coactivated they will exhibit phase coupling between different frequencies. Thus, n:m phase synchronization is a measure that is particularly useful for identifying other assemblies that will be coactivated with the assembly of interest.

In the context of WM and theta, we distinguish between two different binding processes, which we will term within-network and between-network binding. In the first case, we assume that theta power reflects binding processes in one or more different assemblies within a complex network, possibly a cortico-limbic network (Klimesch 1999). We assume that an increase in event-related theta power (i.e. theta ERS) reflects binding of different elements (cues) during the processing of a multidimensional code (see above). In contrast, increased tonic theta power may reflect binding in the sense that different attentional control or central executive processes must be coordinated during the performance of a task. This latter question will be addressed below. Between-network binding is a different type of process referring to the coactivation of different assemblies in different networks. The investigation of the latter cases requires the use of phase sensitive measures and will be considered later in this chapter.

Within-network binding and event-related theta synchronization: evidence for the processing of multidimensional codes?

The hypothesis underlying the following considerations is that the more complex an episodic code, the more components it will have, and hence event-related theta power will increase because of increased binding demands. We proceed from the assumption that the codes that are remembered first will be those that have undergone complex processing during encoding and/or retrieval. We will discuss this hypothesis by considering primarily studies from ERD/ERS research.

A large number of studies have shown that during episodic encoding a pronounced increase in theta is observed within a time window of about 100–300 ms after stimulus presentation (Klimesch *et al.* 1994, 1996, 1997b,c, 2000a–c, 2001a–c; Krause *et al.* 1996, 2001; Burgess and Gruzelier 1997, 2000; reviewed by Klimesch 1996, 1997, 1999). Most interestingly, the increase in theta is significantly larger during the encoding of words that can be remembered in a later recognition or free recall task than during the encoding of words that cannot be remembered (Klimesch *et al.* 1996a,b, 1997c). During recognition, a similar pattern of results was obtained: Correctly identified old words exhibit significantly larger event-related theta power than incorrectly identified or new words (Burgess and Gruzelier 2000). So far, this latter phenomenon indicating a 'repetition effect' for old items (well documented in the ERP literature as a positive component, also termed 'recognition positivity' (e.g. Rugg and Doyle 1992)) has been documented for words only. Burgess and Gruzelier (2000) failed to find a larger increase in theta for old compared with new pictures. However, this may be due to their use of an ERD measure that eliminates the influence of evoked activity (Kalcher and Pfurtscheller 1995; Klimesch *et al.* 1998a,b) and to a possible differential influence of evoked theta during the processing of pictures compared with the processing of words.

In all of these studies the list of items presented during encoding was much too long to be kept in WM. In addition, the phasic increase in theta during retrieval indicates that this type of theta response cannot be related to the active maintenance of information. Instead, the findings imply that an event-related increase in theta is related to the successful encoding and retrieval of episodic information. This interpretation is also supported by experiments that focus on a direct comparison between episodic and semantic processes (Klimesch *et al.* 1994). In a more recent study of sentence processing, it was found that an increase in theta is related to the reading of the first words of a new sentence. If a semantic judgement must also be carried out, there is no additional increase in theta (but a decrease in alpha), indicating that processing of semantic information in WM is not related to changes in theta (Röhm *et al.* 2001; Bastiaansen *et al.* 2002).

One interesting question relates to the nature of those processes that underlie 'successful' encoding and retrieval. Two possible explanations, not necessarily mutually exclusive, seem likely. Successful processing may be related either to fluctuations of attention that influence the strength of a memory trace, or to a 'richer' processing of a code that creates more associations (cues) with already existing knowledge. Memory models assume that at least two different processes, recollection and familiarity, contribute to recognition performance (reviewed by

Yonelinas 2002). Familiarity is a process related to the strength of a trace, whereas recollection is probably also related to the processing of episodic cues. For example, if a subject decides that the word 'wheel' was presented during the study session because of an association with 'car' in the study list or because of a specific personal experience (e.g. flat tyre), this decision would rely on an episodic cue and recognition would be based on recollection. However, a subject may simply feel that an item appears familiar within the context of the study list and makes a decision on the basis of this type of evidence. Thus successful encoding and retrieval may be based primarily on the encoding or representation of episodic cues.

The remember–know (RK) design allows us to distinguish between recollection and familiarity during episodic retrieval. Subjects are asked to indicate whether they consciously recollected the event in which a word was earlier presented (remembering), or whether they recognized it on the basis that it was familiar in the absence of recollection (knowing). We have used this type of task to test the following hypotheses: the time course and extent of an increase in event-related theta are different for the two types of retrieval process; theta is larger during recollection (Klimesch *et al.* 2001b). The first hypothesis could be supported, but not the second.

We have found that an early increase in theta predicted knowing, and a later increase predicted remembering (Figs 5.1 and 5.2). This is in agreement with reaction time experiments which have shown that familiarity is faster than recollection (Hintzman *et al.* 1998). The hypothesis that theta should be larger during recollection was based on the idea that a trace eliciting a remember response is richer with respect to episodic cues. The fact that during remembering theta was actually weaker and exhibited a later onset suggests that retrieval of cues is a distributed and thus less synchronized process that takes some time. In contrast, the early onset and pronounced increase in theta during the processing of familiar items may reflect a retrieval process that is based on early evidence about the existence of a trace without the activation of episodic cues. Evidence about trace strength may be provided by a different (sensory-semantic) network. In other words, the episodic retrieval process may either receive early evidence about the existence of a trace from a different processing system or start to activate episodic cues. The first type of retrieval process is fast, reflected by shorter reaction times and a large evoked activity (Fig. 5.2(b)), and the second is slower, reflected by longer reaction times and a small evoked activity (Fig. 5.2(a)). Thus, in the RK task, theta is largely influenced by the type of retrieval process.

A related interpretation with respect to the influence of retrieval might explain why we and others (e.g. Krause *et al.* 2001) have found repeatedly that an

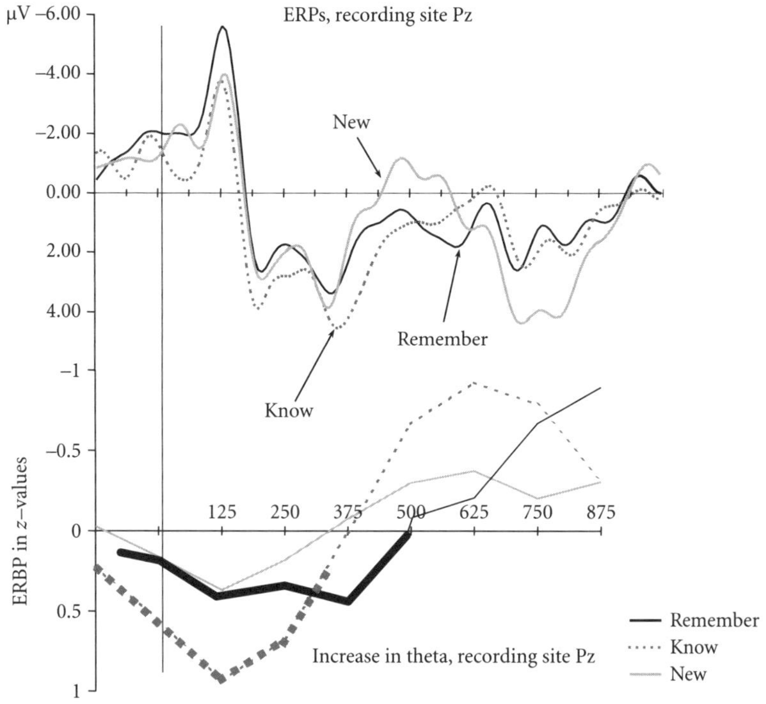

Figure 5.1 Event-related potential (ERP) and event-related band power (ERBP) in the theta frequency range at site Pz for three response types (remember and know responses to target items, and new responses to distractor items). The time course of theta ERBP (transformed to *z*-values) is shown below the respective ERP. Thick bold lines indicate that the increase in theta is statistically significant with respect to a reference interval (baseline) at the beginning of each trial. Remembered items are represented by bold lines, known items by broken lines, and new items by grey lines. (Reproduced from Klimesch *et al.* 2001b.)

event-related increase in theta is generally much stronger during retrieval (regardless of the existence of an episodic trace) than during encoding. For example, in a picture-recognition experiment (Klimesch *et al.* 2001a), we directly compared the increase in theta for correctly remembered pictures (hits) during encoding and later recognition with correctly rejected new pictures (distractors). As expected, we found the largest increase in theta for hits during retrieval. Most interestingly, however, the increase in theta for correctly rejected new pictures (for which no episodic trace exists) was significantly larger than that for pictures during successful encoding (Fig. 5.3). For new pictures, the retrieval process is based on evidence about the lack of an episodic trace and not about the actual processing of a trace. In other words, the increase in theta for new words is

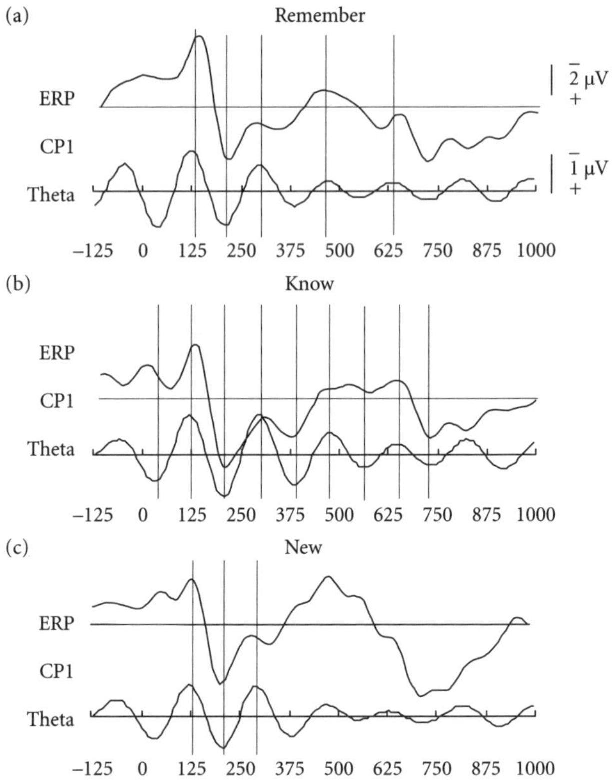

Figure 5.2 Comparison of standard ERP and theta ERP at CP1 for (a) remember, (b) know, and (c) new response. Note that ERP peaks show a close relation to the positive and negative peaks of evoked theta activity (about 4.6–6.6 Hz). Vertical lines connecting the standard and theta ERPs indicate cases where ERP peaks exhibit an obvious correspondence to evoked theta. (Reproduced from Klimesch *et al.* 2001b.)

(retrieval) process specific, not trace specific. Thus we assume that an event-related increase in theta may have at least three explanations, one related to the encoding, one to the access of an episodic trace, and one to the process of episodic retrieval *per se*.

In cases where episodic aspects are irrelevant or of minor importance, theta does not appear to play a selective role. For example, semantic retrieval has no selective effect on theta (Klimesch 1999). Another example is retrieval from short-term (or intermediate) memory in Sternberg (scanning) tasks. In contrast to the tonic load-dependent increase in theta during retention, theta does not increase with load during retrieval. ERP studies have shown that the P300 decreases with load during the retrieval of a probe (Pelosi *et al.* 1992, 1998; Gevins and Smith 2000). Schack and Klimesch (2002) have recently studied this phenomenon by analysing phase locking and evoked power of delta and theta oscillations. It was found that the decrease of the P3 amplitude with increasing load is associated primarily with a large decrease in evoked power and phase

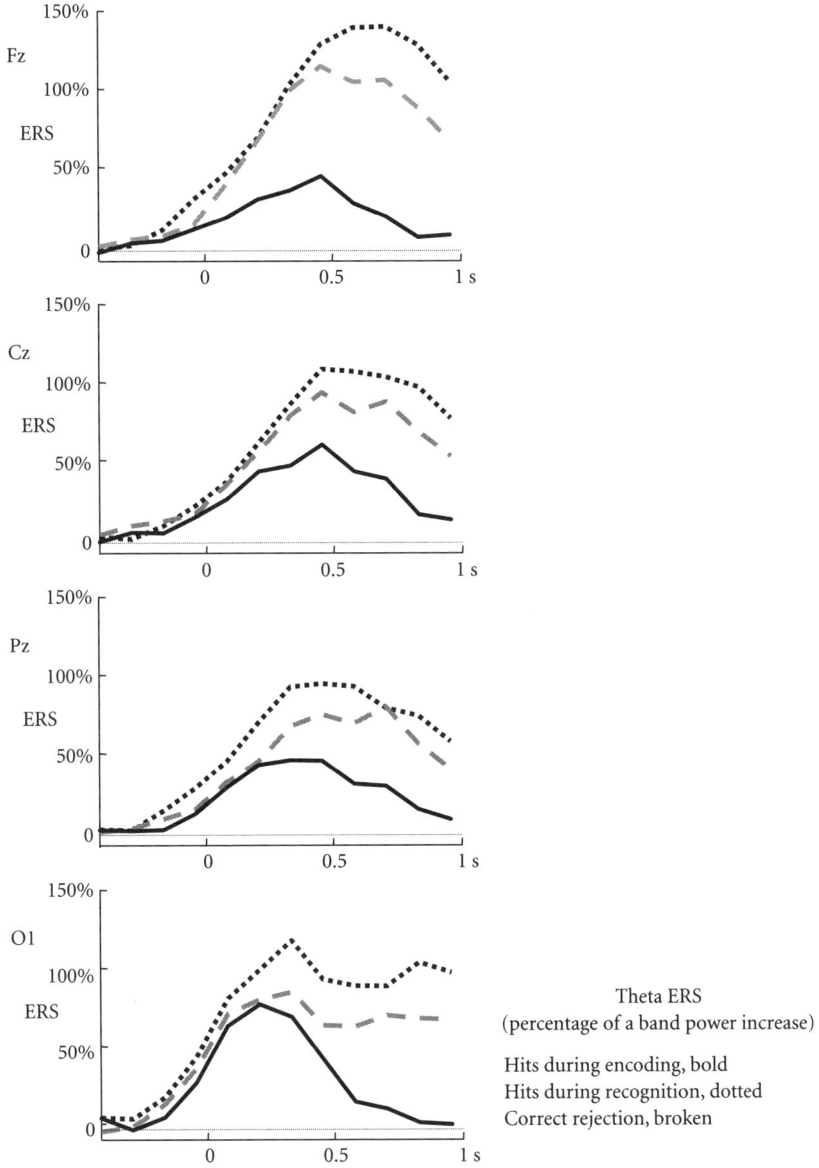

Figure 5.3 Time course of an event-related increase in theta band power (ERS) at midline recording sites and O1 during encoding and recognition of Snodgrass pictures (Snodgrass and Vanderwart 1980). Theta ERS is larger during successful retrieval than during successful encoding. Although the increase in theta is larger for hits than for correct rejections, this difference was not significant (Klimesch *et al.* 2001a). Note that ERS for correctly rejected pictures (for which no episodic trace exists) is larger than for later remembered pictures during encoding.

locking of delta and theta oscillations at posterior sites. We assume that this finding may be due to the lack of episodic processing in this type of task. It may well be argued that, with increasing load, retrieval processes rely more on trace strength and that trace strength decreases with load.

The data reviewed so far show that theta is selectively responsive to some, but not all, types of WM processes. The episodic hypothesis which assumes the establishment of a multidimensional code provides a possible explanation. Nonetheless, one crucial issue which still remains is why theta is also responsive to encoding demands that are typically not episodic, as shown in the following example. In a study with dyslexic children (Klimesch *et al.* 2001c), subjects were presented numbers, number-words, and pseudo-words. They had to read each item and pronounce it after a question mark appeared. Control subjects showed a significant event-related increase in theta band power (compared with a reference interval) at occipital sites that was larger for pseudo-words than for words and numbers. However, dyslexic subjects completely failed to exhibit an increase in theta during pseudo-word processing at occipital sites. Because neither of these stimuli should be specifically related to episodic encoding, the differences in theta may reflect a different, but related, aspect which probably is the encoding of completely new information. Pseudo-words represent new (but meaningless) information, and pseudo-word processing is extremely difficult (or even impossible) for dyslexics. Thus these findings suggest that absence of encoding new information into WM is associated with absence of an event-related increase in theta.

Episodic information must be constantly updated, and thus 'new' and 'episodic' information are closely interrelated terms. Any new information is embedded within the context of personal experience, space, and time. Thus it is likely that any new information is first encoded within an episodic frame until it becomes integrated into or processed in semantic memory.

Under normal circumstances, particularly when mental load is low, the 'default mode' of encoding is episodic. Evidence for this view comes from a study in which pairs of sequentially presented words had to be judged on whether they were semantically congruent or not (Klimesch *et al.* 1997b). An increase in theta power was found only at occipital sites and only during the first 500 ms after presentation of each word. Because the semantic comparison process can be performed only after the second word is presented and (as estimated on the basis of reaction times) is carried out at about 400–600 ms post-stimulus, theta may reflect automatic episodic encoding, but in any case is not related to semantic processes.

Within-network binding and tonic task-related theta synchronization: evidence for central executive functions of varying complexity?

A tonic increase in theta power can be observed in tasks typically requiring sustained focused attention. One well known example is the Sternberg paradigm (Sternberg 1966; reviewed by Cowan 2000) which is a memory scanning task consisting of three parts: encoding, retention, and retrieval (including scanning). The critical factor is the variation of memory load which is defined by the number of items (usually varying between one and seven) presented during encoding. The first study, which reported increased theta power with load, was performed by Mecklinger *et al.* (1992). A series of studies focusing on the retention period (of scanning and n-back style tasks) have also found that theta power increases with load (Gevins *et al.* 1997, 1998; Klimesch *et al.* 1999; Gevins and Smith 2000; McEvoy *et al.* 2001; Raghavachari *et al.* 2001; Fingelkurts *et al.* 2002; Jensen and Tesche 2002). Similar results were also obtained for a haptic memory task (Grunwald *et al.* 1999), thus demonstrating that this type of theta response is independent of modality. This is consistent with cross-modality experiments performed by Basar and colleagues showing that an event-related increase in theta is largely independent of modality (Basar 1999a,b; Basar *et al.* 2001). Finally, it should be noted that a study by Stam (2000) failed to replicate these findings. This may be due to the long retention interval (1 min) and the selection of a comparatively short epoch of 8 s for data analysis.

Studies using subdural electrodes or specific source analysing methods have shown that the length of theta episodes is related to the duration of WM demands in a memory scanning task (Tesche and Karhu 2000; Raghavachari *et al.* 2001) or a spatial WM task (Kahana *et al.* 1999; Araujo *et al.* 2002). These findings suggest that the active maintenance of information in WM (e.g. by rehearsal or focused attention) is reflected by a sustained increase in theta power. It is interesting to note that some studies have found similar effects in the alpha frequency range (Klimesch *et al.* 1999; Jensen *et al.* 2002).

Several studies indicate that rhythmic theta activity over frontal midline sites can be observed in the ongoing EEG. Such rhythmic activity (with a frequency of about 6–7 Hz and consisting of bursts of several seconds that tend to wax and wane) was termed 'frontal midline theta' fmθ (Ishihara and Yoshii 1972). Because fmθ is generated when subjects maintain focused attention by concentrating on a task during an extended period of time, it is assumed that this type of theta reflects attentional processes (Ishii 1999). This interpretation is substantiated by experiments in which subjects had to meditate (Aftanas and Golocheikine

2001; Kubota *et al.* 2001), perform continuous mental calculation tasks (Asada *et al.* 1999; Ishii *et al.* 1999), or perform a visuomotor task under time pressure (Slobounov *et al.* 2000).

It is important to note that the topography of theta during episodic encoding is different and is for visually presented material clearly related to occipital recording sites. This different topography suggests the involvement of different types of theta during encoding and sustained attention.

Source modelling methods indicate that Fmθ is generated by the lateral frontal cortices of both hemispheres (Sasaki *et al.* 1996) or by the medial prefrontal areas including the anterior cingulate gyrus (Asada *et al.* 1999; Ishii *et al.* 1999). Most interestingly, there is also evidence that prefrontal and cingulate sources were activated alternatively with a clear shift in phase during one fmθ cycle. These areas are parts of a complex anterior–posterior attentional network system (reviewed by Corbetta and Shulman 2002; Herrmann and Knight 2001) which also plays an important role in WM.

Between-network binding: the involvement of different brain areas and other frequencies

Results obtained by the traditional methods of analysing power changes are limited in their interpretation. To illustrate this problem let as consider the following hypothesis, which was derived from animal research. Miller (1991) reviewed convincing evidence showing that theta oscillations propagate in a widespread complex network consisting of cortico-limbic/hippocampal re-entrant loops (for more recent evidence and reviews see Buzsáki *et al.* 1992, 1994; Treves and Rolls 1994; Eichenbaum 2000; Kocsis *et al.* 2001; Vertes *et al.* 2001; Wagner, 2001). Based on this hypothesis, it may appear plausible to interpret an event-related increase in EEG theta during episodic processes in terms of theta oscillations propagating in a more widespread cortical network. However, there are two major problems with such an interpretation. First, with the exception of fmθ (which is obtained only under specific conditions), no spectral peak in the theta frequency range can usually be observed. Consequently, based on spectral analysis, there is no evidence for an oscillatory theta activity in the human scalp EEG and it would be premature to conclude that increased theta power reflects increased amplitudes of a network oscillating in a preferred frequency range. Secondly, inferences about the involvement of distributed neural networks or 'assemblies' (Eichenbaum 1993) require the use of appropriate methods.

One way of overcoming these problems (without using subdural or depth electrodes) is the use of phase-sensitive measures such as coherence or 'pure' phase synchronization. Unlike coherence, phase synchronization is not influenced by power. Phase synchronization can be analysed with high time resolution either within the frequency of interest (n:n synchronization) or between different frequencies (n:m synchronization) (reviewed by Varela *et al.* 2001). If, with the help of these methods, it can be shown that the phase of theta responds to memory or other cognitive task demands in a non-random and meaningful way, this will provide a strong argument that theta is indeed an oscillatory processes in distributed cell assemblies beneath the respective recording sites.

The best investigated example (showing n:n synchronization) are local integration processes in the visual cortex which are reflected by coherent gamma oscillations (in the frequency range of about 25–45 Hz). It has been demonstrated (originally on the basis of animal studies) that elementary visual stimulus properties ('features') induce synchronous activity among neurons that are actually involved in sensory processing (for reviews of this classical work see Singer and Gray 1995; König and Engel 1995). Similar findings were also obtained with human EEG (von Stein *et al.* 1995; Müller *et al.*1996). Integration processes are termed 'local' if they occur in a network distributed over an area of about 1 cm or less (Varela *et al.* 2001). Because a scalp electrode records from an area of more than about 1 cm^2 (Lopes da Silva and Pfurtscheller 1999), scalp EEG generally reflects large-scale integration processes.

Convergent evidence reviewed by Tallon-Baudry and Bertrand (1999) and Bertrand and Tallon-Baudry (2000) indicates that an increase in induced gamma band power reflects object presentation and gestalt or object recognition (Herrmann *et al.* 1999; Elliott *et al.* 2000; Herrmann and Mecklinger 2000; Müller *et al.* 2000). Tallon-Baudry *et al.* (1998) have also shown that the maintenance of a single visual target stimulus during the delay period in a matching to sample task is reflected by an increase in induced gamma power (at about 25–30 Hz). The topography of this effect revealed an additional frontal involvement compared with the occipital topography during encoding. Other studies have also found that gamma is related to memory load (De Pascalis and Ray 1998) and associative learning processes (Miltner *et al.* 1999). Thus, whether gamma primarily reflects object presentation, memory processes (Pulvermüller 1999), and/or attention (Keil *et al.* 2001) became an important issue. For a critical review see also Salinas and Sejnowski (2001).

Although these findings nicely underline the functional significance of gamma for the encoding and representation of new information, conclusions cannot be drawn about the involvement of a coherently oscillating network. However, studies measuring n:n synchronization provide clear evidence for such an interpretation. Rodriguez *et al.* (1999) analysed gamma oscillations during the perception of 'mooney faces' (i.e. faces composed of high-contrast black and white shapes that create 'illusionary' contours). They found a topographically widespread phase synchronization centred over posterior recording sites during a brief period of 180–360 ms post-stimulus. Most importantly, this increase in synchronization was found only if the faces were presented upright (and could be recognized) and not if they were presented inverted (and could not be recognized as a face). The implication is that synchronization of neural oscillations acts as an integrative mechanism that 'turns' a highly distributed network into a coherent assembly, thereby enabling the perception of a 'gestalt'. Most interestingly, in a study using depth electrodes in human patients, Fell *et al.* (2001) found that phase synchronization of induced gamma activity between the rhinal cortex and the hippocampus is significantly higher during the encoding of subsequently remembered (recalled) words than the encoding of those that have not been remembered. Phase synchronization occurred at zero time lag and, most interestingly, was accompanied by a decrease in induced power. Together with the fact that gamma power is larger in the hippocampal formation than in neocortical recordings, an increase in phase synchronization (with zero phase lag) and a decrease in induced power during successful encoding reveals a high precision in the timing and a high specificity of local assembly activation.

Coherence has been used in numerous studies as a measure to analyse the topographical pattern of correlated oscillatory activity (Rappelsberger and Petsche 1988; Rappelsberger *et al.* 1991; Petsche *et al.* 1992, 1993a,b; von Stein *et al.* 1995). Some of them have shown that frontopolar regions play a significant role in WM tasks (reviewed by Petsche and Etlinger 1998). A detailed analysis of theta coherence in a WM task was performed by Sarnthein *et al.* (1998). Their subjects had to perform a verbal and visual WM task. In the verbal task, a string of characters, including letters and numbers, was presented and had to be recalled after a retention period of 4 s. In the visual task an abstract line drawing had to be remembered. During the retention interval, a significant increase in theta coherence was found between prefrontal and posterior electrodes. In the verbal task the pattern of coherent theta oscillations showed a network connecting the left occipito-temporal and the bilateral prefrontal regions. In the visual task a more bilateral pattern was observed. The increase in theta coherence (calculated in comparison with a control task in which subjects had to look passively at a computer screen) was pronounced only during retention and was small (consisting of only few interhemispheric connections) during encoding. The authors suggest that coherent theta oscillations are important for the interaction between posterior association cortices (where sensory information is believed to be stored) and prefrontal regions (where relevant current information is held and continuously updated). Supporting this interpretation, similar findings were also reported by Anokhin *et al.* (1999). It is also interesting to note that a global reduction in theta synchronization was found in patients with schizophrenic disorders associated with WM dysfunctions (König *et al.* 2001). Furthermore, decreased theta phase synchronization between anterior sites was found during the onset of propofol anesthesia (Koskinen *et al.* 2001).

One of the questions that arise from these interesting findings is whether other assemblies, operating in different frequencies, are functionally coupled with coherent theta oscillations. Sarnthein *et al.* (1998) have found a widespread pattern of coherent gamma oscillations that was not specific for retention because it could also be observed during encoding. Nontheless, it could be argued that a specific pattern of gamma oscillations is established during encoding and that theta oscillations are necessary to maintain it. The co-occurrence of theta and gamma oscillations during retention, as reported by Sarnthein *et al.* (1998), does not allow us to answer this question. However, if the functional interrelation of these frequencies is analysed by calculating m:n (theta:gamma) phase synchronization, this question can be addressed. This was done in a recent study by Schack *et al.* (2002), which was the first of its kind. On the basis of cross-biamplitude and cross-bicoherence, phase coupling between theta and gamma oscillations during the retention interval of a Sternberg task was analysed. Cross-biamplitude analysis revealed a peak at 5 Hz at Fz and Fp1 and increased amplitudes in the gamma range (about 20–30 Hz) at Fp1. The results of cross-bicoherence analysis proved that there was a significant m:n (theta:gamma) phase synchronization between Fz and Fp1. These findings were interpreted as reflecting the functional linkage between a prefrontal network operating in gamma oscillations and a cortico-limbic network operating in theta oscillations.

The studies of oscillatory assembly activation reviewed here indicate that gamma oscillations play a highly significant role for sensory encoding and higher cognitive processes such as recognition of gestalt-like structures and maintaining a sensory code in short-term memory. In contrast, theta oscillations play a role in the functional coupling of cortical areas that are known to be important for performing a WM task (Sarnthein *et al.* 1998). Furthermore, there is recent evidence that theta is phase coupled with assemblies oscillating in gamma frequency. Thus, theta oscillations may allow the integration of different sensory codes in time by providing an ordered sequential activation of codes (compare the 'nested oscillation' model (Lisman and Idiart 1995; Jensen and Lisman 1998)).

Between-network binding during evoked theta activity

Several studies have reported a resetting of the phase of theta in human EEG (Rahn and Basar 1993a,b; Tesche and Karhu 2000; Makeig *et al.* 2002; Rizzuto *et al.* 2003) and animal studies (Givens 1996). Resetting, demonstrated not only for theta but also for alpha (Brandt 1997; Makeig *et al.* 2002), means that, in a statistical sense, the phase angle (within a narrow time window after stimulus presentation) becomes redistributed and centred at a specific angle. Most interestingly, Rizzuto *et al.* (2003) have shown that in a Sternberg paradigm phase resetting is most clearly seen in response to the presentation of the probe (i.e. at the beginning of the retrieval process). Furthermore, phase resetting was not restricted to theta but was also observed in the alpha frequency range. Because phase resetting is associated with the generation of evoked components, this latter finding raises the question whether resetting of both theta and alpha oscillations leads to a superposition of evoked components such that, within a narrow time window, peaks of the same polarity sum to form a large ERP component. This is a special case of n:m synchronization, reflecting the transient evoked synchronization between different networks (Klimesch *et al.* 2004).

We have investigated this question by studying the superposition of evoked theta and alpha oscillations in a Sternberg task. The basic idea was that during retrieval attempts other frequencies become coactivated with theta. Because several studies indicate that upper alpha oscillations also play an important role for memory (reviewed by Klimesch 1999) and show a memory-load-dependent increase in amplitude during the retention period of a memory scanning task (Klimesch *et al.* 1999; Jensen *et al.* 2002), we investigated whether (i) alpha and theta show a significant phase resetting during retrieval and (ii) exhibit an alignment in absolute phase during retrieval. In a recent study (Schack and Klimesch 2002), we replicated the finding that upper alpha power (at 12 Hz) increases significantly with set size at posterior recording sites (particularly Pz and P4) during retention and found that theta (at about 6 Hz) and upper alpha (at about 12 Hz) undergo a significant phase resetting during retrieval (Fig. 5.4(b)). Furthermore, during retrieval, exactly within these frequency ranges (at 6 and 12 Hz), a significant increase in evoked power could be observed even in the ERP. In addition, the results indicated that the extent of phase locking in upper alpha increased with set size. These findings suggest that oscillatory EEG activity in peak alpha frequency, which is functionally associated with the maintenance of information in WM during retention, is related to evoked activity and increased phase locking during retrieval and memory scanning. Interestingly, the P3b (at Pz and P4) coincides with the last of three evoked alpha peaks. Thus, these findings strongly suggest that alpha oscillations become nested in theta (Fig. 5.4(a)) and play an active role in WM not only during retention, but also during scanning and retrieval. The latter finding implies that alpha oscillations coordinate the encoding of the probe, the scanning process, and the evaluation of the read-out process that most likely is manifested by the P3b. When considering the functional specificity of alpha for semantic long-term memory (Klimesch 1999) and the topography of alpha phase locking and evoked activity over

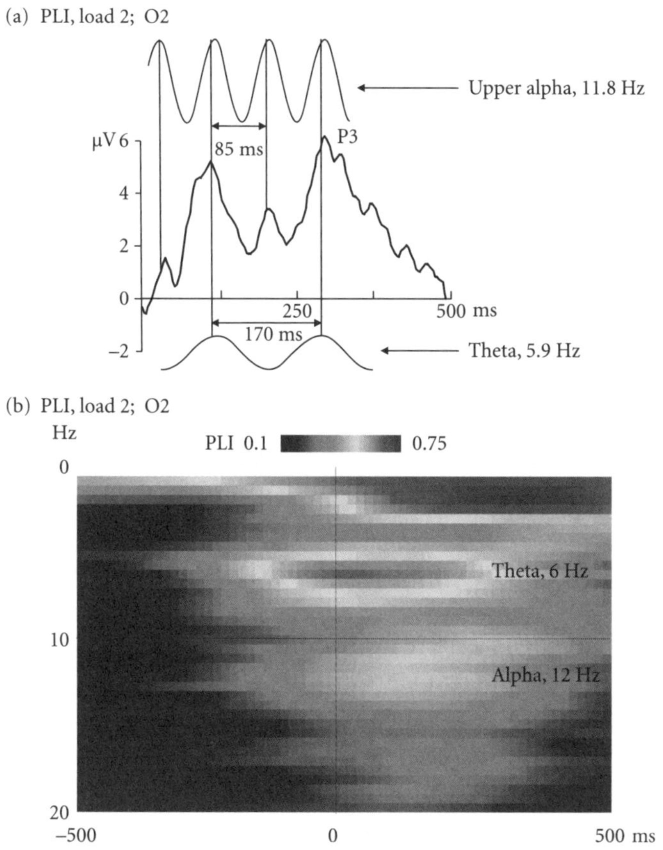

Figure 5.4 (a) ERP and (b) phase locking during successful retrieval (following the presentation of a probe item) in a Sternberg memory scanning task with number-words as items. Early ERP components coincide with evoked theta and upper alpha oscillations as illustrated by the two sine waves, one with a frequency of 6 Hz and the other with a frequency of 12 Hz. Phase locking is particularly large at these frequencies, as indicated by the phase-locking index (PLI), which is a normalized value, ranging between 0 and 1. Results for electrode O2 are from the database reported by Schack and Klimesch (2002). See colour plate section.

parietal areas, we can conclude that phase-locked alpha during scanning and retrieval reflects the 'binding' of storage networks in long-term memory (LTM), where numbers are presented, with a WM network.

A different kind of binding between theta and alpha was investigated by Sauseng *et al.* (2002). In this study, subjects first had to learn a verbal label for a each of eight pictures and then had to retrieve each picture after the label was presented. We assume that the learning and retrieval of a label is guided by executive functions of WM, whereas the imagination and retrieval of a picture represents LTM demands. The reason for this latter assumption is that picture memory is far superior to verbal memory. Thus, the transfer of picture information to LTM occurs much earlier than the transfer of verbal information. The findings indicate that after the presentation of the label, theta behaves like a travelling wave, spreading repeatedly from anterior to posterior sites during a time period of about 700 ms post-stimulus. The travelling wave is reflected by a typical topographical phase relationship, indicating an information flow from frontal to occipital sites. About 700 ms post-stimulus, the direction of the travelling theta wave reverses, indicating an information flow in the opposite direction from occipital to frontal sites. Most interestingly, when the latency of this reversal is determined for each subject and correlated with retrieval success a significant negative correlation can be observed. This indicates that good performers show shorter latencies for the reversal of theta at occipital sites. Furthermore, when the time of reversal is used as trigger (for a 'reversal synchronized' analysis of single EEG epochs) and the extent of band power changes for the lower-1, lower-2, and upper alpha bands is calculated in relation to this trigger, a pronounced desynchronization was found only in the upper alpha band which is also significantly larger than a stimulus synchronized data analysis. These data support the hypothesis that theta guides retrieval attempts, whereas upper alpha, which is functionally related to LTM storage, starts to desynchronize only after the code is actually retrieved. Interestingly, the reversal of the theta wave takes place at posterior recording sites, i.e. at areas that might very well be related to the storage of information. The potential implication for binding is that two different memory networks, one functionally related to WM and the other to LTM, become transiently coactivated during the brief time period of theta 'reversal'.

Between-network binding and the structure of an episodic code: results from animal studies

Pioneering work by O'Keefe and Dostrovsky (1971) (for a summary see Burgess and O'Keefe 1994) has shown that CA1 cells fire when the animal is at a particular place in its environment. Most importantly, these place cells fire at a particular sequence in time that is related to the phase of the ongoing theta rhythm. To explain this relationship, let us consider the following simple example of a rat traversing a cage (Fig. 5.5). Along the path the rat is exploring, three cells *x*, *y*, and *z* (related to places *X*, *Y*, and *Z*) are activated in that sequence. If the rat is at place *Y* at time *t*, cell *y* will fire close to the negative peak of the local field potential oscillating in theta frequency, whereas cell *x* will fire in an earlier phase and cell *z* in a later phase. Thus the phase advance of hippocampal place cells can be interpreted in terms of a temporary contextual code structured in time (past, present, future) and space (different places on a path). If we assume that the place cells fire in gamma oscillations, we observe 'nested oscillations' with a n:m phase synchronization in the theta and gamma frequency range. This concept of 'nested oscillations' was used by Lisman and Idiart (1995)

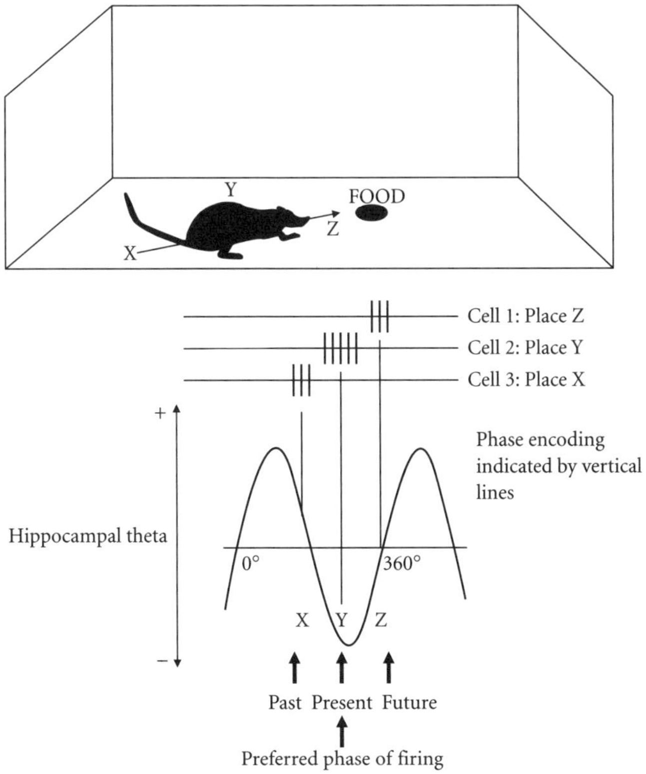

Figure 5.5 Hippocampal place cells. The basic finding is that those cells whose place field the rat is entering will fire late in a theta cycle, whereas those whose place field the rat has traversed will fire earlier in the cycle.

and Jensen and Lisman (1998) to model and explain short-term memory capacity. The idea is that memory codes are represented by different assemblies oscillating in gamma frequency. When several codes have to be kept in the short-term memory at the same time, they become rhythmically activated ('refreshed') on the basis of gamma subcycles in an ordered sequence, triggered by the phase of the ongoing theta rhythm. Because there is limited 'place' to nest gamma cycles into a theta cycle, only a limited number of codes can be kept in mind at the same time. Although this model was designed to explain short-term memory capacity, its formal structure can very well be used to explain the sequential ordering of codes in time, which is one essential aspect of episodic memory.

The assumption underlying the episodic hypothesis is that theta oscillations enable the binding of sensory codes into a coherent context. Context is defined by time, space, and personal experience. One example which we already have discussed is the sequential ordering of different sensory codes in time. A related example is spatial navigation, where different topographical cues of the environment must be integrated to form a coherent episodic trace that enables orientation in space. Finally, personal experience provides orientation within a context that is defined by autobiographical and emotional memories.

Discussion

The most consistent findings are (i) that a short-lasting event-related (phasic) increase in theta can be observed during the encoding and retrieval of episodic information (regardless of modality and stimulus type) and that a task-related (tonic) increase reflects either (ii) the maintenance of information in WM or (iii) a general increase in WM processing demands. Tonic theta is clearly related to effort, as the load-dependent increase in theta during retention and sustained attention indicates (Slobounov *et al.* 2000). In contrast, the increase in phasic theta does not increase with task difficulty or effort, as the following examples suggest.

1. During retrieval in a memory scanning task, posterior theta decreases with load.
2. Dyslexic subjects, who have great difficulties in encoding pseudo-words, completely lack theta synchronization although control subjects show a pronounced increase in theta.
3. In the R-K task, the 'remember' response exhibits a smaller theta increase than the 'known' response although the former is associated with longer reaction times than the latter.

The event-related increase in theta exhibits a nice correspondence to episodic processes. However, there are exceptions, such as an event-related increase in theta during pseudo-word encoding (observed for control but not dyslexic subjects) or during encoding of familiar words in a semantic judgement task (but during semantic comparison, a phasic theta response is absent). These cases may indicate that the 'default mode' of encoding is usually episodic and that the encoding of completely new information elicits an orienting response and episodic integration processes.

When compared with findings about gamma, two facts are interesting. First, during the retention of a target, an increase in induced gamma power can be observed. Secondly, an increase in induced gamma band power is also related to the encoding of new information and, most importantly, gamma phase synchronization between rhinal and hippocampal sites reflects successful episodic encoding. Furthermore, those studies which analysed both frequency domains observed a co-occurrence of theta and gamma activity.

Thus, it appears likely that both frequency domains are functionally interrelated and play a significant role in WM processes. Animal research using depth electrodes has shown consistently that gamma and theta oscillations are coupled in phase during exploratory behaviour (Buzsáki *et al.* 1994; Bragin *et al.* 1995; Chrobak and Buzsáki 1998). Phase coupling between theta and gamma oscillations has now been demonstrated for the human scalp EEG also (Schack *et al.* 2002), supporting the hypothesis that m:n synchronization reflects the coactivation of assemblies in different networks. Because gamma synchronization may reflect sensory encoding, theta synchronization during encoding must play a different role. What is it?

A plausible interpretation is that theta oscillations reflect a basic episodic process that allows the establishment (encoding), and continuous updating of contextual representations that keeps an individual autobiographically oriented in space and time. In other words, theta oscillations reflect a binding process that allows establishment of a structure between sensory codes or, in other words, a multidimensional code. An important aspect of this is that the phase of theta oscillations is a critical factor for triggering the activation of a well-ordered sequence of sensory codes. This argument is based on findings about place cells and theoretical considerations about nested oscillations and short-term memory.

Although the episodic hypothesis appears plausible, the findings reviewed indicate that at least a second type of binding process related to central executive and attentional control processes must be considered. The findings suggest that frontal midline theta is specifically involved in these functions. Increased tonic theta power may reflect binding in the sense that different attentional control or central executive processes must be coordinated during the performance of a task.

Findings about phase resetting suggest that evoked alpha oscillations become nested into an evoked theta cycle during the retrieval of information held in WM. This special case of n:m synchronization probably reflects the transient binding between a WM and LTM network. However, further research is needed to clarify this question.

Acknowledgements

Part of the research reported in this chapter was supported by the Austrian Science Foundation (FWF), project P-13047, and a grant from the University of Salzburg to W.K.

References

Aftanas, L. and Golocheikine, S. (2001). Human anterior frontal midline theta and lower alpha reflect emotionally positive state and internalized attention: high-resolution EEG investigation of meditation. *Neuroscience Letters*, **310**, 57–60.

Anokhin, A., Lutzenberger, W., and Birbaumer, N. (1999). Spatiotemporal organization of brain dynamics and intelligence: an EEG study in adolescents. *International Journal of Psychophysiology*, **33**, 259–273.

Araujo, D., Baffa, O., and Wakai, R. (2002). Theta oscillations and human navigation: a magnetoencephalography study. *Journal of Cognitive Neuroscience*, **14**, 70–78.

Asada, H., Fukuda, Y., Tsunoda, S., Yamaguchi, M., and Tonoike, M. (1999). Frontal midline theta rhythms reflect alternative activation of prefrontal cortex and anterior cingulated cortex in human. *Neuroscience Letters*, **274**, 29–32.

Baddeley, A. (1992). Working memory. *Science*, **255**, 556–559.

Baddeley, A. (2000). The episodic buffer: a new component of working memory? *Trends in Cognitive Sciences*, **4**, 417–422.

Basar, E. (1999a). *Brain Function and Oscillations*. Vol. I: *Principles and Approaches*. Berlin: Springer-Verlag.

Basar, E. (1999b). *Brain Function and Oscillations*. Vol. II: *Integrative Brain Function, Neurophysiology and Cognitive Processes*. Berlin: Springer-Verlag.

Basar, E., Schuermann, M., and Sakowitz, O. (2001). The selectively distributed theta system: functions. *International Journal of Psychophysiology*, **39**, 197–212.

Bastiaansen, M., Berkum, J., and Hagoort, P. (2002). Event-related theta power increases in the human EEG during online sentence processing. *Neuroscience Letters*, **323**, 13–16.

Bertrand, O. and Tallon-Baudry, C. (2000). Oscillatory gamma activity in humans: a possible role for object representation. *International Journal of Psychophysiology*, **38**, 211–223.

Bragin, A., Jando, G., Nadasdy, Z., Hetke, J., Wise, K., and Buzsáki, G. (1995). Gamma (40–100 Hz) oscillation in the hippocampus of the behaving rat. *Journal of Neuroscience*, **15**, 47–60.

Brandt, M.E. (1997). Visual and auditory evoked phase resetting of the alpha EEG. *International Journal of Psychophysiology*, **26**, 285–298.

Burgess, A. and Gruzelier, J.H. (1997). Short duration synchronization of human theta rhythm during recognition memory. *Neuroreport*, **8**, 1039–1042.

Burgess, A. and Gruzelier, J.H. (2000). Short duration power changes in the EEG during recognition memory for words and faces. *Psychophysiology*, **37**, 596–606.

Burgess, R. and O'Keefe, J. (1994). A model of hippocampal function. *Neural Networks*, **7**, 1065–1081.

Buzsáki, G., Horvath, Z., Urioste, R., Hetke, J., and Wise, K. (1992). High frequency network oscillation in the hippocampus. *Science*, **256**, 1025–1027.

Buzsáki, G., Bragin, A., Chrobak, J.J., *et al.* (1994). Oscillatory and intermittent synchrony in the hippocampus: Relevance to memory trace formation. In *Temporal Coding in the Brain* (ed G. Buzsáki, R.R. Llinás, W. Singer, A. Berthoz, and Y. Christen). Berlin: Springer-Verlag, pp. 145–172.

Corbetta, M. and Shulman, G. (2002). Control of goal-directed and stimulus-driven attention in the brain. *Nature Reviews Neuroscience*, **3**, 201–215.

Cowan, N. (2000). The magical number 4 in short-term memory: a reconsideration of mental storage capacity. *Behavioral and Brain Sciences*, **24**, 87–185.

Chrobak, J. and Buzsáki, G. (1998). Gamma oscillations in the entorhinal cortex of the freely behaving rat. *Journal of Neuroscience*, **18**, 388–398.

Cycowicz Y, Friedman D and Snodgrass, J. (2001). Remembering the color of objects: an ERP investigation of source memory. *Cerebral Cortex*, **11**, 322–334.

De Pascalis, V. and Ray, W. (1998). Effects of memory load on event-related patterns of 40-Hz EEG during cognitive and motor tasks. *International Journal of Psychophysiology*, **28**, 301–315.

Doppelmayr, M., Klimesch, W., Pachinger, T, and Ripper, B. (1998a). Individual differences in brain dynamics: important implications for the calculation of event-related band power measures. *Biological Cybernetics*, **79**, 49–57.

Doppelmayr, M., Klimesch, W., Pachinger, T, and Ripper, B. (1998b). The functional significance of absolute power with respect to event-related desynchronization. *Brain Topography*, **11**, 133–140.

Eichenbaum, H. (1993). Thinking about brain cell assemblies. *Science*, **261**, 993–994.

Eichenbaum, H. (2000). A cortical–hippocampal system for declarative memory. *Nature Reviews Neuroscience*, **1**, 41–50.

Elliott, M., Herrmann, C., Mecklinger, A., and Müller, H. (2000). The loci of oscillatory visual-object priming: a combined electroencephalographic and reaction-time study. *International Journal of Psychophysiology*, **38**, 225–241.

Fell, J., Klaver, P., Lehnertz, K., *et al.* (2001). Human memory formation is accompanied by rhinal–hippocampal coupling and decoupling. *Nature Neuroscience*, **4**, 1259–1264.

Fingelkurts, A., Fingelkurts, A., Krause, C., and Sams, M. (2002). Probability interrelations between pre-/post-stimulus intervals and ERD/ERS during a memory task. *Clinical Neurophysiology*, **113**, 826–843.

Gevins, A. and Smith, M. (2000). Neurophysiological measures of working memory and individual differences in cognitive ability and cognitive style. *Cerebral Cortex*, **10**, 829–839.

Gevins, A., Smith, M.E., and McEvoy, L. (1997). High-resolution EEG mapping of cortical activation related to working memory: effects of task difficulty, type of processing, and practice, *Cerebral Cortex* **7**, 374–385.

Gevins, A., Smith, M.E., Leong, H., *et al.* (1998). Monitoring working memory load during computer-based tasks with EEG pattern recognition methods, *Human Factors*, **40**, 79–91.

Givens, B. (1996). Stimulus-evoked resetting of the dentate theta rhythm: relation to working memory, *Neuroreport*, **8**, 159–163.

Gorno-Tempini, M., Price, C., Josephs, O., *et al.* (1998). The neural systems sustaining face and proper-name processing. *Brain*, **121**, 2103–2118.

Grunwald, M., Weiss, T., Krause, W., *et al.* (1999). Power of theta waves in the EEG of human subjects increases during recall of haptic information. *Neuroscience Letters*, **260**, 189–192.

Herrmann, C.S. and Knight, R.T. (2001). Mechanisms of human attention: event-related potentials and oscillations. *Neuroscience and Biobehavioral Reviews*, **25**, 465–476.

Herrmann, C.S. and Mecklinger, A. (2000). Magnetoencephalographic responses to illusory figures: early evoked gamma is affected by processing of stimulus features. *International Journal of Psychophysiology*, **38**, 265–281.

Herrmann, C.S., Mecklinger, A., and Pfeifer, E. (1999). Gamma responses and ERPs in a visual classification task. *Clinical Neurophysiology*, **110**, 636–642.

Hillyard, S.A., Luck, S.J., and Mangun, G.R. (1994). The cuing of attention to visual field locations: analysis with ERP recordings. In *Cognitive Electrophysiology* (ed H.J. Heinze, T.F. Münte, and G.R. Mangun). Boston, MA: Birkhäuser, pp. 1–25.

Hintzman, D.L., Caulton, D.A., and Levition, D.J. (1998). Retrieval dynamics in recognition and list discrimination: further evidence of separate processes of familiarity in recall. *Memory and Recognition*, **26**, 449–462.

Ishihara, T. and Yoshii, N. (1972). Multivariate analytic study of EEG and mental activity in juvenile delinquents. *Electroencephalography and Clinical Neurophysiology*, **33**, 71–80.

Ishii, R., Shinosaki, K., Ukai, S., *et al.* (1999). Medial prefrontal cortex generates frontal midline theta rhythm. *Neuroreport*, **10**, 675–679.

Jensen, O. and Tesche, C. (2002). Frontal theta activity in humans increases with memory load in a working memory task. *European Journal of Neuroscience*, **15**, 1395–1400.

Jensen, O. and Lisman, J. (1998). An oscillatory short-term memory buffer model can account for data on the Sternberg task. *Journal of Neuroscience*, **18**, 10688–10699.

Jensen, O., Gelfand, J., Kounios, J., and Lisman, J. (2002). Oscillations in the alpha band (9–12 Hz) increase with memory load during retention in a short-term memory task. *Cerebral Cortex*, **12**, 877–882.

Kahana, M.J., Sekuler, R., Caplan, J.B, Kirschen, M., and Madsen, J.R. (1999). Human theta oscillations exhibit task dependence during virtual maze navigation. *Nature*, **399**, 781–784.

Kalcher, J. and Pfurtscheller, G. (1995). Discrimination between phase-locked and non-phase locked event-related EEG activity. *Electroencephalography and Clinical Neurophysiology*, **94**, 381–384.

Keil, A., Gruber, T., and Müller, M. (2001). Functional correlates of macroscopic high-frequency brain activity in the human visual system. *Neuroscience and Biobehavioral Reviews*, **25**, 527–534.

Klimesch, W. (1994). *The Structure of Long-Term Memory: A Connectivity Model for Semantic Processing*. Hillsdale, NJ: Erlbaum.

Klimesch, W. (1996) Memory processes, brain oscillations and EEG synchronization. *International Journal of Psychophysiology*, **24**, 61–100.

Klimesch, W. (1997). EEG-alpha rhythms and memory processes. *International Journal of Psychophysiology*, **26**, 319–340.

Klimesch, W. (1999). EEG alpha and theta oscillations reflect cognitive and memory performance: a review and analysis. *Brain Research Reviews*, **29**, 169–195.

Klimesch, W., Schimke, H., and Schwaiger, J. (1994). Episodic and semantic memory: an analysis in the EEG-theta and alpha band. *Electroencephalography and Clinical Neurophysiology* **91**, 428–441.

Klimesch, W., Doppelmayr, M., Schimke, H., and Pachinger, T. (1996a). Alpha frequency, reaction time and the speed of processing information. *Journal of Clinical Neurophysiol.* **13**, 511–518.

Klimesch, W., Schimke, H., Doppelmayr, M., Ripper, B., Schwaiger, J., and Pfurtscheller, G. (1996b). Event-related desynchronization (ERD) and the Dm-effect. Does alpha desychronization during encoding predict later recall performance. *International Journal of Psychophysiology* **24**, 47–60.

Klimesch, W., Doppelmayr, M., Russegger, H., and Pachinger, T. (1996c). Theta band power in the human scalp EEG and the encoding of new information. *Neuroreport*, **7**, 1235–1240.

Klimesch, W., Doppelmayr, M., Pachinger, T., and Ripper, B. (1997a). Brain oscillations and human memory performance: EEG correlates in the upper alpha and theta bands, *Neuroscience Letters*, **238**, 9–12.

Klimesch, W., Doppelmayr, M., Pachinger, T., and Russegger, H. (1997b). Event-related desynchronization in the alpha band and the processing of semantic information. *Cognitive Brain Research*, **6**, 83–94.

Klimesch, W., Doppelmayr, M., Schimke, H., and Ripper, B. (1997c). Theta synchronization in a memory task, *Psychophysiology*, **34**, 169–176.

Klimesch, W., Doppelmayr, M., Russegger, H., Pachinger, T., and Schwaiger, J. (1998a). Induced alpha band power changes in the human EEG and attention. *Neuroscience Letters*, **244**, 73–76.

Klimesch, W., Russegger, H., Doppelmayr, M., and Pachinger, T. (1998b). A method for the calculation of induced band power: implications for the significance of brain oscillations. *Electroencephalography and Clinical Neurophysiology*, **108**, 123–130.

Klimesch, W., Doppelmayr, M., Schwaiger, J., Auinger, P., and Winkler, T. (1999). 'Paradoxical' alpha synchronization in a memory task. *Cognitive Brain Research*, **7**, 493–501.

Klimesch, W., Doppelmayr, M., Röhm, D., Pöllhuber, D., and Stadler, W. (2000a). Simultaneous desynchronization and synchronization of different alpha responses in the human electroencephalograph: a neglected paradox? *Neuroscience Letters*, **284**, 97–100.

Klimesch, W., Vogt, F., and Doppelmayr, M. (2000b). Interindividual differences in alpha and theta power reflect memory performance. *Intelligence*, **27**, 347–362.

Klimesch, W., Doppelmayr, M., Schwaiger, J., Winkler, T., and Gruber, W. (2000c). Theta oscillations and the ERP old/new effect: independent phenomena? *Clinical Neurophysiology*, **111**, 781–793.

Klimesch, W., Doppelmayr, M., Stadler, W., Pöllhuber, D., Sauseng, P., and Röhm D (2001a). Episodic retrieval is reflected by a process specific increase in human electroencepaholographic theta activity. *Neuroscience Letters*, **302**, 49–52.

Klimesch, W., Doppelmayr, M., Yonelinas, A., *et al.* (2001b). Theta synchronization during episodic retrieval: neural correlates of conscious awareness. *Cognitive Brain Research*, **12**, 33–38.

Klimesch, W., Doppelmayr, M., Wimmer, H., *et al.* (2001c). Theta band power changes in normal and dyslexic children. *Clinical Neurophysiology*, **112**, 1174–1185.

Klimesch, W., Schack, B., Schabus, M., Doppelmayr, M., Gruber, W., and Sauseng, P. (2004). Phase locked alpha and theta oscillations generate the P1–N1 complex and are related to memory performance. *Cognitive Brain Research*, **19**, 302–316.

Kocsis, B., Di Prisco, G., and Vertes, R. (2001). Theta synchronization in the limbic system: the role of Guddens' tegmental nuclei. *European Journal of Neuroscience*, **13**, 381–388.

König, P. and Engel, A.K. (1995). Correlated firing in sensory-motor systems. *Current Opinion in Neurobiology*, **5**, 511–519.

König, T., Lehman, D., Saito, N., Kuginuki, T., Kinoshita, T., and Koukku, M. (2001). Decreased functional connectivity of EEG theta-frequency activity in first-episode, neuroleptive-naive patients with schizophrenia: preliminary results. *Schizophrenia Research*, **50**, 55–60.

Koskinen, M., Seppaenen, T., Tuukkanen, J., Yli-Hankala, A., and Jaentti, V. (2001). Propofol anesthesia induces phase synchronization changes in EEG. *Clinical Neurophsysiology*, **112**, 386–392.

Krause, C.M., Lang, H.A., Laine, M., Kuusisto, M.J., and Poern, B. (1996). Event-related EEG desynchronization and synchronization during an auditory memory task, *Electroencephalography and Clinical Neurophysiology*, **98**, 319–326.

Krause, C.M., Salminen, P., Sillanmaeki, L., and Holopainen, I. (2001). Event-related desynchronization and synchronization during a memory task in children. *Clinical Neurophysiology*, **112**, 2233–2240.

Kubota, Y., Sato, W., Toichi, M., *et al.* (2001). Frontal midline theta rhythm is correlated with cardiac autonomic activities during the performance of an attention demanding meditation procedure. *Cognitive Brain Research*, **11**, 281–287.

Lisman, J. and Idiart, M. (1995). Storage of 7 ± short-term memories in oscillatory subcycles. *Science*, **267**, 1512–1514.

Lopes da Silva, F.H. and Pfurtscheller, G. (1999). Basic concepts on EEG synchronization and desynchronization. In *Handbook of Electroencephalography and Clinical*

Neurophysiology. Vol. 6: *Event-Related Desynchronization* (ed G. Pfurtscheller and F.H. Lopes da Silva). Amsterdam: Elsevier, pp. 3–12.

Luck, S.J., Fan, S., and Hillyard, S.A. (1993). Attention-related modulation of sensory-evoked brain activity in a visual search task. *Journal of Cognitive Neuroscience*, **5**, 188–195.

McEvoy, L. ***et al.*** (2001)

Makeig, S., Westerfield, M., Jung, T.P., ***et al.*** (2002). Dynamic brain sources of visual evoked responses. *Science*, **295**, 690–694.

Mangun, G.R. (1994). Orienting attention in the visual fields: an electrophysiological analysis. In *Cognitive Electrophysiology* (ed H.J. Heinze, T.F. Münte and G.R. Mangun). Boston, MA: Birkhäuser, pp. 81–101.

Mecklinger, A., Kramer, A.F., and Strayer, D.L. (1992). Event-related potentials and EEG components in a semantic memory search task. *Psychophysiology*, **29**, 104–119.

Miller, R. (1991). *Cortico-Hippocampal Interplay and the Representation of Contexts in the Brain*. Berlin: Springer-Verlag.

Miltner, W., Braun, C., Arnold, M., Witte, H., and Traub, E. (1999). Coherence of gamma-band EEG activity as a basis for associative learning, *Nature*, **397**, 434–436.

Müller, M.M., Bosch, J., Elbert, T., ***et al.*** (1996). Visually induced gamma band responses in human EEG—a link to animal studies. *Experimental Brain Research*, **112**, 96–112.

Müller, M.M., Gruber, T., and Keil, A. (2000). Modulation of induced gamma band activity in the human EEG by attention and visual information processing. *International Journal of Psychophysiology*, **38**, 283–300.

Neubauer, A., Freudenthaler, H., and Pfurtscheller, G. (1995). Intelligence and spatiotemporal patterns of event-related desynchronization (ERD). *Intelligence*, **20**, 249–246.

O'Keefe, J. and Dostrovsky, J. (1971). The hippocampus as a spatial map. Preliminary evidence from unit activity in the freely moving rat. *Brain Research*, **34**, 171–175.

Otten, L.J. and Rugg, M.D. (2002). The birth of a memory. *Trends in Neuroscience*, **25**, 279–281.

Pelosi, L., Holly, M., Slade, T., Hayward, M., Barrett, G., and Blumhardt, L. (1992). Waveform variations in auditory event related potentials evoked by a memory scanning task and their relationship with tests of intellectual function. *Electroencephalography and Clinical Neurophysiology*, **84**,344–352.

Pelosi, L., Hayward, M., and Blumhardt, L. (1998). Which event-related potentials reflect memory processing in a digit-probe identification task. *Cognitive Brain Research*, **6**, 205–218.

Petsche, H. and Etlinger, S. (1998). *EEG and Thinking: Power and Coherence Analysis of Cognitive Processes*. Vienna: Austrian Academy of Sciences.

Petsche, H., Lacroix, D., Lindner, K., Rappelsberger, P., and Schmidt-Henrich, E. (1992). Thinking with images or thinking with language: a pilot EEG probability mapping study. *International Journal of Psychophysiology*, **12**, 31–39.

Petsche, H., Richter, P., von Stein, A., Etlinger, S., and Filz, O. (1993a). EEG coherence and musical thinking. *Music Percept*, **11**, 117–151.

Petsche, H., Etlinger, S., and Filz, O. (1993b). Brain electrical mechanisms of bilingual speech management: an initial investigation. *Electroencephalography and Clinical Neurophysiology*, **86**, 385–394.

Pfurtscheller, G. (1992). Event-related sychronization (ERS): an electrophysiological correlate of cortical areas at rest. *Electroencephalography and Clinical Neurophysiology*, **83**, 62–69.

Pfurtscheller, G. and Aranibar, A. (1977). Event-related cortical desychronization detected by power measurement of scalp EEG. *Electroencephalography and Clinical Neurophysiology*, **42**, 817–826.

Pfurtscheller, G. and Lopes da Silva, F.H. (ed) (1999). *Handbook of EEG and Clinical Neurophysiology*. Vol. 6: *Event-Related Desynchronization*. Amsterdam: Elsevier

Polich, J. (1997). On the relationship between EEG and P300: individual differences, aging, and ultradian rhythms. *International Journal of Psychophysiology*, **26**, 299–317.

Pulvermüller, F., Keil, A., and Elbert, T. (1999). High-frequency brain activity: perception or active memory? *Trends in Cognitive Sciences*, **3**, 250–252.

Raghavachari, S., Kahana, M., Rizzuto, D., *et al.* (2001). Gating of human theta oscillations by a working memory task. *Journal of Neuroscience*, **21**, 3175–3183.

Rahn, E. and Basar, E. (1993a). Enhancement of visual evoked potentials by stimulation during low prestimulus EEG stages. *International Journal of Neuroscience*, **72**, 123–136.

Rahn, E. and Basar, E. (1993b). Prestimulus EEG-activity strongly influences the auditory evoked vertex response: a new method for selective averaging. *International Journal of Neuroscience*, **69**, 207–220.

Rappelsberger, P. and Petsche, H. (1988). Probability mapping: power and coherence analysis of cognitive processes. *Brain Topography*, **1**, 46–54.

Rappelsberger, P., Lacroix, D., Steinberger, K., Thau, K., and Petsche, H. (1991). EEG probability mapping while listing to a text: a group and a single case study. In *Medical Informatics Europe* (ed K.P. Adlassing, G. Grabner, S. Bengtsson, and R. Hansen). Berlin: Springer-Verlag, pp. 1010–1013.

Rizzuto, D.S., Madsen, J.R., Bromfield, E.R., *et al.* (2003) Reset of human neocortical oscillations during a working memory task. *Proceedings of the National Academy of Sciences of the United States of America*, **100**, 7931–7936.

Rodriguez, E., George, N., Lachaux, J., Martinerie, J., Renault, B., and Varela, F. (1999). Perception's shadow: long-distance synchronization of human brain activity. *Nature*, **397**, 430–433.

Röhm, D., Klimesch, W., Haider, H., and Doppelmayr, M. (2001). The role of theta and alpha oscillations for language comprehension in the human electroencephaologram. *Neuroscience Letters*, **310**, 137–140.

Rugg, M. and Doyle, M. (1992). Event-related potential and recognition memory for low and high-frequency words. *Journal of Cognitive Neuroscience*, **4**, 69–79.

Salinas, E. and Sejnowski T. (2001). Correlated neuronal activity and the flow of neural information. *Nature Reviews Neuroscience*, **2**, 539–550.

Sarnthein, J., Petsche, H., Rappelsberger, P., Shaw, G.L., and von Stein, A. (1998). Synchronization between prefrontal and posterior association cortex during human working memory. *Proceedings of the National Academy of Sciences of the United States of America*, **95**, 7092–7096.

Sasaki, K., Nambu, A., Tsujimoto, T., Matsuzaki, R., Kyuhou, S., and Gemba, H. (1996). Studies on integrative functions of the human frontal association cortex with MEG. *Cognitive Brain Research*, **5**, 165–174.

Sauseng, P., Klimesch, W., Gruber, W., Doppelmayr, M., Stadler, W., and Schabus, M. (2002). The interplay between theta and alpha oscillations in the human electroencephalogram reflects the transfer of information between memory systems. *Neuroscience Letters*, **324**, 121–124.

Schack, B. and Klimesch, W. (2002). Frequency characteristic of the human P300 in a memory scanning task. Submitted for publication.

Schack, B., Rappelsberger, P., Anders, C., Weiss, S., and Möller, E. (2000). Coherence analyses. *International Journal of Bifurcation and Chaos*, **10**, 2565–2586.

Schack, B., Witte, H., Helbig, M., Schelenz, C., and Specht, M. (2001). Time-variant non-linear phase-coupling analysis of EEG burst patterns in sedated patients during electroencephalic burst suppression period. *Clinical Neurophysiology*, **112**, 1388–1399.

Schack, B., Vath, B., Petsche, H., Geissler, H.G., and Möller, E. (2002). Phase coupling of theta-gamma EEG rhythms during short-term memory processing, *International Journal of Psychophysiology*, **44**, 143–163.

Schacter, D. (1977). EEG theta waves and psychological phenomena: a review and analysis. *Biological Psychology*, **5**, 47–82.

Singer, W. and Gray, C.M. (1995). Visual feature integration and the temporal correlation hypothesis. *Annual Review of Neuroscience*, **18**, 555–586.

Slobounov, S.M., Fukada, K., Somin, R., Rearick, M., and Ray, W. (2000). Neurophysiological and behavioral indices of time pressure effects on visuomotor task performance. *Cognitive Brain Research*, **9**, 287–289.

Snodgrass, J.G. and Vanderwart, M. (1980). A standardized set of 260 pictures: norms for name agreement, image agreement, familiarity, and visual complexity, *Journal of Experimental Psychology: Human Learning and Memory*, **6**, 174–215.

Stam, C. (2000). Brain dynamics in theta and alpha frequency bands and working memory performance. *Neuroscience Letters*, **286**, 115–118.

Sterman, M.B., Kaiser, D.A., and Veigel, B. (1996). Spectral analysis of event-related EEG responses during short-term memory performance. *Brain Topography*, **9**, 21–30.

Sternberg, S. (1966). High-speed scanning in human memory. *Science*, **152**, 652–654.

Tallon-Baudry, C. and Bertrand, O. (1999). Oscillatory gamma activity in humans and sit role in object representation. *Trends in Cognitive Sciences*, **3**, 151–162.

Tallon-Baudry, C., Bertrand, O., Peronnet, F., and Pernier, J. (1998). Induced gamma band activity in during the delay of a visual short-term memory task in humans. *Journal of Neuroscience*, **18**, 4244–4254.

Tesche, C. and Karhu, J. (2000). Theta oscillations index human hippocampal activation during a working memory task. *Proceedings of the National Academy of Sciences of the United States of America*, **97**, 919–924.

Tiihonen, J., Hari, R., Kajola, M., Karhu, J., Ahlfors, S., and Tissari, S. (1991). Magnetoencephalographic 10-Hz rhythm from the human auditory cortex. *Neuroscience Letters*, **129**, 303–305.

Treves, A. and Rolls, E. (1994). Computational analysis of the role of the hippocampus in memory. *Hippocampus*, **4**, 374–391

Tulving, E. (1984). Precis of elements of episodic memory. *Behavioral and Brain Sciences*, **7**, 223–268.

Vertes, R., Albo, Z., and Di Prisco, G. (2001). Theta-rhythmically firing neurons in the anterior thalamus: implications for mnemonic functions of Papez's circuit. *Neuroscience*, **104**, 619–625.

von Stein, A. and Sarnthein, J. (2000). Different frequencies for different scales of cortical integration: from local gamma to long range alpha/theta synchronization. *International Journal of Psychophysiology*, **38**, 301–313.

von Stein, A., Sarnthein, J., and Petsche, H. (1995). EEG synchronization seems to reflect functional properties of the underlying cortical networks in the human brain. *European Journal of Neuroscience*, Suppl. 8.

von Stein, A., Rappelsberger, P., Sarnthein, J., and Petsche, H. (1999). Synchronization between temporal and parietal cortex during multimodal object processing in man. *Cerebral Cortex*, **9**, 137–150.

von Stein, A., Chiang, C., and König, P. (2000). Top-down processing mediated by interareal synchronization. *Proceedings of the National Academy of Sciences of the United States of America*, **97**, 14748–14753.

van Essen, D.C., Anderson, C.H., and Felleman, D.J. (1992). Information processing in the primate visual system an integrated systems perspective. *Science*, **255**, 419–423.

Varela, F., Lachaux, J.P., Rodriguez, E., and Martinerie, J. (2001). The brainweb: phase synchronization and large-scale integration. *Nature Neuroscience*, **2**, 229–238.

Wagner, A. (2001). Synchronicity: when you're gone I'm lost without trace? *Nature Neuroscience*, **4**, 1159–1160.

Weiss, S. and Rappelsberger, P. (1996). EEG coherence within the 13–18 Hz band as a correlate of a distinct lexical organisation of concrete and abstract nouns in humans, *Neuroscience Letters*, **209**, 17–20.

Yonelinas, A. (2002). The nature of recollection and familiarity: a review of 30 years of research. *Journal of Memory and Language*, **46**, 441–517.

Yonelinas, A., Hopfinger, J., Buonocore, M., Kroll, N., and Baynes, K (2001). Hippocampal, parahippocampal and occipital-temporal contributions to associative and item recognition memory: an fMRI study. *Neuroreport*, **12**, 359–363.

Chapter 6

Relationship between event-related potentials and oscillatory dynamics in episodic retrieval

Emrah Düzel, Markus Neufang, and Sebastian Guderian

Introduction

Episodic memory allows us to consciously explore and vividly remember events of our past (Tulving 1985). A hallmark of episodic memory is that different types of information about past events, such as time, location, and context, can be remembered as memory contents that belong together. This is a remarkable capability, given that the corresponding neural representations are likely to be distributed across different brain regions (Squire and Zola-Morgan 1991; Nyberg *et al.* 2000; Sutherland and McNaughton 2000; Hoffman and McNaughton 2002) and their integration therefore requires a temporary 'binding' of the activity of the corresponding neural populations (Rolls 1996). The medial temporal lobes (MTLs), particularly the hippocampi, are thought to play a key role in orchestrating such dynamic interactions between distributed neocortical areas during mnemonic processing (Treves and Rolls 1994; McClelland *et al.* 1995). Within this framework, the widespread interconnections of parahippocampal and rhinal cortices provide the anatomical basis for the MTLs to act as convergence zones and associative integrators for information from many unimodal and multimodal cortical association areas (Eichenbaum *et al.* 1996; Murray and Bussey 1999; Lavenex and Amaral 2000).

This chapter is concerned with the large-scale oscillatory population dynamics associated with episodic retrieval that have been suggested to coordinate the binding and integration of distributed neural population activity (Varela *et al.* 2001). Oscillatory fluctuations of neuronal membrane potentials play an important role in the coordination of large-scale interactions of neural assemblies (Sherman and Guillery 1998; Steriade 2000). Such oscillations are caused by the concerted action of long-range afferents, local interneurons, and the intrinsic properties of the neural membrane (Steriade 2000). The fluctuations of local field potentials (LFPs) accompanying oscillations of membrane potentials can be measured at different anatomical scales, ranging from invasive recordings of small neuronal populations to non-invasive recordings of large cortical assemblies from the surface of the scalp using EEG and magnetoencephalography (MEG) (Lopes da Silva 1991).

Oscillatory dynamics and memory

Important insights into the principles that govern the interaction of neural assemblies in the MTL stem from invasive recordings of oscillatory phenomena. Oscillatory rhythms in the MTL, most notably in the theta range (4–12 Hz in rodents, and 4–8 Hz in humans) (Green and Arduini 1954; Vanderwolf 1969), have been studied mostly in relation to spatial navigation and are implicated in the hippocampal coding of an animal's location within a place field (Huxter *et al.* 2003). In humans, invasive recordings in patients with pharmacoresistant epilepsy have shown that neocortical theta oscillations play a role not only during spatial navigation (Kahana *et al.* 1999; Caplan *et al.* 2001, 2003), but also in relation to working memory (Raghavachari *et al.* 2001; Rizzuto *et al.* 2003) and episodic memory encoding (Sederberg *et al.* 2003). These findings provide evidence for the view that human neocortical theta oscillations are involved in the neuronal realization of several memory-related cognitive processes.

Many studies have shown that MTL theta oscillations are accompanied by fast oscillations in the gamma range (30–80 Hz) and that peaks in the gamma oscillations tend to occur at certain phases of the theta rhythm (Chrobak and Buzsáki 1998; Buzsáki 2002). It has been proposed that this theta–gamma phase coupling is a basic mechanism of modifying the rate code of place cells and, in a more general framework, even a basic mechanism of coding episodic memories in the hippocampus (Lisman and Otmakhova 2001). Both theta and gamma rhythms have been recorded non-invasively at a larger anatomical scale in humans (Tallon-Baudry and Bertrand 1999; Klimesch *et al.* 2001; Düzel *et al.* 2003, 2005; Guderian and Düzel 2005), encouraging the study of theta–gamma interactions using non-invasive EEG and MEG recordings in human subjects. Indeed, exploration of such interactions in humans has recently begun (Fell *et al.* 2003; Düzel *et al.* 2005).

Event-related potentials

Much of our knowledge about the electrophysiology of episodic memory in humans stems from the interpretation of EEG and MEG signals averaged across multiple trials, resulting in the so-called event-related potentials (ERPs) and event-related fields (ERFs). Although such averaging leads to a considerable loss of information about oscillatory rhythms, the interpretation of amplitude fluctuations of ERPs/ERFs has provided important insights into the neural mechanisms underlying episodic memory (Rugg *et al.* 1998b; Düzel *et al.* 1999; Dale *et al.* 2000; Tendolkar *et al.* 2000). Certain components of the ERP/ERF are sensitive to relatively selective hippocampal injury and thus seem to reflect an important functional aspect of episodic memory (Düzel *et al.* 2001).

Despite the obvious importance of ERPs/ERFs in the understanding of human memory in both healthy adults and patients, their relationship to the oscillatory phenomena of memory extensively studied in animals is only just being elucidated. Existing views about this relationship have become polarized into theories that emphasize the evoked nature of neural responses to cognitive acts such as perception and attention (Hillyard 1985; Schroeder *et al.* 1995; Shah *et al.* 2004) and theories that favour the dynamic oscillatory nature of neural responses (Makeig *et al.* 2002).

The evoked response view states that a stimulus evokes an additive neural population response in each trial and, because this response is time locked to the onset of stimulus presentation, averaging these evoked responses across trials will preserve them in the ERP. The dynamic response view states that a stimulus induces 'phase resetting' or phase alignment of ongoing oscillatory EEG rhythms in each trial and that averaging these phase-coherent rhythms produces the ERP.

Organization of the chapter

In this chapter we will consider whether ERPs/ERFs elicited during recognition memory occur through phase alignment or reflect evoked neural responses. Further, we will discuss the relationship of theta oscillations to recollection and familiarity-based recognition. Finally, we will address the issue of how the coupling of gamma bursts at certain phases of slow oscillations can be studied in humans and we will present preliminary data on this. Finally, we will speculate on how ERPs/ERFs, slow oscillations, theta oscillations and gamma oscillations might be related to each other and to binding and integration of distributed cortical information during episodic memory retrieval.

ERP indices of episodic memory

Cognitive models of recognition memory, including Tulving's (1985) theory of episodic memory and dual-process models (Jacoby and Kelley 1992; Yonelinas *et al.* 1996), converge on the notion that both episodic and semantic memory contribute to recognition memory. Recollection-based recognition, or 'remembering', is accompanied by contextual information about the episode in which an item was encountered, whereas familiarity-based recognition, or 'knowing', is devoid of such information (Tulving 1985). Remembering and knowing, in turn, characterize episodic and semantic memory, respectively. There is abundant experimental evidence from cognitive studies in healthy adults and in patients with amnesia that recollection-based (or remembering) and familiarity-based judgements (or knowing) cannot be reduced to a quantitative difference, but instead reflect two qualitatively different aspects of recognition memory (Knowlton and Squire 1995; Yonelinas *et al.* 1998; Yonelinas and Levy 2002). This cognitive evidence is supported by ERP findings which have revealed qualitatively distinct brain activity patterns associated with recollection and familiarity (Mecklinger 2000) (see also recent functional imaging evidence for a qualitative distinction (Yonelinas *et al.* 2005)). Remembering or recollecting studied words causes an increased ERP positivity 500–700 ms after the onset of word presentation (Paller and Kutas 1992; Paller *et al.* 1995; Düzel *et al.* 1997; Rugg *et al.* 1998b; Wilding 2000) which is sometimes referred to as the late positive component (LPC) effect. In contrast, knowing or familiarity is associated with an earlier ERP positivity between 300 and 500 ms, which is known as the N400 effect (Curran 1999; Rugg *et al.* 1998b; Düzel *et al.* 1997).

Although the intracerebral generators of the ERP effects recorded from the scalp during recognition memory are not yet precisely established, a consensus is emerging supporting the inference made from topographic analyses of ERPs that the old/new effects in the N400 and LPC time windows are mediated by different neural structures (Elger *et al.* 1997; Rugg *et al.* 1998a; Curran 2000; Düzel *et al.* 2003) rather than just reflecting quantitative amplitude differences. The cortical generators of the N400 ERP/ERF old/new effect have been localized in the left anterior inferior temporal cortex (Düzel *et al.* 2003), compatible with data from invasive ERP recordings in patients with intractable epilepsy which also showed old/new effects in explicit word recognition paradigms (as used here) in the anterior portion of the inferior temporal lobe in the N400 time window (so-called AMTL-N400) (Smith and Halgren 1987; Heit *et al.* 1990; Elger *et al.* 1997; Grunwald *et al.* 1998; Fernandez *et al.* 1999). In the LPC time window, repeated words are associated with stronger sources than new words over posterior regions of the left parietal lobe, the occipital, and the posterior inferior temporal cortices (Düzel *et al.* 2003). In relatively isolated bilateral hippocampal pathology the LPC effect of recognition memory is selectively attenuated, whereas the N400 effect remains largely unaffected (Düzel *et al.* 2001). This suggests that the sources of the LPC effect may reflect modulation of neocortical generators by medial temporal areas (Rugg *et al.* 1998b), a direct contribution from medial temporal generators (Nishitani *et al.* 1999), or a combination of both.

ERP/ERF old/new effects: evoked responses versus phase resetting

To understand the relationship between ERPs/ERFs and the large-scale oscillatory dynamics during recognition memory, it is important to explore the neural basis of recognition-related ERP/ERF generation. Hence we assessed to what extent the N400 and the LPC old/new effects of recognition memory are caused by phase alignment or by evoked responses by determining phase alignment and amplitude values across single trials of a word recognition experiment (Düzel *et al.* 2005). In summary, the experiment was divided into 34 blocks that consisted of a study and test phase. During each study phase, 12 words were presented visually with an inter-stimulus interval of 2 s and a stimulus duration of 1.2 s. Subjects were instructed to make a pleasant–unpleasant judgement on each study word. The test lists comprised 12 studied ('old') words and 12 unstudied ('new') words in a random order, with an inter-stimulus interval of 2 s. Subjects were instructed to indicate via a button press whether each word was old or new. MEG signals (148-channel BTi Magnes 2500 whole-head magnetometer, Biomagnetic Technologies Inc., San Diego, CA) were registered at a digitization rate of 254 Hz and filtered (IIR Butterworth filter) with a bandpass from DC to 50 Hz. Further details of this experiment can be found in Duezel *et al.* (2005).

ERFs were derived by averaging 180–230 artefact-free trials of old and new words (only correct responses were considered). Amplitude and phase alignment of designated frequencies was assessed by wavelet transforming (Morlet wavelets) single trials of MEG recordings separately for old and new words. Taking the frequency resolution of a standard Morlet wavelet into account, 27 wavelets which were logarithmically scaled optimally covered the frequency range of interest (1.0–45.0 Hz) (see Düzel *et al.* (2005) for further details of the methods).

Figure 6.1(a) shows the ERFs elicited by old and new words. It can be seen that in the N400 time window, new words are associated with higher ERF amplitudes than old words over left temporal sensors (e.g. sensor A114 in Fig. 6.1(a)), whereas in the LPC time window, old words are associated with higher amplitudes than new words over left parietal sensors (e.g. sensor A19 in Fig. 6.1(a)). To assess whether these differences are caused by phase alignment or evoked responses across single trials, we first determined the frequency of the ERF differences. To do this, we conducted wavelet transformations of ERFs elicited by old and new words in single subjects, and then averaged these wavelet transforms across subjects and subtracted the results for new words from old words. As can be seen in Figure 6.1(b), the ERF difference in the LPC time window at a left parietal sensor (A19) has a peak frequency of around 2 Hz. In the N400 time

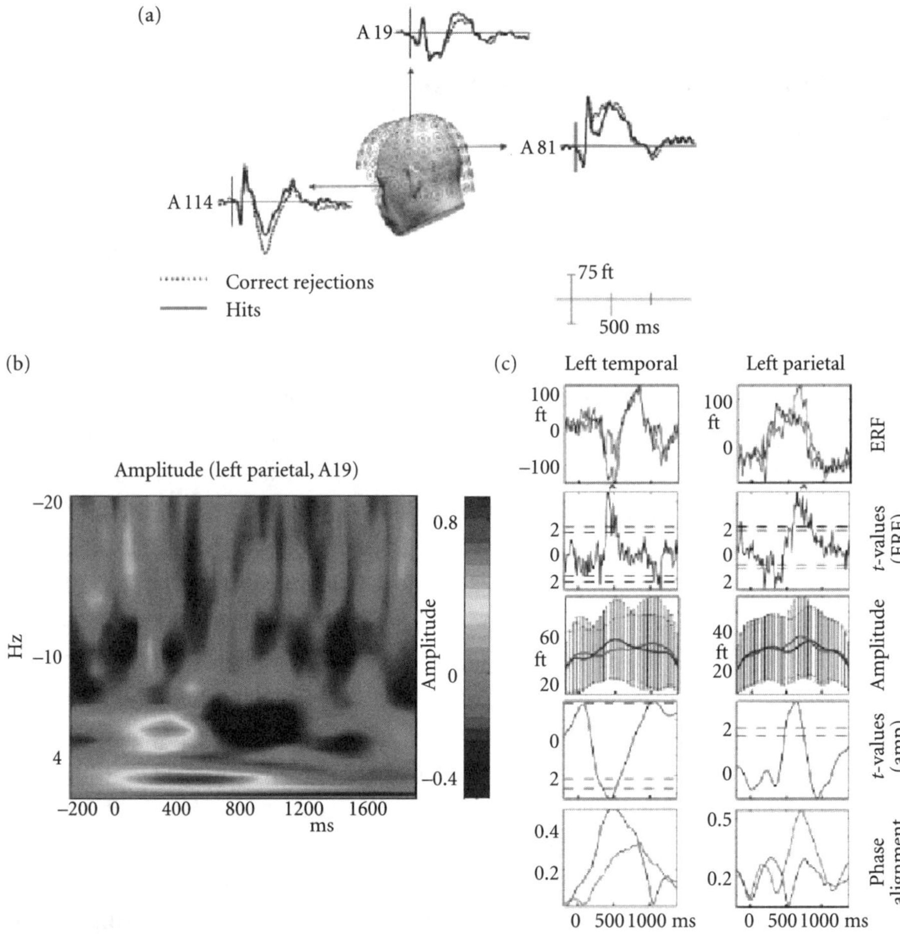

Figure 6.1 (a) Grand average (11 subjects) ERFs elicited by correctly recognized studied (old) words (hits, solid lines) and correctly rejected unstudied (new) words (dotted lines). A114, left temporal sensor; A81, left temporo-parietal sensor; A19, left parietal sensor. The three sensors display differences between old and new words at 275 ms (A81), 400 ms (A114), and 500–600 ms (A19). (b) Time–frequency spectra of the ERF difference between old and new words at sensor A19 obtained by wavelet transformation of the ERF (hence after averaging of single trials). The *x*-axis denotes the time in milliseconds after stimulus onset. The *y*-axis denotes the frequency in hertz. Amplitude is coded as colour. (c) Evidence for evoked responses from single-subject data at a left temporal and a left parietal sensor: comparisons of ERFs, phase alignment, and amplitudes. The left column shows ERF differences and corresponding oscillatory changes in the N400 time window and the right column shows ERF differences and corresponding oscillatory changes in the LPC time window. The first row shows the unfiltered ERFs for hits (red) and correct rejections (blue). The second row displays the time course and the magnitude of *t*-values from serial related measures *t*-tests between the single-trial raw data for hits and correct rejections whose average contributed to the ERFs in the first row. The third row shows the mean of single-trial amplitudes in the dominant frequency of the ERF difference between hits and correct rejections displayed in the first column. The fourth row shows the time course and the magnitude of *t*-values from serial related measures *t*-tests between single-trial amplitudes in the dominant frequency for hits and correct rejections. The fifth row shows phase alignment values across single trials in the same frequency bands. Error bars denote standard deviation. Amplitude values are in fT. See also colour plate section.

window the corresponding difference at a left temporal sensor (A114) also had a peak frequency of around 2 Hz.

If hits and correct rejections differed from each other in evoked neural activity within this frequency range, there should have been parallel differences in the phase alignment and amplitude of delta/theta oscillations between the two stimulus classes. Indeed, a within-subject analysis of single-trial data (Fig. 6.1(c)) revealed clear indices of evoked responses for both N400 and LPC time windows. Of the eight subjects who participated in the study, six showed significant phase alignment differences between hits and correct rejections spatially and temporally related to the ERF differences, and four of these showed parallel differences in phase alignment and amplitude between hits and correct rejections (as exemplified for one subject in Fig. 6.1(c)). More importantly, in these four subjects, the single-trial amplitude differences appeared to be largest over sensors that showed the largest differences in phase alignment (Düzel *et al.* 2005). This is a clear indication that the ERF difference in these subjects can be attributed to an evoked response. Nevertheless, phase alignment differences between hits and correct rejections were the most robust finding in the N400 and LPC time windows as they were found in all six subjects who showed a significant ERF difference between hits and correct rejections (Düzel *et al.* 2005).

It should be noted that rigidly defined concepts such as phase resetting and evoked responses might not fully account for all possible forms of event-related dynamics, such as cases in which the peak latency of an 'evoked' oscillation will vary from trial to trial. Makeig (2002) has recently argued that event-related phenomena may occur anywhere in the whole space of amplitude, phase alignment, and frequency possibilities. Whether there is such a continuum or whether there are classes of neural response patterns as proposed here requires further investigation.

Theta oscillations and binding

In the previous section we have highlighted the contribution of oscillatory phase alignment to the generation of memory-related ERFs. A different type of oscillatory dynamics which is probably not visible in averaged potentials is an induced response. Stimulus-induced neural activity has a loose temporal relationship with stimulus onset (Tallon-Baudry and Bertrand 1999) and consists of oscillations whose latency jitters from trial to trial. Therefore at a given time point after stimulus onset, this type of oscillation will have a different phase in different trials (Tallon-Baudry and Bertrand 1999). This phase variability will cause attenuation of induced oscillations in ERPs and ERFs during averaging of single trials of

EEG and MEG recordings (Varela *et al.* 2001; Düzel *et al.* 2005). Thus induced responses fundamentally differ from evoked responses, which are time-locked additive neural population responses and therefore are adequately represented in ERPs and ERFs (Hillyard 1985; Schroeder *et al.* 1995; Shah *et al.* 2004).

In the study of recognition memory described in the previous section (Düzel *et al.* 2005), we identified prominent amplitude differences between hits and correct rejections in the mid-theta range, thereby faster than the dominant frequency of the ERF differences in the N400 and LPC time windows. These amplitude differences were induced naturally because they were not accompanied by differences in phase alignment.

Induced theta oscillations have been associated with the recollection of personal events (Klimesch *et al.* 2001). A specific role of theta for recollection but not for stimulus familiarity would support links between neocortical theta oscillations and hippocampal functioning, given that a growing body of evidence indicates that the hippocampus is more critical for recollection than for familiarity in the absence of recollection (Mishkin *et al.* 1997; Vargha-Khadem *et al.* 1997; Brown and Aggleton 2001; Düzel *et al.* 2001; Yonelinas *et al.* 2002). During recollection, theta oscillations might mediate a dynamic link between hippocampal and neocortical areas, thereby allowing functional implementation of a reinstatement of retrieved information in distributed neocortical assemblies, which has been postulated in several computational models of memory (e.g. Treves and Rolls 1994; Rolls 2000).

If theta oscillations are related to recruiting and binding distributed cortical representations during recollection, their large-scale cortical dynamics should show two properties. First, their anatomical sources during recollection should be compatible with reactivation of stored representations. Secondly, their temporal dynamics should show phase synchrony between these cortical sites and the MTLs indicative of coupling distributed information with medial temporal processing (Guderian and Düzel 2005). Theoretically, it should be possible to test these two predictions non-invasively in humans by recording theta oscillations during recollection and selectively localizing the sources of only those theta oscillations which show a phase coupling across distant scalp areas. However, this apparently straightforward approach is complicated by the induced nature of theta oscillations which have so far been associated with recollection. Unlike ERPs and ERFs, the localization of induced oscillations requires analyses which are based on single-trial data rather than averaged responses.

We recorded theta oscillations using whole-head MEG while nine healthy subjects made recognition memory judgements on previously studied and unstudied pictures of faces (Guderian and Düzel 2005). For each recognized face, subjects had to indicate whether they also recollected the background image in front of which that face was studied. Trials where subjects succeeded in retrieving the correct background were classified as recollection (correct source judgements (CSJ)). Trials where subjects retrieved the wrong background were classified as reflecting weak recollection or familiarity (wrong source judgements (WSJ)). We observed that theta oscillations were higher in amplitude during recollection than during weak recollection/familiarity as well as during correct rejection of new faces. As expected from previous investigations (Klimesch *et al.* 2000, 2001), the amplitude increase during recollection was observed for induced theta oscillations. We developed a procedure that allowed us to extract the field distribution of induced theta oscillations from single trials by calculating phase differences between sensor pairs at each time point of each single trial. This approach yielded an estimate of the constancy of theta field distributions between trials, irrespective of the timing of theta phase relative to stimulus onset. This information about the phase relationship between sensors was then used to bring oscillatory amplitude information back to the time domain, yielding real fields that incorporate both absolute amplitude and phase information. Since the resulting time course of oscillatory activity retained the single-trial field information after averaging between trials, this information was used to model the sources of non-phase-locked, and hence induced, oscillatory amplitudes. When extracting field information from single trials using the procedure outlined above, only sensors showing a constant phase relation between trials will retain reliable phase information. Sensor groups reflecting activity from a non-synchronous source will show random phase differences between trials. Therefore only activity arising from synchronous sources will yield waveforms that can be localized using inverse source solutions. Hence it can be inferred that the sources obtained reflect synchronous theta activity, without necessarily being time locked to stimulus onset.

Figure 6.2 shows the results of the theta current density reconstructions between 300 and 700 ms. Common to all three experimental conditions were sources of theta activity in bilateral prefrontal as well as right lateral temporal cortices. Sources in bilateral mediotemporal as well as posterior fusiform cortices

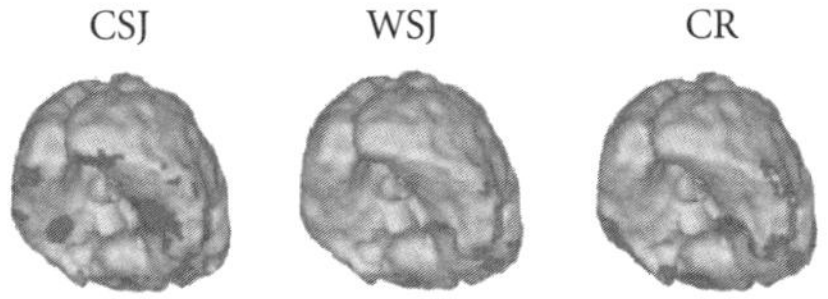

Figure 6.2 Current density distributions of induced theta oscillations for correct source judgements (CSJ), wrong source judgements (WSJ), and correct rejections (CR). See also colour plate section.

were obtained for CSJ only, suggesting that they are related to both the observed item-related increases in theta amplitude as well as the retrieval of contextual information.

Previous functional MRI (fMRI) experiments have shown that the hippocampal formation shows stronger activity for recollected than for familiar items (Eldridge *et al.* 2000; Cansino *et al.* 2002; Yonelinas *et al.* 2005). Additionally, an ERP recognition memory experiment has provided evidence that bilateral hippocampal pathology selectively affects the electrophysiological signature that has been associated with recollection, while suggesting that familiarity-based recognition remains largely intact (Düzel *et al.* 2001). Both lines of functional imaging evidence point to a role of the hippocampal formation in the retrieval of contextual information, but provide no indication of the neuronal realization of a hippocampal contribution to the orchestration of distributed cortical regions during recollection. Our results support the view that theta oscillations might play a role in mediating dynamic interactions between the MTLs and distributed neocortical areas during contextual retrieval. More specifically, the finding of bilateral inferior occipito-temporal sources of theta activity for CSJ is consistent with the recruitment of sensory specific cortices during recollection by means of theta oscillatory dynamics. Corroborating evidence for access to sensory-specific cortical information during recollection comes from fMRI studies which show sensory-specific reactivation during recollection of pictures and sounds (Wheeler *et al.* 2000).

Relationship between phase of delta oscillations and amplitude of gamma oscillations

Numerous interactions between slow and fast oscillations have been observed based on the natural logarithmic frequency scaling in both the animal and the human brain (reviewed by Penttonen and Buzsáki 2003). Evidence for task-related modulations of such relationships originates from intracranial recordings in animals (Basar-Eroglu *et al.* 1991; von Stein *et al.* 2000; Engel *et al.* 2001) and humans (Fell *et al.* 2003) and surface EEG recordings in humans (Burgess and Ali 2002; Schack *et al.* 2002; Düzel *et al.* 2003). In cats, for instance, omitted stimuli evoke a P300 response in the hippocampus which is accompanied by a 40 Hz response (the P300–40 Hz response) (Basar-Eroglu *et al.* 1991). In humans, Schack *et al.* (2002) described an increase in the cross-coherence between theta oscillations and gamma oscillations in a working memory task. Burgess and Ali (2002) have reported increased gamma phase synchrony fluctuating with a slow frequency of 3 Hz during recollection-based, but not familiarity-based, recognition. Although indicative of a relationship between slow and fast oscillations, studies have not yet directly assessed the relationship between the phase of slow oscillations and gamma amplitude.

We postulate that there are two types of relationships between the phase of slow (delta/theta) oscillations and the amplitude of fast (gamma) oscillations that are physiologically relevant for episodic memory. The first type of relationship is temporally extended and cyclic, whereby successive bursts of gamma fall into the same phase of theta cycles over an extended period of time without any need of time locking to stimulus onset. This situation is analogous to the type of theta–gamma coupling observed in rodents during sequential recall of locations (O'Keefe and Recce 1993; Lisman and Otmakhova 2001; Mehta *et al.* 2002). The second type is a temporally limited relationship that is time locked to stimulus onset, whereby an increase of gamma occurs at times of high phase alignment across trials and subjects. Hence this type of situation can be expected to be related to ERP indices of episodic memory.

Our analyses of the ERF old/new effects in the N400 and the LPC time window show that phase alignment of slow oscillations robustly distinguishes old and new words from each other in the dominant frequency of the ERP old/new difference. Given that ERPs reflect increased phase alignment across multiple trials and multiple individuals, there appear to be certain phases of slow oscillations that favourably occur within a given time window after stimulus onset. According to our second postulation, these windows of increased low-frequency phase alignment should be temporally coupled to amplitude changes in gamma oscillations.

In order to address this possibility, a multivariate statistical analysis using partial least-squares (PLS) was performed to assess the relationship of the phase alignment of oscillations in the dominant frequency range of the ERF differences between hits and correct rejections to the corresponding amplitude differences in the gamma frequency range (Düzel *et al.* 2005). This analysis combined phase alignment values in the delta/lower-theta range (1–4.6 Hz) and amplitude values in the gamma range (22–45 Hz) for hits and correct rejections (Fig. 6.3).

Results from this PLS analysis revealed a positive covariance between delta/theta phase alignment (2.9 and 3.4 Hz) and the amplitude of beta and gamma oscillations (29.3 and 33.8 Hz), clearly separating hits and correct rejections ($P < 0.01$, 12 percent of variance explained). The topography of this pattern partly overlapped with the topography of the ERF difference between hits and correct rejections. As can be seen in Figure 6.3, there was higher left temporal phase alignment for correct rejections than for hits in the N400 time window (410 ms). This increase in phase alignment was accompanied by higher left

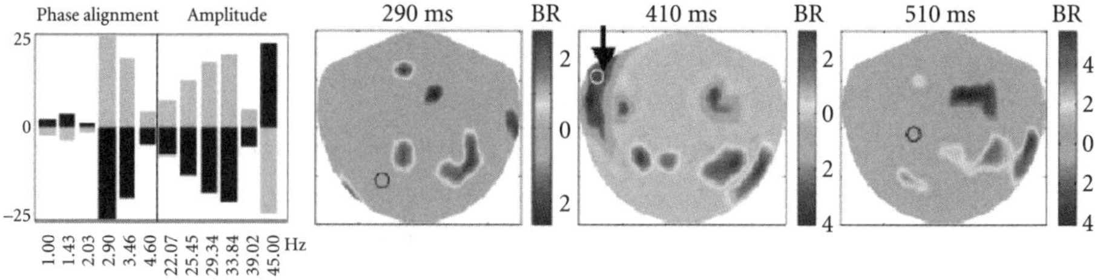

Figure 6.3 Partial least-squares analysis revealing a covariance between phase alignment in the delta and theta range and amplitude in the beta and gamma range. The left panel illustrates how phase alignment of frequencies ranging from 1 to 4.6 Hz and amplitude of frequencies ranging from 22 to 45 Hz jointly distinguish hits (grey bars) and correct rejections (black bars). The topographic maps on the right display the topography of the corresponding frequency patterns at early, N400, and LPC time windows. The values depicted in the topographic maps are bootstrap ratios for the corresponding sensor saliences to their standard error which are similar to *z*-values. Red indicates a positive correlation and blue indicates a negative correlation with the corresponding frequency pattern. For instance, a blue area over the left anterior temporal sensors (black arrow) indicates a stronger phase alignment for correct rejections than for hits and a concomitantly higher amplitude of oscillations between 22 and 34 Hz for correct rejections than for hits. See also colour plate section.

temporal beta and gamma amplitudes (from 29.3 and 33.8 Hz) for correct rejections than for hits.

Summary: ERPs/ERFs, theta oscillations, delta–gamma covariance, and binding

How are distributed neural representations integrated during recollection? We believe that the electromagnetic data presented here are relevant with respect to two aspects of this question: local activation of neural representations, and binding of distributed representations with the MTLs.

The local activation of neural representations could be reflected in the evoked nature of ERF old/new differences in the N400 and LPC time windows, which is commonly interpreted as an addition of neural response amplitude to ongoing background dynamics, together with the associated phase-locked gamma responses. Evidence for the concept of binding of distributed neural activations with MTL regions (Rolls 1996; Vargha-Khadem *et al.* 1997) could be reflected in the induced theta oscillations that are elicited more strongly by recollected old stimuli than by familiar or new stimuli and that are synchronized across different brain regions with mediotemporal areas (Guderian and Düzel 2005). These two aspects together support an influential hypothesis regarding the functional interpretation ERP old/new effects, namely that they reflect the activation of a widespread network controlled by the MTL (Smith and Halgren 1987).

Many issues remain to be addressed in future studies. For instance, what is the anatomical relationship between induced theta responses and ERP/ERF effects of recollection? An anatomical overlap would link the two phenomena and suggest that representations activated via ERPs/ERFs are bound to the MTLs via theta oscillations. Is the low frequency of ERPs/ERFs related to the spatial and temporal summation of synaptic input from many different cortical regions in a way that is compatible with the notion of neuromodulation (Sherman and Guillery 1998; Guillery and Sherman 2002)? That is, do ERPs/ERFs reflect evoked neuromodulatory processing that allows for the temporal integration of information during distributed processing? What is the functional role of beta and gamma oscillations in relation to ERPs/ERFs and theta oscillations? Beta and gamma oscillations are probably too fast to synchronize neural populations over long distances with long conductions delays (Kopell *et al.* 2000) and are more likely to index local information processing (von Stein *et al.* 2000; Engel *et al.* 2001).

We believe that combined approaches using both conventional averaging techniques and detailed analyses of oscillatory dynamics will help to improve our understanding of some of these issues in humans and also to help to bridge the gap between animal studies and electromagnetic studies in humans.

References

Basar-Eroglu, C., Basar, E., and Schmielau, F. (1991). P300 in freely moving cats with intracranial electrodes. *International Journal of Neuroscience*, **60**, 215–226.

Brown, M. and J. P. Aggleton (2001). Recognition memory: What are the roles of the perirhinal cortex and the hippocampus. *Nature Reviews Neuroscience*, **2**, 51–61.

Burgess, A.P. and Ali, E. (2002). Functional connectivity of gamma EEG activity is modulated at low frequency during conscious recollection. *International Journal of Psychophysiology*, **46**, 91–100.

Buzsáki, G. (2002). Theta oscillations in the hippocampus. *Neuron*, **33**, 325–340.

Cansino, S., Maquet, P., Dolan, R.J., and Rugg, M.D. (2002). Brain activity underlying encoding and retrieval of source memory. *Cerebral Cortex*, **12**, 1048–1056.

Caplan, J.B., Madsen, J.R., Raghavachari, S., and Kahana, M.J. (2001). Distinct patterns of brain oscillations underlie two basic parameters of human maze learning. *Journal of Neurophysiology*, **86**, 368–380.

Caplan, J.B., Madsen, J.R., Schulze-Bonhage, A., Aschenbrenner-Scheiber, R., Newman, E.L., and Kahana, M.J. (2003). Human theta oscillations related to sensorimotor integration and spatial learning. *Journal of Neuroscience*, **23**, 4726–4736.

Chrobak, J.J. and Buzsáki, G. (1998). Operational dynamics in the hippocampal–entorhinal axis. *Neuroscience and Biobehavioral Reviews*, **22**, 303–310.

Curran, T. (1999). The electrophysiology of incidental and intentional retrieval: ERP old/new effects in lexical decision and recognition memory. *Neuropsychologia*, **37**, 771–785.

Curran, T. (2000). Brain potentials of recollection and familiarity. *Memory and Cognition*, **28**, 923–938.

Dale, A.M., Liu, A.K., Fischl, B.R., *et al.* (2000). Dynamic statistical parametric mapping: combining fMRI and MEG for high-resolution imaging of cortical activity. *Neuron*, **26**, 55–67.

Düzel, E., Yonelinas, A.P., Mangun, G.R., Heinze, H.J., and Tulving, E. (1997). Event-related brain potential correlates of two states of conscious awareness in memory. *Proceedings of the National Academy of Sciences of the United States of America*, **94**, 5973–5978.

Düzel, E., Cabeza, R., Yonelinas, A.P., *et al.* (1999). Task-related and item-related brain processes of memory retrieval. *Proceedings of the National Academy of Sciences of the United States of America*, **96**, 1794–1799.

Düzel, E., Vargha-Khadem, F., Heinze, H.J., and Mishkin, M. (2001). Brain activity evidence for recognition without recollection after early hippocampal damage. *Proceedings of the National Academy of Sciences of the United States of America*, **98**, 8101–8106.

Düzel, E., Habib, R., Schott, B., *et al.* (2003). A multivariate, spatiotemporal anaylsis of electromagnetic time-frequency data of recognition memory. *NeuroImage*, **18**, 185–1 97.

Düzel, E., Neufang, M., and Heinze, H.J. (2005). The oscillatory dynamics of recognition memory and its relationship to event-related responses. *Cerebral Cortex*, in press.

Eichenbaum, H., Schoenbaum, G., Young, B., and Bunsey, M. (1996). Functional organization of the hippocampal memory system. *Proceedings of the National Academy of Sciences of the United States of America*, **93**, 13500–13507.

Eldridge, L.L., Knowlton, B.J., Furmanski, C.S., Bookheimer, S.Y., and Engel, S.A. (2000). Remembering episodes: a selective role for the hippocampus during retrieval. *Nature Neuroscience*, **3**, 1149–1152.

Elger, C.E., Grunwald, T., Lehnertz, K., *et al.* (1997). Human temporal lobe potentials in verbal learning and memory processes. *Neuropsychologia*, **35**, 657–667.

Engel, A.K., Fries, P., and Singer, W. (2001). Dynamic predictions: oscillations and synchrony in top-down processing. *Nature Reviews Neuroscience*, **2**, 704–716.

Fell, J., Klaver, P., Elfadil, H., Schaller, C., Elger, C.E., and Fernandez, G. (2003). Rhinal–hippocampal theta coherence during declarative memory formation: interaction with gamma synchronization? *European Journal of Neuroscience*, **17**, 1082–1088.

Fernandez, G., Effern, A., Grunwald, T., *et al.* (1999). Real-time tracking of memory formation in the human rhinal cortex and hippocampus. *Science*, **285**, 1582–1585.

Green, J.D. and Arduini, A.A. (1954). Hippocampal electrical activity in arousal. *Journal of Neurophysiology*, **17**, 533–547.

Grunwald, T., Lehnertz, K., Heinze, H.J., Helmstaedter, C., and Elger, C.E. (1998). Verbal novelty detection within the human hippocampus proper. *Proceedings of the National Academy of Sciences of the United States of America*, **95**, 3193–3197.

Guderian, S., and Düzel, E. (2005). Induced theta oscillations mediate large scale synchrony with mediotemporal areas during recollection in humans. *Hippocampus*, **15**, 901–912.

Guillery, R.W. and Sherman, S.M. (2002). Thalamic relay functions and their role in corticocortical communication: generalizations from the visual system. *Neuron*, **33**, 163–175.

Heit, G., Smith, M.E., and Halgren, E. (1990). Neuronal activity in the human medial temporal lobe during recognition memory. *Brain*, **113**, 1093–1112.

Hillyard, S.A. (1985). Electrophysiology of human selective attention. *Trends in Neurosciences*, **8**, 400–405.

Hoffman, K.L. and McNaughton, B.L. (2002). Coordinated reactivation of distributed memory traces in primate neocortex. *Science*, **297**, 2070–2073.

Huxter, J., Burgess, N., and O'Keefe, J. (2003). Independent rate and temporal coding in hippocampal pyramidal cells. *Nature*, **425**, 828–832.

Jacoby, L.L. and Kelley, C.M. (1992). A process-dissociation framework for investigating unconscious influences: Freudian slips, projective tests, subliminal perception, and signal detection theory. *Current Directions in Psychological Science*, **1**, 174–179.

Kahana, M.J., Sekuler, R., Caplan, J.B., Kirschen, M., and Madsen, J.R. (1999). Human theta oscillations exhibit task dependence during virtual maze navigation. *Nature*, **399**, 781–784.

Klimesch, W., Doppelmayr, M., Schwaiber, J., Winkler, T., and Gruber, W. (2000). Theta oscillations and the ERP old/new effect: independent phenomena? *Clinical Neurophysiology*, **111**, 781–793.

Klimesch, W., Doppelmayr, M., Yonelinas, A., *et al.* (2001). Theta synchronization during episodic retrieval: neural correlates of conscious awareness. *Brain Research: Cognitive Brain Research*, **12**, 33–38.

Knowlton, B.J. and Squire, L.R. (1995). Remembering and knowing: two different expressions of declarative memory. *Journal of Experimental Psychology: Learning, Memory, and Cognition*, **21**, 699–710.

Kopell, N., Ermentrout, G.B., Whittington, M.A., and Traub, R.D. (2000). Gamma rhythms and beta rhythms have different synchronization properties. *Proceedings of the National Academy of Sciences of the United States of America*, **97**, 1867–1872.

Lavenex, P. and Amaral, D.G. (2000). Hippocampal–neocortical interaction: a hierarchy of associativity. *Hippocampus*, **10**, 420–430.

Lisman, J.E. and Otmakhova, N.A. (2001). Storage, recall, and novelty detection of sequences by the hippocampus: elaborating on the SOCRATIC model to account for normal and aberrant effects of dopamine. *Hippocampus*, **11**, 551–568.

Lopes da Silva, F. (1991). Neural mechanisms underlying brain waves: from neural membranes to networks. *Electroencephalography and Clinical Neurophysiology*, **79**, 81–93.

McClelland, J.L., McNaughton, B.L., O'Reilly, R.C. (1995). Why there are complementary learning systems in the hippocampus and neocortex: insights from the successes and failures of connectionist models of learning and memory. *Psychological Review*, **102**, 419–457.

Makeig, S. (2002). Response: event-related brain dynamics—unifying brain electrophysiology. *Trends in Neurosciences*, **25**, 390.

Makeig, S., Westerfield, M., Jung, T.P., *et al.* (2002). Dynamic brain sources of visual evoked responses. *Science*, **295**, 690–694.

Mecklinger, A. (2000). Interfacing mind and brain: a neurocognitive model of recognition memory. *Psychophysiology*, **37**, 565–582.

Mehta, M.R., Lee, A.K., Wilson, M.A. (2002). Role of experience and oscillations in transforming a rate code into a temporal code. *Nature*, **417**, 741–746.

Mishkin, M., Suzuki, W.A., Gadian, D.G., and Vargha-Khadem, F. (1997). Hierarchical organization of cognitive memory. *Philosophical Transactions of the Royal Society of London, Series B, Biological Sciences*, **352**, 1461–1467.

Murray, E.A. and Bussey, T.J. (1999). Perceptual–mnemonic functions of the perirhinal cortex. *Trends in Cognitive Sciences*, **3**, 142–151.

Nishitani, N., Ikeda, A., Nagamine, T., *et al.* (1999). The role of the hippocampus in auditory processing studied by event-related electric potentials and magnetic fields in epilepsy patients before and after temporal lobectomy. *Brain*, **122**, 687–707.

Nyberg, L., Persson, J., Habib, R., *et al.* (2000). Large scale neurocognitive networks underlying episodic memory. *Journal of Cognitive Neuroscience*, **12**, 163–173.

O'Keefe, J. and Recce, M.L. (1993). Phase relationship between hippocampal place units and the EEG theta rhythm. *Hippocampus*, **3**, 317–330.

Paller, K.A. and Kutas, M. (1992). Brain potentials during memory retrieval provide neurophysiological support for the distinction between conscious recollection and priming. *Journal of Cognitive Neuroscience*, **4**, 375–391.

Paller, K.A., Kutas, M., and McIsaac, H.K. (1995). Monitoring conscious recollection via the electrical activity of the brain. *Psychological Science*, **6**, 107–111.

Penttonen, M. and Buzsáki, G. (2003). Natural logarithmic relationship between brain oscillators. *Thal Relat Sys*, **2**, 145–152.

Raghavachari, S., Kahana, M.J., Rizzuto, D.S., *et al.* (2001). Gating of human theta oscillations by a working memory task. *Journal of Neuroscience*, **21**, 3175–3183.

Rizzuto, D.S., Madsen, J.R. Bromfield, E.B., *et al.* (2003). Reset of human neocortical oscillations during a working memory task. *Proceedings of the National Academy of Sciences of the United States of America*, **100**, 7931–7936.

Rolls, E.T. (1996). A theory of hippocampal function in memory. *Hippocampus*, **6**, 601–620.

Rolls, E.T. (2000). Hippocampo-cortical and cortico-cortical backprojections. *Hippocampus*, **10**, 380–388.

Rugg, M.D., Fletcher, P.C., Allan, K., Frith, C.D., Frackowiak, R.S., and Dolan, R.J. (1998a). Neural correlates of memory retrieval during recognition memory and cued recall. *NeuroImage*, **8**, 262–273.

Rugg, M.D., Mark, R.E., Walla, P., Schloerscheidt, A.M., Birch, C.S., Allan, K. (1998b). Dissociation of the neural correlates of implicit and explicit memory. *Nature*, **392**, 595–598.

Schack, B., Vath, N., Petsche, H., Geissler, H.G., and Moller, E. (2002). Phase-coupling of theta–gamma EEG rhythms during short-term memory processing. *International Journal of Psychophysiology*, **44**, 143–163.

Schroeder, C.E., Steinschneider, M., Javitt, D.C., *et al.* (1995). Localization of ERP generators and identification of underlying neural processes. *Electroencephalography and Clinical Neurophysiology*, **44** (Suppl), 55–75.

Sederberg, P.B., Kahana, M.J., Howard, M.W., Donner, E.J., and Madsen, E.R. (2003). Theta and gamma oscillations during encoding predict subsequent recall. *Journal of Neuroscience*, **23**, 10809–10814.

Shah, A.S., Bressler, S.L., Knuth, K.H., *et al.* (2004). Neural dynamics and the fundamental mechanisms of event-related brain potentials. *Cerebral Cortex*, **14**, 476–483.

Sherman, S.M. and Guillery, R.W. (1998). On the actions that one nerve cell can have on another: distinguishing drivers from modulators. *Proceedings of the National Academy of Sciences of the United States of America*, **95**, 7121–7126.

Smith, M.E. and Halgren, E. (1987). Event-related potentials elicited by familiar and unfamiliar faces. *Electroencephalography and Clinical Neurophysiology*, **40** (Suppl), 422–426.

Squire, L.R. and Zola-Morgan, S. (1991). The medial temporal lobe memory system. *Science*, **253**, 1380–1386.

Steriade, M. (2000). Corticothalamic resonance, states of vigilance and mentation. *Neuroscience*, **101**, 243–276.

Sutherland, G.R. and McNaughton, B. (2000). Memory trace reactivation in hippocampal and neocortical neuronal ensembles. *Current Opinion in Neurobiology*, **10**, 180–186.

Tallon-Baudry, C. and Bertrand, O. (1999). Oscillatory gamma activity in humans and its role in object representation. *Trends in Cognitive Sciences*, **3**, 151–162.

Tendolkar, I., Rugg, M., Fell, J., *et al.* (2000). A magnetoencephalographic study of brain activity related to recognition memory in healthy young human subjects. *Neuroscience Letters*, **280**, 69–72.

Treves, A. and Rolls, E.T. (1994). Computational analysis of the role of the hippocampus in memory. *Hippocampus*, **4**, 374–391.

Tulving, E. (1985). Memory and consciousness. *Canadian Psychology*, **26**, 1–12.

Vanderwolf, C.H. (1969). *Electroencephalography and Clinical Neurophysiology*, **26**, 407–418.

Varela, F., Lachaux, J.P., Rodriguez, E., and Martinerie, J. (2001). The brainweb: phase synchronization and large-scale integration. *Nature Reviews Neuroscience*, **2**, 229–239.

Vargha-Khadem, F., Gadian, D.G., Watkins, K.E., Connelly, A., Van Paesschen, W., and Mishkin, M. (1997). Differential effects of early hippocampal pathology on episodic and semantic memory [see comments]. *Science*, **277**, 376–380 (Erratum. *Science*, **277**, 1117, 1997).

von Stein, A., Chiang, C., and König, P. (2000). Top-down processing mediated by interareal synchronization. *Proceedings of the National Academy of Sciences of the United States of America*, **97**, 14748–14753.

Wheeler, M.E., Petersen, S.E., and Buckner, R.L. (2000). Memory's echo: vivid remembering reactivates sensory-specific cortex. *Proceedings of the National Academy of Sciences of the United States of America*, **97**, 11125–11129.

Wilding, E. (2000). In what way does the parietal ERP old/new effect index recollection? *International Journal of Psychophysiology*, **35**, 81–87.

Yonelinas, A.P. and Levy, B.J. (2002). Dissociating familiarity from recollection in human recognition memory: different rates of forgetting over short retention intervals. *Psychon Bull Rev*, **9**, 575–582.

Yonelinas, A.P., Dobbins, I., Szymanski, M.D., Dhaliwal, H.S., and King, L. (1996). Signal-detection, threshold, and dual process models of recognition memory: ROCs and conscious recollection. *Consciousness and Cognition*, **5**, 418–441.

Yonelinas, A.P., Kroll, N.E., Szymanski, Dobbins, I., Lazzara, M., and Knight, R.T. (1998). Recollection and familiarity deficits in amnesia: convergence of remember–know, process dissociation, and receiver operating characteristic data. *Neuropsychology*, **12**, 323–339.

Yonelinas, A.P., Kroll, N.E., Quamme, J.R., *et al.* (2002). Effects of extensive temporal lobe damage or mild hypoxia on recollection and familiarity. *Nature Neuroscience*, **5**, 1236–1241.

Yonelinas, A.P., Otten, L.J., Shaw, K.N., and Rugg, M.D. (2005). Separating the brain regions involved in recollection and familiarity in recognition memory. *Journal of Neuroscience*, **25**, 3002–3008.

Chapter 7

Rhinal–hippocampal contribution to declarative memory formation

Guillén Fernández and Jürgen Fell

Background

Declarative memory enables conscious recollection of past events and facts (Gabrieli 1998). Thus it is the kind of memory one ordinarily means when using the term 'memory'. Neuropsychological assessment of patients with circumscribed lesions has firmly linked declarative memory to the medial temporal lobe (MTL) (Scoville and Milner 1957). Indeed, studies of brain-injured patients have formed one of the foundations of cognitive neuroscience, defining different memory systems and their neuroanatomical constituents. However, human lesion studies are usually based on a permanent dysfunction; hence they cannot clearly differentiate between the effects that brain damage has on transient memory processes like encoding (learning), consolidation (storage), and retrieval (recall). Only in recent years has the application of neuroimaging techniques narrowed the gap between knowledge about memory systems and their processes. In particular, considerable progress has been made towards identifying regional brain activity related to the successful building of new memories (Brewer *et al.* 1998; Fernández *et al.* 1998; Wagner *et al.* 1998). An impressive aspect of current developments on this topic is the convergence of evidence from various methods, including neuropsychology, functional brain imaging, and *in vivo* electrophysiology.

Here, we summarize electrophysiological studies of declarative memory formation using depth electrodes implanted in the MTL in epilepsy patients prior to epilepsy surgery. This experimental approach provides a unique opportunity to monitor quasi-normal human brain activity directly, in real time, within distinct MTL subcomponents and with a signal-to-noise ratio far superior to any other neuroimaging technique currently available. Our results reflect that invasive electrophysiology can both localize and characterize brain processes that are important in determining what is remembered and what is forgotten. Thereby we describe insights into the temporal organization of memory formation and the interaction that occurs between substructures of the MTL during this mnemonic operation.

In temporal lobe epilepsy, which is the most common form of drug-resistant focal epilepsy, it is sometimes necessary to insert bilateral depth electrodes into the MTL to define the zone of seizure origin prior to resective surgery. If seizures are proved to originate unilaterally, contralateral electrodes enable MTL activity unrelated to epilepsy to be recorded. Usually depth electrodes with several contacts are implanted, thus enabling separate recordings within the hippocampus and the anterior parahippocampal gyrus (van Roost *et al.* 1998), which is covered by the ento- and perirhinal cortex. This unique approach to the human MTL has been used in memory research since the early 1980s. Initially, mnemonic operations during recognition (Smith *et al.* 1986), perception of stimulus deviance (Halgren *et al.* 1980), and perception of stimulus novelty (Grunwald *et al.* 1998) have been investigated. Recently, mnemonic operations during the formation of new declarative memories have been the subject of depth EEG studies.

How do brain processes that occur during an experience that will be remembered differ from those occurring during an experience that will be forgotten? To address this question directly a comparison between learning events that lead to the successful and unsuccessful formation of memories is required. Such comparisons have been made using event-related potential (ERP) and event-related functional MRI (fMRI) techniques. The experimental logic employed in these studies is identical in each case: brain activity is recorded for every study item, and contrasts are conducted to compare items that are remembered with those that are forgotten as measured by a subsequent memory test. Thus the difference in brain activity between subsequently remembered and forgotten items represents a subsequent memory effect (Sanquist *et al.* 1980) and may be due to memory formation (the dm effect) (Paller 1990).

Medial temporal memory processes

In line with the experimental logic discussed above, Fernández *et al.* (1999a) investigated MTL processes utilizing intra-cerebrally recorded ERPs. During each of 20 study test blocks, patients were initially asked to memorize visually presented words. Following a distraction task, they were required to recall memorized words freely. This procedure makes great demands on declarative memory.

In recordings from within the anterior parahippocampal gyrus, words elicited a large negative potential, peaking about 440 ms after stimulus onset. This potential has been identified in previous studies using verbal stimuli and is referred to as anterior MTL-N400 or AMTL-N400 (McCarthy *et al.* 1995). The AMTL-N400 began to differ about 310 ms after stimulus onset, with subsequently recalled words generating a larger potential than words that were later forgotten. This subsequent memory effect exhibited a steep voltage gradient over the neighbouring electrode contacts and a phase reversal at temporal basal recording sites. Steep voltage gradients and phase reversals indicate that this effect was generated in the cortex covering the anterior parahippocampal gyrus, which is the ento- and perirhinal cortex. Although McCarthy *et al.* (1995) suggested the perirhinal cortex as the generator of the AMTL-N400, we believe that the methods used do not allow a clear distinction between a perirhinal and an entorhinal generator. Hence we suggest using the more general term rhinal cortex.

Within the hippocampus, ERPs elicited by subsequently recalled and unrecalled words separated reliably from about 500 ms to the end of the averaging epoch 2000 ms after stimulus onset. This subsequent memory effect had a positive polarity and was detectable within, but not immediately outside, the hippocampus. Hippocampal neurons are arranged cylindrically. Hence they produce a radially symmetric field that is closed in the sense of being isopotentially zero outside the hippocampus (Klee and Rall 1977). Thus this subsequent memory effect was generated within the hippocampus proper.

A functional connection between the rhinal and hippocampal subsequent memory effects was suggested by the positive correlation between their effect sizes. Together with the sequential onset of the subsequent memory effects, the correlation between their sizes provides compelling evidence for interrelated and sequentially occurring processes related to declarative memory formation within the human MTL. This proposal of a serially organized MTL memory system (Mishkin *et al.* 1997) is also supported by neuroanatomical findings which demonstrate a serial connectivity within the MTL subregions; efferents enter the MTL primarily via the perirhinal and parahippocampal cortices, providing the major input to the entorhinal cortex, which in turn provides the main input to the hippocampus (Witter *et al.* 1989).

Although subsequent memory effects are based on a correlation between brain activity at encoding and subsequent memory performance, the precise nature of the underlying operations remains to be elucidated. Moreover, given the histoanatomical differences between the rhinal cortex and the hippocampus (Amaral and Witter 1989), we cannot assume that the two subsequent memory effects identified within the MTL are correlates of brain processes subserving the very same operation in declarative memory formation.

To explore the specific contribution of the rhinal cortex and the hippocampus to declarative memory formation, Fernández and colleagues performed a follow-up study in which they contrasted MTL depth ERPs during word memorization with high and low word frequency (Fernández *et al.* 2002b). Frequency of word usage is a powerful determinant of the efficiency of its processing in a range of laboratory tasks. For instance, high-frequency words show an advantage over low-frequency words in subsequent free recall tests. In general, accounts of word frequency effects in free recall have assumed that they largely reflect the relative ease with which words of differing frequencies access their stored lexical representation (Gordon 1983). Common words have richer semantic contexts than uncommon words (Gregg 1976) and are more meaningful (Noble 1963); hence they give rise to more associative responses with shorter response times (Cofer and Shevitz 1952; Noble 1963). During memory encoding, high-frequency words are easy to interrelate to one another because they tend to possess more associations with other words in semantic memory (Rubin and Friendly 1986). This relationship between word frequency and semantic associative processing may lead to the free recall advantage of high-frequency words (Gregg 1976). Hence a neural correlate of successful memory formation in a study with a free recall advantage, which occurs for high-frequency but not for low-frequency words, suggests a support operation which is related to item properties, but which is not an exclusively mnemonic operation. However, a subsequent memory effect unrelated to word frequency suggests a difference in the quality of encoding rather than in item properties. Thus it may indicate an exclusively mnemonic operation of declarative memory formation, which is insensitive to item content.

Each patient participated in a direct single-trial word-list learning paradigm similar to the paradigm described (Fernández *et al.* 1999a). In contrast with the initial experiment, the word lists were shorter and consisted of an equal mixture of high- and low-frequency words. High-frequency words tended to be accompanied by a larger AMTL-N400 in the rhinal cortex compared with low-frequency words. The AMTL-N400 exhibited a typical subsequent memory effect for high-frequency words, but not for low-frequency words. In hippocampal recordings, subsequently recalled words were accompanied by a more positive ERP component in the late time window (600 ms after stimulus onset) than forgotten words. This component exhibited neither a main effect nor an interaction with word frequency.

Hence the ERPs associated with high-frequency words replicate the initial findings, also utilizing common words (Fernández *et al.* 1999a). However, the newly introduced manipulation of word frequency broke up the positive correlation between the sizes of the rhinal and the hippocampal subsequent memory effects. Low-frequency words did not trigger a subsequent memory effect at the AMTL-N400. Nevertheless, they were accompanied by a hippocampal subsequent memory effect in the same way as high-frequency words. The interactions between word frequency and recall rates as well as between word frequency and the rhinal subsequent memory effect at the AMTL-N400 indicate that an operation executed by the rhinal cortex facilitates declarative memory formation indirectly. All words, irrespectively of frequency, seem to undergo this operation, because all words were accompanied by an AMTL-N400. However, high-frequency words with a rich semantic context seem to stimulate more elaborate processing in the rhinal cortex, which leads to more effective memory formation. Thus the subordinate rhinal cortex might feed the hippocampus with useful representations of the environment and perform a support operation in the semantic domain during declarative memory formation. This operation appears to make semantic representations of each study item available in the service of comprehension, semantic-associative processing, and memory formation (Craik and Lockhart 1972; Nobre and McCarthy 1995). In contrast, the hippocampal subsequent memory effect did not interact with word frequency. Hence it may be a correlate of an exclusively mnemonic operation within the declarative memory system which might use rhinal input, but which is not influenced by stimulus properties like word frequency or resulting processes. Rather, it might initiate the biochemical cascade underlying synaptic plasticity—the presumed correlate of memory at the cellular level (Huang *et al.* 1996.).

To summarize, evidence was found for specific and interrelated processes within the hippocampus and the rhinal cortex, which together subserve declarative memory formation. At least for high-frequency words, the positive correlation of dm effects suggests an interaction between the two structures (Fernández *et al.* 1999a). However, direct evidence for a mechanism enabling a transient rhinal–hippocampal interaction is still lacking. In the next section we discuss why phase synchronization of gamma EEG activity may provide such a mechanism.

Neural coupling via synchronized gamma activity

Feature binding

Different features of a perceptual object are processed in different submodules of the perceptual systems, for example in the visual system colour in V4 and motion in MT (V5). Hence each sensory submodule contains a complete map of the respective feature. A central neuroscientific problem is how these different aspects are bound together in one coherent representation of the perceived object (feature integration). This problem has been called the binding problem. A more specialized aspect of the binding problem is the question of how visual scenes are spatially segmented into different objects (perceptual segmentation).

Historically, the first hypothesis attempting to explain the binding problem was the model of cardinal neurons. In this model complex information is represented in the brain by convergence of the processing stream to highly specified assemblies or even single neurons. However, this model was unable to explain why objects which are perceived for the first time are obviously processed instantaneously by the brain. Moreover, this kind of representation would be very costly and there would not be enough neurons in the brain to account for the enormous number of possible feature combinations. Similar problems arise when firing rate is added as another coding dimension.

Because of the shortcomings of the cardinal cell hypothesis, at the beginning of the 1980s another binding mechanism was proposed (von der Malsburg 1981; von der Malsburg and Schneider 1986). This model assumes a coding mechanism that relies on time-based coding. The idea is that associated neurons or neural assemblies are characterized by synchronous action potentials. In this way even neurons with the same firing rate could be distinguished by the timing of their discharges. Since neurons could participate in different transient assemblies via slight changes in their action potential timing, this mechanism would be fast and flexible and would enable a very large number of feature combinations. The simultaneous firing of action potentials of associated neurons or assemblies would correspond to phase-synchronous oscillations in the domain of field potentials and EEG.

Experimental evidence supporting the feature-binding hypothesis was first reported at the end of the 1980s. Synchronization of intracranially recorded gamma activity (20–80 Hz) was observed in the visual cortex of anaesthetized cats when they were presented with coherent moving bars rather than independently moving patterns (Eckhorn *et al.* 1988; Gray *et al.* 1989). This effect could not be attributed to local connectivity because the synchronously firing assemblies corresponded to non-overlapping receptive fields. Later, analogous findings were reported for intracranial recordings from awake monkeys (Frien *et al.* 1994; Kreiter and Singer 1996). With similar experimental paradigms an amplitude enhancement of occipital gamma activity was observed in human scalp EEG recordings (Lutzenberger *et al.* 1995; Müller *et al.* 1996). Since it is not possible to separate local synchronization from amplitude effects in scalp recordings, this amplitude enhancement could have been caused by increased phase synchronization in the gamma range. Moreover, correlated firing and synchronized gamma activity has been shown to extend across the border of a single visual area. Phase synchronization of gamma activity related to stimulus features has been reported between V1 and V2 (Frien *et al.* 1994), between V1 and the posterio-medial lateral suprasylvian (PLMS) area, which is an extrastriate motion area (Engel *et al.* 1991a), and between V1 areas belonging to different hemispheres (Engel *et al.* 1991b).

Stimulus-specific phase synchronization of induced gamma oscillations has been observed not only in the visual domain, but also within the somatosensory system (Lebedev and Nelson 1995) and the olfactory system (Freeman 1978; Bressler 1987). Moreover it has been shown that odour discrimination deteriorates in insects when desynchronization is chemically induced in neurons of the olfactory bulb, thus yielding direct proof of the functional synchronization hypothesis (Stopfer *et al.* 1997).

A general mechanism

In principle, two types of gamma-band activity occurring in response to sensory stimuli can be differentiated. First, the evoked response is observed up to 150 ms after stimulus presentation. Since it is precisely time locked to the stimulus it can be analysed by simple averaging in the time domain. The evoked response is followed by induced gamma activity, which occurs in a non-time-locked fashion. In simple visual detection tasks, for example, induced gamma activity can be observed in a time range of up to 400 ms after stimulus onset (Tallon-Baudry and Bertrand 1999). The non-phase-locked jittering induced response cancels out in the time-domain average and therefore has to be analysed by frequency-domain approaches based on evaluation of single trials. The findings of stimulus-specific synchronization described above are related to induced gamma activity.

Induced synchronized gamma activity also appears to be important for perceptual selection, as has been reported in the context of binocular rivalry where the images presented to the two eyes are incoherent and cannot be fused to one percept (Engel *et al.* 1999). Under these conditions only information corresponding to one of the two eyes is selected and perceived, and information from the other eye is suppressed. Thus the perceived image alternates between the two eyes. It was found that firing rate changes, which are correlated with the dominant percept, mainly occur in the higher areas of visual processing, whereas the correlations with discharge rates within the lower visual processing areas are not conclusive (Leopold and Logothetis 1999). However, a pronounced increase of phase synchronization of gamma oscillations has been observed in the lower visual areas (V1 and V2) of cats, which correlates with the dominant percept under binocular rivalry (Fries *et al.* 1997, 2002). This could mean that in a first step synchronized gamma activity emerges in lower visual areas. Afterwards these synchronized assemblies may trigger target neurons in higher visual areas and cause changes in firing rates in these areas.

Several studies suggest an involvement of synchronized gamma activity in attentional processes (reviewed by Fell *et al.* 2003a). With respect to visual selective attention, an enhancement of scalp-recorded gamma activity was reported when subjects attended to a certain stimulus or when they perceived a gestalt (Gruber *et al.* 1999; Müller *et al.* 2000). In intracranial recordings from area V4 in monkeys increased gamma range synchronization and reduced low-frequency synchronization in attended compared with unattended visual stimuli was observed (Fries *et al.* 2001a). The enhancement of gamma synchronization reported in this study was not accompanied by simultaneous increases of firing rates. Therefore synchronization of spike discharges in the gamma range seems to be a mechanism supporting selective attention and perceptual selection, which is independent of firing rate modulation. Increased phase synchronization in the gamma range has also been reported in a selective somatosensory attention task in humans (Desmedt and Tomberg 1994). Moreover, shifts in attention between a visual and a tactile task have been observed to be correlated with changes in the degree of synchronization of neural firing within the somatosensory cortex of monkeys (Steinmetz *et al.* 2000).

Recently, gamma synchronization was reported to be involved in the cognitive integration of visual face perception and task-related motor responses (Rodriguez *et al.* 1999). It was suggested that subsequent phase desynchronization dissolved the connection between two structures and hence terminated perceptual or cognitive operations (Rodriguez *et al.* 1999). To summarize, the above findings point to the view that gamma synchronization is not confined to the visual cortex, nor is its function restricted to object representation and feature binding. Rather, phase synchronization of gamma activity appears to represent a general mechanism enabling a transient association of cortical assemblies (reviewed by Engel and Singer 2001; Varela *et al.* 2001). This mechanism seems to provide effective coupling and decoupling within, as well as between, different subsystems of the brain.

Assembly formation

As early as 1949, Hebb proposed a flexible mechanism for the formation of functional associated neural assemblies. He postulated an increase in synaptic efficacy in the case of correlated activity of the pre- and post-synaptic neurons. In simple terms, he proposed that neurons that fire together, wire together. This kind of

'Hebbian' synaptic plasticity has been experimentally verified and was found to depend on the interaction between post-synaptic potentials and action potentials back propagating into the dendrite of the post-synaptic neuron (Magee and Johnston 1997; Markram *et al.* 1997). The best investigated examples of Hebbian plasticity are long-term potentiation (LTP) and long-term depotentiation (LTD), which provide the basis for most models of learning and memory. Moreover, Hebbian plasticity represents a mechanism for the refinement of initially imprecise neural connections during ontogenetic development. However, different types of spike-timing-dependent synaptic plasticity are now known. Simultaneous firing of pre- and post-synaptic neurons in some types of synapses may even result in a decrease in synaptic efficacy. In other types of synapses potentiation or depotentiation may depend on the sign of the delay between pre- and post-synaptic action potentials (Abbott and Nelson 2000).

In the present case, the dynamics of neurons within the hippocampus and rhinal cortex are of interest, particularly GABA-ergic neurons which are capable of producing gamma oscillations (Traub *et al.* 1999). *In vitro* recordings of GABA-ergic neurons in hippocampal culture exhibited Hebbian potentiation of synaptic connections when pre- and post-synaptic neurons fire simultaneously (Abbott and Nelson 2000). More precisely, the required delay times for effective Hebbian potentiation in this case are of the order of less than ± 10 ms. Synchronization of gamma oscillations has been shown to enable such precise timing of neural action potentials (Engel and Singer 2001; Fries *et al.* 2001b; Varela *et al.* 2001). Thus synchronized high-frequency EEG rhythms like gamma activity could provide optimal conditions for the establishment of Hebbian neural assemblies and may be a crucial mechanism in associative learning and memory formation (Fernández *et al.* 2002a). This view is supported by recent neural network model studies (Sommer and Wennekers 2001). Indeed, in an associative learning experiment increased gamma-band coherence between scalp EEG from visual and somatosensory areas has been reported (Miltner *et al.* 1999).

Hebbian assembly formation also implicates the recruitment of target neurons which have been triggered and forced into synchronous activity. Members of neural assemblies that are synchronized in the gamma range fire action potentials in a highly time-locked manner with a precision of a few milliseconds. When these action potentials are propagated to common target neurons they can cooperate in elevating the membrane potential above firing threshold (von der Malsburg 1999). This cooperation does not occur for incoming action potentials that are not time locked, since the membrane potential decays depending on membrane time constants. Thus synchronized neural assemblies can reliably trigger activity in target neurons. For example, modification of synaptic connections to target neurons owing to synchronized afferent firing has been found to be crucial for the development of ocular dominance columns in the striate cortex (Goodman and Shatz 1993). Thus synchronized gamma activity may also play an important role in the segregation of different paths of neural processing.

Rhinal–hippocampal interaction in memory formation

Because of the significance of synchronized gamma activity for assembly formation and transient assembly coupling (described above) we wondered whether these mechanisms may take part in mediotemporal memory processes. In particular, we hypothesized that a direct interaction between the rhinal cortex and the hippocampus in declarative memory formation may be accomplished by phase synchronization of gamma activity between these two structures.

To test this hypothesis, EEG was acquired from MTL depth electrodes (see above) in nine patients with pharmacoresistant temporal lobe epilepsy while they performed a single-trial word-list learning paradigm with a free recall test (Fell *et al.* 2001). To compare successful and unsuccessful memory encoding EEG was separated offline into segments for subsequently recalled and unrecalled study items. EEG was then wavelet filtered in the gamma frequency range 32–48 Hz (2-Hz steps). Since we investigated induced gamma activity, i.e. gamma activity occurring in a non-time-locked fashion in response to the stimuli, analysis was based on single-trial evaluations (Tallon-Baudry and Bertrand 1999). Phase synchronization values derived from the measure of circular variance (Mardia 1972) between electrode contacts within the rhinal cortex and the hippocampus were calculated from the individual wavelet-transformed EEG segments. The higher the synchronization value, the more constant is the phase difference between the two electrodes over all trials. Additionally, averaged power values were determined separately for rhinal and hippocampal recordings for subsequently recalled and unrecalled words. Finally, synchronization and power values were averaged for consecutive 100-ms time windows from −100 ms to 1500 ms relative to stimulus onset.

Dissociation of phase synchronization curves of subsequently recalled compared with unrecalled words starts within the first 100 ms after stimulus onset. Average gamma synchronization between rhinal and hippocampal recordings was found to be significantly increased by up to 16 per cent for subsequently recalled as opposed to subsequently forgotten words from 100 up to 300 ms. After the early enhancement in gamma synchronization a second increase was detected from 500 to 600 ms, and finally a significant decrease was observed from 1000 to 1100 ms. With respect to the individual analysed frequencies within the gamma band, the early synchronization effect was most pronounced in the frequency range 36–40 Hz (increase of up to 30 per cent for recalled versus unrecalled items). Phase lag distributions for both conditions (subsequently recalled and unrecalled words) had a Gaussian shape and were centred around zero. The difference in synchronization for successful and unsuccessful encoding was based on a narrowing of the phase lag distribution caused by an increased amount of phase differences close to zero. This finding indicates that rhinal and hippocampal neurons oscillate together in a more synchronous rhythm when encoding yields remembering. The observation of a zero phase lag seems to be surprising at the first sight, since a conduction delay between rhinal and hippocampal neurons must be assumed, given the slow speed of axonal conduction. However, oscillatory activity is predictive, and thus a zero phase lag has also been reported in other connectivity studies, for instance in an investigation of long-range synchronization of gamma activity (Rodriguez *et al.* 1999). Indeed, it has been demonstrated that a simple model implementing realistic conditions can produce synchronous gamma oscillations with zero phase lag (Traub *et al.* 1996). This model incorporates a chain of networks of neurons which fire pairs of spikes in rapid succession.

Absolute gamma power values at hippocampal sites were about threefold larger compared with rhinal recordings. At both hippocampal and rhinal sites, gamma power was reduced for subsequently recalled compared with unrecalled words. In rhinal recordings, significant reductions were observed between 600 and 800 ms and between 1300 and 1400 ms after word presentation. In hippocampal recordings, significantly diminished gamma power in EEG segments related to successful as opposed to unsuccessful memory formation was detected between 100 and 400 ms after stimulus onset.

These results represented the first description of EEG activity in the gamma frequency range in field recordings from within the human hippocampus during a memory task. An earlier study (Hirai *et al.* 1999) had revealed a generally higher gamma power in rhinal than neocortical recordings in humans. This knowledge was extended by showing that gamma power in hippocampal recordings is threefold higher than in rhinal recordings, suggesting that high-frequency oscillations of around 40 Hz play a prominent role in medial temporal, and especially hippocampal, information processing. Intracranial EEG recordings allow the reliable separation of synchronization and power effects. In view of the anatomical proximity of the areas inspected (distances in the range of 1 cm), such a separation would be impossible with surface EEG recordings (Bullock *et al.* 1995; Menon *et al.* 1996).

The time course of modulation of gamma synchronization found in this study is consistent with reports of altered firing rates of single MTL neurons within 200 ms after visual object presentation (Kreiman *et al.* 2000). However, it remained unclear whether or not semantic information provided by each stimulus is already available during the initiation of rhinal–hippocampal coupling. If not, directed attention might, in a first step, allocate specific connections necessary for memory formation before actual information transfer takes place. Attention-driven enhancement of gamma-band phase synchronization has been shown in several studies. Here, rhinal–hippocampal coupling might be initiated by a top-down process (LaBerge 1997) mediated by direct anatomical connections between the thalamus and MTL (Amaral and Insausti 1990). The later decrease in synchronization (1000–1100 ms) may occur following information transfer from the rhinal cortex to the hippocampus (Fernández *et al.* 1999a) and terminate the communication between the two structures. Such a functional decoupling has been termed active desynchronization (Rodriguez *et al.* 1999).

Rhinal–hippocampal coupling starts about 200 ms earlier than the ERP subsequent memory effect recorded from the rhinal cortex, but its course fits well with the sequence of processes as monitored by ERPs recorded separately from the rhinal cortex and hippocampus during the same task (Fernández *et al.* 1999a). The early phase of rhinal–hippocampal coupling might be based on a preparatory mechanisms driven by thalamo-cortical connections and under attentional control (LaBerge 1997). Rhinal ERPs to subsequently recalled words start to differ from ERPs to subsequently forgotten words about 300 ms after stimulus onset. This subsequent memory effect in the rhinal cortex is followed by a hippocampal effect some 200 ms later, which lasts until about 2000 ms after stimulus onset (see above). Assuming that rhinal–hippocampal information transfer occurs between the onset of the rhinal and the hippocampal ERP effects, the gamma phase coupling revealed in this study would allow the actual transfer of information after preparation. The decoupling observed follows the end of the rhinal subsequent memory effect at about 900 ms after stimulus onset, the time point when information transfer to the hippocampus might be accomplished. A further interpretation of these findings could be that the early increase of rhinal–hippocampal gamma synchronization may enable the formation of transient Hebbian synaptic connections, which are later dissolved. These transient Hebbian connections may prepare the paths of information transfer between neural assemblies within the rhinal cortex and associated assemblies within the hippocampus.

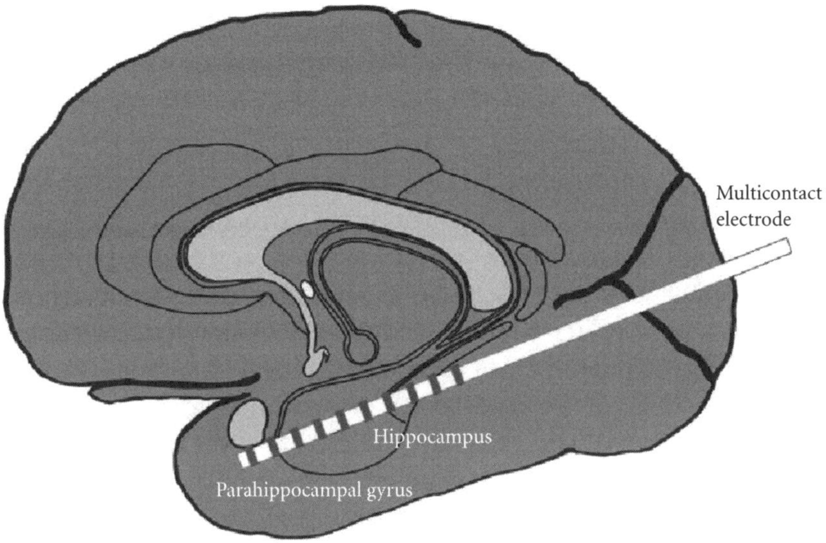

Figure 7.1 Schematic diagram of a parasagittal section at the MTL with a multicontact depth electrode in place.

Efficient medial temporal information processing, leading to successful memory formation, was found to be correlated with reduced gamma power at both recording sites. Together with the previous finding of generally much higher gamma power in the MTL (Hirai *et al.* 1999), the transient reduction of gamma oscillations might be explained by the necessity to suppress noise-like ambient gamma activity unrelated to specific study items. It might be speculated that, in the event of unsuccessful encoding, ongoing background gamma activity interferes with item-related activity and distorts the process of memory formation. Thus reduced gamma power during successful encoding might be a correlate of a higher specificity of local assembly activation.

To summarize, these results suggest that gamma-band noise reduction and appropriate neural coupling and decoupling interact in declarative memory formation within the human MTL. These data do not exclude a third pacemaker site driving phase-locked gamma activity in the rhinal cortex and hippocampus independently from each other. However, the strong anatomical connections between the two structures (Amaral and Insausti 1990) support the hypothesis of a direct rhinal–hippocampal interaction underlying gamma-band phase coupling and decoupling. Thus these findings are in line with models (Buzsáki 1996) proposing that building new declarative memories requires a direct cooperation between the rhinal cortex and the hippocampus.

Cooperation between theta and gamma oscillations in memory formation

In articles discussing the findings on rhinal–hippocampal gamma synchronization described above it has been asked (Wagner 2001; Otten and Rugg 2002) whether the same data show evidence for memory-related coherent theta activity that additionally might functionally bind the two MTL structures together. A significant function of theta oscillations in declarative memory formation has been suggested by previous scalp EEG studies showing an increase in theta power as well as inter- and intra-hemispheric theta coherence in the case of successful word encoding (Klimesch *et al.* 1996, 1997; Weiss *et al.* 2000; Weiss and Rappelsberger 2000; Mölle *et al.* 2002). Moreover, subdural recordings in epilepsy patients and MEG studies have indicated that the occurrence of theta activity is related to spatial learning and working memory tasks (Kahana *et al.* 1999; Tesche and Karhu 2000; Caplan *et al.* 2001; Raghavachari *et al.* 2001; Jensen and Tesche 2002). Experimental animal literature provides substantial evidence connecting hippocampal theta activity with declarative memory (reviewed by Vertes and Kocsis 1997; Berry and Seager 2001; Kahana *et al.* 2001; Lisman and Otmakhova 2001). However, no human data on hippocampal theta during a declarative memory task have yet been reported.

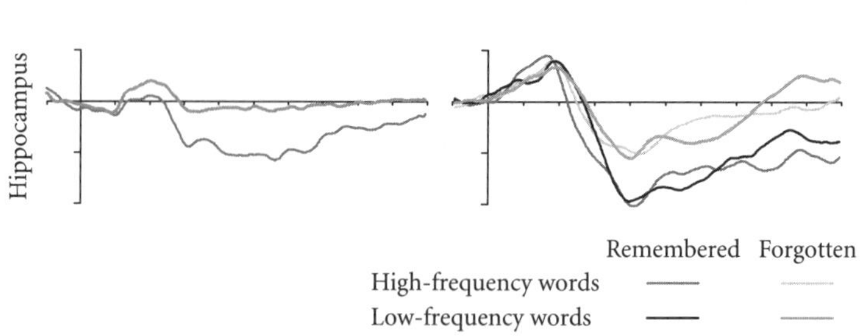

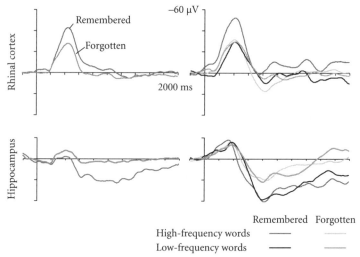

Figure 7.2 ERP data from a contact recording from the rhinal cortex with the maximal AMTL-N400 and from a contact recording from within the hippocampus with the maximal late positive component, separately averaged. ERPs are depicted as grand averages of raw data. Left: remembered versus forgotten words. Right: remembered versus forgotten × high-frequency versus low-frequency words (Fernández *et al.* 1999a, 2002b).

Therefore in a subsequent study (Fell *et al.* 2003b) we investigated whether hippocampal and rhinal theta oscillations contribute to human declarative memory formation (theta hypothesis). We reanalysed the intracranial recordings described above by evaluating rhinal–hippocampal EEG coherence and spectral power at both locations for six frequency bands between 1 and 19 Hz including theta and neighbouring frequency bands. Spectral coherence quantifies the frequency-specific degree of linear relationship between two signals (Challis and Kitney 1991). Two factors may contribute to a high value of spectral coherence: approximately constant phase differences between the two signals across trials (phase synchronization), and parallel variations of signal amplitudes of both signals across trials (amplitude synchronization). EEG characteristics corresponding to subsequently remembered words were again compared with items which were not remembered.

The major result of this investigation was that spectral coherence between the rhinal cortex and the hippocampus exhibited a significant memory-related main effect, but no interaction with the factor frequency band. For all bands rhinal–hippocampal coherence was larger for subsequently remembered than for forgotten words. The memory-related increase in rhinal–hippocampal coherence was most pronounced for the delta and theta bands (relative increase up to 71.5 per cent). In a subanalysis, we evaluated in how much the two aspects of the coherence measure, phase and amplitude synchronization, contributed to the observed coherence enhancement. We found memory effects of similar reliability for both components of the coherence measure (significance values of similar magnitude). In contrast with the coherence results, spectral power was not significantly increased for remembered compared with forgotten words at either the rhinal or the hippocampal recording site.

To explore the regional specificity of the rhinal–hippocampal coherence increase we examined spectral coherence between the hippocampus, the rhinal cortex, and a temporolateral location (superior temporal gyrus) in the vicinity of Wernicke's area where a negative ERP component had been observed under the memorization paradigm, which was attributed to semantic and not to mnemonic processing (Fernández *et al.* 1999a). For identification of the zone of seizure onset, EEG was recorded from this location using subdural strip electrodes in six of the patients. For all frequency bands average rhinal–temporolateral and hippocampal–temporolateral coherence was three to eight times smaller than rhinal–hippocampal coherence, indicating a specifically enhanced connectivity between rhinal cortex and hippocampus. Neither a significant overall memory effect nor memory effects within the delta or theta bands were detected for rhinal–temporolateral or hippocampal–temporolateral coherence estimates.

This result supports the notion that the observed rhinal–hippocampal coherence enhancement is associated with memory-related interaction specifically between the two MTL substructures.

In addition to evidence for memory-related theta activity, several groups have observed a close cooperation between MTL gamma and theta oscillations in rodents. The two rhythms were found to be interwoven, in the sense that hippocampal gamma is amplitude modulated by theta waves (Chrobak and Buzsák 1998a,b). Moreover, it was reported that the firing of hippocampal neurons in rodents during movement through place fields depends on the phase of the theta rhythm (O'Keefe and Recce 1993; Skaggs *et al.* 1996). On the basis of these observations, it was proposed that the interaction between MTL gamma and theta rhythms plays an important role in coding declarative memories (the theta–gamma-hypothesis) (Lisman and Idiart 1995; Jensen *et al.* 1996; Jensen 2001; Lisman and Otmakhova 2001). In particular, it has been hypothesized that memory storage of multiple items is coded by distinct cycles of hippocampal gamma oscillations, as well as by the position of these cycles with respect to the theta phase.

To test the theta–gamma hypothesis, in a second step we evaluated correlations between the memory-related coherence increases in the lower frequency range and the previously reported changes in gamma synchronization, as extracted from the time and frequency range with the most prominent effects (100–200 ms, 36–40 Hz). A positive correlation was detected between memory-related alterations of gamma synchronization and theta coherence ($r = 0.80$, $P = 0.018$), but not for the other frequency bands. This correlation was robust with respect to a jackknife procedure (mean P-value, 0.024 ± 0.026). A stepwise regression analysis with the six coherence measures as independent variables and gamma synchronization as a dependent variable confirmed this result. Variance of gamma synchronization values was explained best when only theta coherence was included in the model (57.5 per cent variance explanation).

Taken together, these results first of all indicate an increase of rhinal–hippocampal connectivity during successful compared with unsuccessful word encoding not only regarding the theta band, but also for the neighbouring frequency bands. Such a memory-related coherence increase has also been reported for scalp EEG data (Weiss *et al.* 2000). Thus our results do not specifically support the theta–gamma hypothesis in humans, but rather support a general memory-related coherence effect spreading across the lower-frequency bands. However, the frequency-band-selective correlation between relative rhinal–hippocampal theta coherence and gamma synchronization changes confirms the theta–gamma-hypothesis postulating that the two oscillations interact in the process of storing representations in declarative memory (Lisman and Idiart 1995; Jensen *et al.* 1996; Chrobak and Buzsáki 1998a,b). In contrast with the rather unspecific memory-related coherence enhancement across the lower-frequency bands, this result supports the hypothesis of a specific function of theta oscillations in declarative memory formation. Owing to their long wavelength, low-frequency oscillations are incapable of enabling transient phase coupling within a time range of the order of 100 ms and precise timing of neural firing, as can be done by gamma oscillations (Engel and Singer 2001; Fries *et al.* 2001b; Varela *et al.* 2001). However, coherent low-frequency activity might accomplish a slowly modulated connectivity between the rhinal cortex and the hippocampus and hence support an encoding state (Fernández *et al.* 1999b). Thus theta-mediated rhinal–hippocampal synchronization may accompany the fast coupling and decoupling processes in the gamma range, which may be more closely related to the actual operation of declarative memory formation.

Rhinal–hippocampal interaction during sleep

The efficiency of declarative formation varies during different states of consciousness. In particular, the formation of new declarative memories during sleep appears to be deficient compared with the waking state (Hobson *et al.* 2000). On the one hand, there is the frequently reported inability to recall dreamed experiences (Goodenough 1991). When dreamed experiences are recalled, they typically contain much less detail than experiences acquired during the waking state. On the other hand, experimentally controlled experiences prior to sleep seem to have little impact on dream content (Fosse *et al.* 2003). Memory also seems to be deficient during sleep, as indicated by the fact that discontinuities and scene shifts within dreams are not recognized by the dreamer and the duration of dreams is usually grossly misestimated (Stickgold *et al.* 1997). Up to now, it has been an open question as to how this deficiency can be explained in terms of electrophysiological correlates of specific mnemonic operations observed during declarative memory formation (Hobson *et al.* 2000). Thus we wondered whether alterations of rhinal–hippocampal connectivity during sleep compared with the waking state might yield an explanation for deficient declarative memory during sleep.

Ongoing rhinal and hippocampal EEG activity recorded during sleep in eight patients with unilateral temporal lobe epilepsy was analysed (Fell *et al.* 2003c). Rhinal–hippocampal EEG coherence and spectral power at both MTL locations were evaluated for eight frequency bands between 1 and 44 Hz and correlated with the different sleep stages as classified by visual scoring based on scalp EEG (positions C3, C4, O1), electro-ocular, and submental electromyographic activity (Rechtschaffen and Kales 1968). Anterior and posterior hippocampal recordings were differentiated because of the evidence for functional dissociation between the two regions (Moser and Moser 1998).

We found a general decrease in both rhinal–hippocampal and intra-hippocampal coherence from waking state via sleep stage 1 towards stage 2, slow-wave sleep (SWS), and rapid eye movement (REM) sleep. Based on the reasoning described above, this result suggests that the deficiency of declarative memory may apply not only to REM sleep, but also to the non-rapid eye movement (NREM) sleep, stage 2, and SWS. The decrease in coherence was significant for the frequency range above 12 Hz and was most pronounced within the gamma band, in particular between 28 and 44 Hz. Within this frequency range, rhinal–hippocampal coherence was reduced on average by up to 56 per cent compared with the waking state. Our coherence findings clearly differ from results reported for surface recordings. An increase of coherence in the lower-frequency range from waking state towards sleep has been observed in several studies using scalp EEG data (Dumermuth *et al.* 1983; Nielsen *et al.* 1990; Achermann and Borbely 1998). Moreover, an MEG study revealed that coherent gamma activity reaches levels similar to waking state during REM sleep (Llinas and Ribary 1993). Thus the sleep-related coherence changes observed in our study appear to be specific to the MTL. Our data support the idea that the deficiency of declarative memory during sleep is associated with reduced rhinal–hippocampal coherence, in particular within the gamma range. However, the analysis of spectral power revealed sleep related changes similar to those reported for scalp EEG recordings, namely an increase in low-frequency and a decrease in high-frequency EEG power with deepness of sleep (Mann and Röschke 1997; Gross and Gotman 1999).

The second remarkable finding was that, in general, coherence between the rhinal cortex and the posterior hippocampus, as well as betwen the rhinal cortex and the anterior hippocampus, was larger than intra-hippocampal coherence. This result underlines the notion of a strong anatomical and functional interaction between the rhinal cortex and the hippocampus (Amaral and Insausti 1990) and supports the hypothesis of a functional dissociation within the hippocampus (Moser and Moser 1998). It has been reported that coherence estimates of intracranial EEG in general decline with increasing distance of the electrode pairs when electrodes are placed within the same brain region (Bullock *et al.* 1995; Shen *et al.* 1999). Our data show that this rule does not necessarily apply when different brain regions are involved, since coherence between the rhinal cortex and the posterior hippocampus was greater than intra-hippocampal coherence despite a larger inter-electrode distance.

Conclusion and outlook

In accord with models of the MTL memory system mainly based on experimental animal work (Mishkin *et al.* 1997; Eichenbaum 2000; Brown and Aggleton 2001) we have initially described a serial processing hierarchy during declarative memory formation within the human MTL. In this hierarchical system, semantic and mnemonic operations are integrated in the first non-relational stage, which may proceed from posterior parahippocampal to anterior rhinal cortices (Fernández *et al.* 2001). Such integration assumes that semantic (and perceptual) information is extracted just in time (i.e. online, as needed) and continuously compared with internal representations, thereby supporting memory formation indirectly (Otten *et al.* 2001; Fernández *et al.* 2002b) and enabling non-relational memory (e.g. recognition memory based on familiarity judgements). This pre-hippocampal processing in the parahippocampal region is superseded by specific mnemonic operations in the hippocampus, utilizing integrated information from prefrontal working memory processes and parahippocampal processes, and thereby enabling relational episodic memory (Düzel *et al.* 2001). Gamma-band phase synchronization appears to be an essential mechanism supporting rhinal–hippocampal interaction within this hierarchy. Enhanced phase synchronization may initiate and decreased phase synchronization may later terminate communication between the two MTL structures. These fast coupling and decoupling processes in the gamma range appear to be acompanied by an increase in rhinal–hippocampal coherence in the lower-frequency range, which possibly supports a slowly modulated encoding state (Fernández *et al.* 1999b).

It is still an open question as to whether rhinal–hippocampal connectivity, in particular, rhinal–hippocampal gamma synchronization, is controlled in a top-down scheme by a third pacemaker area like the thalamus. Indeed, synchronized gamma activity has been reported to be involved in attentional bottom-up, as well as top-down, processes (reviewed by Fell *et al.* 2003a). In the framework of the gamma synchronization hypothesis, bottom-up and top-down mechanisms are believed to be implemented through synchronization-dependent triggering of coincidence-sensitive target neurons (Abeles 1982; König *et al.* 1996). Members of phase synchronized neural assemblies fire action potentials in a highly time-locked manner. When these action potentials are propagated to common target neurons they can cooperate in elevating the membrane potential above the firing threshold (von der Malsburg 1999). Experimental evidence for this kind of activity propagation has been reported for neurons in the visual and the somatosensory cortex, which were triggered by synchronized thalamic

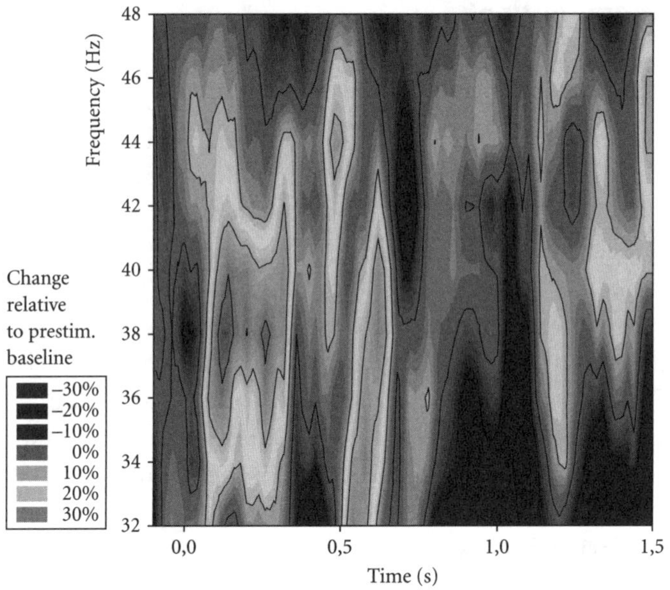

Figure 7.3 Differences of phase synchronization between rhinal cortex and hippocampus (per cent) relative to prestimulus baseline for subsequently recalled versus unrecalled words. The picture shows a colour-coded plot of *S*(recalled)—*S*(unrecalled), where S(recalled) is the phase synchronization (per cent) for subsequently recalled words and *S*(unrecalled) is the phase synchronization (per cent) for subsequently unrecalled words. The different gamma range frequencies (32–48 Hz) are represented on the *y* axis and time is depicted on the *x* axis. Synchronization/desynchronization is coded on a colour scale: red areas show enhancement and blue areas show reduction of synchronization for subsequently recalled versus unrecalled words (Fell *et al.* 2001). See also colour plate section.

afferents (Roy and Alloway 2001; Alonso *et al.* 1996). In the cat geniculocortical pathway the maximal delay times, for which spikes from two different pre-synaptic neurons can cooperatively enhance post-synaptic firing probabilities, were observed to be around 7 ms (Usrey *et al.* 2000). Synchronized oscillations in the gamma range were found to be associated with such precise spike timing (Engel and Singer 2001; Fries *et al.* 2001b; Varela *et al.* 2001). Thus synchronized gamma activity may provide a mechanism of enhancing the impact of lower-order areas onto higher-order areas, as well as propagating influences from higher-order areas responsible for attentional control to lower-order areas. This mechanism may represent the basis for a modulation of rhinal–hippocampal interaction in memory formation by attentional top-down control.

Moreover, synchronized firing in the gamma range may cause Hebbian modification of synaptic efficacy. Hebbian synaptic plasticity was described as depending on the interaction between post-synaptic potentials and action potentials back-propagating into the dendrite of the post-synaptic neuron (Markram *et al.* 1997). The required delay times for effective Hebbian synaptic modifications by correlated firing of the pre- and post-synaptic neurons are of the order of less than $\pm$ 10 ms, as demonstrated by *in vitro* recordings from hippocampal neurons (Abbott and Nelson 2000). Since synchronization of gamma oscillations has been shown to enable such exact timing of neural action potentials (Engel and Singer 2001; Fries *et al.* 2001b; Varela *et al.* 2001), synchronized gamma activity provides optimal conditions for the establishment of Hebbian assemblies. Therefore synchronized gamma activity may enable the formation of Hebbian connections between the rhinal cortex and the hippocampus, as well as within the hippocampus. In this sense, gamma synchronization may provide the initial step for long-term memory formation on the synaptic level. However, cellular *in vivo* data relating hippocampal gamma synchronization to experimental memory performance are still lacking.

During a normal day, some experiences are doomed to be forgotten from the moment we experience them because our brain, and in particular our MTL, has processed these experiences differently from those we remember. Cognitive neuroscience has yielded insights into processes accomplishing declarative memory formation at the system level. Our findings indicate that oscillatory interaction between the rhinal cortex and the hippocampus is a key element in the successful processing of memory items. The deficiency of declarative memory during sleep may be associated with a reduced rhinal–hippocampal connectivity, in particular within the gamma range. An important focus for future investigations is to narrow the gap between these data at the system level and the profound knowledge about the molecular and cellular events at synapses during memory consolidation. Initial investigations have linked *N*-methyl-D-aspartate (NMDA) receptor activity to mnemonic MTL procespses in humans (Grunwald *et al.* 1999; Beck *et al.* 2000), a finding that is in accord with the role of synaptic plasticity assigned to NMDA receptors (Huang *et al.* 1996). Further studies in this direction are needed to reveal an integrated picture of the mechanisms underlying declarative memory formation.

References

Abbott, L.F. and Nelson, S.B. (2000). Synaptic plasticity: taming the beast. *Nature Neuroscience*, **3**, 1178–1183.

Abeles, M. (1982). Role of the cortical neuron: integrator or coincidence detector? *Israel Journal of Medical Science*, **18**, 83–92.

Achermann, P. and Borbely, A.A. (1998). Coherence analysis of the human sleep electroencephalogram. *Neuroscience*, **85**, 1195–1208.

Alonso, J.M., Usrey, W.M. and Reid, R.C. (1996). Precisely correlated firing in cells of the lateral geniculate nucleus. *Nature*, **383**, 815–819.

Amaral, D.G. and Insausti, R. (1990). Hippocampal formation. In *The Human Nervous System* (ed G. Paxinos). San Diego, CA: Academic Press, pp. 711–755.

Amaral, D.G. and Witter, M.P. (1989). The three-dimensional organization of the hippocampal formation: a review of anatomical data. *Neuroscience*, **31**, 571–591.

Beck, H., Goussakov, I.V., Lie, A., Helmstaedter, C. and Elger, C.E. (2000) Synaptic plasticity in the human dentate gyrus. *Journal of Neuroscience*, **20**, 7080–7086.

Berry, S.D. and Seager, M.A. (2001). Hippocampal theta oscillations and classical conditioning. *Neurobiology of Learning and Memory*, **76**, 298–313.

Bressler, S.L. (1987). Relation of olfactory bulb and cortex. I: Spatial variation of bulbocortical interdependence. *Brain Research*, **409**, 285–293.

Brewer, J.B., Zhao, Z., Desmond, J.E., Glover, G.H., and Gabrieli, J.D.E. (1998). Making memories, brain activity that predicts how well visual experience will be remembered. *Science*, **281**, 1185–1187.

Brown, M.W. and Aggleton, J.P. Recognition memory: what are the roles of the perirhinal cortex and hippocampus? *Nature Reviews Neuroscience*, **2**, 51–61.

Bullock, T.H., McClune, M.C., Achimowicz, J.Z., Iragui-Madoz, V.J., Duckrow, R.B., and Spencer, S.S. (1995). EEG coherence has structure in the millimeter domain: subdural and hippocampal recordings from epileptic patients. *Electroencephalography and Clinical Neurophysiology*, **95**, 161–177.

Buzsáki, G. (1996) The hippocampo-neocortical dialogue. *Cerebral Cortex*, **6**, 81–92.

Caplan, J.B., Madsen, J.R., Raghavachari, S., and Kahana, M.J. (2001). Distinct patterns of brain oscillations underlie two basic parameters of human maze learning. *Journal of Neurophysiology*, **86**, 368–380.

Challis, R.E. and Kitney, R.I. (1991). Biomedical signal processing. Part 3: The power spectrum and coherence function. *Medical and Biological Engineering and Computing*, **29**, 225–241.

Chrobak, J.J. and Buzsáki, G. (1998a). Operational dynamics in the hippocampal–entorhinal axis. *Neuroscience and Biobehavioral Reviews*, **22**, 303–310.

Chrobak, J.J. and Buzsáki, G. (1998b). Gamma oscillations in the entorhinal cortex of the freely behaving rat. *Journal of Neuroscience*, **18**, 388–398.

Cofer, C.N. and Shevitz, R. (1952). Word-association as a function of word-frequency. *American Journal of Psychology*, **65**, 75–79.

Craik, F.I.M. and Lockhart, R.S. (1972). Levels of processing: a framework for memory research. *Journal of Verbal Learning and Verbal Behaviour*, **11**, 671–684.

Desmedt, J.E. and Tomberg, C. (1994) Transient phase-locking of 40 Hz electrical oscillations in prefrontal and parietal human cortex reflects the process of conscious somatic perception. *Neuroscience Letters*, **168**, 126–129.

Dumermuth, G., Lange, B., Lehmann, D., Meier, C.A., Dinkelmann, R., and Molinari, L. (1983). Spectral analysis of all-night sleep EEG in healthy adults. *European Neurology*, **22**, 322–339.

Düzel, E., Vargha-Khadem, F., Heinze, H.J., and Mishkin, M. (2001). Brain activity evidence for recognition without recollection after early hippocampal damage. *Proceedings of the National Academy of the United States of America*, **98**, 8101–8106.

Eckhorn, R., Bauer, R., Jordan, W., *et al.* (1988). Coherent oscillations: a mechanism of feature linking in the visual cortex? Multiple electrode and correlation analyses in the cat. *Biological Cybernetics*, **60**, 121–130.

Eichenbaum, H. (2000). A cortical-hippocampal system for declarative memory. *Nature Reviews Neuroscience*, **1**, 41–50.

Engel, A.K. and Singer, W. (2001). Temporal binding and the neural correlates of sensory awareness. *Trends in Cognitive Sciences*, **5**, 16–25.

Engel, A.K., Kreiter, A.K., König, P., and Singer, W. (1991a). Synchronization of oscillatory neuronal responses between striate and extrastriate visual cortical areas of the cat. *Proceedings of the National Academy of the United States of America*, **88**, 6048–6052.

Engel, A.K., König, P., Kreiter, A.K., and Singer, W. (1991b). Interhemispheric synchronization of oscillatory neuronal responses in cat visual cortex. *Science*, **252**, 1177–1179.

Engel, A.K., Fries, P., König, P., Brecht, M., and Singer, W. (1999). Temporal binding, binocular rivalry, and consciousness. *Consciousness and Cognition*, **8**, 128–151.

Fell, J., Klaver, P., Lehnertz, K., *et al.* (2001). Human memory formation is accompanied by rhinal–hippocampal coupling and decoupling. *Nature Neuroscience*, **4**, 1259–1264.

Fell, J., Fernández, G., Klaver, P., Elger, C.E., and Fries, P. (2003a). Is synchronized gamma activity relevant for selective attention? *Brain Research: Brain Research Reviews*, **42**, 265–272.

Fell, J., Klaver, P., Elfadil, H., Schaller, C., Elger, C.E., and Fernández, G. (2003b). Rhinal–hippocampal theta coherence during declarative memory formation: interaction with gamma synchronization? *European Journal of Neuroscience*, **17**, 1082–1088.

Fell, J., Städtgen, M., Burr, W., *et al.* (2003c). Rhinal–hippocampal EEG coherence is reduced during sleep. *European Journal of Neuroscience*, **18**, 1711–1716.

Fernández, G., Weyerts, H., Schrader-Bölsche, M., *et al.* (1998). Successful verbal encoding into episodic memory engages the posterior hippocampus: a parametrically analyzed functional magnetic resonance imaging study. *Journal of Neuroscience*, **18**, 1841–1847.

Fernández, G., Effern, A., Grunwald, T., *et al.* (1999a). Real-time tracking of memory formation in the human rhinal cortex and hippocampus. *Science*, **285**, 1582–1585.

Fernández, G., Brewer, J.B., Zhao, Z., Glover, G.H., and Gabrieli, J.D. (1999b). Level of sustained entorhinal activity at study correlates with subsequent cued-recall performance: a functional magnetic resonance imaging study with high acquisition rate. *Hippocampus*, **9**, 35–44.

Fernández, G., Heitkemper, P., Grunwald, T., *et al.* Inferior temporal stream for word processing with integrated mnemonic function. *Human Brain Mapping*, **14**, 251–260.

Fernández, G., Fell, J., and Fries, P. (2002a). Response: the birth of a memory. *Trends in Neurosciences*, **25**, 281–282.

Fernández, G., Klaver, P, Fell, J., Grunwald T., and Elger, C.E. (2002b). Human declarative memory formation: segregating rhinal and hippocampal contributions. *Hippocampus*, **12**, 514–519.

Fosse, M.J., Fosse, R., Hobson, J.A., and Stickgold, R.J. (2003). Dreaming and episodic memory: a functional dissociation? *Journal of Cognitive Neuroscience*, **15**, 1–9.

Freeman, W.J. (1978) Spatial properties fo an EEG event in the olfactory bulb and cortex. *Electroencephalography and Clinical Neurophysiology*, **44**, 586–605.

Frien, A., Eckhorn, R., Bauer, R., Woelbern, T., and Kehr, H. (1994). Stimulus-specific fast oscillations at zero phase between visual areas V1 and V2 of awake monkey. *Neuroreport*, **5**, 2273–2277.

Fries, P., Roelfsema, P.R., Engel, A.K., König, P., and Singer, W. (1997). Synchronization of oscillatory responses in visual cortex correlates with perception in interocular rivalry. *Proceedings of the National Academy of the United States of America*, **94**, 12699–12704.

Fries, P., Reynolds, J.H., Rorie, A.E., and Desimone, R. (2001a). Modulation of oscillatory neuronal synchronization by selective visual attention. *Science*, **291**, 1506–1507.

Fries, P., Neuenschwader, S., Engel, A.K., Goebel, R., and Singer, W. (2001b). Rapid feature selective neuronal synchronization through correlated latency shifting. *Nature Neuroscience*, **4**, 194–200.

Fries, P., Schroder, J.H., Roelfsema, P.R., Singer, W., and Engel, A.K. (2002). Oscillatory neuronal synchronization in primary visual cortex as a correlate of stimulus selection. *Journal of Neuroscience*, **22**, 3739–3754.

Gabrieli, J.D. (1998). Cognitive neuroscience of human memory. *Annual Review of Psychology*, **49**, 87–115.

Goodenough, D.R. (1991). Dream recall: history and current status of the field. In *The Mind in Sleep: Psychology and Psychophysiology* (ed S.J. Ellman and J.S. Antrobus). New York: John Wiley, pp.143–171.

Goodman, C.S. and Shatz, C.J. (1993). Developmental mechanisms that generate precise patterns of neuronal connectivity. *Cell*, **72**, 77–98.

Gordon, B. (1983). Lexical access and lexical decision: mechanisms of frequency sensitivity. *Journal of Verbal Learning and Verbal Behaviour*, **22**, 24–44.

Gray, C.M., König, P., Engel, A.K., and Singer, W. (1989). Oscillatory responses in cat visual cortex exhibit inter-columnar synchronization which reflects global stimulus properties. *Nature*, **338**, 334–337.

Gregg, V. (1976). Word frequency, recognition and recall. In *Recall and Recognition* (ed J. Brown). London: John Wiley, pp. 183–216.

Gross, D.W. and Gotman, J. (1999). Correlation of high-frequency oscillations with the sleep-wake cycle and cognitive activity in humans. *Neuroscience*, **94**, 1005–1018.

Gruber, T., Müller, M.M., Keil, A., and Elbert, T. (1999) Selective visual–spatial attention alters induced gamma band responses in the human EEG. *Clinical Neurophysiology*, **110**, 2074–2085.

Grunwald, T., Lehnertz, K., Heinze, H.J., Helmstaedter, C., and Elger, C.E. (1998). Verbal novelty detection within the human hippocampus proper. *Proceedings of the National Academy of the United States of America*, **95**, 3193–3197.

Grunwald, T., Beck, H., Lehnertz, K., *et al.* (1999). Evidence relating human verbal memory to hippocampal *N*-methyl-D-aspartate receptors. *Proceedings of the National Academy of the United States of America*, **96**, 12085–12089.

Halgren, E., Squires, N.K., Wilson, C.L., Rohrbauch, J.W., Babb, T.L., and Crandall, P.H. (1980). Endogenous potentials generated in the human hippocampal formation and amygdala by infrequent events. *Science*, **210**, 803–805.

Hebb, D.O. (1949). *The Organisation of Behavior*. New York: John Wiley.

Hirai, N., Uchida, S., Maehara, T., Okubo, Y., and Shimizu, H. (1999). Enhanced gamma (30–150 Hz) frequency in the human medial temporal lobe. *Neuroscience*, **90**, 1149–1155.

Hobson, J.A., Pace-Schott, E.F., and Stickgold, R. (2000). Dreaming and the brain: toward a cognitive neuroscience of conscious states. *Behavioral and Brain Sciences*, **23**, 793–842.

Huang, Y.Y., Nguyen, P.V., Abel, T., and Kandel, E.R. (1996). Long-lasting forms of synaptic potentiation in the mammalian hippocampus. *Learning and Memory*, **3**, 74–85.

Jensen, O. (2001). Information transfer between rhythmically coupled networks: reading the hippocampal phase code. *Neural Computation*, **13**, 2743–2761.

Jensen, O. and Tesche, C.D. (2002). Frontal theta activity in humans increases with memory load in a working memory task. *European Journal of Neuroscience*, **15**, 1395–1399.

Jensen, O., Idiart, M.A.P., and Lisman, J.E. (1996). Physiologically realistic formation of autoassociative memory in networks with theta–gamma oscillations: role of fast NMDA channels. *Learning and Memory*, **3**, 243–256.

Kahana, M.J., Sekuler, R., Caplan, J.B., Kirschen, M., and Madsen, J.R. (1999). Human theta oscillations exhibit task dependence during virtual maze navigation. *Nature*, **399**, 781–784.

Kahana, M.J., Seelig, D., and Madsen, J.R. (2001) Theta returns. *Current Opinion in Neurobiology*, **11**, 739–744.

Klee, M. and Rall, W. (1977). Computed potentials of cortically arranged populations of neurons. *Journal of Neurophysiology*, **40**, 647–666.

Klimesch, W., Doppelmayr, M., Russegger, H., and Pachinger, T. (1996). Theta band power in the human scalp EEG and the encoding of new information. *Neuroreport*, **7**, 1235–1240.

Klimesch, W., Doppelmayr, M., Schimke, H., and Ripper, B. (1997). Theta synchronization and alpha desynchronization in a memory task. *Psychophysiology*, **34**, 169–176.

Kreiman, G., Koch, C., and Fried, I. (2000) Imagery neurons in the human brain. *Nature*, **408**, 357–361.

Kreiter, A.K. and Singer, W. (1996). Stimulus-dependent synchronization of neuronal responses in the visual cortex of the awake macaque monkey. *Journal of Neuroscience*, **16**, 2381–2396.

König, P., Engel, A.K., and Singer, W. (1996). Integrator or coincidence detector? The role of the cortical neuron revisited. *Trends in Neurosciences*, **19**, 130–137.

LaBerge, D. (1997). Attention, awareness, and the triangular circuit. *Consciousness and Cognition*, **6**, 149–181.

Lebedev, M.A. and Nelson, R.J. (1995) Rhythmically firing (20–50 Hz) neurons in monkey primary somatosensory cortex: activity patterns during initiation of vibratory-cued hand movements. *Journal of Computational Neuroscience*, **2**, 313–334.

Leopold, D.A. and Logothetis, N.K. (1999). Multistable phenomena: changing views in perception. *Trends in Cognitive Sciences*, **3**, 254–264.

Lisman, J.E. and Idiart, M.A.P. (1995). Storage of 7 ± 2 short-term memories in oscillatory subcycles. *Science*, **267**, 1512–1515.

Lisman, J.E. and Otmakhova, N.A. (2001). Storage, recall, and novelty detection of sequences by the hippocampus: elaborating on the SOCRATIC model to account for normal and aberrant effects of dopamine. *Hippocampus*, **11**, 551–568.

Llinas, R. and Ribary, U. (1993). Coherent 40-Hz oscillations characterized dream state in humans. *Proceedings of the National Academy of the United States of America*, **90**, 2078–2081.

Lutzenberger, W., Pulvermüller, F., Elbert, T., and Birbaumer, N. (1995) Visual stimulation alters local 40-Hz responses in humans: an EEG-study. *Neuroscience Letters*, **183**, 39–42.

McCarthy, G., Nobre, A.C., Bentin, S., and Spencer, D.D. (1995). Language-related field potentials in the anterior-medial temporal lobe. I: intracranial distribution and neural generators. *Journal of Neuroscience*, **15**, 1080–1089.

Magee, J.C. and Johnston, D. (1997) A synaptically controlled, associated signal for Hebbian plasticity in hippocampal neurons. *Science*, **275**, 209–213.

Mann, K. and Röschke, J. (1997). Different phase relationships between EEG frequency bands during NREM and REM sleep. *Sleep*, **20**, 753–756.

Mardia, K.V. (1972). *Probability and Mathematical Statistics: Statistics of Directional Data.* London: Academic Press.

Markram, H., Lubke, J., Frotscher M. and Sakmann, B. (1997). Regulation of synaptic efficacy by coincidence of postsynaptic APs and EPSPs. *Science*, **275**, 213–215.

Menon, V., Freeman, W.J., Cutillo, B.A., *et al.* (1996). Spatio-temporal correlations in human gamma band electrocorticograms. *Electroencephalography and Clinical Neurophysiology*, **98**, 89–102.

Miltner, W.H., Braun, C., Arnold, M., Witte, H., and Taub, E. (1999). Coherence of gamma-band EEG activity as a basis for associative learning. *Nature*, **397**, 434–436.

Mishkin, M., Suzuki, W.A., Gadian, D.G., and Vargha-Khadem, F. (1997). Hierarchical organization of cognitive memory. *Philosophical Transactions of the Royal Society of London, Series B, Biological Sciences*, **352**, 1461–1467.

Mölle, M., Marshall, L., Fehm, H.L., and Born, J. (202). EEG theta synchronization conjoined with alpha desynchronization indicate intentional encoding. *European Journal of Neuroscience*, **15**, 923–928.

Moser, M.-B. and Moser, E.I. (1998). Functional differentiation in the hippocampus. *Hippocampus*, **8**, 608–619.

Müller, M.M., Bosch, J., Elbert, T., *et al.* (1996). Visually induced gamma-band responses in human electroencephalographic activity—a link to animal studies. *Experimental Brain Research*, **112**, 96–102.

Müller, M.M., Gruber, T., and Keil, A. (2000) Modulation of induced gamma band activity in the human EEG by attention and visual information processing. *International Journal of Psychophysiology*, **38**, 283–299.

Nielsen, T., Abel, A., Lorrain, D., and Montplaisir, J. (1990). Interhemispheric EEG coherence during sleep and wakefulness in left- and right-handed subjects. *Brain and Cognition*, **14**, 113–125.

Noble, C.E. (1963). Meaningfulness and familiarity. In *Verbal Behavior and Learning: Problems and Progress* (ed C.N. Cofer and B.S. Musgrave). New York: McGraw-Hill, pp. 76–119.

Nobre, A.C. and McCarthy, G. (1995). Language-related field potentials in the anterior-medial temporal lobe. II: Effects of word type and semantic priming. *Journal of Neuroscience*, **15**, 1090–1098.

O'Keefe, J. and Recce, M.L. (1993). Phase relationship between hippocampal place units and the EEG theta rhythm. *Hippocampus*, **3**, 317–330.

Otten, L.J. and Rugg, M.D. (2002). The birth of a memory. *Trends in Neurosciences*, **25**, 279–281.

Otten, L.J., Henson, R.N., and Rugg, M.D. (2001). Depth of processing effects on neural correlates of memory encoding: relationship between findings from across- and within-task comparisons. *Brain*, **124**, 399–412.

Paller, K.A. (1990). Recall and stem-completion have different electrophysiological correlates and are modified differentially by directed forgetting. *Journal of Experimental Psychology: Learning, Memory, and Cognition*, **16**, 1021–1032.

Raghavachari, S., Kahana, M.J., Rizzuto, D.S., *et al.* (2001). Gating of human theta oscillations by a working memory task. *Journal of Neuroscience*, **21**, 3175–3183.

Rechtschaffen, A. and Kales, A. (1968). *A Manual of Standarized Terminology, Techniques, and Scoring System for Sleep Stages of Human Subjects.* NIH Publication No. 204. Washington, DC: US Government Printing Office.

Rodriguez, E., George, N., Lachaux, J.P., Martinerie, J., Renault, B., and Varela, F.J. (1999). Perception's shadow: long-distance synchronization of human brain activity. *Nature*, **397**, 430–433.

Roy, S.A. and Alloway, K.D. (2001). Coincidence detection or temporal integration? What the neurons in somatosensory cortex are doing. *Journal of Neuroscience*, **21**, 2462–2473.

Rubin, D.C. and Friendly, M. (1986). Predicting which words get recalled: measures of free recall, availability, goodness, emotionality, and pronounciability for 925 nouns. *Memory and Cognition*, **14**, 79–94.

Sanquist, T.F., Rohrbaugh, J.W., Syndulko, K., and Lindley, D.B. (1980). Electrocortical signs of levels of processing, perceptual analysis and recognition memory. *Psychophysiology*, **17**, 568–576.

Scoville, W.B. and Milner, B. (1957). Loss of recent memory after bilateral hippocampal lesions. *Journal of Neurology, Neurosurgery and Psychiatry*, **20**, 11–21.

Shen, B., Nadkarni, M., and Zappulla, R.A. (1999). Spectral modulation of cortical connections measured by EEG coherence in humans. *Clinical Neurophysiology*, **110**, 115–125.

Skaggs, W.E., McNaughton, B.L., Wilson, M.A., and Barnes, C.A. (1996). Theta phase precession in hippocampal neuronal populations and the compression of temporal sequences. *Hippocampus*, **6**, 149–172.

Smith, M.E., Stapleton, J.M., and Halgren, E. (1986) Human medial temporal lobe potentials evoked in memory and language tasks. *Electroencephalography and Clinical Neurophysiology*, **63**, 145–159.

Sommer, F.T. and Wennekers T. (2001). Associative memory in networks of spiking neurons. *Neural Networks*, **14**, 825–834.

Steinmetz, P.N., Roy, A., Fitzgerald, P.J., Hsiao, S.S., Johnson, K.O., and Niebur, E. (2000). Attention modulates synchronized neuronal firing in primate somatosensory cortex. *Nature*, **404**, 187–190.

Stickgold, R., Pace-Schott, E.F., and Hobson, J.A. (1997). Subjective estimates of dream duration and dream recall process. *Sleep Research*, **26**, 279.

Stopfer, M., Bhagavan, S., Smith, B.H., and Laurent G. (1997). Impaired odour discrimination on desynchronization of odour-encoding neural assemblies. *Nature*, **390**, 70–74.

Tallon-Baudry, C. and Bertrand, O. (1999). Oscillatory gamma activity in humans and its role in object representation. *Trends in Cognitive Sciences*, **3**, 151–162.

Tesche, C.D. and Karhu, J. (2000) Theta oscillations index human hippocampal activation during a working memory task. *Proceedings of the National Academy of the United States of America*, **97**, 919–924.

Traub, R.D., Whittington, M.A., Stanford, I.M., and Jefferys, J.G. (1996). A mechanism for generation of long-range synchronous fast oscillations in the cortex. *Nature*, **383**, 621–624.

Traub, R.D., Jeffereys, J.G.R., and Whittington, M.A. (1999). *Fast Oscillations in Cortical Circuits*. Cambridge MA: MIT Press.

Usrey, W.M., Alonso, J.M., and Reid, R.C. (2000). Synaptic interaction between thalamic inputs to simple cells in cat visual cortex. *Journal of Neuroscience*, **20**, 5461–5467.

van Roost, D., Solymosi, L., Schramm, J., van Oosterwyck, B., and Elger, C.E. (1998). Depth electrode implantation in the length axis of the hippocampus for the presurgical evaluation of medial temporal lobe epilepsy: A computed tomography-based stereotactic insertion technique and its accuracy. *Neurosurgery*, **43**, 819–826.

Varela, F., Lachaux, J.P., Rodriguez, E., and Martinerie, J. (2001). The brainweb: phase synchronization and large-scale integration. *Nature Reviews Neuroscience*, **2**, 229–239.

Vertes, R.P. and Kocsis, B. (1997). Brainstem–diencephalo-septohippocampal systems controlling the theta rhythm of the hippocampus. *Neuroscience*, **81**, 893–926.

von der Malsburg, C. (1981). *The Correlation Theory of Brain Function*. Internal Report 81–2, MPI Biophysical Chemistry.

von der Malsburg, C. (1999). The what and why of binding: the modeler's perspective. *Neuron*, **24**, 95–104.

von der Malsburg C, Schneider W. A neural cocktail-party processor. *Biological Cybernetics* 1986; 54, 29–40.

Wagner, A.D. (2001). Synchronicity: when you're gone I'm lost without a trace? *Nature Neuroscience*, **4**, 1159–1160.

Wagner, A.D., Schacter, D.L., Rotte, M., *et al.* (1998). Building memories, remembering and forgetting of verbal experiences as predicted by brain activity. *Science*, **281**, 1188–1191.

Weiss, S. and Rappelsberger, P. (2000). Long-range EEG synchronization during word encoding correlates with successful memory performance. *Brain Research: Cognitive Brain Research*, **9**, 299–312.

Weiss, S., Müller, H.M., and Rappelsberger, P. (2000). Theta synchronization predicts efficient memory encoding of concrete and abstract nouns. *Neuroreport*, **11**, 2357–2361.

Witter, M.P., Groenewegen, H.J., Lopes da Silva, F.H., and Lohman, A.H.M. (1989). Functional organization of the extrinsic and intrinsic circuitry of the parahippocampal region. *Progress in Neurobiology*, **33**, 161–253.

Section 2

A computational approach to mechanisms of binding

Chapter 8

Neural mechanisms of binding in the hippocampus and neocortex: insights from computational models

Daniel M. Cer and Randall C. O'Reilly

Introduction

Nearly all cognitive phenomena explicitly or implicitly entail some degree of binding. For instance, visual perception involves correctly binding features such as the shape, colour, and location of the objects currently being perceived. Similarly, auditory perception implies binding temporally extended acoustic information to facilitate the interpretation of such acoustic sequences by downstream systems as particular sounds or phones. Finally, higher-level cognitive processes such as abstract reasoning and planning appear to require flexible variable/value binding whereby various operations are defined over variable-like entities and are then flexibly applied to any valid values that a given variable can take on.

Accordingly, the development of accurate models of the neural mechanisms underlying binding represents a critical step in the understanding of the mechanisms that give rise to most cognitive processes. In this chapter we discuss two distinct approaches to the binding problem. The first, which enjoys significant popularity, is **temporal synchrony** (von der Malsburg 1981; Engel *et al.* 1992; Gray *et al.* 1992; Hummel and Biederman 1992; Zemel *et al.* 1995). Abstractly, theories following this approach solve the binding problem by proposing that when neurons that represent various features fire together, the given features are bound together. The representation of multiple sets of bindings (e.g. to represent two distinct objects) is supported by the system alternating between representing each of the appropriate sets of bindings. Accordingly, the representations for the different sets can be said to fire out of phase with each other.

While temporal synchrony does have many attractive properties, such as being relatively easy to understand, it also has several drawbacks that motivate exploring a different approach to the binding problem. The alternative approach that we will present is based on a theoretical framework which postulates that different regions of neural tissue are specialized to provide solutions to particular types of computational problems (O'Reilly *et al.* 1999, 2003; O'Reilly and Munakata 2000; O'Reilly and Norman 2002). We refer to this framework as the specialized neural regions for global efficiency (SNRGE, pronounced 'synergy') framework (Fig. 8.1). The specializations associated with different brain areas represent computational trade-offs that are inherent in the neurobiological implementation of cognitive processes, i.e. the trade-offs are a direct consequence of what computational processes can be easily implemented in the underlying biology. The specializations correspond anatomically to the hippocampus, the prefrontal cortex, and all of the neocortex that is posterior to prefrontal cortex (posterior cortex). An overview of the computational properties and phenomena that can be associated with each of these three areas is presented next, followed by a more in-depth assessment of the temporal synchrony approach. Then we explore in more detail each of the three binding mechanisms involved in the SNRGE approach.

Posterior cortex

The posterior cortex is heavily involved in any given cognitive task, contributing everything from sensory processing up to higher-level semantic and associative processes. Indeed, it is often striking how much of cognition remains intact with frontal and hippocampal lesions. Essentially, the prefrontal cortex and the hippocampus appear to serve as memory areas that dynamically and interactively

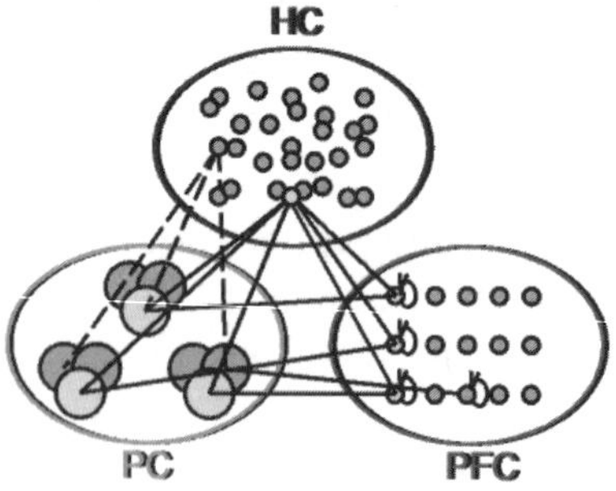

Figure 8.1 The components of the specialized neural regions for global efficiency (SNRGE) framework, including the posterior cortex (PC), hippocampus (HC) and prefrontal cortex (PFC) (the motor frontal cortex constitutes a blend between PFC and PC specializations, and is included conceptually in PC). Large overlapping circles in PC represent overlapping distributed representations used to encode semantic and perceptual information. Small separated circles in HC represent sparse pattern-separated representations used to rapidly encode ('bind') entire patterns of information across the cortex while minimizing interference. Isolated self-connected representations in FC represent isolated stripes (columns) of neurons capable of sustained firing (i.e. active maintenance or working memory).

support the computation that is being performed by posterior brain areas. To be able perform such computation, the posterior cortex requires flexible representations that both encode semantic information about the world and facilitate efficient processing of novel information in the context of such previously learned material. These representations should also be relatively robust to both noise in the system and traumatic insult. One such class of representations that fit this criteria, and the one that will be examined here, is the coarse-coded distributed representation (CCDR) (Wickelgren 1969; Hinton *et al.* 1986; Seidenberg and McClelland 1989; St John and McClelland 1990; Mozer 1991; Mel and Fiser 2000).

In a CCDR, neural units each encode a particular set of low-order conjunctions of features in a graded manner. For example, a unit in the visual system could be active in the presence of any one of the following: something that is round and blue, something that is square and red, or something that is triangular and green. Given that the conjunctions are low order and each unit can code for multiple conjunctions, a large number of such units will generally be used to represent any given object. In other words, binding of features to objects is represented by distributed representations over a population of neural units.

The intuition behind why CCDR are desirable is twofold. First, CCDR can allow for efficient information processing by downstream neurons such that the formation of the representations themselves from the input features performs a variety of useful computations. That is, in neural network models of cognitive processes, the intermediate representations that are developed within the network's internal layers (i.e. its hidden layers), are not just an efficient encoding of the network's inputs, but are also a re-representation of such inputs that is computationally useful for the task that the network was being trained on. Secondly, CCDR supports a flexible, but compact, manner of encoding information. For instance, as will be demonstrated later in this section, CCDRs allow for representations that can economically support a large number of possible binding relationships. Further, modelling has demonstrated the flexibility of CCDR in that such representations can support a great variety of computational tasks. Notably, for the purposes of this chapter, they support a very compact way of encoding binding information. However, CCDRs are limited in that they take a substantial amount of training experience to form, and thus cannot be used to encode novel information rapidly. Further, CCDRs are driven by the current input to the system and thus cannot actively maintain task-relevant information unless such information is readily cued by some aspect of the environment. These limitations are directly addressed by the specializations seen in the two other regions described below.

Hippocampus

The hippocampus is known to play a critical role in the formation of episodic memories as well as in the rapid encoding of novel information. Accordingly, this entails an underlying mechanism which can quickly form persistent representations that bind a large number of arbitrary pieces of information into a collective whole. Additionally, the hippocampus seems to operate as a sort of content-addressable memory system. That is, a chunk of stored information is retrieved by giving the system, as a retrieval cue, some subset of the information in the chunk that is to be retrieved. For example, passing a grocery store on the way home may serve as a cue for a memory formed earlier that day of running out of milk. Computationally, this sort of retrieval behaviour can be described as pattern completion. Further, a neural mechanism that accounts for the behaviour of this memory system is one in which neural units with high learning rates (i.e. the connection strength between units can change rapidly) and sparse activation across a layer are used to form large-scale conjunctive representations of stimuli (Marr 1971; O'Reilly and McClelland 1994; O'Reilly and Rudy 2001; O'Reilly and Norman 2002).

As will be explored later in this chapter, the sparse conjunctive nature of hippocampal representations has the desired properties of being able to encode new memories rapidly and retrieve such memories via pattern completion. Additionally, it also maintains existing memories in a way that is highly robust to interference from the encoding of new ones. This latter property is due to the low degree of representational overlap between any two memories in the system. However, this low degree of overlap significantly limits the amount of arbitrary computation that can be done by this system since any such computation would exhibit little to no generalization. Further, the hippocampus, like the posterior cortex, is largely driven by input from other systems. As such, it cannot actively maintain a representation, i.e. provide as output some memory, unless the retrieval cue for the memory is continuously provided as input. Of course, the computational limitations of the hippocampus are not a problem since the CCDRs of the posterior cortex facilitate general information processing in the brain. Also, as will be seen below, the prefrontal cortex facilitates the active maintenance of information that is not readily available/computable from the immediate information.

Prefrontal cortex

The prefrontal cortex (PFC) has long been thought to support working memory in the form of active maintenance of task-relevant information (Fuster and Alexander 1971; Kubota and Niki 1971; Goldman-Rakic 1987). This ability to actively maintain task-relevant information is critical for the rapid adaptation to novel situations and tasks. As demonstrated by patients with PFC damage, the lack of an intact PFC leads to perseveration when such patients are trained to do one task and then are subsequently required to perform another similar but not identical task (Milner 1963; Weinberger *et al.* 1991; Stuss *et al.* 2000). That is, these patients take far longer than normal subjects to learn the behaviour that is appropriate for the second task. A critical observation for these experiments is found in that the patients and the normal participants take a more comparable amount of time to learn the first task. Accordingly, the patients' deficit is generally not accounted for by a learning deficit, but rather by an inability to adjust their behaviour flexibly.

Computationally, a model of the PFC must not only account for the active maintenance of relevant information but also for the rapid updating of this information as circumstances change (O'Reilly *et al.* 1999). Further, the model must account for the interaction between the PFC and other cortical areas such that the PFC can strongly bias the processing that occurs in such areas (Miller and Cohen 2001). We suggest that rapid and transient binding of task-relevant information can emerge from the biological mechanisms that support these PFC functions. Unlike the hippocampus, information is only transiently stored in the PFC. Of course, since the PFC's transient storage can be actively maintained and hippocampus's long-term storage cannot, these two regions serve as complementary memory systems.

Summary of binding in the SNRGE model

As outlined above, the SNRGE approach entails partitioning the binding problem into three distinct subproblems. The first involves the occurrence of binding in long-term semantic memory and how such a binding mechanism can facilitate processing of novel stimuli in the context of existing knowledge. The second involves how separate aspects of an experience are bound in order to form a single episodic memory. This second subproblem also includes how novel information is rapidly learned. Such learning necessarily requires binding the individual components of the learned information together. Finally, the third subproblem involves how task-relevant information is bound with such bindings being actively maintained by the system. The motivation behind this decomposition is found in both the empirically observed functional specialization of the corresponding three brain areas and the theoretical observation that computational specialization can alleviate tensions that would exist in a mechanism that tries to 'do it all'. This latter observation is particularly critical when the medium used to implement the computational system poses significant constrains on the solution space.

Temporal synchrony and its limitations

As described above, temporal synchrony is a popular way of accounting for how the brain flexibly preforms binding. In summary, the temporal synchrony account of binding is that when populations of neurons that represent various features fire together, those features are considered to be bound together. If the system needs to represent multiple distinct sets of bindings simultaneously, it alternates between representing each set of bindings. For instance, consider the case where the system is asked to represent three objects. To do this, first all of the neurons that represent features of the first object would fire simultaneously, or nearly simultaneously. Subsequently, all the neurons representing the features of the second object would fire. Then the same would happen for the third object. Finally, after representing the third object, the system would loop and represent the first object again. Accordingly, the simultaneous binding of the features for each of the three objects would be represented in the system by the neural representation of each the distinct set of bindings firing out of phase with the other representations.

A more concrete example is shown in Figure 8.2. Here, there are two objects: a blue square and a red triangle. Further, the observer has four neuronal units. For our purposes, it does not matter whether these units represent individual neurons or populations of neurons. Perception of the two objects would be represented by oscillation between the red and triangle units firing together and then the square and blue units firing together. Thus, the time course of firing serves to disambiguate which feature becomes bound to what object. Part of the appeal of temporal synchrony is that it appears to solve the binding problem trivially. Additionally, it appears to offer a general process that can account for all instances of binding during any given cognitive process. Accordingly, as a unitary mechanism, it also initially appears to be a very parsimonious account of binding. Further, we do not have any issue with admitting that the simultaneous firing of populations

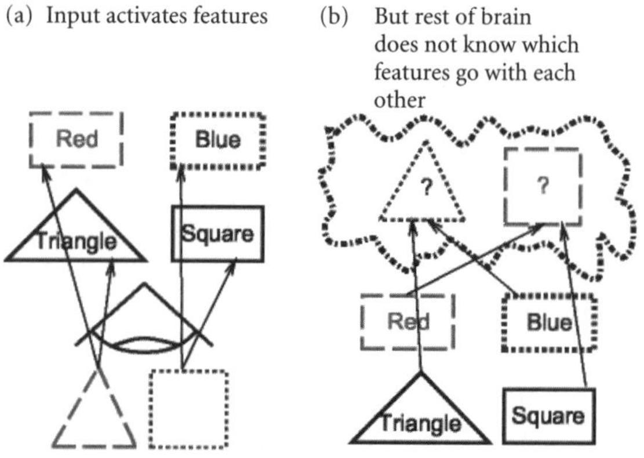
(a) Input activates features
(b) But rest of brain does not know which features go with each other
Red
Blue
Triangle
Square
?
?
Red
Blue
Triangle
Square

Figure 8.2 Illustration of the binding problem. (a) Visual inputs (red triangle, blue square) activate separate representations of colour and shape properties. (b) However, the mere activation of these features does not distinguish for the rest of the brain the alternative scenario of a blue triangle and a red square.

of neurons is important for facilitating binding. However, there are significant issues inherent in the proposition that simultaneously representing different sets of bindings is primarily done via oscillation between the representations for each set of bindings. Specifically, three important criticisms of this mechanism, which are addressed below, are the transience of the binding relationships, the difficulties inherent in downstream systems decoding a set of objects encoded via out-of-phase firing, and the apparent fragility of this mechanism.

Transience

Initially, the transience of the bindings associated with temporal synchrony could be seen as an asset, i.e. with this mechanism computation involving bringing various features together need not induce additional structure within the system. Since, in any given day, an individual probably performs a large number of cognitive processes that collectively require billions if not trillions of elementary binding operations, it would seem that transient bindings are a good thing as they significantly lower the storage requirements of the system. However, the disadvantage of this is that once a stimulus is removed there is no memory of it. Therefore, returning to Figure 8.2, if the red square and the blue triangle were removed from the subject's field of vision, he or she would have no memory of ever seeing the two objects. Of course, proponents of temporal synchrony have taken steps to explain how a lasting trace could be generated from within a temporal synchrony framework. They account for such long-term traces by postulating a complementary memory system that can form persistent representations of sets of features previously bound together via synchronized firing.

For example, Hummel and Holyoak (1997) propose that such a memory system operates by forming a simple conjunctive representation of the features that are to be bound together. While, initially, this may seem like a workable solution, there is a significant body of empirical evidence that all experiences leave a lasting trace in the brain. Accordingly, following the approach proposed by Hummel and Holyoak (1997), a conjunctive representation would need to be formed for all items that were ever represented by the system. Even over a very short period of time, this could result in the system requiring a very large number of units to sort all of its conjunctive memories. Further, one of the most significant criticisms of systems that do not use temporal synchrony has been an intuition that such systems require an enormous number of units in order to arbitrarily bind any non-trivial set of features. As will be analytically demonstrated below, this criticism of such an alternative models is in principle unfounded.

If a temporal synchrony model does use an efficient encoding system that can statically represent a large number of binding relationships, the question arises as to what is additionally to be gained by postulating that bindings are done through temporal synchrony. Proponents of temporal synchrony would point out that this modelling framework provides an unmatched level of systematicity in its representations (Hummel and Holyoak 2003). Further, such systematicity is critical for generalization. Nonetheless, as will be discussed later, models using CCDRs do exhibit a promising degree of generalization. Temporal synchrony also complicates various computational processes, and it is not clear whether the benefits added to systematicity are worth the cost of this added complexity.

Decoding by downstream systems

Returning to Figure 8.2, imagine that the subject was involved in a task which required integrating information about both objects presented. For instance, if a red triangle and a blue square are presented, the subject should push a button on the left. However, if a blue triangle and a red square are presented, the subject should push the button on the right. Finally, if any other pair of objects is presented (e.g. two red triangles), the subject should do nothing at all. Since success at this task entails both binding features to objects and then in some downstream process computing some function over multiple distinct bindings, it is not immediately obvious what is the best way to represent this process within a temporal synchrony framework.

Specifically, a system that simply combines the two representations so that all the relevant features can be simultaneously presented to the downstream system will not work. In this case, the downstream system will not be able to distinguish between the case where it is presented with a red triangle and a blue square and the case where it is presented with a blue triangle and a red square (Fig. 8.3). An alternative workable approach would be to intelligently integrate the individual

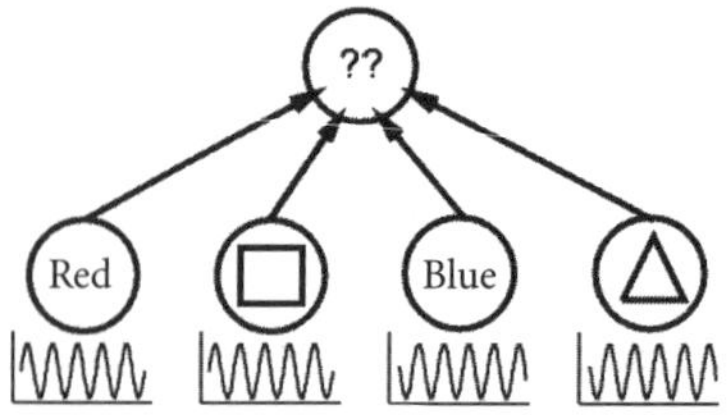

Figure 8.3 Decoding problem for temporal synchrony. Two sets of features are each firing in phase with each other and out of phase with the other set (as indicated by the sine wave plots below the features). Without additional mechanisms, it is unclear how a downstream neuron can decode this information to determine what is actually present; it is being uniformly driven by synaptic input at all phases, and its activation would be the same for any combination of synchrony in the input features. One solution is to build in preferential weights for one set of features (e.g. 'red square'), but this amounts to a conjunctive representation which the temporal synchrony approach is designed to avoid in the first place.

representations of the two objects into a combined non-temporally extended representation which maintains the appropriate binding information. However, once again, if the system must create such a representation in order to facilitate downstream processing, why should temporal synchrony be used in the first place. Why not just go directly to the unified representation? Of course, there are other possible solutions to facilitating downstream processing in a system based on temporal synchrony, but these involve sophisticated cognitive machinery which not only detracts from the apparent elegance of the temporal synchrony framework, but also raises significant questions as to how learning would occur in such systems.

Fragility

The temporal synchrony approach to binding requires a precise timing mechanism that could coordinate the out-of-phase representation of different sets of bindings. Further, such precise timing would depend on the the exact firing behaviour of individual neurons. If this timing system were to fail, the results could be catastrophic. Features involved in different sets of bindings would be randomly mixed to create new sets of bindings that would make little or no sense. Accordingly, it appears that any system based on temporal synchrony would be necessarily fragile in that any small perturbation in timing would cause serious problems for the system. This runs counter to the observation that the brain is rather robust both to insult and to interference with normal neurological processes by psychoactive agents such as alcohol. Specifically, under such conditions not only does performance degrade gracefully but there is also no selective early failure of the binding system. Finally, electrophysiological recordings strongly suggest that the brain is a relatively noisy environment. Therefore it appears that supporting temporal synchrony in such a context would be necessarily very difficult. Further, the electrophysiological recordings that do support the concept of temporal synchrony only emerge after averaging over many trials. Thus they may just be artefacts of some other neurological process.

As will be illustrated in the following section, the weaknesses of temporal synchrony are actually the strengths of the SNRGE approach. That is, through the CCDRs of the posterior cortex and the large-scale conjunctive representations of the hippocampus, the system naturally supports non-transient bindings and accounts for all experiences to leave some trace in the computational machinery. Also, unlike temporal synchrony, simultaneously representing multiple sets of bindings is assumed to be represented as a single unitary representation. Accordingly, downstream systems have no difficulty in decoding the bindings for use in some cognitive task that depends on two or more sets of binding relationships.

Additionally, since there is no need for a precise timing mechanism, the system intuitively appears more robust than one based on temporal synchrony. This intuition is supported by evidence from computation simulations whereby systems based on the representations that we are advocating degrade gracefully on injury or insult (O'Reilly and Munakata 2000).

Coarse-coded distributed representations of low-order conjunctions

One trivial solution to the binding problem is to use conjunctive representations to represent each binding that the system needs to perform. For example, returning to Figure 8.2, there would be a particular unit that codes for a blue square and another that codes for a red triangle. While it is intuitively easy to understand how such conjunctive representations solve the binding problem, they are intractable because they produce a combinatorial explosion in the number of units required to code for all possible bindings as the number of features to be bound increases. For example, assume that all objects in the world can be described by 32 different dimensions (shape, size, colour, etc.), each of which contains 16 different feature values. To encode all possible bindings using the naive approach, we would need 16^{32} or 35×10^{38} units. If the system needed to bind features for four objects simultaneously, four times as many units would be needed. Of course, the brain binds many more types of features and does so with far less units. This combinatorial explosion problem for simple conjunctive representations is an important reason why they have been largely ignored as a solution to the binding problem.

However, there are far more efficient ways of implementing conjunctive representations which, as we show below, have very modest lower bounds in terms of the number of units required to encode a large number of possible bindings. The efficient conjunctive encoding we advocate is CCDR of low-order conjunctions. As described earlier, we believe that this type of representation is used in the posterior cortex to facilitate efficient binding in the immediate service of information processing. In summary, in CCDR each unit can code in a graded fashion for multiple low-level conjunctions, and thereby achieve much greater efficiency. Table 8.1 shows a simple example of this kind of representation (O'Reilly and Munakata 2000). Localist units are used to encode either one of three shape features or one of three colour features. Clearly, the use of these localist units alone does not allow the system to bind pairs of features together (e.g. blue binds with square, red binds with triangle, and circle binds with green). However, by adding just one additional unit that codes for three low-level conjunctions, the system now has a unique representation for each possible binding of the feature types to three objects.

Table 8.1 Solution to the binding problem by using representations that encode combinations of input features (i.e. colour and shape), but achieve greater efficiency by representing multiple such combinations

obj1	obj2	R	G	B	S	C	T	RC GS BT
RS	GC	1	1	0	1	1	0	0
RC	GS	1	1	0	1	1	0	1
RS	GT	1	1	0	1	0	1	0
RT	GS	1	1	0	1	0	1	1
RS	BC	1	0	1	1	1	0	0
RC	BS	1	0	1	1	1	0	1
RS	BT	1	0	1	1	0	1	1
RT	BS	1	0	1	1	0	1	0
RC	GT	1	1	0	0	1	1	1
RT	GC	1	1	0	0	1	1	0
RC	BT	1	0	1	0	1	1	1
RT	BC	1	0	1	0	1	1	0
GS	BC	0	1	1	1	1	0	1
GC	BS	0	1	1	1	1	0	0
GS	BT	0	1	1	1	0	1	1
GT	BS	0	1	1	1	0	1	0
GC	BT	0	1	1	0	1	1	1
GT	BC	0	1	1	0	1	1	0

obj1 and obj2 show the features of the two objects. The first six columns show the responses of a set of representations that encode the separate colour and shape features: R, red, G, green, B, blue, S, square, C, circle, T, triangle. Using only these separate features causes the binding problem; observe that the two configurations in each pair are equivalent according to the separate feature representation. The final unit encodes a combination of the three different conjunctions shown at the top of the column, and this is enough to disambiguate the otherwise equivalent representations.

Analysis of efficient conjunctive binding representations

We now present some results that demonstrate the high level of representational efficiency that can in principle be obtained by CCDRs. The key insight is that we can represent the efficiency of a distributed representation, which comes from representing a large number of possibilities using different combinations of a much smaller number of units, by using an optimal binary encoding of bits. Thus the number of bits required to encode all the different binding combinations gives an optimal lower-bound estimate for the number of binary thresholded units that would be required to distinguish the different binding cases.

This lower bound does not account for whether a fixed set of neural weights could actually achieve the necessary pattern of firing required for such a maximally efficient representation. In addition, it does not take into account the kind of graded activations that are more consistent with the typical description of CCDRs (which are typically much more efficient than binary units). Nevertheless, this analysis provides an easily calculated lower bound that makes it clear that the combinatorial explosion issue for conjunctive binding representations should not pose a problem for CCDRs.

To parametrize the analysis, we consider D sets of mutually exclusive feature dimensions (e.g. shape, colour, size, etc.). Each feature dimension has a number of features D (e.g. square, triangle, circle, etc. for the shape dimension). We could easily consider different numbers of features per dimension, but this is not necessary for a basic analysis. Also, the feature set can contain a null element that represents no feature from the given set being bound to a given object. The system can represent (bind) N different items composed of these dimensions and features at a time.

Using this notation, the number of ways that features from each dimension can be bound to N objects is given by

$$(F^D)^N. \tag{1}$$

This is a very large number even for small values of F, D, and N. However, taking $\log_2$ of this quantity produces a much smaller number, which reflects the number of bits (i.e. binary thresholded units) required to represent each possible set of bindings. This simplifies to the following expression:

$$\text{min bits} = ND \log_2 F. \tag{2}$$

Note that this expression is linear in the number of objects N and dimensions D, and even more efficient as the number of features per dimension F increases.

As an example of this efficiency, we return to the example given earlier regarding a system that must be able to represent all arbitrary bindings of 32 different dimensions (i.e. $D = 32$), each of which has 16 distinct features ($F_i = 16$), to four separate objects ($N = 4$). As noted earlier, a simple conjunctive encoding for such a system would require 136×10^{39} units. However, 512 units would be required with an optimal binary distributed representation. Again, the actual number of units required for an actual graded neural network encoding will probably be different, but should be roughly of the same order and nowhere near as many as the simple conjunctive encoding.

Tuple binding and combinatorial generalization

As a complement to the above analytical results, the remainder of this section focuses on empirical results for models that make use of CCDR. These results further demonstrate both that CCDR can efficiently represent binding information, and that such representations can be learned by a model. Furthermore, we focus on the generalization performance of these models (i.e. their ability to process novel inputs in a systematic manner consistent with training), which has been raised as an important problem for CCDR networks as contrasted with temporal synchrony models (Hummel and Holyoak 2003). Indeed, some would argue that generalization is a greater problem than that of capacity. In this respect, the arguments from temporal synchrony advocates strongly resemble those levelled at neural networks from the perspective of traditional symbolic cognitive models (Fodor and Pylyshyn 1988; Pinker and Prince 1988). This makes sense given that many extant temporal synchrony models can be characterized as essentially more elaborate implementations of these traditional symbolic architectures, particularly in their ability to leverage arbitrary symbol binding for producing systematic behaviour. Furthermore, these temporal synchrony models suffer many of the same limitations as earlier symbolic models, particularly with respect to the difficulty of incorporating powerful learning mechanisms that can develop new knowledge and processing representations from initially undifferentiated neural tissue.

Therefore, to show that an approach based on CCDR offers a competitive alternative to temporal synchrony models, it is vital to demonstrate that they generalize sufficiently well. Below, we discuss a number of generalization tests with relatively generic posterior cortex models employing CCDR which demonstrate that these representations are indeed capable of high levels of generalization in the context of tasks that have extensive binding demands. Other related results are given by Edelman and Intrator (2003). We then return to these issues in the section on prefrontal cortex, where we discuss recentresults showing how rule-like representations in the prefrontal cortex, learned in the context of task performance, can promote even more systematic behaviour in neural networks (Rougier *et al.* 2005).

Tuple reordering task

We have explored a variation of a widely explored test of generalization in neural networks called either the *N*-tuple or the combinatorial generalization task (Brousse and Smolensky 1989; Phillips and Wiles 1993; O'Reilly 2001) (Fig. 8.4). Although the basic task does not require much in the way of binding, we were able to extend it to do so. This task has the form of a simple auto-associative network where the input is a tuple of *N* items and the target output is the same tuple of *N* items. Early work with this task suggested that feedforward back-propagation neural networks could not adequately generalize to this task, supporting the need

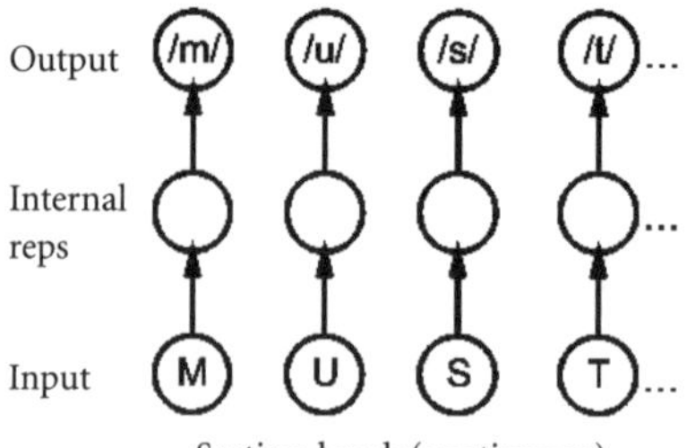

Figure 8.4 Illustration of the *N*-tuple or combinatorial generalization task in the more naturalistic context of systematically pronouncing letter inputs. In the combinatorial extreme represented by this task, each letter position is mapped to a corresponding output in a way that does not depend on any of the other letters. Thus the most efficient solution is to develop internal representations that encode each input/output tuple mapping separately. Clearly, this level of combinatoriality is too extreme in the case of letter pronunciation, but nevertheless it serves as a convenient benchmark task.

in cognitive modelling for alternative more systematic architectures (Brousse and Smolensky 1989). However, subsequent work demonstrated that such neural networks could in fact generalize well to this task (Phillips and Wiles 1993; O'Reilly 2001). Successful networks learned to develop separate mapping pathways between input and output tuples, as illustrated in Figure 8.4.

We have developed a straightforward extension of the *N*-tuple auto-associative task that requires a much more demanding solution, involving the binding and remapping of input features in slots (Cer and O'Reilly, in preparation) (Fig. 8.5). Specifically, we introduced an additional input to the model that indicates how the items in the input tuple should be reordered when they are output by the model. That is, rather than mapping the *i*th element of the input tuple directly to the *i*th element of the output tuple, the mapping instruction given to the network will indicate the *j*th element in the output to which any given *i*th element in the input should be mapped. While superficially this may appear to be a trivial extension of the *N*-tuple task, the current task represents a significant extension in terms of the computation that must be performed by the model. Specifically, note that the mapping operations that the model is instructed to perform are defined over the input and output slots. However, to perform the task the network must operate on the values represented within these slots. Thus success at this task would indicate that the model can not only bind values to variable-like entities but can also systematically perform operations defined over the variables on the values held by those variables.

To explore how successful a neural network that performed binding via CCDR would be at this task, we constructed the model shown in Figure 8.5. Both input and output slots consist of six units, with the values represented within these

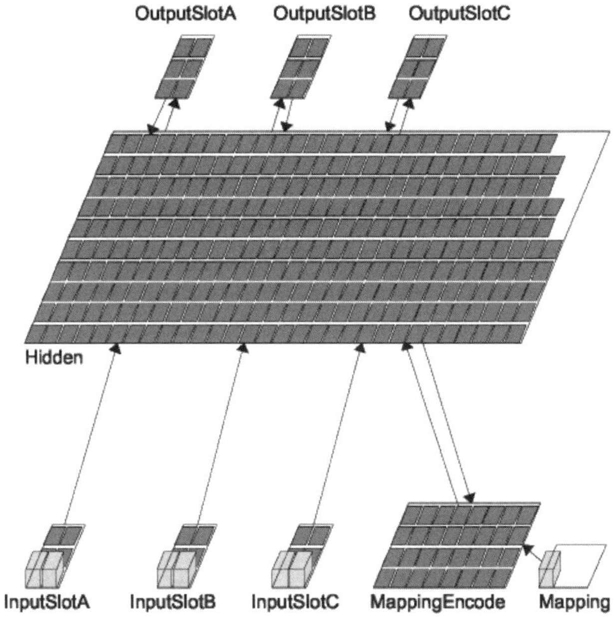

Figure 8.5 The tuple reordering network. Input patterns are presented across three slots, and the mapping input layer provided a transformation signal for reordering the presentation of these inputs across the three output slots.

slots by activating two of the six units. While this representation allows the slots to take on up to 15 different values, only six values were used in our experiment. The mapping instructions are presented using a localist representation, i.e. each of the six units in the mapping layer corresponds to one of the six possible ways that three slots can be rearrange. Finally, the hidden layer consists of 300 units.

The model is implemented in the Leabra framework (O'Reilly 1998; O'Reilly and Munakata 2000), which includes a biologically plausible form of error back-propagation, Hebbian learning, and inhibitory competition. The inhibitory competition and Hebbian learning in Leabra have been shown to produce improved generalization relative to plain back-propagation in a range of different tasks (O'Reilly 2001; O'Reilly and Busby 2002). Standard Leabra parameters were used in all parts of the network, except in the mapping encode layer where the kwta percentage was decreased from 0.25 to 0.20. Biologically, this roughly corresponds to increasing the degree of lateral inhibition in this layer.

The model's training set consisted of 432 examples of how to perform the tuple mapping operation. This training set represents 33 per cent of the total problem space. The test set consisted of 138 randomly selected tuple mappings that did not occur in the training set. After training for 25 epochs (where each epoch consisted of presenting every item in the training set once), the model was able to obtain perfect performance. Further, at this point the network only made two errors out of the entire test set, i.e. its generalization performance as measured by the test set is 98.7 per cent.

These results appear to indicate that CCDR can facilitate binding values to variable-like entities and then perform operations defined over the variables on the appropriate values. Again, the good generalization performance of the model indicates that it has not simply learned some degenerate associative mapping such as a holistic mapping of various patterns presented on the input layers to certain patterns of activity on the output layer. Rather, since the network is able to generalize well, its representations must have largely captured the abstract computational operation that was being requested.

Spatial relationship binding model

A more sophisticated binding task, in which a network was trained to encode and report a number of relationships between items that were presented on its inputs, was explored by O'Reilly and Busby (2002). The model (Fig. 8.6) roughly represents a simplified model of the early visual system. During training the model is presented with a pair of input items in a simulated visual field and one of four corresponding questions. Two of the questions, 'what?' and 'where?', only required the network to report information pertaining to one of the two objects. For the 'what?' question, the Location layer was used as an additional input to the network indicating the location of the input item it was being asked about. In response to this question, the model was trained to present in the Object layer the item at the given location in the input field. In the case of the 'where?' question, the Object layer acted as an additional input, and the network was trained to output in the Location layer the input position corresponding to the item presented in the Object layer. The two remaining questions require the network to identify relationships between the two items presented in the input layer. The 'relation-obj?' question is similar to the 'what?' question in that the Location layer is used as an input that indicates the location in the input field of the object that the network should output in the Object layer. However, for this question the network must also output in the Relation layer the relative relationship between the queried item and the other item presented in the input field. Similarly, the 'relation-loc?' question is like the 'where?' question in that the Object layer is used as an input that indicates the identity of the item in the input field whose location the network should output in the location layer. As with the'relation-obj?' question, the network must also identify the relative location of the other item presented in the input field relative to the queried item and report this information in the Relation layer.

Like the model described in the last section, the current model was implemented as a recurrent neural network. In addition to a Leabra implementation, a model using only contrastive Hebbian (CHL) error-driven learning and another

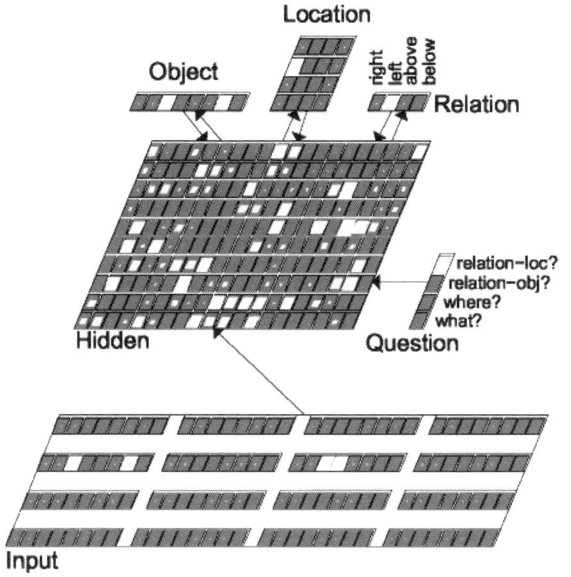

Figure 8.6 Spatial relationship binding model of O'Reilly and Busby (2002). Objects are represented by distributed patterns of activation over eight feature values in each location, with the input containing a 4 × 4 array of object locations. Input patterns contain two different objects arranged either vertically or horizontally. The network answers different questions about the inputs based on the activation of the Question input layer. For the 'what?' question, the location of one of the objects is activated as an input in the Location layer, and the network must produce the correct object features for the object in that location. For the 'where?' question, the object features for one of the objects are activated in the Object layer, and the network must produce the correct location activation for that object. For the 'relation-obj?' question, the object features for one object are activated, and the network must activate the relationship between this object and the other object, in addition to activating the location for this object. For the 'relation-loc?' question, the location of one of the objects is activated, and the network must activate the relationship between this object and the other object, in addition to activating the object features for this object (this is the example shown in the network, responding that the target object is to the left of the other object). Thus the hidden layer must have bound object, location, and relationship information in its encoding of the input.

model using the Almedia–Pineda recurrent back-propagation algorithm were also run. It was found that Almedia–Pineda model was unable to learn to perform the task successfully, while both the Leabra and CHL networks were able to do so. The additional constraints in Leabra (Hebbian learning and inhibitory competition) produced almost twice as good generalization as CHL (Fig. 8.7).

These experiments demonstrate both that CCDRs can systematically perform binding relationships, and that not all mechanisms for developing such relationships are equivalent. Specifically, by incorporating additional biologically motivated constraints on the development of internal representations in the network,

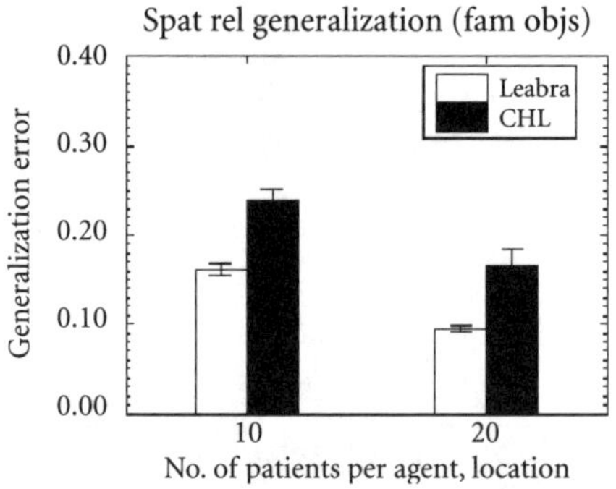

Figure 8.7 Generalization results for different algorithms on the spatial relationship binding task (testing on familiar objects in novel locations; similar results also hold for novel objects). Only the 400 Agent, Location × 10 or Location × 20 Patient, Location cases are shown. It is clear that Leabra performed roughly twice as well as the CHL algorithm, consistent with earlier results on other tasks. (Reproduced from O'Reilly 2001.)

the Leabra model is able to achieve more systematicity in its representations, which subsequently give rise to better generalization performance.

Language surface form transformations

The models presented above strongly suggest that CCDRs can not only bind various features together, but also facilitate systematic operations over these bindings. However, the tasks given so far were designed explicitly to be pure investigations of binding. Thus the possibility remains that such tasks biased the learning that occurred in the network in such a way that the binding performance of the system was exaggerated over and above what can typically be expected of similar networks applied to more realistic cognitive tasks. That is, it is possible that a more complex task would make it harder for the network to identify the abstract computational process that it is being asked to perform and thus bias the system towards finding degenerate solutions.

In order to explore this issue further, we constructed a task involving sentence surface form transformations (Cer and O'Reilly, in preparation). Specifically, the task involves giving the network a sentence one word at a time during the encoding part of the task. Then, during the decoding part of the task, the network is asked to repeat either the sentence that it was given during encoding or some transformation of it. The transformations we selected were active to passive, or passive to active. Further, when asked to perform a transformation, the model is not told explicitly what sort of transformation it should perform (i.e. active to passive versus passive to active). Rather, during decoding, it is just told whether or not it should transform the sentence. This complicates the task, because the network must condition its transformation on the type of the current sentence.

The linguistic environment used for this task was a simple English-like grammar that supports the two constructions given below:

Active construction: [Det] [Noun] [Verb] [Det] [Noun]

Passive construction: [Det] [Noun] was [Verb] by [Det] [Noun]

For the experiment reported here, this simple language included 32 nouns, eight verbs and two determiners. All verbs had the same form in the active and passive constructions. Additionally, when such sentences are given to the model, they are enclosed in start and end of sentence markers.

Notably, this task requires binding words into some structure that represents their relative positions in the sentence. Additionally, the network must be able to flexibly extract information from this structure such that both the active and the passive forms of a sentence can be reconstructed. Further, since the task is more computationally complex than those described above, the added complexity should be such that it is not trivially easy to identify that a good solution to the task involves such binding.

The network that was trained to perform this task is illustrated in Figure 8.8. This network was originally developed to examine some psycholinguistic phenomena, although it was easily adapted for the task at hand. During encoding, words are presented one at a time in the layer labelled 'in_current_prev'. For each

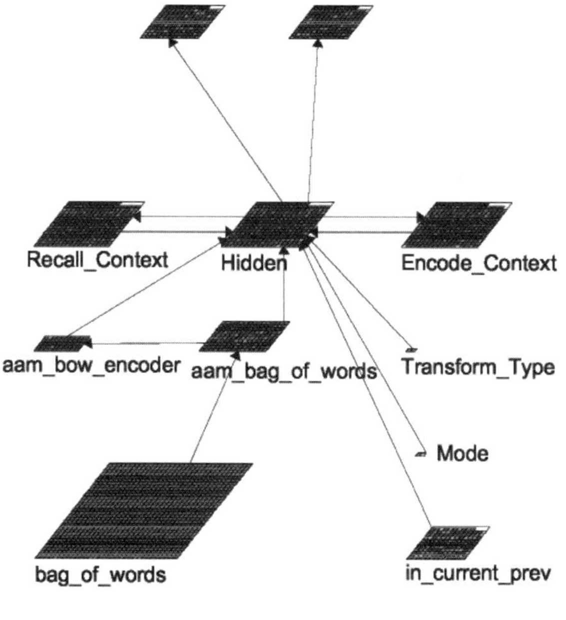

Figure 8.8 Language transformation network. See text for details on the role of each layer and the nature of the input/output patterns used.

word that is presented as input, the network is trained to produce the same word in the 'out_current_prev' layer. Additionally, the network must reproduce the word that was presented immediately before the current word in the 'out_prev_current' layer. The representations of words used within these three layers correspond to distributed representations developed during training using forming global representations with extended back-propagation (FGREP) (Miikkulainen 1993). After the presentation of each word, the activation values for the units in the hidden layer are copied to the units in the 'Encode_Context' layer. Also, after each word is presented to the network, the unit in the 'bag_of_words' layer which corresponds to that word is activated (if it is not already active from a previous presentation of the same word in the current sentence). Once activated, the units in the 'bag_of_words' layer remain active for the rest of the encoding and decoding process for the current sentence. Finally, the fact that a sentence is being presented for encoding is cued by the activation of the first unit in the mode layer.

During decoding, the second unit in the mode layer is activated. Additionally, if the network should reproduce the exact sentence it was given during encoding, the first unit in the transformation layer is activated. If the network should transform the encoded sentence, the second unit in the transformation layer is activated. The first item presented in the 'in_current_prev' layer during decoding is the beginning of sentence marker. In response to this, the network must reproduce the beginning of sentence marker in the 'out_current_prev' layer and the first word from the appropriate form of the sentence in the 'out_prev_current' layer. Similarly, during the next time step, the network is given the first word in the sentence as input in the 'in_current_prev' layer and must produce the second word in the sentence in the 'out_prev_current' layer. Note that the type of sentence production scheme used here is similar to the constrained production paradigm given by Rohde (2002). Between each time step, the activations of the units in the hidden layer are copied over to the units in the 'Decode_Context' layer. Also, note that during decoding the 'Encode_Context' layer is frozen to whatever the last pattern of activation was in the hidden layer at the end of the encoding process.

The hidden layer and the two context layers each comprise 250 units, and the three FGREP layers each comprise 140 units. The 'bag_of_words' layer comprises 1024 units, although only 46 of these are used for the given task. The 'aam_bag_of_words' layer comprises 150 units. It should be noted that the connections from the 'bag_of_words' input layer and the 'aam_bag_of_words' layer are pretrained in an autoencoder network over all representations that the 'bag_of_words' layer can take on in the training set. These connections are then fixed during the training of the larger network. This pretraining allows for a stable CCDR distributed representation of each pattern that is presented in the 'bag_of_words' layer (which would otherwise use localist representations all words). The 'bag_of_words_encoder' layer comprises 50 units. Finally, the model was implemented as a standard back-propagation network. A learning rate of 0.1 and momentum of 0.9 were used.

The network was trained on 4000 transformations, which represented 6.1 per cent of the total problem space. Testing was done using 100 randomly selected transformations of sentences that did not occur in the training set. Network performance was evaluated by scoring the representations produced by the network during decoding. Accordingly, scoring was restricted to the network's ability to construct/reconstruct the appropriate surface form of the previously presented sentence. The representations were scored by identifying the word whose representation most closely matched the representation produced by the network as measure by the Euclidean distance between the two.

After training, the network was able to obtain 84.2 per cent generalization performance over the test set. While this is not close to the perfect generalization performance of the models presented previously, it is still relatively good given the dramatically more difficult task. Accordingly, these results suggest that the network was able to form CCDRs that overall served to perform the binding necessary to encode the sequential order of the words in the sentence, and then systematically transform them during decoding.

Summary

As demonstrated in the three models we have presented and the analytical results, CCDRs represent an efficient means of encoding binding relationships. However, such representations both take a substantial amount of time to develop and are always driven by inputs from other systems. Accordingly, they do not account for how people rapidly form episodic memories or learn new material such that a large number of arbitrary features are durably bound together. CCDR also do not account for how people actively maintain bindings that are not directly driven by the immediate environment. As will be shown below, these two variants of the binding problem are addressed by the hippocampus and the prefrontal cortex, respectively.

Hippocampal conjunctive binding

The role of the hippocampus in binding can be contrasted with the posterior cortex models just discussed along several dimensions. First, the hippocampus has sparser activity levels than the posterior cortex (approximately 5 per cent to less than

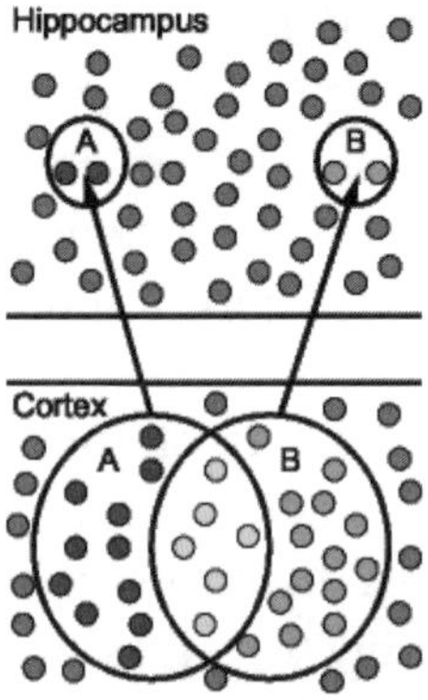

Figure 8.9 Sparse representations in the hippocampus relative to the cortex leads to pattern separation (less probability of activation patterns overlapping, as is evident in the figure), and to units in hippocampus representing larger conjunctions of features in the cortex. This means that the hippocampus performs higher-order conjunctive binding than the cortex. See colour plate section.

1 per cent in different regions of the hippocampus, compared with approximately 15–25 per cent for cortex). These sparse hippocampal representations cause units to respond only to specific patterns of activity across the cortex (Fig. 8.9). Therefore the hippocampal representations encode more specific *high-order* conjunctions of many features, which contrasts with the relatively *low-order* conjunctions (i.e. conjoining relatively few features) in the posterior cortical representations.

Thus the hippocampal units encode specific events more uniquely, while the cortical units encode smaller recurring subsets of events. Therefore the cortical representations support similarity-based generalization to novel situations, whereas the hippocampal representations are better able to avoid interference between similar events, especially when rapid learning is required to encode fleeting episodes. The details of the hippocampal models have been published in a number of papers, and so are not repeated here (O'Reilly and Munakata 2000; O'Reilly and Rudy 2001; Norman and O'Reilly 2003). These models have demonstrated the ability to explain a wide range of data from animal and human experiments.

In one example, experiments with rats and corresponding models showed that the hippocampus is essential for rapidly binding together the stimulus features that define an environment (Rudy *et al.* 2002). In the experiments, the rats were repeatedly transported in a distinctive black ice bucket to a pre-exposure environment. Then the rats were brought in this bucket into a different conditioning environment, where they were shocked. One day later, the rats were transported in a distinct cage to either the original pre-exposure environment or the conditioning environment. We found that the rats expressed fear conditioning (freezing behaviour) to the pre-exposure environment, but not to the conditioning environment.

We interpreted this result as reflecting the rapid binding of the pre-exposure environment features, together with the bucket, into a conjunctive hippocampal representation. This representation was reactivated by the bucket cue just prior to the conditioning, causing the rat to associate the shock with a memory of the pre-exposure environment instead of the actual environment in which it was shocked. This interpretation was supported by a computational model, and confirmed by hippocampal lesions in the rats which abolished the fear responding to the pre-exposure environment.

In summary, the results reviewed here, and many more like them, suggest that the hippocampus is specialized for rapidly binding together the features or elements of episodes and environments. The resulting conjunctive representations are distinctive from those in the cortex by virtue of being highly specific (i.e. higher order), in contrast with the low-order conjunctive representations found in cortex. Both types of representations have their costs and benefits, and thus the SNRGE model suggests that different brain areas are specialized for each of these functions.

Prefrontal cortex

As noted earlier, the prefrontal cortex is thought to be specialized for the active maintenance and updating of information, commonly referred to as working memory. This specialization has several implications for binding. Generally speaking, actively maintained information can be used to perform transient forms of binding needed only for a short time during the performance of a given task. This contrasts with the relatively long-lasting forms of binding represented by both the low-order and high-order conjunctive representations associated with the cortex and the hippocampus, respectively. For example, the phonological loop is a working memory system that can actively maintain a short chunk of phonological (verbal) information (Baddeley 1986; Baddeley *et al.* 1998; Burgess and Hitch 1999; Emerson and Miyake 2003). This actively maintained verbal information is often used to maintain bindings necessary for solving a given task.

An example of this form of transient phonologically dependent binding comes from a task studied by Miyake and Soto (in preparation). In this task, participants saw sequentially presented coloured letters one at a time on a computer display, and had to respond to targets of a red X or a green Y, but not to any other colour–letter combination (e.g. green X and red Y, which were also presented). After an initial series of trials with this set of targets, the targets were switched to be a green X and a red Y. Thus the task clearly requires binding of colour and letter information, and updating these bindings after the switch condition. Miyake and Soto (in preparation) found that if they simply asked participants to repeat the word 'the' continually during the task (i.e. articulatory suppression), it interfered significantly with performance. In contrast, performing a similar repeated motor response which did not involve the phonological system (repeated foot tapping) did not produce interference (but this task did interfere at the same level as articulatory suppression in a control visual search task, so that one cannot argue that the interference was simply a matter of differential task difficulty). Miyake and Soto (in preparation) interpret this pattern of results as showing that the phonological loop supports the binding of stimulus features (e.g. participants repeatedly say to themselves 'red X, green Y', which is supported by debriefing reports), and that the use of this phonological system for unrelated information during articulatory suppression leads to the observed performance deficits.

This transient binding function of the PFC was simulated in a model that reproduces (in a simplified fashion) several of the biological specializations associated with the PFC (O'Reilly and Soto 2002). Specifically, this model included separate 'stripes' (columns) in the PFC, with each stripe receiving a separate updating signal from a simulated basal ganglia system (O'Reilly and Munakata 2000; Frank *et al.* 2001). These features enabled the PFC to use dedicated stripes for each sequential position in a stream of phonemes. This is possible because phonemes are a small closed class, and thus each stripe can have representations for all possible phonemes. Taken together, these specializations enable this phonological loop model to maintain arbitrary phonological sequences in active memory. Furthermore, the network exhibited high levels of generalization after training on a small subset (10 per cent) of possible phonological sequences. Thus this model suggests how the PFC can maintain arbitrary bindings in a phonological code; these phonological sequences will then impact on semantically associated representations throughout the cortex to support task-appropriate processing (Cohen *et al.* 1990; Miller and Cohen 2001).

Another critical contribution of the PFC to supporting task-relevant processing in a flexible generalizable manner comes from abstract rule-like representations that can develop through an interaction between biological specializations of the PFC and broad experience across different tasks. Rougier *et al.* developed a model that addresses this fundamental question: How is information represented in the PFC and, critically, how does this develop? We showed that PFC-specific mechanisms interact with the breadth of training experience to produce abstract rule-like representations that support generalization of performance in novel task circumstances. We also showed that these rule-like representations support patterns of performance characteristic of neurologically intact and frontally damaged subects on benchmark tasks of cognitive control (Stroop Test and Wisconsin Card Sort Test). Although the rule-like representations that developed in the model of PFC support flexible cognitive control, they did so in a way that is fundamentally different from symbolic representations characteristic of more traditional unified theories of cognition. Therefore these results bear on both the organization and development of PFC at the neurobiogical level, as well as debates regarding the nature of cognitive flexibility and rule-like behaviour at the psychological level. Specifically, this model demonstrates that systematic generalization of the sort emphasized by symbolic approaches (Fodor and Pylyshyn 1988; Pinker and Prince 1988; Hummel and Holyoak 2003) can emerge from biological specializations in neural network models.

Conclusions

In summary, we have presented a range of computational models based on the biological specializations associated with different brain areas that support a range of different contributions to binding. The posterior cortex can learn CCDRs of low-order conjunctions which can efficiently and systematically bind information in the service of many different forms of cortical information processing. However, these representations are learned slowly over experience; in contrast, the hippocampus is specialized for rapidly binding novel information into high-order conjunctive representations (e.g. episodes or locations). Finally, the prefrontal cortex can actively maintain dynamic bindings in working memory and, through more abstract rule-like representations, support more flexible generalization of behaviour across novel task contexts. Taken together, we believe that this overall biologically based cognitive architecture represents a more plausible framework for understanding binding than that provided by temporal synchrony approaches.

Acknowledgements

This work was supported by ONR grants N00014–00–1–0246 and N00014–03–1–0428, and NIH grants MH613 16–01 and MH64445.

References

Baddeley, A.D. (1986). *Working Memory*. New York: Oxford University Press.

Baddeley, A., Gathercole, S., and Papagno, C. (1998). The phonological loop as a language learning device. *Psychological Review*, **105**, 158.

Brousse, O. and Smolensky, P. (1989). Virtual memories and massive generalization in connectionist combinatorial learning. In *Proceedings of the 11th Annual Cognitive Science Society Conference*. Hillsdale, NJ: Erlbaum, pp. 26–33.

Burgess, N. and Hitch, G.J. (1999). Memory for serial order: a network model of the phonological loop and its timing. *Psychological Review*, **106**, 551–581.

Cer, D.M. and O'Reilly, R.C., in preparation.

Cohen, J.D., Dunbar, K., and McClelland, J.L. (1990). On the control of automatic processes: a parallel distributed processing model of the Stroop effect. *Psychological Review*, **97**, 332–361.

Edelman, S. and Intrator, N. (2003). Towards structural systematicity in distributed, statically bound visual representations. *Cognitive Science*, **27**, 73–109.

Emerson, M.J. and Miyake, A. (2003). The role of inner speech in task switching: a dual-task investigation. *Journal of Memory and Language*, **48**, 148–168.

Engel, A.K., Konig, P., Kreiter, A.K., Schillen, T.B., and Singer, W. (1992). Temporal coding in the visual cortex: new vistas on integration in the nervous system. *Trends in Neurosciences*, **15**, 218–226.

Fodor, J.A. and Pylyshyn, Z.W. (1988). Connectionism and cognitive architecture: a critical analysis. *Cognition*, **28**, 3–71.

Frank, M.J., Loughry, B., and O'Reilly, R.C. (2001). Interactions between the frontal cortex and basal ganglia in working memory: a computational model. *Cognitive, Affective, and Behavioral Neuroscience*, **1**, 137–160.

Fuster, J.M. and Alexander, G.E. (1971). Neuron activity related to short-term memory. *Science*, **173**, 652–654.

Goldman-Rakic, P.S. (1987). Circuitry of primate prefrontal cortex and regulation of behavior by representational memory. *Handbook of Physiology: The Nervous System*, **5**, 373–417.

Gray, C.M., Engel, A.K., Konig, P., and Singer, W. (1992). Synchronization of oscillatory neuronal responses in cat striate cortex: temporal properties. *Visual Neuroscience*, **8**, 337–347.

Hinton, G.E., McClelland, J.L., and Rumelhart, D.E. (1986). Distributed representations. In *Parallel Distributed Processing*. Vol. 1: *Foundations* (ed D.E. Rumelhart, J.L. McClelland, and PDP Research Group). Cambridge, MA: MIT Press, pp. 77–109.

Hummel, J.E. and Biederman, I. (1992). Dynamic binding in a neural network for shape recognition. *Psychological Review*, **99**, 480–517.

Hummel, J.E. and Holyoak, K.J. (1997). Distributed representations of structure: A theory of analogical access and mapping. *Psychological Review*, **104**, 427–466.

Hummel, J.E. and Holyoak, K.J. (2003). A symbolic-connectionist theory of relational inference and generalization. *Psychological Review*, **110**, 220–264.

Kubota, K. and Niki, H. (1971). Prefrontal cortical unit activity and delayed alternation performance in monkeys. *Journal of Neurophysiology*, **34**, 337–347.

Marr, D. (1971). Simple memory: a theory for archicortex. *Philosophical Transactions of the Royal Society of London, Series B, Biological Sciences*, **262**, 23–81.

Mel, B.A. and Fiser, J. (2000). Minimizing binding errors using learned conjunctive features. *Neural Computation*, **12**, 73 1–762.

Miikkulainen, R. (1993). *Subsymbolic Natural Language Processing: An Integrated Model of Scripts, Lexicon, and Memory*. Cambridge, MA: MIT Press.

Miller, E.K. and Cohen, J.D. (2001). An integrative theory of prefrontal cortex function. *Annual Review of Neuroscience*, **24**, 167–202.

Milner, B. (1963). Effects of different brain lesions on card sorting. *Archives of Neurology*, **9**, 90–100.

Miyake, A. and Soto, R. (in preparation). The role of the phonological loop in executive control.

Mozer, M.C. (1991). *The Perception of Multiple Objects: A Connectionist Approach.* Cambridge, MA: MIT Press.

Norman, K.A., and O'Reilly, R.C. (2003). Modeling hippocampal and neocortical contributions to recognition memory: a complementary learning systems approach. *Psychological Review*, **110**, 611–646.

O'Reilly, R.C. (1998). Six principles for biologically-based computational models of cortical cognition. *Trends in Cognitive Sciences*, **2**, 455–462.

O'Reilly, R.C. (2001). Generalization in interactive networks: the benefits of inhibitory competition and Hebbian learning. *Neural Computation*, **13**, 1199–1242.

O'Reilly, R.C. and Busby, R.S. (2002). Generalizable relational binding from coarse-coded distributed representations. In *Advances in Neural Information Processing Systems (NIPS)*, Vol. 14 (ed T.G. Dietterich, S. Becker, and Z. Ghahramani). Cambridge, MA: MIT Press.

O'Reilly, R.C. and McClelland, J.L. (1994). Hippocampal conjunctive encoding, storage, and recall: avoiding a tradeoff. *Hippocampus*, **4**, 661–682.

O'Reilly, R.C. and Munakata, Y. (2000). *Computational Explorations in Cognitive Neuroscience: Understanding the Mind by Simulating the Brain.* Cambridge, MA: MIT Press.

O'Reilly, R.C. and Norman, K.A. (2002). Hippocampal and neocortical contributions to memory: advances in the complementary learning systems framework. *Trends in Cognitive Sciences*, **6**, 505–510.

O'Reilly, R.C. and Rudy, J.W. (2001). Conjunctive representations in learning and memory: Principles of cortical and hippocampal function. *Psychological Review*, **108**, 311–345.

O'Reilly, R.C. and Soto, R. (2002). A model of the phonological loop: generalization and binding. In *Advances in Neural Information Processing Systems (NIPS)*, Vol. 14 (ed T.G. Dietterich, S. Becker, and Z. Ghahramani). Cambridge, MA: MIT Press.

O'Reilly, R.C., Braver, T.S., and Cohen, J.D. (1999). A biologically based computational model of working memory. In *Models of Working Memory: Mechanisms of Active Maintenance and Executive Control* (ed A. Miyake and P. Shah). New York: Cambridge University Press, pp. 375–411.

O'Reilly, R.C., Busby, R.S., and Soto, R. (2003). Three forms of binding and their neural substrates: Alter-natives to temporal synchrony. In *The Unity of Consciousness: Binding, Integration, and Dissociation* (ed A. Cleeremans). Oxford: Oxford University Press, pp. 168–192.

Phillips, S. and Wiles, J. (1993). Exponential generalizations from a polynomial number of examples in a combinatorial domain. In *Proceedings of the International Joint Conference on Neural Networks (IJCNN93), Nagoya, Japan*, pp. 505–508.

Pinker, S. and Prince, A. (1988). On language and connectionism: analysis of a parallel distributed processing model of language acquisition. *Cognition*, **28**, 73–193.

Rohde, D.L.T. (2002). A connectionist model of sentence comprehension and production. PhD Thesis, Computer Science Department, Carnegie–Mellon University, Pittsburgh, PA.

Rougier, N.P., Noelle, D., Braver, T.S., Cohen, J.D., and O'Reilly, R.C. (2005). Prefrontal cortex and the flexibility of cognitive control: rules without symbols. *Proceedings of the National Academy of Sciences*, **102**, 7338–7343.

Rudy, J.W., Barrientos, R.M., and O'Reilly, R.C. (2002). Hippocampal formation supports conditioning to memory of a context. *Behavioral Neuroscience*, **116**, 530–538.

Seidenberg, M.S. and McClelland, J.L. (1989). A distributed, developmental model of word recognition and naming. *Psychological Review*, **96**, 523–568.

St John, M.F. and McClelland, J.L. (1990). Learning and applying contextual constraints in sentence comprehension. *Artificial Intelligence*, **46**, 217–257.

Stuss, D.T., Levine, B., Alexander, M.P., *et al.* (2000). Wisconsin Card Sorting Test performance in patients with focal frontal and posterior brain damage: effects of lesion location and test structure on separable cognitive processes. *Neuropsychologia*, **38**, 388–402.

von der Malsburg, C. (1981). The correlation theory of brain function. In *Models of Neural Networks I* (ed E. Domany, J.L. van Hemmen and K. Schulten). Berlin: Springer-Verlag.

Weinberger, D.R., Berman, K.F., and Daniel, D.G. (1991). Prefrontal cortex dysfunction in schizophrenia. In *Frontal Lobe Function and Dysfunction* (ed H.S. Levin, H.M. Eisenberg, and A.L. Benton). New York: Oxford University Press, pp. 276–285.

Wickelgren, W.A. (1969). Context-sensitive coding, associative memory, and serial order in (speech) behavior. *Psychological Review*, **76**, 1–15.

Zemel, R.S., Williams, C.K., and Mozer, M.C. (1995). Lending direction to neural networks. *Neural Networks*, **8**, 503.

Chapter 9

Binding in working memory and long-term memory: towards an integrated model

Jaap M.J. Murre, Gezinus Wolters, and Antonino Raffone

Introduction

There is a long tradition of viewing memory as associative (James 1890; Hebb 1949; Willshaw *et al.* 1969; Raaijmakers and Shiffrin 1981; Hinton and Anderson 1989), assigning it a fundamental role in retrieving some information on the basis of a cue: someone's name springs to mind when we see her face, or when we read a film title we remember the storyline and the principal actors. Memory is an active process, especially in humans. For instance, Bartlett (1932) showed that the retrieval process often takes the form of an active reconstruction. Processes of schematization that continue to influence the contents of memory over time also are at work during storage. During initial encoding, the combined effects of attention, perception, interpretation, and context all influence what will be stored, limiting for example what search cues can later elicit the information (Tulving and Thompson, 1973). In this chapter, we will focus on what we believe are the most fundamental binding processes of associative encoding, storage, and retrieval.

The past 20 years have seen a giant leap forward in our knowledge about the neural mechanisms that transiently or permanently bind information in memory. We will review some of this work on the basis of existing connectionist models and propose an integrated model. First, we will delineate four different binding mechanisms that we believe are important in memory. Then we will present a network model of working memory based on synchronized neuronal activation patterns that can be actively maintained and manipulated in recurrent loops between posterior and prefrontal cortical areas. We will also review some work on the modelling of storage and consolidation in long-term memory. In the final section we will integrate the two approaches.

Four neurodynamic binding mechanisms

Binding is the process that determines the structure of representations in the brain (Damasio 1989a,b). During the binding process neurons become bound into a coherent representation corresponding to actual objects or concepts in the world. Here, we distinguish four neural binding processes that allow flexible compositional operations in perceptual working memory and long-term memory representations. The processes do not exclude each other, but cooperate in various ways during encoding, storage, and retrieval.

Coactivation-based binding

In general, coactivation through simultaneously high-frequent firing of neurons does not imply binding. Nor does such a high firing rate imply a causal link between active neurons. However, when coactive neurons both exchange excitation and are part of a larger cell assembly (Hebb 1949) their activation states are interdependent and functionally related. For instance, the activation of the complete cell assembly may be triggered by a external input to a subset of its neurons, owing to mutual associative connections. Local and non-local (global) assemblies for coactive binding can be inscribed in brain activity, supported by intra-regional and inter-regional (long-range) connectivity between pyramidal cells or via cortico-thalamic loops.

In neural networks, these cell assemblies or neural coactivation dynamics have been formalized in terms of attractor dynamics (Hopfield 1982; Amit 1989). In attractor dynamics, after a transient period, self-reinforcing synaptic excitation reaches a stationary state (attractor) in which the assembly pattern of activation remains persistent. To clarify what we mean by this, consider the small model in Figure 9.1, which demonstrates some design principles of the model proposed by McClelland and Rumelhart (1981). In this model for context effects in letter perception, there are word nodes (artificial neurons) and letter nodes. When a four-letter word such as LAP is activated through its constituent letter nodes L, A, and P, this pattern of coactivated nodes remains stable over time because the letter nodes excite the word node. The word node in turn activates the letter nodes, thus reinforcing and maintaining its own source input: The coactivated letter nodes and word node are bound into an attractor.

In general, we define two coactivated neurons as being bound if they are part of a neural assembly (attractor) and thus reinforce each other's activation state, either directly (e.g. letter and word nodes in Fig. 9.1) or indirectly (letter nodes via a word node), or if they are activated by some external source, (e.g. a visual input). In the latter case, it is the input pattern that causes node coactivation. In the visual system, this input-driven coactivation is achieved via feedforward converging

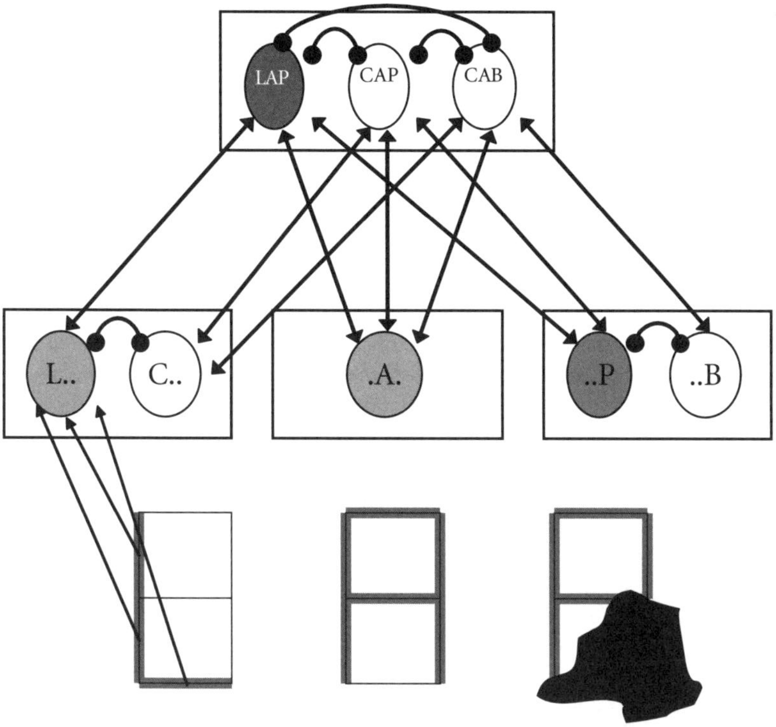

Figure 9.1 Binding by coactivation. See text for explanation. (After McClelland and Rumelhart 1981.)

connections (Felleman and van Essen 1991). This bottom-up binding will not persist when the input source is removed, but plays a crucial role in the ignition of attractor dynamics at a higher representational stage. Attractor-driven binding, in contrast, will persist over time and also past the offset of external input.

Both feedforward and attractor-based forms of coactive binding are involved in cortical information processing. An interesting functional MRI (fMRI) study (Courtney *et al.* 1997) showed a progressive increase in selectivity and stability (persistence) of neural activity from posterior (occipital) to more anterior (prefrontal) cortical areas involved in visual processing. Coactivation may initially be based on feedforward input volleys in more posterior visual cortical areas with progressively dominant attractor dynamics in high-level visual processing areas and the prefrontal cortex.

Synchrony-based binding

Perceptual binding based on coactivation or firing rates has some limitations that may be overcome by a richer short-term binding mechanism. In particular, it has difficulty explaining how multiple objects can be segregated in a given

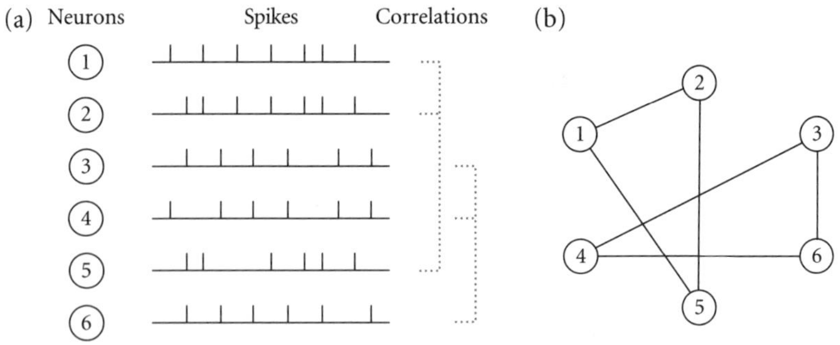

Figure 9.2 Binding by synchronization: (a) neurons 1, 2, and 5 fire in synchrony and so do neurons 3, 4, and 6; (b) a connectivity pattern that could underlie the correlations shown in (a).

visual scene (von der Malsburg 1981). The same segregation problem can be observed in a working memory representation of multiple patterns (Luck and Vogel 1997). For example, if six neurons are coactivated, it will not be clear whether or not they represent one, two, or more objects or events, whereas if the spiking times and synchronization–desynchronization patterns between the six neurons are considered, there may be two or more groups of neurons with high within-group temporal correlations of firing but low between-group correlations. In this way multiple objects can be represented simultaneously (von der Malsburg 1981; Engel *et al.* 1992).

In Figure 9.2(a), spiking of neurons 1, 2, and 5 is temporally correlated and so is that of neurons 3, 4, and 6. However, spiking of two neurons from different groups, such as neurons 2 and 3, is only weakly correlated. In this form of binding, when two neurons are highly correlated in their time-resolved firing, there is a strong indication that they are bound into a common representation.

The mechanisms for synchronization-based binding may be similar to the mechanisms for coactive binding: (i) forming part of an attractor in the presence of fast synchronizing connections, or (ii) temporary synchronization by some outside source (e.g. correlated noise). However, faster synaptic processes of lateral excitation and inhibition are demanded. We will discuss this form of neural binding below with reference to perceptual and working memory representations.

Interactive or ecphoric binding

Interactive binding refers to the interaction of two or more partly overlapping or convergent representations. For example, two input streams to a given brain area may each activate a large number of neurons. The neurons that receive support from both streams are most strongly activated (Fig. 9.3). If there is suitably calibrated inhibition or a multiplicative combination of neural inputs, only the

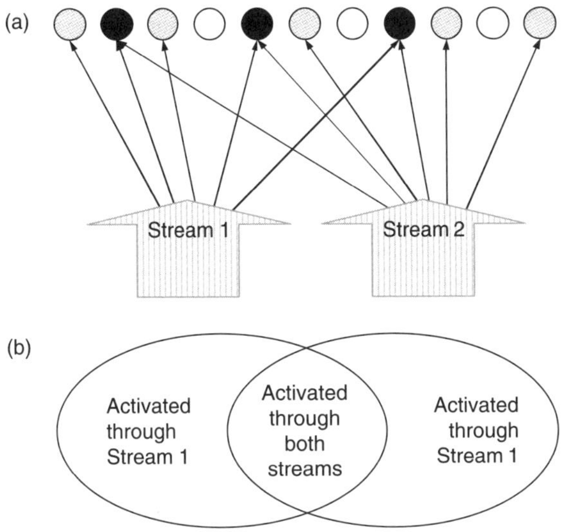

Figure 9.3 Interactive binding. (a) Two streams of activation patterns converge on a single layer in which three neurons receive inputs from both streams. Through a suitably calibrated inhibitory mechanism these three neurons remain active, suppressing the rest. (b) Illustration of how this mechanism can be viewed as the intersection of two sets of activated neurons.

strongly activated neurons will remain activated. In neural networks, this is typically modelled by some form of inhibition that drives a competition process so that it selects the 'winning' neurons, or by a mechanism in which neurons remain active only if two (or more) inputs arrive in close succession. Interactive binding decorrelates the winning neurons from the losing neurons, resulting in a concise representation coded by a subset of the total set of activated neurons. For example, if a set of neurons represents a broad concept such as GROUND, selection of a subset (e.g. by combining it with a particular context input) can be viewed as a process of interpretation, for example GROUND as 'the top layer of a garden'. Similarly, the combination of goal-relevant top-down signals with a bottom-up perceptual input may produce a selective attention effect.

Interactive binding may work in tandem with other types of binding, as can be seen in the small network in Figure 9.1. The letter nodes deliver a broad range of coactivations to the word nodes, which through inhibitory processes are reduced to a single interpretation, the winning word node. Interactive binding can occur in two ways. One is to combine different streams multiplicatively. The other is to feed different successive inputs to the same receptive units. Funnelling a rich stream of neural activations through a single node is an extreme form of interactive binding. Nonetheless, it can be a very powerful coding process that binds multiple subordinate representations into a single superordinate representation (Page 2000).

Interactive binding can explain Tulving's 'ecphoric' processes that are responsible for encoding specificity. Thus, if during list learning, a word pair COFFEE–GROUND is presented, COFFEE will later be able to function as a retrieval cue for GROUND. In fact, the newly learned association may be even more effective than pre-existing associations like COLD (Tulving and Thompson 1973). This can be understood in terms of the interactive binding, whereby from the many neurons activated by COFFEE and GROUND only a small set is selected and associated, creating a highly specific episodic representation.

A similar mechanism operates during any type of retrieval that involves a reference to some context. This includes practically all forms of explicit memory. Modellers have frequently noticed that in order for a context cue *C* to retrieve only the items encoded in context *C*, but not those encoded in other possibly similar contexts C_1, C_2, etc., it is necessary to have a very selective cueing process. Thus, in the SAM model of associative memory, context and items interact in a multiplicative manner, allowing context *C* to 'let through' or select only those items that were associated with the cued context (Raaijmakers and Shiffrin 1981). Interactive binding can be viewed as a multiplicative interaction, in this case the interaction of two sets of active neurons from which some highly coactivated intersection remains active. Taking the intersection of two sets is often referred to in mathematics as set multiplication. Thus, item–item interactions and context–item interactions must be highly selective for memory retrieval to operate in accordance with known phenomena in memory psychology.

Recent evidence suggest that the entorhinal cortex might carry out a form of interactive binding of context and item (or object) information, with context information being carried by the parahippocampal area and item information by the perirhinal area, both of which converge on the entorhinal cortex, which in turn is the main gateway to and from the hippocampus. A recent implementation indicates that such a model might also explain selective impairments of memory typically found in patients with schizophrenia. In schizophrenia, the parahippocampal area tends to be reduced in volume so that one might hypothesize that context cues fail to select items learned, causing a noticeably reduced free recall performance. However, recognition remains largely intact, as this is much less dependent on the contextual cues. A recent simulation of such a mechanism confirms these intuitions (Talamini *et al.* 2005).

Associative long-term binding

Hebb's learning rule (Hebb 1949) echoes early ideas about association of 'brain processes' (James 1890). This rule is often summarized as 'neurons that fire together, wire together'. Formulated in this manner, Hebbian learning is the long-term encoding of representations that are bound coactively. Connections will grow stronger between coactive neurons, binding them associatively. Also, representations that have been formed through interactive binding process may be associated into long-term memory in this manner by strengthening the connections between both the neurons within a representation (Fig. 9.4) and the neurons in streams that feed into a representation.

The relationship between associative and synchronous binding is more complicated. If connections exist between coincidently firing neurons (i.e. neurons that fire at the same time), a rich pattern of correlations can be encoded in the network, and these can be reproduced when the network is stimulated suitably at some later time. Thus, in Figure 9.2(b), connections have developed between neurons 1 and 2, 1 and 5, and 2 and 5, creating a small network. A similar network has developed between neurons 3, 4, and 6. In principle, associative binding is thus also suitable for the long-term encoding of synchronously bound representations.

Suppose that a network such as that in Figure 9.2(b) is stimulated by a diffuse input that affects all neurons equally and suppose that the neural firing is a chance process, such that the more input they receive the higher is the firing probability. Then, firing neurons will tend to contribute to the (simultaneous) firing of other neurons in the network, causing the network as a whole to exhibit a high degree of synchronous firing. If, as in Figure 9.2(b), a network consists of two subnetworks or assemblies, the neurons within such an assembly will fire synchronously, but the correlations in firing between the assemblies will be low. In this way, long-term encoded synchronous firing patterns can be read out.

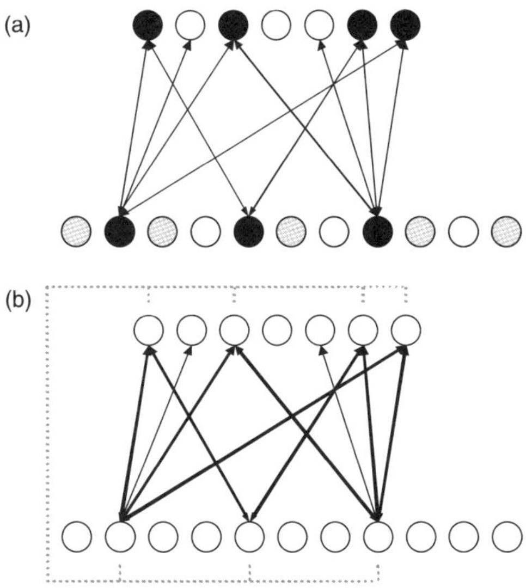

Figure 9.4 Associative binding. (a) Bidirectional connections have developed between strongly activated nodes. (b) During read-out (not shown) the connected neurons will exhibit synchronous (or correlated) firing.

If additionally, there are both inhibitory and refractory processes, only a small number of neurons can remain active for only a short time. The inhibition limits the size of an active (synchronously firing) assembly and the refractoriness causes an assembly to be silent for a brief period after firing, perhaps allowing another assembly to become active. In this way, a set of assemblies encoded in the same neural network can be read out consecutively. In engineering, the mechanism whereby simultaneously encoded representations are activated sequentially is known as time multiplexing.

Recently, it has been observed that if pre-synaptic firing precedes the post-synaptic spike within a small time window, the synapse is potentiated, whereas if it follows the post-synaptic spike, the synapse is depressed (Markram *et al.* 1997; Bi and Poo 1998). This phenomenon corresponds to spike-timing-dependent Hebbian plasticity (STDP). The temporal window for inducing such synaptic changes is on the order of 10 ms. Therefore spike timing appears to be crucial for Hebbian associative binding. A near-synchrony state with a small positive time lag of firing between post- and pre-synaptic neurons appears to be optimal for long-term synaptic strengthening. A larger time lag between neurons coding for different patterns may be used to cue sequence recall between subsequent assemblies, for example in serial recall in working memory. Such a representational differentiation cannot be achieved in terms of pure firing rates or coactivation-based binding.

Multiple binding processes in memory

The four neurodynamic binding processes may be associated with different memory processes. Synchronous binding and coactive binding structure neural representations in working memory. Interactive binding allows highly specific episodic (event) codes to become active during encoding, whereas during retrieval it allows selective activation of memory items on the basis of specific search cues-in-context. Associative binding is responsible for long-term storage. In the following sections, we will review in more detail how these binding processes operate in memory and how their integration is accomplished by large-scale brain architectures.

From perception to working memory

One of the most salient attributes of neural representations in perception is their spatial and temporal discontinuity at different scales. Therefore an important problem to solve is how coherent perceptual interpretations arise from these discontinuities. The perception of coherent entities (i.e. discretely categorizable real-world objects or sounds) in complex scenes implies the dynamic linking (binding) and separation (segregation) of active neural representations corresponding to these entities. Several solutions to this problem have been suggested. One solution is to assume higher-order representations (e.g. cardinal cells (Barlow 1972, 1989)) onto which signals from neurons coding for to-be-bound features converge. It is clear that some form of higher-order representation is stored in long-term memory, but given the variability of retinal projections and the multitude of ways in which discrete features can be combined, this solution is often considered implausible since it ultimately would lead to a combinatorial explosion of the number of cells that represent all possible feature combinations.

However, this combinatorial problem can be resolved if the concept of high-level representations is combined with the idea that binding can also be accomplished by selective synchronization of time-resolved neuronal responses (von der Malsburg 1981, 1999; Eckhorn *et al.* 1988; Engel *et al.* 1992; Gray 1999). According to this view, the action potentials of neurons coding features of the same object are synchronized, while being uncorrelated to neurons that code for the features of other objects. Although such neural synchrony may be supported by the existence of conjunctive codes at a high level, it may also be decoded by means of categorizing units in a read-out layer without requiring a pre-established mapping onto 'cardinal' representations covering the full combinatory spectrum.

As an elaboration of the temporal coding hypothesis, Raffone and Van Leeuwen (2002, 2003) suggested that feature binding with multiple active perceptual patterns may be mediated by a dynamic (e.g. chaotic) rather than a static synchronization, as is typically observed with coupling of sinusoidal neural oscillators. For instance, given a visual scene with a red circle, a red square, and a green square, neurons coding for red would be intermittently synchronized with neurons coding for circle and neurons coding for square without necessarily implying spurious synchronization of the neurons coding for disjoint features. As was shown in computer simulations, this dynamic and graded synchrony may enable the flexible encoding of multiple active patterns in associative memory networks. Read-out of this dynamic synchronization may take place efficiently by means of a fast self-organizing network layer.

The end result of perception is the selection and conscious awareness of a small part of the information that is present in our environment at any moment in time. What is selected and what is in conscious awareness forms the content of working memory. According to Baddeley (Baddeley 1986; Baddeley and Hitch, 1974), the concept of working memory refers to a system for temporarily holding and manipulating information that is required for performing cognitive tasks such as comprehension, learning, and reasoning. Note that this definition is much broader than is customary in the neuroscience literature, where working memory mainly refers to a maintenance function that is distinguished from other functions like attention and executive control (Duncan 2001).

It is generally accepted that the prefrontal cortex (PFC) is of cardinal importance for behaviour guided by internal states and intentions, including behaviour requiring the selective maintenance of earlier information, the suppression of automatic responses, and the establishment of new or rapidly changing mappings between perception and action (Cohen and Servan-Schreiber 1992; Duncan 2001; Miller and Cohen 2001; Wood and Grafman 2003). Anatomically, the PFC is well positioned to coordinate and control processing in the rest of the brain. It consists of a large number of interconnected areas that collectively have reciprocal connections with almost all other neocortical and subcortical structures. It is also an area that shows late development, both phylogenetically and ontogenetically (Fuster 2001).

Based on these anatomical considerations, it can be argued that executive control functions of working memory have developed as a consequence of an evolutionary development of the anterior parts of the brain that allow neural processes to control primary perception–action relations in the rest of the brain (Phaf and Wolters 1997). In this view, the role of PFC in controlling behaviour is modulatory rather than transmissive (Norman and Shallice 1986; O'Reilly *et al.* 1999; Miller and Cohen 2001). Whereas simple adaptive behaviour rests on an external control loop between perception, action, and perception of action results, the extended PFC may have created the possibility of an internalization of this loop. More specifically, it created the possibility of maintaining information in an activated state by recurrent connections (loops) between the PFC and other areas of the cortex (Phaf and Wolters 1997).

Apart from maintenance, two other executive functions are top-down control of selective attention and large-scale integration of multisource information into a unitary episodic representation, i.e. an episodic buffer (Baddeley 2000). Large-scale integration may be realized as an attractor state in a high-level system that receives input from all other subsidiary systems in the PFC and from long-term memory. Interactions between this integrative PFC area and modality-specific reverberating loops may modulate the feedback of maintained information to posterior cortical areas, thus allowing top-down control over the selection of actions and over selective attention to sensory input by biasing neural processing in these lower cortical areas. This top-down control may take the form of interactive or ecphoric binding.

Neuroscientific evidence substantiates these theoretical considerations. For example, single-cell studies have shown persistent firing during delayed matching tasks in both the PFC and other cortical areas like the inferotemporal and parietal cortex (Goldman-Rakic 1988; Ungerleider *et al.* 1998; Fuster 2001; Sakai *et al.* 2002). Evidence for top-down attentional modulation of neural activity (i.e. relative enhancement of neuronal responses) to task-relevant stimuli and relative suppression of responses to task-irrelevant stimuli has been shown as early as the primary visual cortex (Chelazzi *et al.* 1993; Reynolds *et al.* 2000; O'Connor *et al.* 2002). In addition, task-specific activity in PFC may also generate top-down biasing signals involved in long-term memory retrieval (Hasegawa *et al.* 1998) and storage (Wagner *et al.* 1998; Kydd and Bilkey 2003). These findings have led to the biased competition model (Desimone and Duncan 1995), suggesting that top-down control activates relevant representations which are then in a better position to compete with irrelevant information for perceptual awareness and motor control. Within PFC, the occurrence of interaction and integration is suggested by findings showing that individual cells in lateral PFC adapt their responsiveness to different combinations of stimulus attributes according to changing task demands (Asaad *et al.* 2000; Rushworth and Owen 1998; Wallis *et al.* 2001). A possible location of a large-scale binding system is the anterior PFC, which appears to play a specific role in integrating the outcomes of multiple cognitive operations in the pursuit of higher behavioural goals (Ramnani and Owen, 2004).

A connectionist model of binding in working memory

On the basis of the previous considerations a network model was developed that aimed at demonstrating how core functions of working memory, such as its limited capacity for maintenance, binding (chunking), and modulation of selective attention, can be unitarily accounted for in terms of cortical circuit dynamics involving a recurrent interaction between the PFC and other cortical areas (Raffone and Wolters 2001; Raffone *et al.* 2001). Although the model concerns visual working memory, the basic mechanisms of maintenance and binding can be generalized to other working memory systems.

The model (Fig. 9.5) consists of a cortical module, located in the inferotemporal cortex (ITC) and a prefrontal module (e.g. dorsolateral/ventrolateral PFC). Pre-existing cell assemblies within the ITC module are assumed. These are defined by strong intra-assembly connections and weak inter-assembly connections. Assemblies are assumed to code for simple features; multifeature objects are coded by sets of coupled (i.e. strongly interassociated) assemblies. A global inhibition (competition) mechanism between cell assemblies is implemented within the ITC module. Smaller assemblies, reciprocally connected to corresponding ITC assemblies, are assumed in the PFC module. The units of the model are

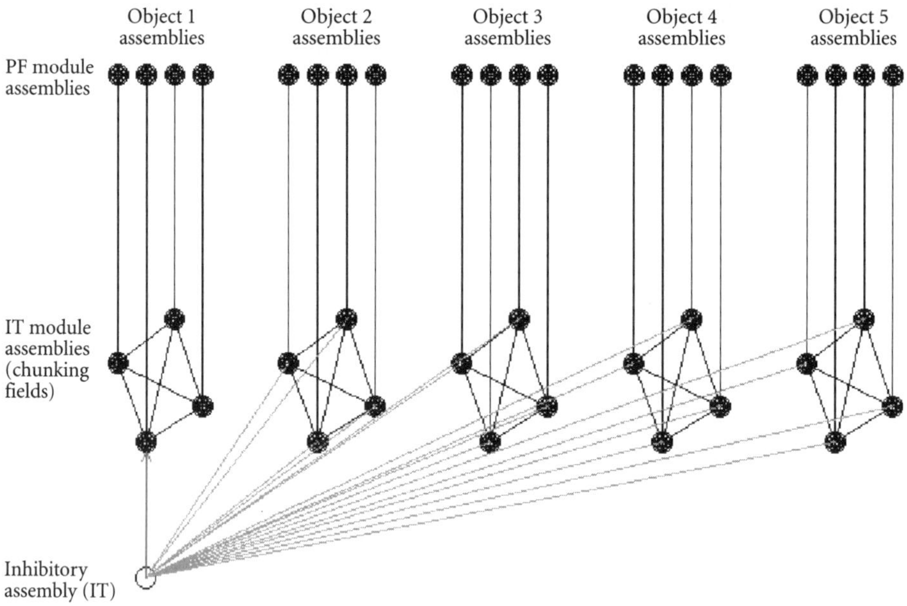

Figure 9.5 Scheme of the working memory model. In the ITC module, 20 neural assemblies of 100 neurons (not shown individually) code for 20 hypothetical visual features. Assemblies are activated by input from unspecified lower areas. The figure shows the situation with five four-feature objects with strong (synchronizing) connections (the diamond-shaped configurations). The ITC module also contains small assemblies of inhibitory neurons. Inhibitory input to each object assembly equals the number of firing neurons of the other ITC assemblies coding for competing features or objects. The PFC module consists of a set of 20 assemblies of 50 neurons 'matching' the ITC module structure.

spiking neurons modelled after MacGregor and Oliver (1974). Transmission times between connected cells within a module are assumed to be much faster than between cells of different modules. Stimulus input to the ITC module is given by stochastic spike trains to specific assemblies coming from lower level visual areas during a limited onset–offset period.

Figure 9.6 shows the working of the model when a single cell assembly input was presented. During stimulus input, average activity of the ITC assembly (and the matching PFC module after a conduction delay) shows an oscillation with a gamma-band frequency (around 35 Hz). These oscillations are due to the fast synaptic coupling within the assembly. After a certain critical number of its neurons has fired as a consequence of enhanced input, the fast positive activation spreading through the assembly entrains most neurons to fire almost simultaneously. After firing, neurons fall into a collective refractory period. Synchronous firing also occurs in the PFC module. This is generated by the synchronized feedforward input form the ITC module. Feedback form the PFC to the ITC

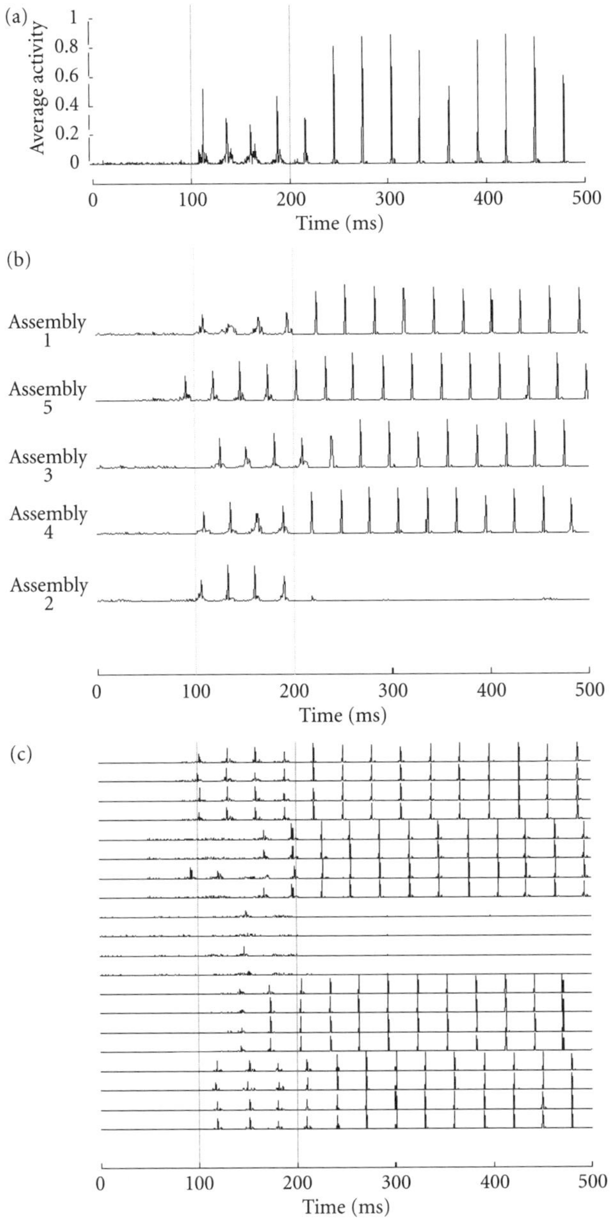

Figure 9.6 (a) Dynamic behaviour of one assembly activated by stimulus input to ITC and with active feedback from PFC. Stimulus onset (at 100 ms) and offset (at 200 ms) times are marked by vertical lines. The panel shows the evolution and continuation of the average spiking activity of one ITC assembly (100 interconnected nodes coding a single feature). (b) Phase segregation of ITC assemblies coding for independent features. Four out of five assemblies remain active. Because of mutual inhibitory activity, the assemblies become optimally spaced in the oscillatory phase. (c) Phase segregation of objects (chunks) consisting of four interconnected assemblies. Four out of five objects are retained in terms of internally synchronized and mutually desynchronized chunks, whereas all features coding the fifth object are suppressed.

module suffices to maintain the modules in an oscillatory state after stimulus offset. The matched ITC and PFC assemblies reverberate trough delayed mutual excitation. In realistic cortical networks, PFC is autonomous and stable against interference in working memory activity, whereas maintenance in posterior cortical areas is PFC-dependent and interference-sensitive (Miller *et al.*, 1996). Raffone and Wolters' (2001) model can accommodate this evidence by the addition of another reverberatory loop within the PFC module, probably mediating a working memory rehearsal process.

In this model, the limited capacity of (visual) working memory emerges due to the interactions via inhibitory interneurons between independent assemblies. Once an assembly becomes oscillatory, the enhancement of its average spike rate will exert a fast, strong, and transient inhibitory action on other assemblies. However, after producing a synchronized spike burst this inhibitory effect dissipates quickly, allowing another assembly to gain activation. The capacity of the model was tested by presenting simultaneous inputs to multiple assemblies. Owing to the stochastic nature of the model, the number of stored items varied realistically from trial to trial, but an average capacity to maintain about three or four assemblies after stimulus offset was observed (Fig. 9.6). This simulated storage capacity is remarkably similar to recent estimations of working memory capacity (Luck and Vogel 1997; Cowan 2001). As can be seen in Figure 9.6, the inhibitory mechanism caused oscillating assemblies to become spaced optimally in time.

In Figure 9.6, the limited storage capacity in the model, both in computational and functional terms, depends on the functional balance of a sufficiently high oscillation frequency (firing rate), enabling a good signal-to-noise ratio, and sufficient phase segregation between firing of neural assemblies coding for different objects (minimizing interference). The same desynchronizing mechanism that enables phase segregation between assemblies coding for separate items imposes a limit on the number of oscillatory reverberations. In other words, a reduced phase-lag would increase interference between the maintained items and a lower firing rate would reduce the strength or resolution of the neural responses coding for a given item. Both interference and reduced resolution would make access or read-out in terms of association to response codes or higher-order conjunctive units more difficult.

In a classic paper, Miller (1956) argued that the capacity of working memory has to be expressed in terms of coherent units or 'chunks' of information, instead of some formal measure of amount of information. Working memory handles higher-order chunks, where large amounts of organized information can become integrated as one chunk or one single unit of capacity (Ericsson and Kintsch 1995). Luck and Vogel (1997) showed that the storage capacity of working memory is about four objects, and that this capacity limit is indeed independent of the number of features making up the objects. We simulated this chunking capacity by assuming multifeature objects to be represented as strongly interconnected feature assemblies (assuming mutual synchronizing associations between different assemblies). From these simulations, it appeared that multi-assembly units show the same within-object synchronization and between-object segregation as single assemblies, and that the modelled capacity is largely unaffected by the size or number of features of integrated representations. Therefore the model can potentially account for chunking based on the strength and stability of composite representations in long-term memory.

The theoretical solution to the problem of limited capacity of short-term memory proposed by Raffone and Wolters (2001) makes the neurophysiological constraints considered in earlier theoretical work (Lisman and Idiart 1995; Cowan, 2001) computationally explicit. The role of oscillations and neural synchrony in working memory suggested by these computational investigations is supported by neurophysiological and EEG data (Nakamura *et al.* 1992; Villa and Fuster 1992; Tallon-Baudry *et al.* 2001).

This basic recurrent architecture between the PFC and the posterior cortex also suggests a possible scheme for implementing a top-down biased competition mechanism for controlling selective attention via interactive or ecphoric binding. As shown by Rainer *et al.* (1998), the prefrontal neurons of monkeys performing a delayed matching-to-sample task exhibited a higher firing rate when they coded for a target object. It was suggested that such neurons were involved in both the maintenance and selection of behaviourally relevant information. A top-down selective biasing effect may be assumed to originate from PFC areas presumably involved in supervisory control (Rushworth and Owen 1998). It has been shown that both additive and multiplicative modulatory inputs to simulated PFC maintenance modules can be effective in selecting and selectively maintaining biased inputs (Deco and Rolls 2003; Raffone *et al.* 2003).

So far, maintenance, capacity, and chunking effects have been realized by a binding principle based on synchronous firing mediated by pre-existing representations in long-term memory. Binding within reverberating assemblies may also be possible in the absence of pre-existing associative representations, because correlated spikes from areas at early processing stages may be used to generate synchronous firing in assemblies in higher-level areas, as was suggested by Abeles (1991) and Roelfsema *et al.* (1996). Raffone and Wolters (2001) showed that even weak connections between ITC assemblies can synchronize their reverberatory activities with strongly correlated inputs. It is likely that early perceptual grouping and long-term memory guidance in terms of pre-existing assemblies with strong connections (i.e. chunks) may cooperate in the formation of integrated entities to be maintained in working memory (Jensen and Lisman 1996).

Thus, with structured input to the system, coherent and synchronized activation patterns representing aspects of the input are constructed and can be maintained over time, allowing subsequent operations to be performed. We suggest that one of these subsequent operations is the creation of novel associations between the maintained patterns via the hippocampus (interactive and associative binding), which creates a conjunctive episodic code. Such a code wil, in turn, recursively contribute to further structuring of the elements (chunks) that appear in the assemblies activated in working memory.

Connectionist models of long-term memory and consolidation

Most recent connectionist models of the neural basis of long-term memory emphasize the associative binding role of the hippocampus (Alvarez and Squire 1994; McClelland *et al.* 1995; Murre 1996; Nadel and Moscovitch 1997; Nadel *et al.* 2000). These models implement and extend earlier theorizing along similar lines, assuming that long-term memories are initially, and sometimes also subsequently, bound by the hippocampus (Milner 1957, 1989; Marr 1971; O'Keefe and Nadel 1978; Wickelgren 1979, 1987; Mishkin 1982; Squire *et al.* 1984; Teyler and DiScenna 1986; McNaughton and Nadel 1990; Squire and Zola-Morgan 1991; Gluck and Meyers 1993; Treves and Rolls 1994; Squire and Alvarez 1995; Nadel *et al.* 2000).

At least three of the models that have simulated cortico-hippocampal interactions (Alvarez and Squire 1994; McClelland *et al.* 1995; Murre 1996) share the basic assumption that there is a fast-learning hippocampal memory system and a neocortical memory system in which representations are gradually built up in a consolidation phase which follows the initial learning episode. This consolidation phase is implemented as a process of reactivation, in which stored patterns are strengthened by rehearsal of the original patterns (McClelland *et al.* 1995) or as 'pseudorehearsal' in which patterns are generated from the network from random cues (Alvarez and Squire 1994; Meeter and Murre 2004a; Murre 1996). Those patterns are then interleaved with new patterns to protect, repair, or strengthen old ones.

In the TraceLink model of long-term memory and consolidation (Murre 1996; Meeter and Murre 2004a,b), for example, the neocortical memory system is a large layer in which only weak connections are laid down between nodes (artificial neurons) belonging to one pattern. Consolidation is simulated by letting the model relax from an initially random state into an attractor (i.e. retrieving an existing memory) and then updating the weights with a Hebbian learning rule (Fig. 9.7). Eventually, the connections between neocortical nodes built up during

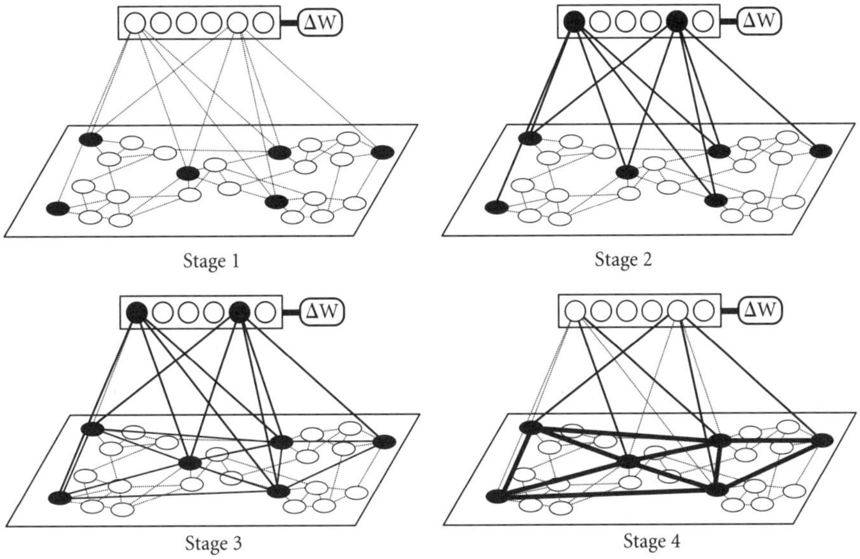

Figure 9.7 Associative binding in long-term memory as modelled by TraceLink: stage 1, coactive or synchronous neurons represent the contents of an experience; stage 2, through Hebbian learning they are bound indirectly into a representation via neurons in the link system; stage 3, direct cortico-cortical connections have developed; stage 4, the neurons are now associatively bound through direct interconnections at a cortical level. The representation has become independent of the link system.

consolidation allow the patterns to be retrieved without the support of the hippocampal system. TraceLink and the models of Alvarez and Squire (1994) and McClelland *et al.* (1995) all assume that neocortical learning is very slow compared with hippocampal learning. It is this assumption that assigns a binding role to the hippocampus in the time period following initial learning of a novel episode.

The consolidation stage that follows this first stage is modelled as the strengthening of connections within a neocortical pattern that is retrieved through the hippocampal system. This implies that there must be consolidation phases in which the hippocampal system reinstates patterns in neocortical memory areas. Such a consolidation mechanism is sensitive to 'runaway consolidation', a vicious circle in which one pattern becomes stronger through consolidation, then becomes more likely to be consolidated in the next trial, and finally monopolizes all consolidation resources while crowding out other memories (Meeter 2003). In the models runaway consolidation is avoided through the dominance of the hippocampal system, helping to reactivate patterns in the neocortex that have not yet benefited from consolidation (Alvarez and Squire 1994; McClelland *et al.* 1995; Murre 1996; Meeter and Murre 2005). If learning occurs within the hippocampal system during the reactivation, runaway consolidation immediately rears its head as consolidated memories now become stronger in both the hippocampus and the neocortex (Meeter and Murre 2004a). Therefore consolidation should take place during a period when the hippocampus is not very plastic.

A different view of the consolidation process was proposed by Nadel and Moscovitch (1997). They call the approach taken by the above models the Standard Theory of Consolidation; a principal characteristic of this approach is that, in the course of the consolidation process, successful retrieval requires less and less hippocampal involvement. In contrast, Nadel and Moscovitch (1997) argue that the hippocampus always remains involved in the retrieval of memories and that consolidation occurs through a gradual increase in the strength of the hippocampal trace, rather than the neocortical trace. A connectionist implementation of their model was presented by Nadel *et al.* (2000).

The models mentioned above differ in detail and motivation but they share several crucial assumptions central to the subject matter of this chapter.

- They assume a binding role of the hippocampus, at least in the initial stages of acquisition.
- They assume that there is a neural hierarchy in the sense that the hippocampus receives inputs from a large portion of the cerebral cortex while being able to influence processes, via recurrent connections, in these areas.
- They assume a slower formation of cortico-cortical connections than of (cortico-)hippocampal connections.
- They assume a long-term consolidation process in which learned memories continue to evolve well after initial acquisition (see also Murre et al. 2001; Meeter and Murre 2004b).

Trace binding role of the hippocampus

If the hippocampus has a binding role, we may ask ourselves: What is being bound? An early model by O'Keefe and Nadel (1978) is based on experiments with rats. With these animals, single-cell recordings reveal many place-sensitive cells in the hippocampus, and therefore the model stresses the role of the hippocampus in navigation. One might assume that whatever is important for an organism and occurs frequently enough will tend to be represented in the hippocampus. For the rat, learning new locations quickly appears to be important, for example to seek shelter in case of danger. To remember places of shelter, it is necessary to bind the representation for 'safe spot' to certain locations in the current context. More generally, we might view the binding process as one where one or more objects or attributes (e.g. safe places, boxes with cereal) in a given context (e.g. an experimental maze or my backyard) are bound together.

A functional model proposed by Gluck and Meyers (1993) emphasizes the integration of context- and task-related objects by a compression mechanism regulated by the hippocampus. An important observation that emerges from this work is that even tasks that can be performed without a hippocampus (e.g. after lesioning) may still show differences when comparing experimental results before and after lesioning. One example of how their model deals with this involvement is the explanation of context effects in simple conditioning. When a task is moved into a different context, normal animals will show a marked decrease in responding. Animals that undergo lesioning of the hippocampus after having learned the task do not show such a decrease; they respond equally well before and after context shifts (Penick and Solomon 1991). These and other phenomena are explained by Gluck and Meyers (1993) by assuming that the hippocampus controls a compression mechanism that is automatic and always operative. This mechanism integrates the context and object in a manner akin to the integrative binding mechanism above, thus filtering out irrelevant aspects of the context.

After prolonged training the context will be strongly compressed. Stimuli that are central to the task remain prominently represented but those that are coincidental are 'squeezed out'. Thus task aspects such as the lever to be pressed and its consequences will be well represented (many neurons firing), whereas the colour of the floor or any objects that have nothing to do with the task will come to be represented by fewer and fewer neurons. Compression of irrelevant inputs, or attention to relevant aspects of the input, has been part of many theories of cortical functioning. For example, Barlow (1989) has argued that an important function of unsupervised learning in the cortex is to extract redundancy by filtering out irrelevant stimuli. One way in which such extraction can take place is by merging similar stimuli; if stimulus variations are irrelevant, it is not necessary to represent them. This leads to categorization or clustering of representations, possibly, but not necessarily, in a topological organization. Many connectionist approaches to unsupervised learning have been proposed, and most of these use similar hypothesized processes in the cortex as a justification (Grossberg 1976, 1987; Rumelhart and Zipser 1985; Kohonen 1989; Murre 1992; Murre *et al.* 1992; Linsker 1996 a–c). These have in common that categories emerge through mutual inhibition of a limited set of categorizing nodes (artificial neurons). This funnels an elaborate representation through just a few nodes. These mechanisms are effective in extracting statistical regularities from the input, and thus compressing it. This resembles the mechanism whereby regularities of a computer file (e.g. repeated words or sentence fragments) are utilized by compression algorithms to reduce their size.

McClelland *et al.* (1995) emphasize yet another possible role of the hippocampus. They point out that purely sequential learning may not lead to useful internal representations and that a case can be made for the necessity of a more interleaved mode of learning. In particular, newly learned deviant patterns may disturb already learned representations. Thus there are also good behavioural reasons for a slow (interleaved) learning process, i.e. a learning process whereby occasionally an old pattern is given an extra learning trial, amongst newly arrived learning patterns. This mechanism can be interpreted as binding of related patterns that occur at disparate moments in time, a form of interactive binding in time.

Thus we see that the hippocampus may take part in several binding processes. The most prevalent is associative binding, which is very prominent initially, before consolidation to the neocortex has taken place. Additionally, the hippocampus is probably involved in interactive binding of context and task-central items or objects with progressive compression of irrelevant aspects of these representations over time, binding them into a compact representation suitable for efficient long-term storage. It is also likely that the long-term consolidation mechanism, in which the hippocampus is the central area, executes a form of dynamic interactive binding, integrating new representations with similar ones already in long-term memory.

An integrated architecture for binding in working memory and long term-memory

In the previous sections, we have presented four basic neurodynamic binding mechanisms operating with a different spatial and temporal resolution. We have presented essential computational desiderata for flexible representational compositions in perceptual and working memory processing. We have also discussed a model of working memory based on short-term binding for maintenance of integrated information chunks. We have also discussed how transiently active representations in the posterior cortex can be quickly bound for intermediate-term storage via the hippocampus with interactive and associative binding processes and how these episodic representations may transfer to the posterior cortex in the form of permanent associative binding.

Based on these neurodynamic and structural constraints for memory binding, we suggest as an integrative architecture a tripartite system with cooperative interactions between the posterior cortex and the PFC and between the posterior cortex and the hippocampal or medial temporal lobe (MTL) area. Unfortunately, it is still not known what kind of signalling occurs between the PFC and the MTL; the anatomical connections between these areas and their possible functional interaction have only recently come under consideration (Simons and

Spiers 2003). Some of these memory binding interactions are summarized in the architecture shown in Figure 9.8.

Of course, many interactions between the PFC and the MTL can be explained by their connections with a common posterior cortex system. For instance, the PFC may provide top-down control of encoding processes by selecting, modifying, and elaborating the representations in the posterior cortex that are subsequently stored via MTL. Similarly, the PFC may control memory search and the selection of retrieval cues or strategies via its interaction with the posterior cortex and without direct interaction with the MTL. However, the presence of direct anatomical links between subsystems in the MTL and the PFC (Simons and Spiers, 2003) suggests direct interactions as well. For example, there are strong reciprocal connections between the prefrontal cortex and the perirhinal and entorhinal cortices (Groenewegen and Uylings 2000). A possible functional interpretation of this direct link is that it plays a role in the integration and association of the spatial and temporal contexts of events. Recent suggestions on the role of PFC have stressed its ability to integrate the outcomes of separate cognitive operations (Kroger *et al.* 2002; Ramnani and Owen 2004) and to control processing according to spatial or temporal context demands (Koechlin *et al.* 2003). If it is assumed that the spatial–temporal context of events is integrated in the PFC, direct inputs from PFC to MTL may provide the contextual information that is combined with event-specific information to create a spatio-temporal

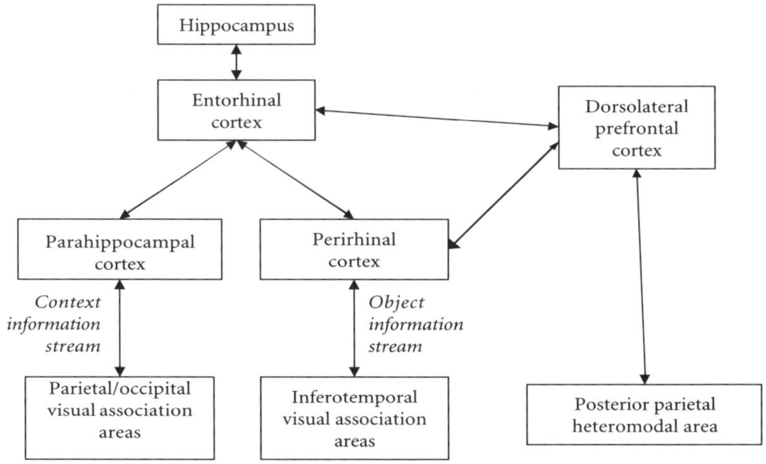

Figure 9.8 Simplified neural hierarchy of some principal areas implicated in short- and long-term memory.

specific episodic trace (Kydd and Bilkey 2003). However, these suggestions are clearly in need of further substantiation.

The tripartite architecture involves all four forms of neurodynamic binding considered above, with a differential involvement depending on the level and timescale of neural representation and processing. For instance, attractor dynamics or coactivation-based binding may take place in the inferotemporal cortex, the prefrontal cortex, and field CA3 of the hippocampus (Rolls and Treves 1998). These attractor dynamics may be qualitatively different, for example because of the differential involvement of fast (AMPA-mediated) and slow (NMDA-mediated) excitatory currents. At a functional level, coactive binding in the prefrontal cortex is likely to be associated with executive control processes, probably mediated by NMDA voltage-dependent currents (Wang 1999; Raffone *et al.* 2003). Attractor dynamics in posterior cortical areas may be supported by both local intra-regional cooperation and non-local feedback from the prefrontal cortex, and it may be sensitive to feedforward input (Miller *et al.* 1996; Courtney *et al.* 1997). Multimodal coactive binding in the hippocampus may take place in CA3 because of dense recurrent collateral excitation, in terms of both AMPA- and NMDA-mediated currents, with theta oscillation modulation.

Synchrony-based binding is likely to take place at different representational levels in posterior cortical areas related to perceptual processing (Singer 1999). Because of technical recording problems, the role of synchrony in higher-level attentional and working memory processing has been supported by only a few studies (Villa and Fuster 1992; Fries *et al.* 2001). Single-cell recording evidence against the role of synchrony in these cognitive functions is not available. Neural synchrony at a system level may also play a crucial role in cooperation between the prefrontal cortex, posterior cortical networks, and MTL neural assemblies, as indicated by a recent magnetoencephalography (MEG) study with a complex attentional task (Gross *et al.* 2004). Finally, temporal coding may play an important role in hippocampal sequence coding in terms of nested theta/gamma oscillations (Jensen and Lisman 1996).

As considered above, interactive or ecphoric binding of object and multimodal episodic context information may take place in the MTL, specifically in the entorhinal cortex. Ecphoric binding may also take place in the prefrontal cortex, where attentional-biased competition is primarily mediated (Deco and Rolls 2003). The convergence of top-down biasing inputs from target-coding prefrontal assemblies and bottom-up input from temporal and parietal networks is likely to give rise to competitive neural dynamics, selecting the neural assemblies with the highest level of activation in the PFC. Multiplicative effects in this ecphoric binding may be mediated by NMDA currents present in the PFC (Wang

1999). Interactive binding in terms of voltage-dependent synapses may also take place at lower levels of perceptual processing, to mediate context effects via horizontal connections, in the absence of spurious activation spreading that could be caused by coactivation-based binding (Tononi *et al.* 1992).

As discussed above, associative long-term binding may take place in the MTL and neocortical areas at different stages. However, a relative division of labour may exist between neocortical and hippocampal systems, as rats with hippocampal lesions can still learn tasks such as non-linear discrimination problems. Similar evidence has been gained with amnesic patients. Therefore there may be a relative independence between cortical and hippocampal binding processes. In our framework, this relative independence in non-episodic learning tasks may be supported by the presence of the four neurodynamic binding mechanisms in both hippocampal and neocortical areas. Differential processing and learning at neocortical and hippocampal networks may depend upon architectural and encoding (mapping) properties emphasizing either idiosyncratic or common features and feature conjunctions making up entities and events. However, in a proper episodic memory, hippocampal binding is likely to be a prerequisite for a subsequent neocortical binding.

A major unknown aspect concerns the relative role of PFC and posterior cortical areas in episodic information storage and retrieval. It is currently unclear whether the PFC stores and retrieves information about object and events or, rather, operates on posterior and motor cortical areas by means of task-adaptive codes (Duncan 2001; Wood and Grafman 2003). In a functional imaging study conducted by Prabhakaran *et al.* (2000), the activation of prefrontal cortex was greater for maintaining integrated rather than unintegrated representations. These results suggest that the PFC is involved in integrating verbal and spatial information in working memory, i.e. in mediating the function of the episodic buffer suggested by Baddeley (2000). Therefore it can be assumed that the transfer of episodic codes from the hippocampus to the neocortex during the consolidation process may differentially involve neocortical areas. Associative neocortical binding may be governed by higher-order convergence codes in PFC, which can be related to goals, plans, and encoding of task setting. PFC may play a role similar to the hippocampus after the consolidation process, in terms of multimodal integration, with access to action-related codes.

To conclude, perception and action do not occur in a vacuum. Perceptual input enters a neural system that is already in an activated state, representing lasting effects of previous inputs and short- and long-term goals and intentions. Which aspects of a momentary input are selectively attended is determined as much (and sometimes even more) by the present activation state of the system as by the actual input itself. Activation states, in turn, are determined in large part by the pre-existing neural structures that have been shaped by years of experience making up what is referred to as long-term memory, containing semantic knowledge of concepts, episodic memory of specific events, conditioned stimulus-response associations, and perceptual, conceptual, and motor skills.

The general scheme we have presented here is that the versatility of the brain in coping with continuously changing environments and demands is due to the capacity to store coherent patterns of input and output in long-term memory and the capacity to control the processing of input by selecting and maintaining task-relevant information in working memory. These processes require the possibility of transiently and permanently binding neural assemblies representing elements of input and output. These binding processes continuously interact. What is transiently bound in working memory governs what is temporarily and eventually permanently bound in long-term memory. In turn, what is permanently bound affects transient binding in working memory. The interplay of these binding processes determines how the brain develops into a structured system that is cumulatively correlated with its environment, thus implementing a process that is able to lift itself to higher levels of cognitive functioning.

References

Abeles, M. (1991). *Corticonics: Neural Circuits of the Cerebral Cortex.* Cambridge: Cambridge University Press.

Alvarez, R. and Squire, L.R. (1994). Memory consolidation and the medial temporal lobe: a simple network model. *Proceedings of National Academy of Sciences of the United States of America*, **91**, 7041–7045.

Amit, D.J. (1989). *Modeling Brain Function*. Cambridge: Cambridge University Press.

Asaad, W.F., Rainer, G., and Miller, E.K. (2000). Task-specific neural activity in the primate prefrontal cortex. *Journal of Neurophysiology*, **84**, 451–459.

Baddeley, A.D. (1986). *Working Memory*. Oxford: Oxford University Press.

Baddeley, A.D. (2000). The episodic buffer: a new component of working memory? *Trends in Cognitive Sciences*, **4**, 417–423.

Baddeley, A.D. and Hitch, G.J. (1974). Working memory. In *The Psychology of Learning and Motivation* (ed G.A. Bower). London: Academic Press, 47–89.

Barlow, H.B. (1972). Single units and sensation: a neuron doctrine for perceptual psychology? *Perception*, **1**, 371–394.

Barlow, H.B. (1989). Unsupervised learning. *Neural Computation*, **1**, 295–311.

Bartlett, F.C. (1932). *Remembering*. Cambridge: Cambridge University Press.

Bi, G.Q. and Poo, M.M. (1998). Synaptic modifications in cultured hippocampal neurons: dependence on spike timing, synaptic strength, and postsynaptic cell type. *Journal of Neuroscience*, **18**, 10464–10472.

Chelazzi, L., Miller, E.K., Duncan, J., and Desimone, R.A. (1993). A neural basis for visual search in inferior temporal cortex. *Nature*, **363**, 345–347.

Cohen, J.D. and Servan-Schreiber, D. (1992). Context, cortex and dopamine: a connectionist approach to behavior and biology in schizophrenia. *Psychological Review*, **99**, 45–77.

Courtney, S.M., Ungerleider, L.G., Keil, K., and Haxby, J.V. (1997). Transient and sustained activity in a distributed neural system for human working memory. *Nature*, **386**, 608–611.

Cowan, N. (2001). The magical number 4 in short-term memory: a reconsideration of mental storage capacity. *Behavioral and Brain Sciences*, **24**, 87–114.

Damasio, A.R. (1989a). The brain binds entities and events by multiregional activation from convergence zones. *Neural Computation*, **1**, 123–132.

Damasio, A.R. (1989b). Time-locked multiregional retroactivation: a systems-level proposal for the neural substrates of recall and recognition. *Cognition*, **33**, 25–62.

Deco, G. and Rolls, E.T. (2003). Attention and working memory: a dynamical model of neuronal activity in the prefrontal cortex. *European Journal of Neuroscience*, **18**, 2374–2390.

Desimone, R. and Duncan, J. (1995). Neural mechanisms of selective visual attention. *Annual Review of Neurosciences*, **18**, 193–222.

Duncan, J. (2001). An adaptive coding model of neural function in prefrontal cortex. *Nature Reviews Neuroscience*, **2**, 820–829.

Eckhorn, R., Bauer, R., Jordan, W., *et al.* (1988). Coherent oscillations: a mechanism of feature linking in the visual cortex? *Biological Cybernetics*, **60**, 121–130.

Engel, A.K., König, P., Kreiter, A.K., Schillen, T.B., and Singer, W. (1992). Temporal coding in the visual cortex: new vistas on integration in the nervous system. *Trends in Neuroscience*, **15**, 218–226.

Ericsson, K.A. and Kintsch, W. (1995). Long-term working memory. *Psychological Review*, **102**, 211–245.

Felleman, D.J. and van Essen, D.C.V. (1991). Distributed hierarchical processing in the primate visual cortex. *Cerebral Cortex*, **1**, 1–47.

Fries, P., Reynolds, J.H., Rorie, A.E, and Desimone, R. (2001). Modulation of oscillatory neuronal synchronization by selective visual attention. *Science*, **291**, 1560–1563.

Fuster, J.M. (2001). The prefrontal cortex—an update: time is of the essence. *Neuron*, **30**, 319–333.

Gluck, M.A. and Meyers, C.E. (1993). Hippocampal mediation of stimulus representation: a computational theory. *Hippocampus*, **3**, 491–516.

Goldman-Rakic, P.S. (1988). Topography of cognition: parallel distributed networks in primate association cortex. *Annual Review of Neuroscience*, **11**, 137–156.

Gray, C.M. (1999). The temporal correlation hypothesis of visual feature integration: still alive and well. *Neuron*, **24**, 31–47.

Gray, C. M., König, P., Engel, A. K., and Singer, W. (1989). Oscillatory responses in cat visual cortex exhibit inter-columnar synchronization which reflects global stimulus properties. *Nature*, **338**, 334–337.

Groenewegen, H.J.U. and Uylings, H.B.M. (2000). The prefrontal cortex and the integration of sensory, limbic and autonomic information. *Progress in Brain Research*, **126**, 3–28.

Gross, J., Schmitz, F., Schnitzler, I., *et al.* (2004). Modulation of long-range neural synchrony reflects temporal limitations of visual attention in humans. *Proceedings of the National Academy of Sciences of the United States of America*, **101**, 13050–13055.

Grossberg, S. (1976). Adaptive pattern classification and universal recoding. II: Feedback, expectation, olfaction, and illusions. *Biological Cybernetics*, **23**, 187–202.

Grossberg, S. (1987). Competitive learning: from interactive activation to adaptive resonance. *Cognitive Science*, **11**, 23–63.

Hasegawa, I., Fukushima, T., Ihara, T., and Miyashita, Y. (1998). Callosal window between prefrontal cortices: cognitive interaction to retrieve long-term memory. *Science*, **281**, 814–818.

Hebb, D.O. (1949). *The Organization of Behavior*. New York: John Wiley.

Hinton, G.E. and Anderson, J.A. (ed) (1989). *Parallel Models of Associative Memory*. Hillsdale, NJ: Erlbaum.

Hopfield, J.J. (1982). Neural networks and physical systems with emergent collective computational abilities. *Proceedings of the National Academy of Sciences of the United States of America*, 79, 2554–2558.

Horn, D. and Usher, M. (1991). Parallel activation of memories in an oscillatory neural network. *Neural Computation*, **3**, 31–43.

James, W. (1890). *Principles of Psychology*. New York: Dover Publications, 1950.

Jensen, O. and Lisman, J.E. (1996). Novel lists of 7 ± 2 known items can be reliably stored in an oscillatory short-term memory network: interaction with long-term memory. *Learning and Memory*, **3**, 257–263.

Koechlin, E., Ody, C., and Kouheiner, F. (2003). The architecture of cognitive control in the human prefrontal cortex. *Science*, **302**, 1181–1185.

Kohonen, T. (1989). *Self-Organization and Associative Memory* (3rd edn). Berlin: Springer-Verlag.

Kroger, J.K., Sabb, F.W., Fales, C.L., Bookheimer, S.Y., Cohen, M.S., and Holyoak, K.J. (2002). Recruitment of anterior dorsolateral prefrontal cortex in human reasoning. *Cerebral Cortex*, **12**, 477–485.

Kydd, R.J. and Bilkey, D.K. (2003). Prefrontal cortex lesions modify the spatial properties of hippocampal place cells. *Cerebral Cortex*, **13**, 444–451.

Linsker, R. (1986a). From basic network principles to neural architecture: emergence of spatial-opponent cells. *Proceedings of the National Academy of Sciences of the United States of America*, **83**, 7508–7512.

Linsker, R. (1986b). From basic network principles to neural architecture: emergence of orientation-selective cells. *Proceedings of the National Academy of Sciences of the United States of America*, **83**, 8390–8394.

Linsker, R. (1986c). From basic network principles to neural architecture: emergence of orientation columns. *Proceedings of the National Academy of Sciences of the United States of America*, **83**, 8779–8783.

Lisman, J.E. and Idiart, M.A.P. (1995) Storage of 7 ± 2 short-term memories in oscillatory subcycles. *Science*, **267**, 1512–1515.

Luck, S.J. and Vogel, E.K. (1997). The capacity of visual working memory for features and conjunctions. *Nature*, **390**, 279–281.

McClelland, J.L. and Rumelhart, D.E. (1981). An interactive activation model of context effects in letter perception. Part I: An account of basic findings. *Psychological Review*, **5**, 375–407.

McClelland, J.L., McNaughton, B.L., and O'Reilly, R.C. (1995). Why there are complementary learning systems in the hippocampus and neocortex: insights from the successes and failures of connectionist models of learning and memory. *Psychological Review*, **102**, 419–457.

MacGregor, R.J. and Oliver, R.M. (1974). A model for repetitive firing in neurons. *Kybernetik*, **16**, 53–64.

McNaughton, B.L. and Nadel, L. (1990). Hebb–Marr networks and the neurobiological representations of action in space. In *Neuroscience and Connectionist Theory* (ed M.A. Gluck and D.E. Rumelhart). Hillsdale, NJ: Erlbaum, pp. 1–63.

Markram, H., Lubke, J., Frotscher, M., and Sakmann, B. (1997). Regulation of synaptic efficacy by coincidence of postsynaptic APs and EPSPs. *Science*, **275**, 213–215.

Marr, D. (1971). Simple memory: a theory for archicortex. *Philosophical Transactions of the Royal Society of London, Series B, Biological Sciences*, **262**, 23–81.

Meeter, M. (2003). Control of consolidation in neural networks: avoiding runaway effects. *Connection Science*, **15**, 45–61.

Meeter, M. and Murre, J.M.J. (2004a). Simulating episodic memory deficits in semantic dementia with the TraceLink model. *Memory*, **12**, 272–287.

Meeter, M. and Murre, J.M.J. (2004b). Consolidation of long-term memory: evidence and alternatives. *Psychological Bulletin*, **130**, 843–857.

Meeter, M. and Murre, J.M.J. (2005). TraceLink: a model of consolidation and amnesia. *Cognitive Neuropsychology*, **22**, 559–587.

Meeter, M., Talamini, L.M., and Murre, J.M.J. (2004). Mode shifting between storage and recall based on novelty detection in oscillating hippocampal circuits. *Hippocampus*, **14**, 722–741.

Miller, G.A. (1956). The magical number seven, plus or minus two: some limits on our capacity for processing information. *Psychological Review*, **63**, 81–97.

Miller, E.K. and Cohen, J.D. (2001). An integrative theory of prefrontal cortex function. *Annual Review of Neuroscience*, **24**, 167–202.

Miller, E.K., Erickson, C.A., and Desimone, R. (1996). Neural mechanisms of visual working memory in prefrontal cortex of the macaque. *Journal of Neuroscience*, **16**, 5154–5167.

Milner, P.M. (1957). The cell assembly: Mark II. *Psychological Review*, **64**, 242–252.

Milner, P.M. (1989). A cell assembly theory of hippocampal amnesia. *Neuropsychologia*, **6**, 215–234.

Mishkin, M. (1982). A memory system in the monkey. *Philosophical Transactions of the Royal Society of London, Series B, Biological Sciences*, **298**, 85–95.

Murre, J.M.J. (1992). *Categorization and Learning in Modular Neural Networks*. Hillsdale, NJ: Erlbaum.

Murre, J.M.J. (1996). TraceLink: A model of amnesia and consolidation of memory. *Hippocampus*, **6**, 675–684.

Murre, J.M.J., Phaf, R.H., and Wolters, G. (1992). CALM: Categorizing And Learning Module. *Neural Networks*, **5**, 55–82.

Murre, J.M.J., Graham, K., and Hodges, J. (2001). Semantic dementia: new constraints on computational models of long-term memory. *Brain*, **124**, 647–675

Nadel, L. and Moscovitch, M. (1997). Memory consolidation, retrograde amnesia and the hippocampal complex. *Current Opinion in Neurobiology*, **7**, 217–227.

Nadel, L., Samsonovitch, A., Ryan, L., and Moscovitch, M. (2000). Multiple trace theory of human memory: Computational, neuroimaging and neuropsychological results. *Hippocampus*, **10**, 352–368.

Nakamura, K., Mikami, A., and Kubota, K. (1992) Oscillatory neuronal activity related to visual short-term memory in monkey temporal pole. *Neuroreport*, **3**, 117–120.

Norman, D.A. and Shallice, T. (1986). Attention to action: willed and automatic control of behaviour. In *Consciousness and Self-Regulation*, Vol. 4 (ed R.J. Davidson, G.E. Schwartz, and D.E. Shapiro). New York: Plenum Press, 1–18.

O'Connor, D.H., Fukui, M.M., Pinsk, M.A., and Kastner, S. (2002). Attention modulates responses in the human lateral geniculate nucleus. *Nature Neuroscience*, **5**, 1203–1209.

O'Keefe, J. and Nadel, L. (1978). *The Hippocampus as a Cognitive Map*. Oxford: Clarendon Press.

O'Reilly, R.C., Braver, T.S., and Cohen, J.D. (1999). A biologically based computational model of working memory. In *Models of Working Memory* (ed A. Miyake and P. Shah). Cambridge: Cambridge University Press, pp. 375–411.

Page, M. (2000). Connectionist modelling in psychology: a localist manifesto. *Behavioral and Brain Sciences*, **23**, 443–512.

Penick, S. and Solomon, P. (1991). Hippocampus, context and conditioning. *Behavioral Neuroscience*, **105**, 611–617.

Phaf, R.H. and Wolters, G. (1997). A constructivist and connectionist view on conscious and nonconscious processes. *Philosophical Psychology*, **10**, 287–307.

Prabhakaran, V., Narayanan, K., Zhao, Z., and Gabrieli, J.D.E. (2000). Integration of diverse information in working memory within the frontal lobe. *Nature Neuroscience*, **3**, 85–90.

Raaijmakers, J.G.W. and Shiffrin, R.M. (1981). Search of associative memory. *Psychological Review*, **88**, 454–457.

Raffone, A. and van Leeuwen, C. (2002). Activation and coherence in memory processes: revisiting the parallel distributed processing approach to retrieval. *Connection Science*, **13**, 349–382.

Raffone A. and van Leeuwen, C. (2003). Dynamic synchronization and chaos in an associative neural network with multiple active memories. *Chaos*, **13**, 1090–1104.

Raffone, A. and Wolters, G. (2001). A cortical mechanism for binding in visual working memory. *Journal of Cognitive Neuroscience*, **13**, 766–785.

Raffone, A., Wolters, G., and Murre, J.M.J. (2001). A neurophysiological account of working memory limited capacity: within-chunk integration and between-item segregation. *Behavioral and Brain Sciences*, **24**, 139–141.

Raffone, A., Murre, J.M.J., and Wolters, G. (2003). NMDA synapses can bias competition between object representations and mediate attentional selection. *Behavioral and Brain Sciences*, **26**, 100–101.

Rainer, G., Asaad, W.F., and Miller, E.K. (1998). Selective representation of relevant information by neurons in the primate prefrontal cortex. *Nature*, **393**, 577–579.

Ramnani, N. and Owen, A.M. (2004). Anterior prefrontal cortex: Insights into function from anatomy and neuroimaging. *Nature Reviews Neuroscience*, **5**, 184–194.

Reynolds, J.H., Pasternak, T., and Desimone, R. (2000). Attention increases sensitivity of V4 neurons. *Neuron*, **26**, 703–714.

Roelfsema, P.R., Engel, A.K., König, P., and Singer, W. (1996). The role of neuronal synchronization in response selection: a biologically plausible theory of structured representations in the visual cortex. *Journal of Cognitive Neuroscience*, **8**, 603–625.

Rolls, E.T. and Treves, A. (1998). *Neural Networks and Brain Function*. Oxford: Oxford University Press.

Rumelhart, D.E. and Zipser, D. (1985). Feature discovery by competitive learning. *Cognitive Science*, **9**, 75–112.

Rushworth, M.F.S. and Owen, A.M. (1998). The functional organization of the lateral frontal cortex: conjecture or conjuncture in the neurophysiological literature? *Trends in Cognitive Sciences*, **2**, 46–53.

Sakai, K., Rowe, J.B., and Passingham, R.E. (2002). Active maintenance in prefrontal area 46 creates distractor-resistant memory. *Nature Neuroscience*, **5**, 479–484.

Simons, J.S. and Spiers, H.J. (2003). Prefrontal and medial temporal lobe interactions in long-term memory. *Nature Reviews Neuroscience*, **4**, 637–648.

Singer, W. (1999) Neuronal synchrony: a versatile code for the definition of relations? *Neuron*, **24**, 49–65.

Squire, L.R. (1992). Memory and the hippocampus: a synthesis from findings with rats, monkeys, and humans. *Psychological Review*, **99**, 195–231.

Squire, L.R. and Alvarez, P. (1995). Retrograde amnesia and memory consolidation: a neurobiological perspective. *Current Opinion in Neurobiology*, **5**, 169–177.

Squire, L.R. and Zola-Morgan, S. (1991). The medial temporal lobe memory system. *Science*, **253**, 1380–1386.

Squire, L.R., Cohen, N.J., and Nadel, L. (1984). The medial temporal region and memory consolidation: a new hypothesis. In *Memory consolidation* (ed H. Weingarter and E. Parker). Hillsdale, NJ: Erlbaum.

Talamini, L.M., Meeter, M., Elvevåg, B., Murre, J.M.J., and Goldberg, T.E. (2005). Reduced parahippocampal connectivity produces schizophrenia-like memory deficits in simulated neural circuits. *Archives of General Psychiatry*, **62**, 485–493.

Tallon-Baudry, C., Bertrand, O., and Fischer, C. (2001). Oscillatory synchrony between human extrastriate areas during visual short-term memory maintenance. *Journal of Neuroscience*, **21**, 1–5.

Teyler, T.J. and DiScenna, P. (1986). The hippocampal memory indexing theory. *Behavioral Neuroscience*, **100**, 147–154.

Tononi, G., Sporns, O., and Edelman, G.M. (1992). Reentry and the problem of integration of multiple cortical areas: simulation of dynamic integration in the visual system. *Cerebral Cortex*, **2**, 310–335.

Treves, A. and Rolls, E.T. (1994). Computational analysis of the role of the hippocampus in memory. *Hippocampus*, **4**, 374–391.

Tulving, E. (1972). Episodic and semantic memory. In *Organisation of Memory* (ed E. Tulving and W. Donaldson). New York: Academic Press, pp. 381–403.

Tulving, E. and Thomson, D.M. (1973). Encoding specificity and retrieval processes in episodic memory. *Psychological Review*, **80**, 352–373.

Ungerleider, L.G., Courtney, S.M., and Haxby, J.V. (1998). A neural system for human visual working memory. *Proceedings of the National Academy of Sciences of the United States of America*, **95**, 883–890.

Villa, A.E.P. and Fuster, J.M. (1992). Temporal correlates of information processing during visual short-term memory. *Neuroreport*, **3**, 113–116.

von der Malsburg, C. (1981). *The Correlation Theory of Brain Function*. Internal Report 81–2, Max Planck Institute for Biophysical Chemistry, Göttingen.

von der Malsburg C. (1999). The what and why of binding: the modeler's perspective. *Neuron*, **24**, 95–104.

Wagner, A.D., Desmond, J.E., Glover, G.H., and Gabrieli, J.D. (1998). Prefrontal cortex and recognition memory: functional-MRI evidence for context-dependent retrieval processes. *Brain*, **121**, 1985–2002.

Wallis, J.D., Anderson, K.C., and Miller, E.K. (2001). Single neurons in prefrontal cortex encode abstract rules. *Nature*, **411**, 953–956.

Wang, X.J. (1999). Synaptic basis of cortical persistent activity: the importance of NMDA receptors to working memory. *Journal of Neuroscience*, **19**, 9587–9603.

White and Wise (1999).

Wickelgren, W.A. (1979). Chunking and consolidation: a theoretical synthesis of semantic networks, configuring in conditioning, S-R versus cognitive learning, normal forgetting, the amnesic syndrome, and the hippocampal arousal system. *Psychological Review*, **86**, 44–60.

Wickelgren, W.A. (1987). Site fragility theory of chunking and consolidation in a distributed associative memory. In *Neuroplasticity, Learning, and Memory* (ed N.W. Milgram, C.M. MacLeod and T.C. Petit). New York: Liss, pp. 301–325.

Willshaw, D.J., Buneman, O.P., and Longuet-Higgins, H.C. (1969). Non-holographic associative memory. *Nature*, **222**, 960–962.

Wood, J.N. and Grafman, J. (2003). Human prefrontal cortex: processing and representational perspectives. *Nature Reviews Neuroscience*, **4**, 139–147.

Zipser, D. and Anderson, R.A. (1988). A back-propagation programmed network that simulates response properties of a subset of posterior parietal neurons. *Nature*, **331**, 679–684.

Chapter 10

The role of time in human memory and binding: a review of the evidence

Gordon D. A. Brown and Teresa McCormack

Introduction

In this chapter we review evidence for the temporal memory binding hypothesis—the suggestion that temporal coordinates play a privileged role in the maintenance and retrieval of associative binding relations in human memory. More specifically, we address two particular questions concerning the role of time in human memory and binding.

One important theoretical issue is whether temporal coordinates are essential components of human memories. It has been argued that temporal and spatial coordinates are central to memory records because they enable maintenance of the unity of remembered experiences (Gallistel 1990). Our first question concerns whether (and in what sense) temporal coordinates are an important part of human memories. Is memory chronologically organized? If there is no sense in which memory is chronologically organized, it would seem unlikely that the stronger claim that temporal coordinates are involved in binding could be sustained. We argue for an affirmative answer to this first question, although data are limited. Our second question is whether, as Gallistel has suggested, temporal and/or spatial coordinates link components of human memories together over the medium to long term. We will argue that the answer to the second question is less clear, given current evidence.

We begin with the hypothesis described and explored in detail by Gallistel (1990). Gallistel argues that temporal and spatial coordinates are obligatory components of animal memory records because such coordinates play a crucial role in unifying and interrelating the records. He argues that temporal and spatial dimensions are privileged in this unifying function that they serve. There are various functional and adaptive reasons for entertaining such a hypothesis; here we can only summarize some of the reasons given by Gallistel. For example, evolutionary and biological considerations converge on the view that much of the brain is modular in organization (Fodor 1983). That is, different brain regions are specialized for performing different functions and/or representing different stimulus dimensions (such as shape and colour). Given a modular organization, a problem arises. This problem is a form of the binding problem; although it has been investigated primarily in the domain of visual perception, a related problem arises in retrieval from memory. For example, suppose that I am looking at a visual display containing a picture of a red herring and a picture of a green ham. It may be desirable both to perceive and remember the fact that what is being viewed is a red herring and a green ham, rather than a red ham and a green herring. One way in which such a problem might be solved is by representing the spatial and/or temporal locations of the various features (here, object identity and colour). Co-location could then provide the basis for feature binding. Note that according to such a view there is no direct association between 'red' and 'herring' or between 'green' and 'ham'. Instead, the object–colour associations are indirect in the sense that they are mediated through common spatial and/or temporal coordinates. Such accounts have been widespread within theories of visual attention and perception. For example, Nissen (1985) argues that separate properties, such as the shape and colour of an object, are not directly integrated but are linked simply in terms of their association with a common spatial location (see also Isenberg *et al.* 1990). As evidence, Nissen (1985) and others report that object colour cannot be used a direct probe for object shape; instead a successful memory of object location is required if shape is to be retrieved from colour (see also Treisman and Gelade 1980). Temporal co-location has also been implicated in perceptual binding (Treisman 1977; but see Keele *et al.* 1988). There is ample evidence that such coding schemes operate in the domain of short-term visual processing. Gallistel (1990) reviews much of the early evidence (more recent work is reviewed by Heathcote *et al.* 2001). However, such assumptions are at present not widely incorporated into models of human memory, despite the considerations raised by Gallistel and others. Instead, models of human memory typically assume that direct associative links are formed, either between separate items (e.g. pairs of words) or between fragments of items.

For now, we take as a given the idea that spatial location and perhaps also temporal location play an important unifying role in the perceptual/attentional processing of visually presented stimuli over the short term. Our concern in the present chapter is with the more controversial claim that similar mechanisms may underpin the maintenance and retrieval of binding relations in established memories. There is ample evidence that different features of objects may be represented separately in memory (Stefurak and Boynton 1986; reviewed by Heathcote *et al.* 2001). As Heathcote *et al.* note, a major challenge is establish the mechanisms responsible for maintaining associative binding relations in memory.

While Heathcote *et al.* focus on the possible role of spatial location, here we garner evidence for and against the proposition that temporal coordinates play a role in the representation of associative relationships in human memory over the longer term (i.e. minutes, hours, and days or longer). We emphasize temporal rather than spatial memory in order to preserve a focus on the temporal memory binding hypothesis. The approach we adopt is both empirical and theoretical. First, we briefly discuss the relation between binding problems in perception and in memory. We then describe evidence consistent with the claim that temporal coordinates form an important part human memory records, i.e. that memory is in some sense chronologically organized. We then review current formal models of human memory to examine the role that time plays or might play in such models and, more specifically, the role that time plays in binding together human memories and their components. Although some recent models of free recall and serial recall ascribe an important role to time as a dimension underpinning memory, models of associative memory have not generally made the same assumption. Finally, we review studies that bear directly on the role of time in binding in human long-term memory. Most of these studies examine whether binding errors in associative memory, such as memory conjunction errors, respect temporal factors. Some evidence consistent with this claim is found, although at present the evidence is weak and many of the results cannot unambiguously be attributed to storage and retrieval processes rather than to initial encoding.

Is there a binding problem in human memory analogous to that in perception?

The existence of a binding problem in visual perception is often motivated by appeal to the fact that neuropsychological evidence points clearly to the existence of neuroanatomically distinct brain regions for processing different aspects of objects (Treisman 1977). The binding problem is often conceived of as being a problem about perceptual experience itself: How is that our visual experience is of a world with discrete objects, given that the features of such objects are in fact processed separately?

Setting up a 'binding problem' in memory that closely parallels that in visual perception is not straightforward. First, it is by no means obvious what we should take to be the relevant properties that need to be bound together. Even in the perceptual case, there may be debate over which attributes of the object actually constitute the 'component properties' that Treisman refers to. The memory case appears to be even more complex. For example, in a list-learning task involving visual presentation of words, which properties of the word should we assume are separately processed? Do aspects of the context in which the word appeared need to be considered as component properties, or are the relevant properties simply perceptual features of the words themselves? What about semantic properties? Specifying the 'component properties' becomes even more difficult if we consider episodic memories outside the laboratory (e.g. memories of different summer holidays one has taken). Indeed, although as we review below there are numerous experimental studies of conjunction errors in memory, the separable features that participants may erroneously conjoin in such studies are often not ones that it makes sense to believe are processed by separate modules (e.g. different components of faces or different syllables of words).

These difficulties in isolating the relevant components can be seen in part as arising from a more general problem in specifying the 'objects' of memory experience. Although episodic memory is commonly described as involving memory for events, there have been few attempts actually to describe what events actually are, and, importantly, how we should individuate them. Given these issues, rather than taking a direct memory parallel of the binding problem in visual perception for granted, it may be more fruitful to consider the more general issue that suggests itself by considering the visual case. As Gallistel puts it, spatial location is, in Treisman's theory, a 'privileged variable'. Are there variables that are in some sense 'privileged' in memory because they serve as a means of linking together a number of event features? We can consider whether some variables are privileged without drawing a full-blown analogy to the binding problem in perception, i.e. without attempting to identify a variable or variables whose processing underpins memory experiences for discrete events. Further, we need not assume that the event features that are linked together via the variable in question are processed in different neural pathways or in different modules. We can simply ask whether certain variables have a privileged status by virtue of their being used to link together different event features.

The underlying assumption of much research on memory and cognition is that memory involves the formation of associative links. These associative links are assumed to be formed at many different levels between many different types of features. For example, these links may be between separate perceptual attributes of a single to-be-remembered item (e.g. colour and shape), between different components of the item (e.g. syllables of a word), between different items (e.g. in paired associate learning), between items and contextual features in episodic memory, or between different events. As we discuss below, it is often tacitly assumed that associative links are made directly between the features in question. However, Gallistel argues that time plays a privileged role in memory—that many event features are linked together not directly but via a representation of spatio-temporal location. It is possible to make versions of the claim that temporal location is privileged that differ in strength. The strongest possible claim is that *all* links between *all* event features are indirect, occurring only via a mediating specification of spatio-temporal location. However, temporal location may play a privileged role in linking some types of event features but not others, or may play a role in memory by linking together diverse sets of event features that may have within-set direct associative links. We assess the evidence for these claims below, after a review of evidence for more general claims about the chronological organization of memory.

The chronological organization of human memory

Is memory chronologically organized? Positive evidence for this suggestion will form the backdrop for consideration of the rather stronger claim that temporal relations mediate associations and binding in memory. Indeed, if temporal coordinates of memories are never encoded and remembered, they can hardly form the basis of associative binding. We first review some theoretical considerations, and then consider evidence for and models of time-based memory for free recall and memory for serial order. We conclude that such models have (perhaps paradoxically, given the current concern) been more inclined to assign a major role for time than have the models of associative memory that we consider in a separate section.

Claims about the chronological organization of human memory could be interpreted in a number of different ways. For example, current conceptions of episodic memory (Wheeler *et al.* 1998), following on from Tulving (1983), emphasize the role of 'mental time travel' in episodic remembering. The remembering of an event as having occurred in the past (as well as having been experienced by the rememberer) seems to be an important part of our conception of episodic memory, and hence the ability to represent time and temporal relations in particular (and perhaps human-like) ways seems to be a prerequisite for truly episodic memory (see McCormack (1999, 2001), McCormack and Hoerl (1999), Hoerl (2001), and Martin (2001) for recent discussion of the nature of episodic memory). Suddendorf and Corballis (1997) argued that mental time travel is what separates humans from animals (see also Roberts 2002). However, these conceptions of episodic remembering, while emphasizing the notion of 'pastness', do not seem to mandate strong conclusions regarding the role of time in associative binding in memory. In any case, many of the studies we review below rely on data from recognition and serial recall memory tasks, and the performance of such tasks need not always involve episodic memory as traditionally conceived.

One way to interpret the claim that memory is chronologically organized is developed and critiqued by Friedman (2001). Friedman explores the possibility that every memory is associated with a temporal code, perhaps through involvement of a specialized mechanism. On the basis of an extensive review of the empirical literature, Friedman concludes that there is little evidence for the consistent and obligatory operation of such a mechanism. However, it is important to be clear about the type of claim regarding the chronological organization of memory that Friedman dismisses. Friedman is concerned primarily with the capacity that enables us to remember the time of past events, and he presents compelling evidence that reconstructive processes, such as the use of temporal landmarks (Shum 1998), underpin such abilities. There is little evidence that temporal distance or temporal location information are remembered and used directly to date past events. However, the evidence that Friedman convincingly reviews does not seem incompatible with the claim that, for example, event memories are located in a multidimensional space where one of the dimensions is temporal. We describe such a model below, but note here that such models need carry no implication that past events are datable in terms of their position along such a dimension.[1] Thus the position we defend is considerably weaker than the one Friedman rejects.

Here we argue that (a) there are evolutionary considerations to suggest that it might be adaptive to organize memory chronologically, (b) there is considerable empirical evidence consistent with the claim that temporal information can be and often is encoded memorially, and (c) several recent models of both human and animal memory have time at their core and moreover time is central to their explanation of several empirical phenomena (Gallistel and Gibbon 2000; Brown *et al.* 2002; Fairhurst *et al.* 2003). Following Gallistel (1990), these arguments are developed in more detail by Brown and Chater (2001) (see also Brown and Vousden 1998) and below.

Evolutionary and adaptive considerations

Events in the world that have occurred recently are more likely to be relevant in the immediate future than are events that have not occurred so recently (Anderson and Milson 1989). Anderson and Schooler (1991) develop this perspective and show that the 'need probability' of an event in memory (i.e. the probability that information about that event will have to be retrieved) is related in systematic ways to the recency of last occurrence of that event. They show that the form of human memory forgetting curves, which typically show that the rate of forgetting is initially rapid and then levels off over time (Rubin and Wenzel 1996) can be explained on the assumption that the memory system is adaptive in the sense that it allocates greater retrievability to more recent memories. Arguably, this could be viewed as a form of adaptive chronological organization in memory (Brown and Chater 2001).

Gallistel (1990) reviews evidence that it may be adaptive to represent memories in terms of the phase of different temporal oscillators, such as circadian rhythms, with which they were associated. For example, circadian oscillators can be used to represent the fact that the source of food is available at a particular time every day (see also Brown and Vousden 1998). It is possible that temporal oscillators, which may have a memory function even in simple organisms, have become adapted to provide the foundation for complex human temporal and sequential behaviour such as speech production (Vousden *et al.* 2000) and short-term memory for serial order (Brown *et al.* 2000; Burgess and Hitch 1992, 1999); for applications to music and attention see Large and Jones (1999) and Large and Palmer (2002). A final argument concerns what may be termed trace uniqueness. As Gallistel emphasizes, the fact that time never repeats has the consequence that representations of items in terms of their position along an episodic/temporal continuum guarantees a unique tag for every memory trace.[2]

In summary, there are a variety of reasons to entertain the hypothesis that there is at least some sense in which human memory is chronologically organized. Fortunately, there is some relevant empirical evidence available and it is to this that we now turn.

Empirical evidence

Many of the experimental methods traditionally used to explore human memory could require participants to retrieve and use temporal information, although direct evidence on whether or not temporal information is actually used is surprisingly limited. One relevant observation is that humans can reliably distinguish temporal recency from familiarity, although such abilities may be compromised in amnesic patients (Mayes *et al.* 1989). Such an ability seems to suggest that humans have access to information in memory about at least the relative time of occurrence of particular items and that experimental participants are not, for example, simply relying on some non-temporal quantity such as global familiarity or trace strength to perform the task (Brown and Chater 2001). We now consider a number of specific memory tasks.

Recognition memory

In a typical recognition memory experiment, participants view a list of 30 or 40 words and subsequently, after list presentation is complete, are presented with a series of test items. Each test item must be classified as 'old' or 'new' according to whether or not it occurred in the list. A typical experiment will involve presentation of many such lists. One way of interpreting such tasks is as a type of temporal judgement (Brown *et al.* 2000): when faced with a test item, the participant must decide whether that item occurred within the temporal window defined by the presentation of the test list. Indeed, much current controversy surrounding models of human recognition memory (Dennis and Humphreys 2001; Criss and Shiffrin 2004) revolves around a contextual interpretation of the recognition memory task. Is recognition performance limited primarily by interference arising from other contexts within which the test item has appeared, or by the other items within the test list? Initial suggestions that recognition memory performance reflects the operation of some global familiarity computation suffer from a number of problems (Clark and Gronlund 1996). More recent models, such as that of Dennis and Humphreys (2001), emphasize instead the retrieval of the episodic contexts associated with a given test item, and time plays an important role in the contextual component of the Dennis and Humphreys model. Some model-based approaches to explaining temporal recency effects in recognition (Corballis 1967; Shiffrin 1970a) have emphasized the possible role of temporal distinctiveness in explaining such recency (Neath 1993; Brown *et al.* 2000). However, rather little direct evidence is available, and current comprehensive models of recognition memory do not ascribe a major role to the temporal coordinates of to-be-remembered items.

Free recall

Free recall tasks could also (although again need not) be interpreted as indirect tests of memory for time of occurrence. In free recall, the participant is normally, although not always (Shiffrin 1970b), required to retrieve as many of the items that occurred within the most recent list as possible. Indeed, the temporal recency of an item's most recent presentation or rehearsal is an excellent predictor of the probability of successful recall in such experiments (Rundus 1971; Tan and Ward 2000). However, comprehensive research on the influence of time, as opposed to dimensions correlated with time, such as ordinal position or number of item occurrences (see below), remains limited.

Effects of temporal proximity can be observed in free recall. A detailed analysis of free recall protocols shows two clear relevant tendencies. The recall of an item tends to be followed by recall of an item that was temporally close in the presented list, and during recall there is a generally forward bias such that items that followed one another during list presentation tend to be recalled in corresponding order at output (see Howard and Kahana (1999, 2002), Kahana (1996), and Laming (1999) for extensive analysis and discussion).

In response to observations of this type, many recent models of serial recall, free recall, and recency judgements have incorporated a strong temporal component. For example, the model of Howard and Kahana (2002) has at its heart a temporal context vector. The learning context for a given item is made up partly from this temporal context and partly from pre-experimental associations, and retrieval of a given item leads to concomitant recall of the learning contexts originally associated with the recalled item. Howard and Kahana show that their time-based model of free recall can accommodate many classic free recall data.

Memory for serial order

Traditional serial recall tasks of the type used to assess short-term memory for serial order have often been interpreted as temporal order memory tasks although, as we shall see below, recent evidence questions this interpretation. A rich source of potential evidence concerns the nature of errors made in human memory for serial order. A widely replicated finding is that items that are temporally adjacent at the time of learning are more likely to be confused in memory than are temporally more distant items. Such effects can be seen in speech production (MacKay 1970; Vousden *et al.* 2000), judgements of relative recency (Hacker 1980), and serial recall (Healy 1974; reviewed by Brown *et al.* 2000). For example, the sequence A B C D is more likely to be recalled (incorrectly) as A C B D than as A D C B, and items that occurred two seconds ago and three seconds ago will have their relative recency judged less accurately than will items that occurred two seconds ago and five seconds ago.

Such data have motivated recent models in the domain of serial recall. The temporal oscillator-based models of Burgess and Hitch (1992, 1999) and Brown *et al.* (2000) assume that successive items of a to-be-recalled list become associated with successive states of a time-varying oscillator-based context signal of some kind. Reinstatement of the temporal context of learning allows dynamic reinstatement of successive cues for successive items. Such models offer a comprehensive account of a number of phenomena, including in particular the tendency for temporally adjacent items to be recalled in the wrong relative order with greater than chance probability. However, non-temporal accounts of the same basic phenomena are also available (Henson 1998; Page and Norris 1998).

Can the success of these time-based models be used to support claims about temporal encoding in memory? The temporal mechanisms that are central to recent models of serial and free recall are responsible for crucial aspects of the model's behaviour, and, given that models can be seen as an attempt at a shorthand description of a range of empirical data, the important role ascribed to time in such models buttresses claims about the importance of time in memory.

However, the fact that both temporal and non-temporal models of serial recall can account for confusions of temporally adjacent items highlights a general methodological problem that we now consider in detail. In a typical human memory experiment, temporal and positional information are highly confounded (Crowder and Greene 1987). Items that have similar positional representations are also temporally closer to one another than are more positionally distant items. Therefore the results described above concerning the confusion of temporally adjacent items cannot be taken as unambiguous evidence for the chronological organization of memory. Evidence for the role of temporal rather than positional influences is crucial for hypotheses concerning the temporal organization of memory.

In order to address this issue directly, a number of recent studies have attempted to deconfound temporal and positional information. These studies fall into two categories. First, experiments have examined whether it is the temporal or the positional location of items within a list (or within-list group) that determines the probability of their erroneous recall in an equivalent location in a subsequent list or group (Henson 1999; Ng and Maybery 2002). For example, when two lists of six letters are learned and recalled successively, the fifth letter in the first list may incorrectly appear in the fifth position of the recall of the second list. But do these order errors respect temporal or positional constraints? The experimental studies have converged on the conclusion that, at least in serial recall tasks, items are represented and retrieved in terms of their location along a positional dimension as well as or instead of their position along a temporal dimension. Additional data, problematic for purely time-based accounts of serial recall, are consistent with a role for position rather than time. For example, Lewandowsky *et al.* (2004) found that the degree of forgetting that occurred during the time course of serial recall was essentially uninfluenced by the speed of recall and hence independent of the changing retention intervals for successively recalled items. They showed that these results were inconsistent with several time-based models of memory for serial recall, but were consistent with a model in which a positional dimension was more important for representing order (see also Maybery *et al.* 2002).

A second source of evidence comes from attempts to separate temporal and positional information at presentation. This has been done in various ways, although we argue that at present a clear conclusion is only possible for the case of serial recall. For example, Neath and Crowder (1990) (see also Corballis 1966; Welte and Laughery 1971; Crowder and Neath 1991; Neath and Crowder 1996) used a varying rate of presentation for items in free recall and serial recall tasks. Increasing and decreasing rates of presentation are illustrated in Figure 10.1. Note that this procedure allows the temporal proximity of items to be varied

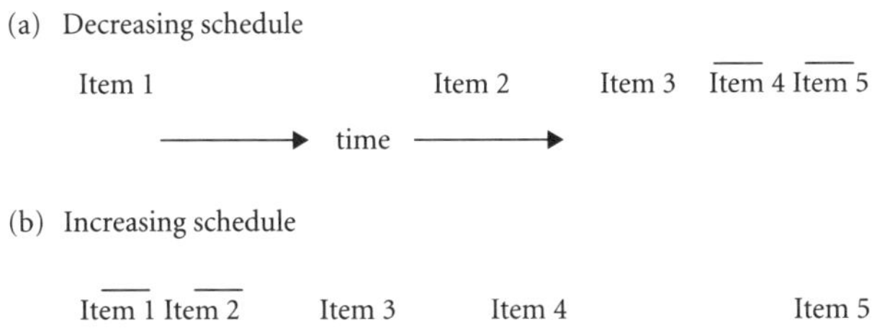

Figure 10.1 Illustration of increasing and decreasing presentation schedules for a list of items in a memory task.

without a confounding change in the item's location along a positional dimension. For example, in the increasing rate of presentation condition, the sixth and seventh items occur in close temporal proximity while in the decreasing presentation rate condition, the items occupying the same ordinal positions (sixth and seventh) are more widely separated in time. Any effect of increasing versus decreasing rate of presentation would therefore seem to implicate representation of items along a temporal dimension. Neath and Crowder (1990; 1996) indeed found that items in more temporally crowded regions of the list were less well recalled. These results appear to offer clear evidence for the importance of temporal as opposed to positional distinctiveness.

The deconfounding methodology has been applied to both serial and free recall. However, one problem of interpretation of the serial recall results arises from the predictability of the presentation schedules. Using a serial recall task, Lewandowsky *et al.* (2006) found that the recall advantage for temporally isolated items disappeared when the increasing and decreasing presentation schedules were embedded in a series of lists in which the inter-item presentation times were random. More generally, Lewandowsky *et al.* found that the serial recall of an item is not independently predicted by the temporal isolation of that item, and concluded that the location of items along a positional rather than temporal dimension is the main influence in determining serial recall probability (see also Lewandowsky and Brown 2005). Therefore there is little evidence in serial recall for effects of temporal closeness over and above positional closeness. In other tasks, such as free recall or recognition memory, the temporal dimension may be more salient. As we note below, a hallmark of many time-based and temporal distinctiveness models of memory is pronounced and extended recency effects when recall is immediate. Therefore the fact that temporally extended recency effects are generally observed in immediate probed recall, free recall, and recognition memory, but not in serial recall, is consistent with a reduced role of temporal coding in the serial recall task compared with other memory tasks. Consistent with this interpretation, Duncan and Murdock (2000) found that recency effects in recognition memory disappear if the memory task may be serial recall or recognition and is post-cued rather than pre-cued (i.e. participants did not know whether they would face a recognition task or a serial recall task until after the list was presented). Just this pattern of results would be expected if a temporal dimension is useful in recognition but cannot support serial recall, because participants appear to be using the temporal dimension (and hence producing recency effects) only when they are sure that a recognition task will follow. Given the present state of the evidence, we tentatively conclude that a temporal (rather than positional) dimension is more likely to be important in free recall, and perhaps recognition, than in serial recall. This may be due to the differing task requirements. A serial recall task highlights the positional rather than the temporal dimension; the task is explicitly to recall the 'first' item, then the 'second' item, and so on. There is little or no advantage in, and perhaps a cost of, encoding order with such precision in free recall or recognition tasks. Furthermore, shorter lists are normally, although not invariably, employed in serial recall than in recognition or recall. If only a small number of positional markers can be remembered, use of a positional dimension may be more adaptive when lists are short.

A final source of evidence comes the use of interference methodology. If memory for serial order relies on an oscillator-based timing signal of some kind, as suggested by the models of Brown *et al.* (2000) and Burgess and Hitch (1999), then it might be possible to interfere selectively with memory for order information (as opposed to memory for item information) by requiring participants to remember information while at the same time performing a secondary task designed to engage timing mechanisms. Henson *et al.* (2003) adopt just this approach, finding *inter alia* that temporal grouping manipulations and a temporally paced tapping task both interfered more with memory for order than with memory for items. Furthermore, concurrent speech production (articulatory suppression), which has been hypothesized to rely on oscillator-based timing signals of the same type that underpin memory for serial order (Vousden *et al.* 2000), is well known to impair short-term memory for serial order. As Henson *et al.* themselves note, alternative explanations for their interference effects may be possible. However, the approach clearly offers considerable potential for addressing questions of the type under consideration here.

Summary

There are some theoretical considerations to support the hypothesis that human memory is chronologically organized. There is some empirical evidence consistent with the hypothesis, although not for serial recall data. Given this conclusion, we can turn to our second question: Do temporal coordinates play a privileged role in memory binding?

Temporal binding in memory hypothesis

In this second part of the chapter, we directly address the hypothesis that temporal coordinates play a privileged role in the storage and retrieval of associative and binding relations in human memory. We refer to the general hypothesis as the temporal memory binding hypothesis. We contrast it with the traditional assumption that item representations or features may be associated directly. These two contrasting possibilities are illustrated, in simplified form, in Figure 10.2.

Evidence for the temporal memory binding hypothesis would not, of course, mandate the conclusion that direct item–item associations (or associations of within-item features) cannot be formed. (Following Cohen *et al.* (1997), we think of an 'item' as the object identified by the output of a well-defined processing module.) For example, it could be that subjects in memory experiments can form such associations but choose not to do so, perhaps because this is more computationally efficient given the combinatorial explosion that would otherwise result. As we noted above, the hypothesis that temporal coordinates are important in memory binding can be interpreted in a number of ways, depending on the level of units involved. The binding may involve linking together features of object representations (e.g. colour, shape, and size of an object), the association of items that would normally be regarded as separate objects in themselves (e.g. pairs of words), or the particular configuration of several objects that together form a rich episodic memory. Most of the relevant research has focused on the first two possibilities, and therefore we also focus on these.

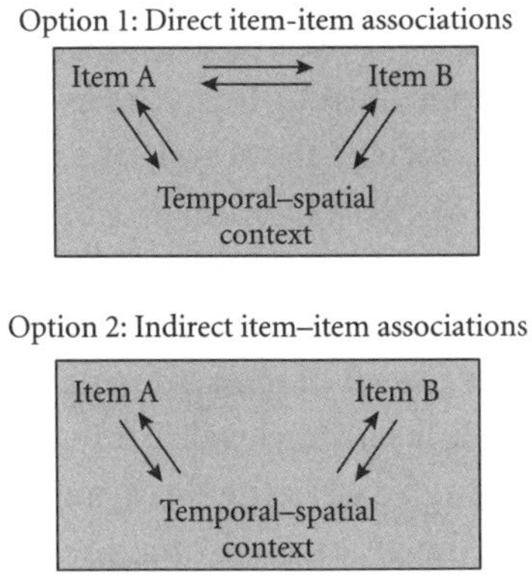

Figure 10.2 Illustration of possible models for associative binding relations in memory.

Models of memory

What predictions do existing mathematical and computational models of human associative memory make for the role of time in associative binding? To anticipate: our conclusion will be that most such models, in contrast with several models of serial and free recall, do not currently assign a major role to the representation of temporal or spatial coordinates in memory. Even models that do assume such a role for time do not generally assume that such coordinates are used to mediate binding relations such as item–item associations.

As we have already noted, various of models of free recall (Howard and Kahana 1999, 2002), serial recall (Burgess and Hitch 1999; Brown *et al.* 2000, 2002), and some small-scale approaches to recognition memory (Neath 1993; Brown *et al.* 2000) rely on the assumption of a temporal dimension in memory. However, many recent models of free recall, associative learning, and recognition, including the most comprehensive extant accounts, do not ascribe a central role to time. Although many early accounts could incorporate the idea that contemporaneously occurring items would become associated, time was not seen as major part of context, and experiment-specific item–item associations were mediated through linking nodes (Anderson and Bower 1973, 1974). Most models we consider are applicable to memory processes operating at the item level (e.g. recognition or association of pairs of words or pictures). However, accounts that focus on the storage and retrieval of featural configurations in memory, such as fragmentation theory (e.g. Jones 1976; see below), also have typically not assumed a role of time in binding. In particular, models that involve the formation of item–item associations almost invariably assume that such associations can be formed directly between item representations rather than through a mediating location along some spatial or temporal continuum. One influential model of this type is Murdock's theory of distributed associative memory (TODAM) (Murdock 1982, 1983, 1993; Lewandowsky and Murdock 1989). Such models typically represent items as vectors of features, and use mechanisms such as convolution or vector multiplication to form the associations between items. Some well-developed accounts, such as the search of associative memory (SAM) model (Raaijmakers and Shiffrin 1981; Gillund and Shiffrin 1984; Mensink and Raaijmakers 1988), do allow for contextual information to be represented as part of memory representations, but although this contextual information may play an important role in memory retrieval of item information, it does not normally mediate item–item associative links at retrieval, although temporal overlap may be involved in associative coding (e.g. in the SAM model associative strengths between items will depend on the amount of time they are co-present in a limited-capacity buffer). Mensink and Raaijmakers (1988) introduce a temporal–contextual component into the SAM model. In the model of Sikstrom (2000), bidirectional item–item links and item–temporal context links are both available, with the balance between them depending on task demands.

In another popular class of model, connectionist models, it is generally assumed that the formation of item–item associations, often mediated by layers of hidden units but nonetheless direct in the sense that the representation of one item (e.g. a pattern of activation on a set of input units), can be used as a probe to retrieve the representation of another item (a pattern of activation over a set of output units) without the intervening retrieval of information about temporal or spatial coordinates.

In summary, most current models of human associative memory assume that direct item–item associations can be formed. In other words, they implicitly deny the temporal memory binding hypothesis. Therefore we turn to consideration of a recent model that does place time at the heart of memory, and consider the types of prediction such a model would make for experiments on binding relations in memory. The behaviour of the model is then used to motivate discussion of experiments that have directly examined the role of time in memory binding.

A time-based memory model

The model we describe, which is known as the scale-invariant memory, perception, and learning (SIMPLE) model (Brown *et al.* 2002), implements the hypothesis that the representation and retrieval of memories (over both short and long timescales) is dependent on the amount of time that has elapsed since that memory was laid down—the temporal distance of the memory. The model is intended to apply to serial and free recall over a number of different timescales, and to account within a unified framework for empirical phenomena that have previously been ascribed to separate short- and long-term memory systems. Brown *et al.* summarize several strands of evidence for scale invariance in human memory.

The temporal component at the heart of the SIMPLE model is motivated by the influential 'telephone pole' analogy introduced by Crowder (1976) (see also Bjork and Whitten 1974). Crowder suggested that the items in a regularly presented list could be seen as analogous to evenly spaced telephone poles passed by a moving train:

> The crucial assumption is that just as each telephone pole in the receding distance becomes less and less distinctive from its neighbours, likewise each item in the memory list becomes less distinctive from the other list items as the presentation episode recedes into the past. Therefore, retrieval probability is assumed to depend on discriminability of traces from each other. (Crowder 1976, p. 462)

The analogy suggests that recent items are more discriminable from one another along a temporal distance dimension, and hence more retrievable from memory, for the same kind of reason that the spatially close ('recent') telephone poles are more discriminable from one another. The SIMPLE model instantiates a very similar idea by assuming that (a) every item in memory is represented in a multidimensional psychological space, (b) one of the dimensions is logarithmically transformed temporal distance into the past, and (c) items in more crowded regions of multidimensional psychological space (i.e. items with many similar neighbours) will be harder to retrieve. The mathematical principles assumed to underpin memory retrieval in the model are essentially the same as those used in models of simple categorization tasks (e.g. Nosofsky 1986), with the main difference being the addition of a temporal distance dimension and the application of the model to traditional memory paradigms such as free recall and serial recall. In other words, SIMPLE suggests that memories can be discriminated from one another in terms of their distance along the dimension of 'time elapsed' just as a set of tones can be discriminated from one another in terms of their position along a frequency dimension, or objects may be discriminated from one another in terms of their position along a weight dimension (Murdock 1960). More generally, SIMPLE is an exemplar model that conforms to many of the principles outlined by Gallistel (1990); temporal and other coordinates of items are represented separately for each encounter with an item, and the location of items along the temporal dimension is always encoded (although it may not always be attended at retrieval).

It should be emphasized that temporal distance is not the only dimension along which items are represented in the model, and that the relative attention paid to each dimension, including the temporal one, is assumed to depend on experimental circumstances. Whether or not location along a remembered temporal dimension forms the primary retrieval-relevant dimension, all items in memory are located in terms of their position along a temporal dimension even though location information along this dimension may be increasingly less accurate and available as items recede into the past. Full implementation details are given in Brown *et al.* (2002); see also Brown and Chater (2001), Lewandowsky *et al.* (2004), and Lewandowsky and Brown (2005) where it is argued that the model can account for many empirical results from the study of free recall, serial recall, and perceptual identification. Furthermore, an essentially similar model has been successfully applied to the performance of children and adults on temporal interval estimation tasks (McCormack *et al.* 2002), consistent with the suggestion that memory retrieval can be seen in part as a process of temporal discrimination.

One possible advantage of incorporating a logarithmically compressed temporal distance dimension into a multidimensional memory model is that it offers a potential solution to one of the general problems faced by any model of memory, which we call the episodic generalization problem. In brief, an adaptive memory system has two conflicting demands placed on it. On the one hand, the memory system must be able to represent episodes as distinct from one another, even if the events are similar, and to learn them after a single exposure. In other words, similar events must sometimes be kept episodically distinct. On the other hand, the memory must be able to generalize, i.e. to represent memories in terms of their similarities to one another in order to permit inference and generalization. This second type of learning may require gradual incremental learning, as in connectionist models. These two complementary requirements of a memory system motivated models that ascribe computationally different (very roughly, episodic and semantic) memory functions to different areas of the brain—the hippocampus and the neocortex, respectively (McClelland *et al.* 1995). Many more recent models are motivated by this same basic distinction, and have been linked in detailed ways to neuroscience level evidence. However, we note here that a temporal distance model like SIMPLE can offer an alternative perspective on the distinction. This can be seen by an extension of the telephone pole analogy.

Following Crowder (1976), we can imagine retrieval from memory as analogous to standing at the end of a line of evenly spaced telephone poles receding into the past. The spatial dimension along which the telegraph poles are represented is analogous to the temporal distance dimension; recency effects occur because recent items have more discriminable representations in memory just as do the spatially close telephone poles. Memories, like the telephone poles, become harder to distinguish from one another as they recede into the distance. However, in the SIMPLE model temporal distance is only one of the many dimensions along which items may be represented. To introduce additional non-temporal dimensions into the telephone pole analogy, we can imagine that the telephone poles have horizontal bars on each side at different heights as shown in Figure 10.3. Figure 10.3(a) illustrates the basic unidimensional telephone pole analogy, but with the telephone poles augmented by bars on each side. These additional features are intended to be analogous to additional dimensions along which memories might be represented (such as size or colour). The side of the telephone pole on which the bar appears is a dimension, and the height of the bar on that side represents a value on that dimension. The mean values of items on these non-temporal dimensions will not change as the items recede into the distance.

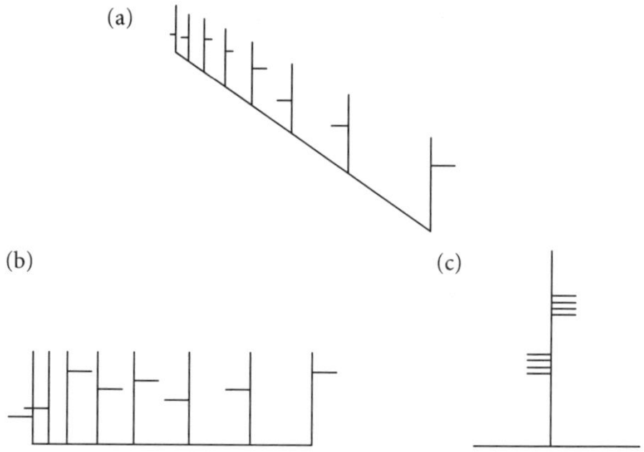

Figure 10.3 Illustration of the telephone pole analogy extended to two dimensions.

The point of the analogy is to show that the use of a logarithmically compressed temporal distance dimension allows memories to be represented in a way that allows them to be kept episodically distinct but also allows generalization. For example, the recent telegraph poles are clearly distinct from one another; their representations are unlikely to be confused. However, generalization along the other dimensions is difficult because the commonalities between sidebar heights is not directly represented, especially for recent items. As items recede into the past (as the telephone poles become more distant), it becomes more difficult to represent items as distinct events. However, the advantage is that generalization occurs automatically for the more distant items. As they recede and blur together, the items become indistinct and merge into one another, but they can still be distinguished in terms of the positions of the sidebars. Now generalization can occur more easily. For example, it becomes explicit in the representation that poles tend to have high bars on the right-hand side or lower bars on the left-hand side. Thus generalization across items will become easier as the items recede into the past, but at the same time their individual representations become merged together, somewhat akin to the transition from episodic to semantic memory.

An alternative way of achieving the generalization is to pay less attention at retrieval to the temporal dimension, corresponding to greater attention to the other dimensions. Differential attention to dimensions is central to the account offered by SIMPLE and by models of categorization, and a number of categorization studies have shown that subjects are adaptive in the sense that they can pay selective attention to the dimensions that are most useful for performing the task at hand. In the analogy, the extreme case of allocating no attention to the temporal dimension, thus allowing maximum generalization, is illustrated by the situation of standing right at the end of the telephone poles in line with them. This is effectively like collapsing over the temporal dimension—items are no longer episodically distinct, but commonalities can thus be more readily discerned (this is like cueing the memory system in a different way; see Humphreys *et al.* (1989)). This case is illustrated in Figure 10.3(c).

In summary, a unitary time-based model may allow in a complementary way both semantic-like generalization and episodic-like distinct event representations, with the balance between them depending on temporal distance in the past and on the weight given to the temporal distance dimension in retrieval.

The model is relevant to the temporal memory binding hypothesis in two ways. First, it provides an example of how a model of temporally organized memory may account for a number of memory phenomena. Secondly, although SIMPLE has not been applied to paradigms such as paired associate learning, it needs little extension to see how a basic temporal memory binding hypothesis could be implemented within such a model. Consider the case when the hypothesis is applied to paired associate learning of items (e.g. words). The task is to learn pairs of words that appear simultaneously: A–B, C–D, E–F, etc. A memory test could take place in one of two ways. Either, as in a traditional paired associated learning task, participants are presented with one item of the pair (A) and required to respond with the other member of the pair (B). Alternatively, participants view pairs of items and indicate whether the test pair occurred together, as a pair, in the presented list (i.e. the task is associative recognition). Many of the studies we describe below adopt the latter technique. Therefore we implemented the most basic kind of this model possible in the SIMPLE framework.

A simple model

We assumed that the probability of correctly recognizing that two pairs of items had occurred together in the presented list, rather than as separate pairs, depends on the similarity of their locations along the temporal distance dimension. In the SIMPLE model, the similarity of two locations along the temporal dimension is given by their ratio raised to some power (Brown *et al.* 2002). More specifically,

$$\eta_{ij} = (TD_i/TD_j)^c$$

where η_{ij} is the similarity between locations i and j, TD_i is the temporal distance (from the point of recall) of the more recent location, TD_j is the temporal distance of the less recent location, and c is a free parameter. However, this measure does not take account of similarity on hierarchically organized temporal dimensions, as is the case for the full SIMPLE model. For example, all items within some list may have similar representations at the list level of temporal representation.

A full implementation of this idea (as applied to serial and free recall) is given by Brown *et al.* (2002). Here, we simply augment the expression above by a constant L:

$$\eta_{ij} = (TD_i/TD_j)^c + L$$

where L represents similarity due to list context (McGovern 1964). We emphasize that this is not intended as more than an exploratory 'toy' model; we use it here purely illustratively.

Of particular interest is the role of temporal proximity in producing 'memory illusions' in such a model. If fragments of memories, or pairs of items such as words, are bound together by virtue of common temporal locations, as the temporal memory binding hypothesis suggests, it might be expected that items that occur nearby in time would be more likely to participate in conjunction errors. For example, consider the item pairs illustrated in Figure 10.4. Each column represents a list, and each pair of letters represents a trial. Letters represent either items that co-occur within a trial (e.g. whole words) or fragments of a single object (e.g. syllables within words, or facial features). At the end of each list, participants are asked whether AD occurred on the list. A positive response indicates a memory conjunction error, and will (subject to appropriate control conditions) indicate that within-trial bindings have been lost such that A and D, which did not occur together, are falsely remembered as having co-occurred. Will false conjunctions be more likely after the sequence of items shown in the first column has been seen, compared with the second column? The presented pairs (AB and CD) containing the components of the conjunction error item (AD) occur closer together, temporally, in the first column than in the second column. Evidence that false conjunction memory errors are more likely when the intact items that contain the conjoined components occur in close temporal proximity would seem consistent with the temporal memory binding hypothesis.

We examined the predictions of the basic model we described for the paradigm illustrated in Figure 10.4. It was assumed for simplicity that the probability

	Condition 1	Condition 2
	A — B	A — B
	C — D	E — F
	E — F	G — H
	G — H	C — D
	I — J	I — J
Test	A — D ?	A — D ?

Figure 10.4 Lists of items for paired associate recognition memory task to illustrate predictions of temporal memory binding hypothesis.

of responding 'yes' to a conjunction pair was simply proportional to the similarity between the temporal locations of the individual items. (Such a process could be implicated in either familiarity-based or recall-based processes.) Figure 10.5(a) shows the 'yes' response probability given by the model as a function of the temporal separation of the individual items in the presented list. As expected, the probability of responding 'yes' to a conjunction decreases as a function of temporal separation. The three lines on the graph represent the performance of the model using three different values of parameter *c*, which effectively governs the rate at which temporal separation decreases with temporal distance. Figure 10.5(b) shows the behaviour of the model when $L = 0.5$ (i.e. under the assumption that there is some fixed non-zero level of similarity for all items associated with the same list context). There it can be seen that, especially for low values of *c*, the probability of a false conjunction error declines rapidly as a function of temporal proximity, and then remains at a significant level. Thus the exact effect of temporal proximity on conjunction errors that even this simplistic implementation of the temporal memory binding hypothesis predicts will depend on detailed aspects of the implementation of whatever model of memory is assumed to underlie the memory conjunction errors. As we will see, such considerations are relevant to interpretation of the empirical evidence to which we now turn.

As illustrated by the simple simulation, a key prediction of the temporal memory binding hypothesis would seem to be that false conjunction errors will be affected by temporal factors. Although many studies have examined memory conjunction errors, only a few have directly examined the role of temporal proximity in giving rise to such errors. We review some of these below. A second key prediction is that the encoding of binding relations may depend on the temporal conjunction of items or features at encoding, and we briefly review these encoding stage approaches first.

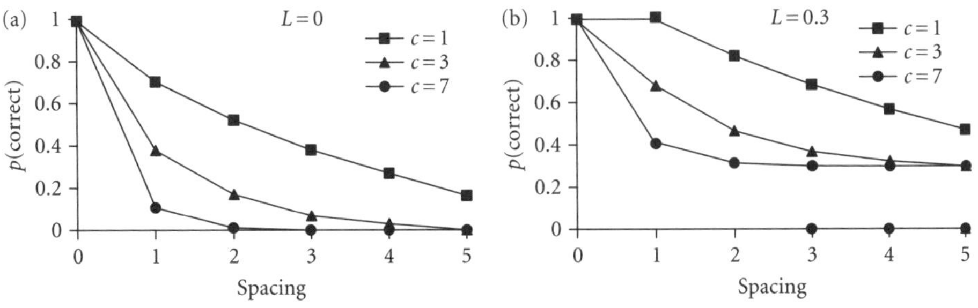

Figure 10.5 Predictions of the simple temporal proximity model.

Time and encoding of binding relations

Conjunction errors could clearly occur either at encoding or at retrieval, and we discuss encoding stages first. Memory binding phenomena of the type discussed here are often ascribed to processes such as memory cohesion (Moscovitch 1994) in which newly perceived information is transformed into more permanent storage and consolidation (assumed to occur over longer timescales). As we noted earlier, such processes can be treated as distinct from binding processes which are assumed to happen at perception.

Some evidence for the role of temporal co-occurrence in the formation of binding links in memory comes from the findings of Ceraso *et al.* (1998). As these authors note, there is a longstanding distinction between models of memory which assume memories are encoded as fragments and accounts that emphasize holistic pattern storage. They reason that the nature of memory representations can be assessed by looking at the coherence of recall of the different properties of a given display. For example, if two properties of a display are recalled, they may either be recalled together or separately (i.e. on different recall occasions). To the extent that properties are likely to recalled separately (low recall coherence), the suggestion is that memory representations are fragmented and only integrated with repeated trials of learning. Ceraso *et al.*'s initial experiment confirmed earlier results in finding that when the display of properties was unitary rather than separate (e.g. when the display contained a coloured shape, rather than containing a separate shape and colour patch) recall coherence was higher. Of particular interest in the present context was their Experiment 2, where they examined the relative importance of spatial co-occurrence and temporal co-occurrence in determining the coherence of recall. When object form and shape were presented at the same time and in the same location, recall coherence was high (forms and shapes that had co-occurred tended to be recalled together). When form and shape were presented in different locations but at the same time, coherence was again high. However, when form and shape were presented at the same location but at different times, recall coherence was much lower. (Note that in the latter two cases participants were instructed to recall temporal or spatial conjunctions, respectively).

Thus the findings of Ceraso *et al.* provide good evidence consistent with the importance of temporal proximity in leading to coherent memory representations. Other evidence is consistent. For example, locations that were learned nearby in time tend to be recalled together by both adults and children (Clayton and Habibi 1991; McNamara *et al.* 1992; Curiel and Radvansky 1998; Hund *et al.* 2002). However, as a number of studies suggest, attention at encoding is also necessary; temporal proximity is not sufficient in itself (Ceraso 1985; Reinitz and

Demb 1994; Walker and Cuthbert 1998; Wheeler and Treisman 2002). Consistent with this, dividing attention at encoding increases the level of conjunction errors (Reinitz *et al.* 1994), as does prevention of verbal labelling (Stefurak and Boynton 1986), although it is difficult to prove that the effect is selective (Rubin *et al.* 1999; Jones and Jacoby 2001).

Memory conjunction errors

We now review evidence from the study of memory conjunction errors (Underwood and Zimmerman 1973; Murdock 1974; Underwood *et al.* 1976; Reinitz and Demb 1994; Kroll *et al.* 1996; Reinitz and Alexander 1996; Reinitz and Hannigan 2001). Memory conjunction errors are normally examined using recognition memory paradigms and occur when 'false conjunctions', made up of newly combined fragments of previously presented items, are incorrectly recognized as previously seen items. One can think of conjunction errors as involving either within-item features (e.g. blending of faces) or whole items. Stimuli typically used have included drawings of faces (Reinitz *et al.* 1992; Kroll *et al.* 1996; Hannigan and Reinitz 2000), abstract figures (Kroll *et al.* 1996) whole words (Murdock 1974; Underwood *et al.* 1976), and sublexical segments (Underwood and Zimmerman 1973; Underwood *et al.* 1976; Reinitz and Demb 1994; Kroll *et al.* 1996; Reinitz *et al.* 1996).

To borrow an example from Underwood and Zimmerman (1973), if the words 'inside' and 'consult' occurred in the presented list, a conjunction error would occur if subjects incorrectly responded 'yes' when they were asked whether 'insult' had occurred on the list. Following common usage, we refer to the items or pairs of items whose components may lead to a false conjunction memory error ('inside' and consult' in the example above) as 'parents'. We will often be concerned with the temporal separation between parent items. In the false memory literature the term 'lag' is sometimes used to refer to the retention interval, i.e. the time or number of items elapsed between the second parent and the false conjunction lure (Jones and Atchley 2002), and sometimes used to refer to the number of items between parent items (Underwood *et al.* 1976). Therefore we use the terms 'retention interval' and 'temporal spacing' respectively.

Many studies have examined the incidence of conjunction errors in both normal and impaired populations. For example, Kroll *et al.* (1996) used a continuous recognition paradigm, in which a recognition decision (whether the item had appeared previously in the list) was made about each individual word in a presented sequence. If the words 'valley' and 'barter' appeared in the list, the subsequent presentation of the item 'barley' would test for a conjunction error. Kroll *et al* found that students and older adults made several conjunction errors (incorrectly responding 'old' to items such as 'barley'), and patients with left or bilateral hippocampal lesions made many more conjunction errors than the control groups. The particular difficulty that hippocampal patients have with such tasks is of course consistent with the widespread notion that the hippocampus plays a key role on the binding or contextual linking of episodic memories (Cohen *et al.* 1997).

Theoretical interpretation of conjunction errors

We argue that plausible instantiations of the temporal memory binding hypothesis would predict an effect of the temporal lag between parent items on the probability of occurrence of memory conjunction errors. Alternative theoretical accounts of conjunction errors could not readily accommodate such a finding except by reference to temporal processes occurring at encoding (such as co-rehearsal of adjacent items). In theoretical terms, if there is no temporal binding, and simple associative links between items or item attributes are formed instead, links that are formed and subsequently lost must be lost in a manner that does not respect the temporal relations between the parent items.

One obvious source of conjunction errors is familiarity. To the extent that the recognition decision is based on the familiarity of a test item, a test item that is familiar because it is made up of fragments seen previously (albeit separately) will lead to incorrect response for false conjunctions. As a number of authors have noted, an unmodified familiarity hypothesis cannot account for the fact that false conjunction errors are not invariably made, and hence familiarity-based accounts need to be supplemented with additional processes such as configural-associative representations or recall-based recognition (Jones and Jacoby 2001; Kelley and Wixted 2001). Therefore a key issue is whether associative recognition (i.e. recognition of pairs of items) involves familiarity-based as well as recall-based processes. Some evidence that it does is given by Yonelinas *et al.* (1999) (see also Kelley and Wixted 2001; Jones and Atchley 2002). Importantly, however, Yonelinas *et al.* used rearranged faces (rather than pairs of items) and found a role for familiarity-based recognition only for faces in normal orientation. Thus the extent to which familiarity is used in associative recognition is at best uncertain, and may depend on factors such as the nature of the stimuli used and the retention interval (Jones and Atchley 2002). However, it is clear that memory for items and memory for associations can be dissociated, including in the relative extent to which they make use of familiarity-based and recollection-based memory processes (Hockley 1992; Yonelinas 1997; Hockley and Consoli 1999; Jones *et al.* 2001).

Thus verbally expressed familiarity-based accounts do not predict temporal spacing effects. Various mathematical models have examined possible sources of memory conjunction errors or blending errors (Metcalfe 1990; Busey and Tunnicliff 1999; Zaki and Nosofsky 2001) but have not generally predicted spacing effects.

Data on temporal proximity in conjunction errors

An effect of the temporal proximity of parents on conjunction error probability could take a number of different forms. The experiments reviewed below have adopted a wide variety of methodologies, and therefore it is important to be clear about the theoretical significance of different types of effect. The observation of conjunction errors (relative to an appropriate control condition) does not itself provide evidence for the temporal memory binding hypothesis. A necessary (although not sufficient) condition would be the observation of temporally graded errors. Even these can take a number of forms. Consider a presented sequence A–B, C–D, E–F, G–H, where pairs of letters represent pairs or items. Some experiments present pairs of faces, and look for within-pair feature exchanges. One possible result of such experiments is an effect just of **simultaneity**, such that the features of A and B become miscombined more often than do the features of (say) A and D, but A–D conjunction errors are as likely as A–F conjunction errors. A similar result is possible if the items are simultaneously presented words whose sublexical segments can be recombined. An effect of simultaneity alone, while consistent with the temporal memory binding hypothesis, would provide only weak evidence for it as more natural encoding-stage explanations might be available.

An alternative outcome would be what we call an effect of **adjacency** only. If A–D errors are more likely than A–F errors, but A–F errors are no more likely than A–H errors, the evidence is only that exchanges are more likely to occur between adjacent pairs than between non-adjacent pairs, again consistent with the temporal memory binding hypothesis but susceptible to alternative encoding-stage or co-rehearsal explanations. Finally, we say that a **temporally graded** effect occurs when the effect of temporal proximity extends beyond adjacency. Such an effect (e.g. A–F conjunction errors being more likely than A–H errors) would provide the strongest evidence for the temporal memory binding hypothesis, although encoding-stage explanations would still need to be excluded. The possible outcomes are listed in Table 10.1. We can now classify observed findings in the light of this table.

Table 10.1 Different spacing effects in associative recognition

Effect	A–B	A–D	A–F	A–H
Simultaneity only	High	Baseline	Baseline	Baseline
Adjacency only		High	Baseline	Baseline
Temporally graded		High	Medium	Baseline

Although Underwood and Zimmerman (1973) did not examine the effects of temporal spacing on conjunction error rate, Underwood *et al.* (1976) did. In a presentation phase, both individual items and pairs of items were presented. In the test phase, pairs of items were presented, some of which were false conjunctions made up of words presented individually during exposure. Across two experiments, the parent items were separated by zero, one, five, ten, or twenty items. Although a high rate of false conjunction errors was observed overall, there was no graded tendency for the proportion of conjunction errors to reduce with increasing separation between parents. Instead, there was a higher rate of conjunction errors to pairs made up of items presented adjacently, and a lower but roughly constant rate of false conjunction errors to items made up from parent pairs with all other separations. In our terms (Table 10.1), this is an effect of adjacency only. Underwood *et al.* argue that these are most likely to represent a special case, perhaps due to co-rehearsal of immediately adjacent items. An alternative account might be given in terms of the simple model implementation we described above: if some similarity between the temporal coordinates of parent pairs is due to common list location, and further similarity arises due to within-list temporal proximity but drops off rapidly with lag, the observed pattern would be predicted. This is essentially the position shown in Figure 10.5(a). Such an account is post hoc, but suggests the cautious conclusion of 'not proven either way' for the temporal memory binding hypothesis.

Kroll *et al.* (1996) also examined temporal proximity effects. As described above, these authors used a continuous recognition paradigm and examined conjunction errors in students, older participants, and patients with hippocampal lesions. The spacing between the items contributing to potential conjunction errors could be either one or five words, i.e. following the words 'valley'/'barter'/'barley' example above, either one word or five words intervened between 'valley' and 'barley'. The temporal binding hypothesis would predict a greater number of conjunction errors when the spacing is small. There was no clear effect of spacing on the number of conjunction errors produced by young participants, older participants, or patients with right hippocampal lesions. However, patients with left hippocampal lesions and a patient with a bilateral lesion produced more conjunction errors for the parent items separated by a small spacing than for more widely spaced parents. Thus these results, which illustrated a temporally graded effect, are consistent with the role of the left hippocampus in binding for language materials, but provide no specific support for the hypothesis more generally.

Hannigan and Reinitz (2000) directly address the role of temporal proximity on the frequency of memory conjunction errors. They examined false memory effects for faces, and varied the spacing between parent face pairs. The pairs of parent faces were separated by either zero presentations (i.e. the false conjunction pair of faces was made up of composites of two faces that had previously been presented simultaneously), one presentation (i.e. the parent faces were presented in adjacent pairs), or two presentations (one presentation intervened between the pairs of parent faces). In their first experiment, where a retention interval of 15 min was used, there was a strong tendency for conjunction errors to reduce as the spacing between the parent face pairs increased. In our terms, there were effects of simultaneity and adjacency. In a second experiment, otherwise identical but with a retention interval of 24 h, there was an effect of simultaneity only. Overall, then, the results obtained by Hannigan and Reinitz appear to provide partial support for the temporal memory binding hypothesis.

Reinitz and Hannigan (2001) again aimed to provide some evidence for a temporal proximity effect on conjunction errors. In a series of experiments they found a simultaneity effect: conjunction errors are more likely when items in parent pairs are presented simultaneously rather than sequentially. An adjacency effect may also be found when items are presented sequentially but alternating. They concluded that conjunction errors occur due to attention switching at input. Therefore this study is consistent with the general possibility that *any* effects of temporal proximity on memory conjunction errors might reflect the temporal spread of attention at encoding, perhaps in tandem with strategic processes such as co-rehearsal of adjacent items or item pairs. It would be necessary to exclude such a possibility if the idea that maintenance and retrieval of binding relations in memory is mediated by temporal coordinates.

Busey and Tunnicliff (1999) described a series of face recognition studies in which parent faces were presented adjacently (one after the other) or widely separated. Test items included items that were blends of the parent faces. In three out of the four relevant comparisons, they found no effect of adjacency at all, although one effect was found.

As we have noted, temporal spacing effects on conjunction errors could be attributed to encoding-stage processes. Some evidence that false conjunction errors can occur at retrieval as well as (or instead of) at encoding is given by an event-related potential (ERP) study conducted by Rubin *et al.* (1999). They found that the electrical brain potentials generated by false conjunction test items resembled the potentials generated by new items rather than by old items, consistent with a retrieval-based locus for false conjunction errors. Further evidence for a retrieval-based account of false conjunction errors could come from evidence of temporal scale invariance in memory conjunction errors, as are seen in output ordering effects in free recall (Howard and Kahana 1999, 2002), or proximity effects observed under incidental learning conditions.

One study that employed a situation analogous to that in Figure 10.4 is described by Murdock (1974). Murdock presented lists of six word pairs to participants. At the end of the list presentation, participants were given various test pairs. Some of the pairs had occurred in the list, and some were novel combinations of words that had occurred in separate presented pairs (conjunctions). Participants were required to rate, on a six-point scale, their confidence (from 'sure-no' to 'sure-yes') as to whether each test pair had occurred in the presented list. Murdock gives the mean ratings for each possible conjunction as a function of the positions of the each member of the conjunction. We calculated the confidence ratings associated with conjunctions as a function of the separation between the parents of each possible conjunction, and these are presented in Figure 10.6.

As Murdock himself notes, the temporal gradients are not strong. However, it is evident that there was a small but clear trend for participants' confidence that a false conjunction was presented in the list to be higher when the components of the conjunction occurred in relatively close temporal proximity, i.e. there appears to be evidence for a temporally graded proximity effect, consistent with the temporal memory binding hypothesis.[3] However, serial position effects render the results of our reanalysis of Murdock's study difficult to interpret. For example, if participants were presented with a false conjunction when one of the parents was from the last serial position (for which performance was relatively high in Murdock's results), it is likely that a recall-to-reject process would enable participants to remember the correct pairing of the sixth parent member, and hence reject the false conjunction (Rotello and Heit 2000). Because the end pairs would contribute disproportionately to long-distance conjunction errors, reduced confidence ratings for the longest separations could partly reflect greater accuracy for end pairs. Indeed, the trend illustrated in Figure 10.6 is considerably

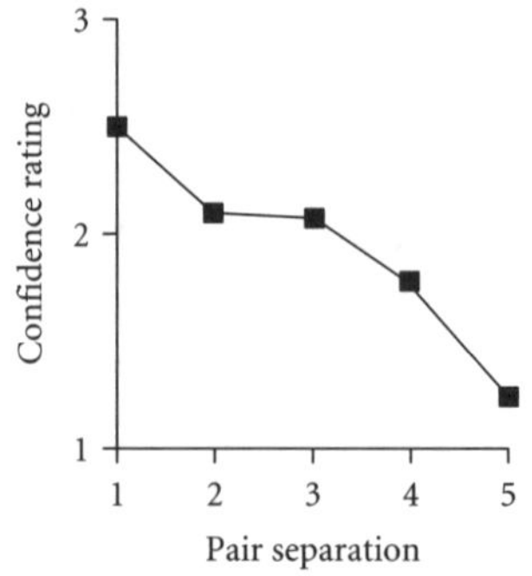

Figure 10.6 Separation effect in data reported by Murdock (1974).

weakened, becoming an effect of adjacency rather than a temporally graded effect, when results from conjunctions involving the most recently presented pair are excluded. Thus Murdock's own conclusion (Murdock 1974)appears to be sustained: there is little evidence for temporally mediated associations.

Jones (1976) reported an additional type of experiment that allows us to assess whether particular properties of an object presentation play a privileged role in binding. Jones presented lists of nine displays (photographs) to participants in a sequence. Each photograph depicted an object in a given location and in a particular colour. Thus each display can be seen as having four attributes: shape, colour, spatial location, and temporal/sequential position. No attribute values were repeated within a list (there were nine different colours, shapes, and spatial locations). After list presentation and a filled delay of 25 s, participants were given one, two, or three of the item attributes, and were required to recall the remaining attributes of the cued object. Although the central aim of the experiment was to assess the fragmentation hypothesis of memory developed by Jones (1976), the experimental procedure allows test of the predictions of the temporal memory binding hypothesis. If temporal location can be equated with serial position, serial position should have a privileged role in binding together the different attributes of memory, and this should be evident in the pattern of cued recall performance.

For example, an extreme view of the temporal binding hypothesis might suggest that object shape and object colour are only bound together by virtue of their common association to a given temporal location. If so, there would be no possibility of recalling the colour of an object when provided with the shape of the object unless via a mediating recall of the position of the object (cf Fig. 10.2). Such a position is probably too extreme. Given a cue of object colour, it could happen that some temporal information is retrieved but not with sufficient precision to allow for a correct overt recall of serial position (because the mapping between temporal location and serial position of presentation is not straightforward). However, the partial retrieval of temporal location information might nevertheless be sufficient to allow retrieval of object identity information.[4]

It is probably unrealistic to expect a clear derivation of recall probabilities (analogous to that analysis of Nissen (1985) in visual perception) such that, for example,

$$P(\text{shape}|\text{colour}) = P(t\text{-position}|\text{colour}) \times P(\text{shape}|t\text{-position})$$

where t-position is the temporal position of an item in the sequence, $P(\text{shape}|\text{colour})$ is the probability of recalling item identity given its colour. Nevertheless, evidence consistent with the temporal binding hypothesis would seem to be provided if $P(\text{shape}|\text{colour})$ and $P(\text{colour}|\text{shape})$ are small relative to $P(\text{shape}|t\text{-position})$, $P(\text{colour}|t\text{-position})$, $P(t\text{-position}|\text{shape})$, and $P(t\text{-position}|\text{colour})$. (We ignore for now the spatial location attribute, while acknowledging that it might also serve a binding role.) Evidence against a mediating role for t-position would be given if $P(\text{shape}|\text{colour})$ and/or $P(\text{colour}|\text{shape})$ were greater than $P(\text{colour}|t\text{-position}) \times P(\text{shape}|t\text{-position})$.

Initial examination of the data appears to provide evidence against the hypothesis of temporal binding in memory. The observed probability of retrieving shape given colour as a cue (0.42) is much greater than the product of the probability of retrieving t-position given colour (0.12) and the probability of retrieving shape given t-position (0.37). The same is true for the reverse retrieval:

$$P(\text{colour}|\text{shape}) < P(t\text{-position}|\text{shape}) \times P(\text{colour}|t\text{-position}).$$

A similar pattern is seen when object location is treated as a potential binding variable. Furthermore, $P(\text{colourandshape}|t\text{-position}) = 0.04$, which is greater than $P(\text{colour}|t\text{-position}) \times P(\text{shape}|t\text{-position})$ ($= 0.004$).

Although these initial analysis are inconsistent with the simplest possible interpretation of the temporal binding hypothesis, a more sophisticated interpretation can be given. As we noted above, the ability explicitly to recall the serial position of a list item may not be an accurate reflection of the ability to retrieve partial information about the temporal–positional location of the item's occurrence. Consistent with this, Jones (1976) observed that attempts to retrieve the serial position of an item (given other attributes as cues) often led to approximately correct retrievals (e.g. if the blue cup occurred as the sixth item, and 'blue' was provided as a retrieval cue but the serial position was not recalled correctly as six, incorrect recall as five or seven was more likely than incorrect recall as four or eight. If partial temporal location information can indeed mediate retrieval of item properties, without at the same time permitting correct recall of serial position information, the analyses we describe above would not permit clear conclusions (see also Ward *et al.* (1997) for response bias considerations).

Therefore we developed a simple model to explore the possibility that partial retrieval of temporal context might mediate the recall of binding relations in Jones's (1976) data. The model is shown in Figure 10.7. The logic behind the modelling is as follows. We first examine the ability of a simple model without direct colour–shape associations to account for the data, and then compare that model with a one that is identical but also includes direct colour–shape associations.

Figure 10.7(a) shows the version of the model that assumes no associative links between colours and shapes. We ignore the spatial location attribute for the purposes of illustration. The letters on the lines represent retrieval probabilities.

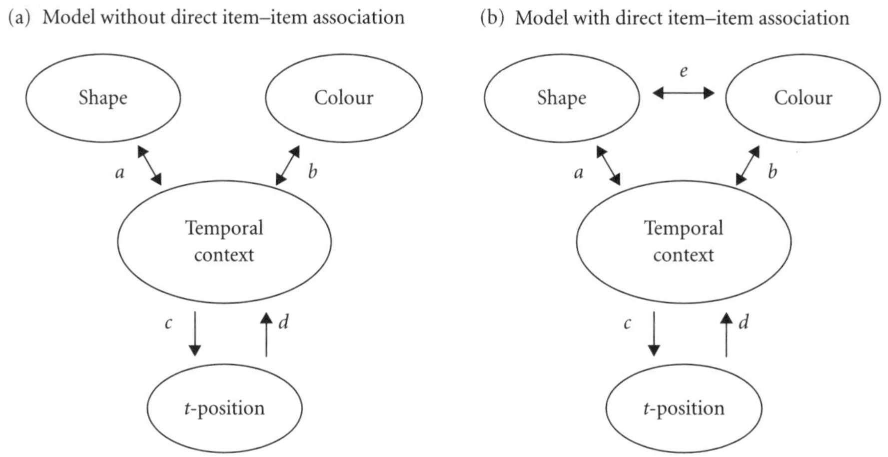

Figure 10.7 Model proposed as a possible account of data from Jones (1976).

Thus $a = P(t\text{-position}|\text{shape}) = P(\text{shape}|t\text{-position})$ and $b = P(t\text{-position}|\text{colour}) = P(\text{colour}|t\text{-position})$. These probabilities are assumed to be symmetrical; *c* represents the probability of successfully recalling serial position information given that temporal information is available, and *d* represents the probability of reconstructing temporal–contextual information given sequential position as a retrieval cue. We ignore the complications due to asymmetry of associations (Ward *et al.* 1997) to avoid over-parameterization.

Given the data reported by Jones (1976) for the cases where a single attribute (colour, shape, or sequential position) is used as a retrieval cue, we can estimate the values for *a*, *b*, *c*, and *d* that give the best-fitting account to the relevant retrieval probabilities. There were nine empirically observed retrieval probabilities to be accounted for, corresponding to the probability of recalling colour, shape, or both, given *t*-position as a retrieval cue, the probability of recalling colour, *t*-position, or both, given shape as a retrieval cue; and the probability of recalling shape, position, or both, given colour as a retrieval cue.

The model without a direct colour–space retrieval pathway produced estimated $a = 0.61$, $b = 0.71$, $c = 0.31$, and $d = 0.53$. With retrieval probabilities expressed as percentages, the mean absolute error of prediction was 1.072 per cent. Of more interest for present purposes is comparison with the model in Figure 10.7(b). This model has an additional probability *e* of retrieving colour from shape directly, or vice versa. The best-fitting value for *e* turned out to be almost exactly zero, and the mean absolute error of prediction was 1.070%.

In summary, no better prediction of the data was achieved by inclusion of a direct recall pathway linking colour and shape. Although the model is far from complete, the results illustrate that Jones's (1976) data can be interpreted in a manner consistent with the temporal memory binding hypotheses. However, the analysis cannot be said to provide strong evidence for the view that object attributes are linked together via common temporal location.

It is possible that the formation of direct (as opposed to indirect) item–item associations is task dependent or at least partly under strategic control. For example, we might expect binding via temporal context to be most useful when other cues (such as semantic relationships between items which do not co-occur) are misleading. Conversely, if the items to be associated are semantically related, there would appear to be little advantage in using additional temporal cues to mediate the association.

Conclusion

We began the chapter with the question of whether temporal coordinates are essential components of human memories, and with the temporal memory binding hypothesis. The initial review focused on the relatively weak claim that (in some sense) human memory is temporally organized. It was concluded that there are various adaptive and empirical conclusions in favour of the suggestion that memory is chronologically organized, although the evidence is far from compelling overall. Current evidence suggests that when short-term serial recall is required of subjects, more attention is paid to a positional than to a temporal dimension. In the case of other widely used memory tasks, evidence is either lacking or favours the role of a temporal dimension in retrieval.

The main part of the review examined direct evidence for the temporal memory binding hypothesis. Temporal proximity effects in memory conjunction errors were identified as a key source of possible data. However, a consideration of several such studies found little effect for a temporally graded effect of temporal proximity. Instead, there are widespread observations of adjacency (such that members of adjacent pairs are more likely to give rise to conjunction errors than are members of more distant pairs) and simultaneity. Although such results can be interpreted as consistent with a temporal memory binding hypothesis, most of the empirical results are susceptible to alternative explanations in terms of processes happening at encoding.

Overall, then, we found little convincing evidence either for or against the temporal memory binding hypothesis in the form we have considered. Given the central role that time plays in recent models of both human (Brown *et al.* 2000) and animal (Gallistel and Gibbon 2000) learning and memory, it is perhaps surprising that so little attention has been paid to this issue. We identify it as a key area for further research. Use of new methodologies may shed more light on the issue. For example, Rubin *et al.* (1999) describe one of the few attempts to demonstrate that memory conjunction errors occur at retrieval rather than encoding; more attention to the retrieval versus encoding issue will clearly be necessary if further evidence for the temporal memory binding hypothesis is to be gained. Other methodological details, such as the method of presentation, may be influential. For example, Sohn *et al.* (1996) found that illusory conjunctions were eliminated when presentation of parent items was made to separate hemispheres. Furthermore, both familiarity-based and recollection-based memory processes may be involved in retrieval of memory for associative relations between pairs of items. Temporal proximity may have differential effects on the different modes of remembering. Dosher (1984) found that when short response latencies were required, false conjunction errors were particularly likely to occur to semantically related items that had appeared separately in the list. For example, if presented pairs were 'king–house' and 'queen–pear', 'king–queen' would be an attractive lure at short response latencies (perhaps predominantly reflecting a familiarity-based associative recognition process). This tendency reduced as more response time became available. Rotello and Heit (2000) found that rearranged pairs were increasingly rejected relative to new pairs at longer response deadlines, and interpreted their results as consistent with a role for recall-to-reject processing in associative recognition. Thus effects of temporal proximity, if they are related to familiarity-based retrieval processes, might only occur at short response deadlines. Therefore there is clearly scope for further research to shed light on the temporal memory binding hypothesis.

Notes

1. To anticipate later discussion, such models typically embody scale-invariant dimensional representations of temporal distance, and such representations would be particularly unsuited to the purpose of dating remembered events in absolute chronological space.
2. Note that representing events as distinct through their unique location on a non-repeating temporal continuum is not sufficient for episodic memory. One might (non-episodically) remember that every event in memory occurred at a unique date and time, but this would be different from remembering the events as events (Hoerl 2001).
3. We note that this result does not exclude the possibility that it is positional, rather than temporal, closeness that gives rise to the effect. To separate these possibilities it would be necessary to use an irregular schedule of temporal presentation, as with serial recall and free recall in studies reviewed earlier.

4. Consistent with this, Jones (1976) found that sequential position was more likely to be a successful retrieval cue than to be retrieved itself (although see Ward *et al.* (1997) for a discussion of cue asymmetry).

Acknowledgements

This research was supported by grants from the Economic and Social Research Council (R000 23 9002) and the Biotechnology and Biological Sciences Research Council (88/S 15050). We thank Evan Heit and Murray Maybery for useful discussions.

References

Anderson, J.R. and Bower, G.H. (1973). *Human Associative Memory.* Washington, DC: Winston.

Anderson, J.R. and Bower, G.H. (1974). A propositional theory of recognition memory. *Memory and Cognition*, **2**, 406–412.

Anderson, J.R. and Milson, R. (1989). Human memory: an adaptive perspective. *Psychological Review*, **96**, 703–7 19.

Anderson, J.R. and Schooler, L.J. (1991). Reflections of the environment in memory. *Psychological Science*, **2**, 396–408.

Bjork, R.A. and Whitten, W.B. (1974). Recency-sensitive retrieval processes in longterm free recall. *Cognitive Psychology*, **6**, 173–189.

Brown, G.D.A. and Chater, N. (2001). The chronological organization of memory: common psychological foundations for remembering and timing. In *Time and Memory: Issues in Philosophy and Psychology* (ed C. Hoerl and T. McCormack). Oxford: Oxford University Press, pp. 77–110.

Brown, G.D.A. and Vousden, J.I. (1998). Adaptive analysis of sequential behavior: oscillators as rational mechanisms. In *Rational Models of Cognition* (ed M. Oaksford and N. Chater). Oxford: Oxford University Press, pp. 165–193.

Brown, G.D.A., Preece, T., and Hulme, C. (2000). Oscillator-based memory for serial order. *Psychological Review*, **107**, 127–181.

Brown, G.D.A., Neath, I., and Chater, N. (2002). A ratio model of scale-invariant memory and identification. Submitted for publication.

Burgess, N. and Hitch, G.J. (1992). Towards a network model of the articulatory loop. *Journal of Memory and Language*, **31**, 429–460.

Burgess, N. and Hitch, G.J. (1999). Memory for serial order: a network model of the phonological loop and its timing. *Psychological Review*, **106**, 551–581.

Busey, T.A. and Tunnicliff, J.L. (1999). Accounts of blending, distinctiveness, and typicality in the false recognition of faces. *Journal of Experimental Psychology: Learning, Memory, and Cognition*, **25**, 1210–1235.

Ceraso, J. (1985). Unit formation in perception and memory. *Psychology of Learning and Motivation: Advances in Research and Theory*, **19**, 179–210.

Ceraso, J., Kourtzi, Z., and Ray, S. (1998). The integration of object properties. *Journal of Experimental Psychology: Learning, Memory, and Cognition*, **24**, 1152–1161.

Clark, S.E. and Gronlund, S.D. (1996). Global matching models of recognition memory: how the models match the data. *Psychonomic Bulletin and Review*, **3**, 37–60.

Clayton and Habibi (1991).

Cohen, N.J., Poldrack, R.A., and Eichenbaum, H. (1997). Memory for items and memory for relations in the procedural/declarative memory framework. *Memory*, **5**, 131–178.

Corballis, M.C. (1966). Memory span as a function of variable presentation speeds and stimulus durations. *Journal of Experimental Psychology*, **71**, 461–465.

Corballis, M.C. (1967). Serial order in recognition and recall. *Journal of Experimental Psychology*, **74**, 99–105.

Criss, A.M. and Shiffrin, R.M. (2004). Context Noise and Item Noise Jointly Determine Recognition Memory: a comment on Dennis and Humphreys (2001). *Psychological Review*, **111**, 800–807.

Crowder, R.G. (1976). *Principles of Learning and Memory*. Hillsdale, NJ: Erlbaum.

Crowder, R.G. and Greene, R.L. (1987). On the remembrance of times past: the irregular list technique. *Journal of Experimental Psychology: General*, **116**, 265–278.

Crowder, R.G. and Neath, I. (1991). The microscope metaphor in human memory. In *Relating Theory and Data: Essays on Human Memory in Honor of Bennet B. Murdock* (ed W.E. Hockley and S. Lewandowsky). Hillsdale, NJ: Erlbaum, pp. 111–125.

Curiel, J.M. and Radvansky, G.A. (1998). Mental organization of maps. *Journal of Experimental Psychology*, **24**, 202–214.

Dennis, S. and Humphreys, M.S. (2001). A context noise model of episodic word recognition. *Psychological Review*, **108**, 452–478.

Dosher, B.A. (1984). Discriminating preexperimental (semantic) from learned (episodic) associations: a speed accuracy study. *Cognitive Psychology*, **16**, 519–555.

Duncan, M. and Murdock, B. (2000). Recognition and recall with precuing and postcuing. *Journal of Memory and Language*, **42**, 301–313.

Fairhurst, S., Gallistel, C.R., and Gibbon, J. (2003). Temporal landmarks: proximity prevails. *Animal Cognition*, **6**, 113–120.

Fodor, J. (1983). *The Modularity of Mind*. Cambridge, MA: MIT Press.

Friedman, W.J. (2001). Memory processes underlying humans' chronological sense of the past. In *Time and Memory: Issues in Philosophy and Psychology* (ed C. Hoerl and T. McCormack). Oxford: Oxford University Press, pp. 139–167.

Gallistel, C. (1990). *The Organization of Learning*. Cambridge, MA: MIT Press.

Gallistel, C.R. and Gibbon, J. (2000). Time, rate, and conditioning. *Psychological Review*, **107**, 289–344.

Gillund, G. and Shiffrin, R.M. (1984). A retrieval model for both recognition and recall. *Psychological Review*, **91**, 1–67.

Hacker, M.J. (1980). Speed and accuracy of recency judgments for events in shortterm memory. *Journal of Experimental Psychology: Human Learning and Memory*, **6**, 651–675.

Hannigan, S.L. and Reinitz, M.T. (2000). Influences of temporal factors on memory conjunction errors. *Applied Cognitive Psychology*, **14**, 309–321.

Healy, A.F. (1974). Separating item from order information in short-term memory. *Journal of Verbal Learning and Verbal Behavior*, **13**, 644–655.

Heathcote, D., Walker, P., and Hitch, G.J. (2001). Feature independence and the recovery of feature conjunctions. *Journal of General Psychology*, **121**, 253–266.

Henson, R.N.A. (1998). Short-term memory for serial order: the Start-End Model. *Cognitive Psychology*, **36**, 73–137.

Henson, R.N.A. (1999). Positional information in short-term memory: relative or absolute? *Memory and Cognition*, **27**, 915–927.

Henson, R., Hartley, T., Burgess, N., Hitch, G., and Flude, B. (2003). Selective interference with verbal short-term memory for serial order information: a new paradigm and tests of a timing-signal hypothesis. *Quarterly Journal of Experimental Psychology, Section A, Human Experimental Psychology*, **56**, 1307–1334.

Hockley, W.E. (1992). Item versus associative information: further comparisons of forgetting rates. *Journal of Experimental Psychology: Learning, Memory, and Cognition*, **18**, 1321–1330.

Hockley, W.E. and Consoli, A. (1999). Familiarity and recollection in item and associative recognition. *Memory and Cognition*, **27**, 657–664.

Hoerl, C. (2001). The phenomenology of episodic recall. In *Time and Memory: Issues in Philosophy and Psychology* (ed C. Hoerl and T. McCormack). Oxford: Oxford University Press, pp. 315–335.

Howard, M.W. and Kahana, M.J. (1999). Contextual variability and serial position effects in free recall. *Journal of Experimental Psychology: Learning, Memory, and Cognition*, **25**, 923–941.

Howard, M.W. and Kahana, M.J. (2002). A distributed representation of temporal context. *Journal of Mathematical Psychology*, **46**, 269–299.

Humphreys, M.S., Bain, J.D., and Pike, R. (1989). Different ways to cue a coherent memory system: a theory for episodic, semantic, and procedural tasks. *Psychological Review*, **96**, 208–233.

Hund, A.M., Plumert, J.M., and Benney, C. (2002). Experiencing nearby locations together in time: the role of spatial-temporal contiguity in children's memory for location. *Journal of Experimental Child Psychology*, **82**, 200–225.

Isenberg, L., Nissen, M.J., and Marchak, L.C. (1990). Attentional processing and the independence of color and orientation. *Journal of Experimental Psychology: Human Perception and Performance*, **16**, 869–878.

Jones, G.V. (1976). A fragmentation hypothesis of memory: cued recall of pictures and of sequential position. *Journal of Experimental Psychology: General*, **105**, 277–293.

Jones, T.C. and Atchley, P. (2002). Conjunction error rates on a continuous recognition memory test: little evidence for recollection. *Journal of Experimental Psychology: Learning, Memory, and Cognition*, **28**, 374–379.

Jones, T.C. and Jacoby, L.L. (2001). Feature and conjunction errors in recognition memory: evidence for dual-process theory. *Journal of Memory and Language*, **45**, 82–102.

Jones, T.C., Jacoby, L.L., and Gellis, L.A. (2001). Cross-modal feature and conjunction errors in recognition memory. *Journal of Memory and Language*, **44**, 131–152.

Kahana, M.J. (1996). Associative retrieval processes in free recall. *Memory and Cognition*, **24**, 103–109.

Keele, S.W., Cohen, A., Ivry, R., Liotti, M., and Yee, P. (1988). Tests of a temporal theory of attentional binding. *Journal of Experimental Psychology: Human Perception and Performance*, **14**, 444–452.

Kelley, R. and Wixted, J.T. (2001). On the nature of associative information in recognition memory. *Journal of Experimental Psychology: Learning, Memory, and Cognition*, **27**, 701–722.

Kroll, N.E.A., Knight, R.T., Metcalfe, J., Wolf, E.S., and Tulving, E. (1996). Cohesion failure as a source of memory illusions. *Journal of Memory and Language*, **35**, 176–196.

Laming, D. (1999). Testing the idea of distinct storage mechanisms in memory. *International Journal of Psychology*, **34**, 419–426.

Large, E.W. and Jones, M.R. (1999). The dynamics of attending: how people track time-varying events. *Psychological Review*, **106**, 119–159.

Large, E.W. and Palmer, C. (2002). Perceiving temporal regularity in music. *Cognitive Science*, **26**, 1–37.

Lewandowsky, S. and Brown, G.D.A. (2005). Serial recall and presentation schedule: a micro-analysis of local distinctiveness. *Memory*, **13**, 283–292.

Lewandowsky, S. and Murdock, B.B. (1989). Memory for serial order. *Psychological Review*, **96**, 25–57.

Lewandowsky, S., Duncan, M., and Brown, G.D.A. (2004). Time does not cause forgetting in short-term serial recall. *Psychonomic Bulletin and Review*, **11**, 771–790.

Lewandowsky, S., Brown, G.D.A., Wright, T., and Nimmo, L.M. (2006). Timeless memory: evidence against temporal distinctiveness models of short-term memory for serial order. *Journal of Memory and Language*, **54**, 20–38.

McCormack, T. (1999). Temporal concepts and episodic memory: a response to Hoerl. *Mind and Language*, **14**, 252–262.

McCormack, T. (2001). Attributing episodic memory to animals and children. In *Time and Memory: Issues in Philosophy and Psychology* (ed C. Hoerl and T. McCormack). Oxford: Oxford University Press, pp. 285–313.

McCormack, T. and Hoerl, C. (1999). Memory and temporal perspective: the role of temporal frameworks in memory development. *Developmental Review*, **19**, 154–182.

McCormack, T., Brown, G.D.A., Maylor, E.A., Richardson, L.B.N., and Darby, R.J. (2002). Effects of aging on absolute identification of duration. *Psychology and Aging*, **17**, 363–378.

McGovern, J.B. (1964). Extinction of associations in four transfer paradigms. *Psychological Monographs*, **78**(16).

McClelland, J.L., McNaughton, B.L., and O'Reilly, R.C. (1995). Why there are complementary learning-systems in the hippocampus and neocortex: insights from the successes and failures of connectionist models of learning and memory. *Psychological Review*, **102**, 419–457.

MacKay, D. (1970). Spoonerisms: the structure of errors in the serial order of speech. *Neuropsychologia*, **8**, 323–350.

McNamara, T.P., Halpin, J.A., and Hardy, J.K. (1992). Spatial and temporal contributions to the structure of spatial memory. *Journal of Experimental Psychology: Learning, Memory, and Cognition*, **18**, 555–564.

Martin, M.G.F. (2001). Out of the past: episodic memory as retained acquaintance. In *Time and Memory: Issues in Philosophy and Psychology* (ed C. Hoerl and T. McCormack). Oxford: Oxford University Press, pp. 257–284.

Maybery, M.T., Parmentier, F.B.R., and Jones, D.M. (2002). Grouping of list items reflected in the timing of recall: implications for models of serial verbal memory. *Journal of Memory and Language*, **47**, 360–385.

Mayes, A.R., Baddeley, A.D., Cockburn, J., Meudell, P.R., Pickering, A. and Wilson, B. (1989). Why are amnesic judgements of recency and frequency made in a qualitatively different way from those of normal people? *Cortex*, **25**, 479–488.

Metcalfe, J. (1990). Composite holographic associative recall model (CHARM) and blended memories in eyewitness testimony. *Journal of Experimental Psychology: General*, **119**, 145–160.

Mensink, G.J. and Raaijmakers, J.G.W. (1988). A model for interference and forgetting. *Psychological Review*, **95**, 434–455.

Moscovitch, M. (1994). Memory and working with memory: evaluation of a component processing model and comparisons with other models. In *Memory Systems* (ed D.L. Schacter and E. Tulving). Cambridge, MA: MIT Press, pp. 269–319.

Murdock, B.B. (1960). The distinctiveness of stimuli. *Psychological Review*, **67**, 16–31.

Murdock, B.B. (1974). *Human Memory: Theory and Data*. Potomac, MD: Erlbaum.

Murdock, B.B. (1982). A theory for the storage and retrieval of item and associative information. *Psychological Review*, **89**, 609–626.

Murdock, B.B. (1983). A distributed memory model for serial-order information. *Psychological Review*, **90**, 316–338.

Murdock, B.B. (1993). TODAM2: a model for the storage and retrieval of item, associative, and serial-order information. *Psychological Review*, **100**, 183–203.

Neath, I. (1993). Distinctiveness and serial position effects in recognition. *Memory and Cognition*, **21**, 689–658.

Neath, I. and Crowder, R.G. (1990). Schedules of presentation and distinctiveness in human memory. *Journal of Experimental Psychology: Learning, Memory, and Cognition*, **16**, 316–327.

Neath, I. and Crowder, R.G. (1996). Distinctiveness and very short-term serial position effects. *Memory*, **4**, 225–242.

Ng, M.L.H. and Maybery, M.T. (2002). Grouping in short-term verbal memory. Is position coded temporally? *Quarterly Journal of Experimental Psychology*, **55**, 391–424.

Nissen, M.J. (1985). Accessing features and objects. Is location special? In *Attention and Performance XI* (ed M.I. Posner and O.S. Marin). Hillsdale, NJ: Erlbaum, pp. 205–219.

Nosofsky, R.M. (1986). Attention, similarity and the identification–categorization relationship. *Journal of Experimental Psychology: General*, **115**, 39–57.

Page, M.P.A. and Norris, D. (1998). The primacy model: a new model of immediate serial recall. *Psychological Review*, **105**, 761–781.

Raaijmakers, J.G.W. and Shiffrin, R.M. (1981). Search of associative memory. *Psychological Review*, **88**, 93–134.

Reinitz, M.T. and Alexander, R. (1996). Mechanisms of facilitation in primed perceptual identification. *Memory and Cognition*, **24**, 129–135.

Reinitz, M.T. and Demb, J.B. (1994). Implicit and explicit memory for compound words. *Memory and Cognition*, **22**, 687–694.

Reinitz, M.T. and Hannigan, S.L. (2001). Effects of simultaneous stimulus presentation and attention switching on memory conjunction errors. *Journal of Memory and Language*, **44**, 206–219.

Reinitz, M.T., Lammers, W.J., and Cochran, B.P. (1992). Memory conjunction errors: Miscombination of stored stimulus features can produce illusions of memory. *Memory and Cognition*, **20**, 111.

Reinitz, M.T., Morrisey, J., and Demb, J. (1994). Role of attention in face encoding. *Journal of Experimental Psychology: Learning, Memory, and Cognition*, **20**, 161–168.

Reinitz, M.T., Verfaellie, M., and Milberg, W.P. (1996). Memory conjunction errors in normal and amnesic subjects. *Journal of Memory and Language*, **35**, 286–299.

Roberts, W.A. (2002). Are animals stuck in time? *Psychological Bulletin*, **128**, 473–489.

Rotello, C.M. and Heit, E. (2000). Associative recognition: a case of recall-to-reject processing. *Memory and Cognition*, **28**, 907–922.

Rubin, D.C. and Wenzel, A.E. (1996). One hundred years of forgetting: a quantitative description of retention. *Psychological Review*, **103**, 734–760.

Rubin, S.R., Van Petten, C., Glisky, E.L., and Newberg, W.N. (1999). Memory conjunction errors in younger and older adults: event-related potential and neuropsychological data. *Cognitive Neuropsychology*, **16**, 459–488.

Rundus, D. (1971). Analysis of rehearsal processes in free recall. *Journal of Experimental Psychology*, **89**, 63–77.

Shiffrin, R.M. (1970a). Memory search. In *Models of Memory* (ed D.A. Norman). New York: Academic Press, pp. 375–447.

Shiffrin, R.M. (1970b). Forgetting, trace erosion or retrieval failure? *Science*, **168**, 1601–1603.

Shum, M.S. (1998). The role of temporal landmarks in autobiographical memory processes. *Psychological Bulletin*, **124**, 423–442.

Sikstrom, S. (2000). The TECO theory and lawful dependency in successive episodic memory tests. *Quarterly Journal of Experimental Psychology, Section A, Human Experimental Psychology*, **53**, 693–728.

Sohn, Y.S., Liederman, J., and Reinitz, M.T. (1996). Division of inputs between hemispheres eliminates illusory conjunctions. *Neuropsychologia*, **34**, 1057–1068.

Stefurak, D.L. and Boynton, R.M. (1986). Independence of memory for categorically different colors and shapes. *Perception and Psychophysics*, **39**, 164–174.

Suddendorf and Corballis, M.C. (1997)

Tan, L. and Ward, G. (2000). A recency-based account of the primacy effect in free recall. *Journal of Experimental Psychology: Learning, Memory, and Cognition*, **26**, 1589–1625.

Treisman, A. (1977). Focused attention in the perception and retrieval of multidimensional stimuli. *Perception and Psychophysics*, **22**, 1–11.

Treisman, A. and Gelade, G. (1980). A feature integration theory of attention. *Cognitive Psychology*, **12**, 97–136.

Tulving, E. (1983). *Elements of Episodic Memory*. Oxford: Oxford University Press.

Underwood, B.J. and Zimmerman, J. (1973). The syllable as a source of error in multisyllable word recognition. *Journal of Verbal Learning and Verbal Behavior*, **12**, 701–706.

Underwood, B.J., Kapelak, S.M., and Malmi, R.A. (1976). Integration of discrete verbal units in recognition memory. *Journal of Experimental Psychology: Human Learning and Memory*, **2**, 293–300.

Vousden, J.I., Brown, G.D.A., and Harley, T.A. (2000). Serial control of phonology in speech production: a hierarchical model. *Cognitive Psychology*, **41**, 101–175.

Walker, P. and Cuthbert, L. (1998). Remembering visual feature conjunctions: visual memory for shape-colour associations is object-based. *Visual Cognition*, **5**, 409–455.

Ward, G., Churchill, E.F., and Musgrave, P. (1997). An investigation of cued recall of multiattribute stimuli. *Journal of Experimental Psychology: Learning, Memory, and Cognition*, **23**, 1247–1260.

Welte, J.W. and Laughery, K.R. (1971). Short-term memory: the effects of inter-item time distribution and recall procedure. *Canadian Journal of Psychology*, **25**.

Wheeler, M.A., Stuss, D.T., and Tulving, E. (1997). Toward a theory of episodic memory: the frontal lobes and autonoetic consciousness. *Psychological Bulletin*, **121**, 331–354.

Wheeler, M.E. and Treisman, A.M. (2002). Binding in short-term visual memory. *Journal of Experimental Psychology: General*, **131**, 48–64.

Yonelinas, A.P. (1997). Recognition memory ROCs for item and associative information: the contribution of recollection and familiarity. *Memory and Cognition*, **25**, 747–763.

Yonelinas, A.P., Kroll, N.E.A., Dobbins, I.G., and Soltani, M. (1999). Recognition memory for faces: when familiarity supports associative recognition judgments. *Psychonomic Bulletin and Review*, **6**, 654–661.

Zaki, S.R. and Nosofsky, R.M. (2001). Exemplar accounts of blending and distinctiveness effects in perceptual old–new recognition. *Journal of Experimental Psychology: Learning, Memory, and Cognition*, **27**, 1022–1041.

Chapter 11

Ageing deficit in neuromodulation of representational distinctiveness and conjunctive binding: computational explorations of possible links

Shu-Chen Li and Ulman Lindenberger

Introduction

> The mind is a kind of theatre, where several perceptions successively make their appearance; pass, repass, glide away, and mingle in an infinite variety of postures and situations.
>
> What we call a mind is nothing but a heap or collection of different perceptions, united together by certain relations and suppos'd, tho' falsely, to be endow'd with a perfect simplicity and identity.
>
> To me, there appear to be only three principles of connexion among ideas, namely, resemblance, contiguity in time or place, and cause or effect.
>
> (David Hume, *A Treatise of Human Nature*, Book I, Part 4, Section 6, and Part 1, Section 7; *An Enquiry Concerning Human Understanding*, Section 3.)

Although David Hume, the eighteenth-century Scottish empiricist philosopher, was sceptical about the veracity with which human perceptual and memory processes capture and store the manifold world and our experiences in it, he was certain that the mind works by combining assorted aspects of experienced reality and that such combinatory processes pose a task for the mind to solve. What modern students of mind and brain are still uncertain about are, indeed, the details of so-called 'binding mechanisms'. How—or, in Hume's term, by what relations—are multiple features of the experiential world and the stored memory episodes bound together to produce coherent neurocognitive representations? Hume himself proposed three relational principles: resemblance, spatial and temporal contiguity, and causality. Parallel to, although not necessarily motivated by, Hume's contention, much of current cognitive and neuroscience research on the issues of binding focuses on mechanisms for flexible coding of conjunctive relations between multiple attributes of objects and complex memory events, or both. Put more generally, the research on perceptual and memory binding aims at understanding the neurocognitive mechanisms that afford dynamic versatile implementations of representations, so that the mind can fluently integrate information across time, space, attributes, or ideas (reviewed by Treisman 1999).

Apart from investigating mechanisms supporting flexible combinatorial information processing in young adults, ontogenetic changes in the brain (Sowell *et al.* 2003) and cognitive functions (Li *et al.* 2004) across the lifespan can be expected to affect the efficacy of binding mechanisms. Understanding ontogenetic factors operating during either child development or ageing that strengthen or weaken, respectively, our capacity to handle perceptual and cognitive combinatorial complexity may shed light on basic mechanisms of binding. The question of how ageing may affect the mechanisms subserving conjunctive integration of information has gained increasing research attention (Spencer and Raz 1995; Chalfonte and Johnson 1996; Mitchell *et al.* 2000; Naveh-Benjamin 2000; Naveh-Benjamin *et al.* 2003). In this chapter, and based on earlier work (Li and Lindenberger 1999; Li 2002), we present a neurocomputational model that formalizes the disproportionate deficits in conjunctive feature binding in older adults. First, we provide a brief and selective review of the empirical literature on adult age differences in conjunctive feature binding. Secondly, we present the general neurocomputational framework adopted in the present and earlier simulations of adult age changes in information processing efficiency. Thirdly, we present a series of simulations that are specifically aimed at relating age-associated conjunctive binding differences to a triad consisting of deficient neuromodulation, less efficient distributed conjunctive coding, and reduced representational distinctiveness. Finally, we relate our findings to other models of binding, and discuss their generality.

Ageing and conjunctive memory binding

Ageing affects different aspects of memory function to varying degrees (reviewed by Zacks *et al.* 2000). Overall, memory for explicitly encoded event information (i.e. episodic memory) and online memory processing capacity (i.e. working memory) show greater ageing deficits than memory for general facts (i.e. semantic memory), personal history (i.e. autobiographic memory), or incidentally encoded events (i.e. implicit memory). With respect to episodic memory, complex memory events often involve various kinds of information, such as the persons involved in the events, the time or place at which the events took place, and other general background contextual information. Various researchers have suggested that mechanisms for binding together multiple details of a memory episode may be compromised by ageing (MacKay and Burke 1990; Light 1991; Chalfonte and Johnson 1996; Naveh-Benjamin 2000).

Thus far, three aspects of ageing-related memory binding deficits have been identified: memory for contextual information, memory for feature combinations of a given event, and memory for associations between events. Regarding context and source memory (Johnson *et al.* 1993; McIntyre and Craik 1987), older adults experience greater difficulty than younger adults in remembering contextual details of memory episodes, such as whether the remembered actions were imagined or performed, whether the information was presented visually or aurally, whether the remembered event happened before or after other events, and whether the memory episode happened in one or other possible locations (reviewed by Spencer and Raz 1995). Concerning feature combinations, older adults show poorer memory performance than younger adults when different features of the studied items (e.g. objects and locations, objects and colours, or words and font types) need to be combined (Chalfonte and Johnson 1996; Naveh-Benjamin 2000). As for associations between items or events, negative age differences in cued recall for paired associates, revealing a deficit in retrieving associative information, have been found in many studies (Kliegl and Lindenberger 1993; reviewed by Kausler 1994). More recent studies have also shown that older adults have disproportional difficulties relative to young adults in encoding and storing associations between memory items (Naveh-Benjamin 2000; Naveh-Benjamin *et al.* 2003).

In summary, cognitive ageing appears to adversely affect some, if not most, aspects of conjunctive binding in the domain of episodic memory. Older adults exhibit disproportional performance deficits relative to younger adults under task conditions that require conjunctive associations between multiple features (e.g. the contexts and contents of the memory events, stimulus attributes, or the associations between events). Ageing-related memory encoding and binding deficits have been attributed to frontal hippocampal circuitry (Mitchell *et al.* 2000; Grady *et al.* 2003) but have not been linked formally to impaired neuromodulation involving this circuitry. We now review a theory that relates cognitive ageing to deficient neuromodulation of representational distinctiveness and then demonstrate through simulations that less efficient distributed conjunctive coding may underlie ageing-related deficits in conjunctive memory binding.

Deficient neuromodulation and cognitive ageing

The factors contributing to cognitive ageing deficits cut across behavioural, cognitive, and neurobiological levels. Therefore integrative theories facilitating cross-level data synthesis and hypothesis testing (Churchland and Sejnowski 1988) are necessary for a comprehensive understanding of neurocognitive ageing. Building on various approaches for modelling neuromodulation from computational neuroscience, few recent computational theories have explored computational principles that relate ageing-related decline of neuromodulation to behavioural manifestations of cognitive ageing. For instance, with respect to the ability of monitoring the valence of behavioural consequences, a recent model relates weakened phasic activity of the mesencephalic dopamine system to ageing-related deficits in error processing (Nieuwenhuis *et al.* 2002). Another theory has focused on functional interactions between dopaminergic modulation and the dorsal lateral prefrontal cortex (PFC) to capture the effect of ageing on context representation and maintenance (Braver *et al.* 2001). Below, we briefly summarize ageing-related decline in neuromodulatory systems, and then focus on a cross-level theory that elucidates a potential sequence of functional relations from deficient dopaminergic modulation to reduced neural information processing fidelity, with ensuing consequences for cortical representational distinctiveness that may underlie various behavioural manifestations of cognitive ageing (Li *et al.* 2000). As will be demonstrated in later sections, this approach can also be used to model the effects of deficits in conjunctive feature binding on episodic memory for associated events.

Ageing and neuromodulation

Brain ageing involves structural losses in neurons and the connections between them (reviewed by Schneider *et al.* 1996). Severe progressive neuroanatomical degeneration resulting from cell death and reduced synaptic density is typical of pathological ageing (e.g. Alzheimer's disease). In normal ageing, the volumes of various cortical regions also show slightly declining trends. The most substantial shrinkage is observed in the PFC (Raz 2000; Head *et al.* 2002). Parallel to the less severe neuroanatomical changes, the milder cognitive declines that occur during normal ageing are likely to be due to neurochemical shifts in still relatively intact neural circuitry (Morrison and Hof 1997). Such neurochemical shifts affect the efficacy of signal transmission, which, in turn, regulates neural activity within and across cell assemblies. Various transmitter systems are affected by ageing and have implications for cognitive declines associated with pathological and normal ageing. For instance, the transmitter acetycholine (Ach) is important for long-term memory consolidation. It plays a specific role in the memory deficit for retaining new information seen in Alzheimer's patients (Hasselmo 1995). Furthermore, for an understanding of the neurochemical circuits of the ageing brain, it is important to consider both the effects of various transmitters independently and the interactions between multiple transmitters, such as the recently discovered interaction of glutamate with other transmitters (e.g. dopamine, GABA, and acetylcholine) (Segovia *et al.* 2001).

Among various neuromodulatory systems, the monoamines (e.g. serotonin and the catecholamines, particularly dopamine) are promising neurochemical correlates of normal cognitive ageing. There is evidence of a reduction in dopamine D_2 receptors of about 7–11 per cent per decade during normal ageing, starting at about age 20 years in the nigrostriatal region (Wong *et al.* 1997). There is now also evidence of D_2 receptor loss in various other extrastriatal regions (Kaasinen *et al.* 2000; reviewed by Bäckman and Farde 2005), such as the anterior cingulate cortex (13 per cent), the frontal cortex (11 per cent), the hippocampus (10 per cent), and the amydgala (7 per cent). In addition, D_1 receptor loss has been observed in the striatum (Giorgi *et al.* 1987) and the frontal cortex (de Keyser 1990, Zahrt *et al.* 1997).

In addition to the trends of ageing-related declines of dopamine receptors in different brain regions across the adult lifespan, there is also more direct experimental evidence for functional relationships between deficient dopaminergic modulation and cognitive deficits. For instance, deficient dopaminergic modulation was found to be associated with increased fluctuation in response speed and reaction time in old rats (MacRae *et al.*1988). Drugs that facilitated dopaminergic modulation were found to alleviate working memory deficits in old monkeys (Arnsten and Goldman-Rakic 1985; Arnsten *et al.* 1994). In humans, ageing-related attenuation of the striatal D_2 receptor binding mechanism was found to be statistically associated with age differences in processing speed and episodic memory (Bäckman *et al.* 2000).

From deficient neuromodulation to increased neuronal noise and less distinctive representation

Although ample evidence indicates that deficient dopaminergic modulation has implications for cognitive ageing, many details of this neuromodulation–cognition link await further explication. At the cellular level, empirical and theoretical work on how dopaminergic modulation affects the memory field and signal integration of PFC neurons has only recently begun (Camperi and Wang 1998; Durstewitz *et al.* 1999; Goldman-Rakic *et al.* 2000). At a higher level of abstraction, a general feature of the net effect of dopamine in decreasing background firing rate and enhancing the excitability of target neurons has been modelled as the regulation of the signal-to-noise ratio of neural information processing by altering the gain parameter *G* of the neural network's activation function (Servan-Schreiber *et al.* 1990). It has also been demonstrated recently that simulating ageing-related decline of dopaminergic neuromodulation by attenuating the parameter *G* in neural networks suggests a possible chain of mechanisms that relate deficient neuromodulation to increased neuronal noise and less distinctive cortical representations both within and across processing pathways (Li *et al.* 2001; Li and Sikström 2002).

Reduced responsivity and increased neuronal noise

Reducing the parameter *G* simulates ageing-related attenuation of dopaminergic modulation by decreasing the slope and flattening the non-linearity of the S-shaped logistic activation function (i.e. making it more linear), such that a unit's average response to excitatory and inhibitory input signals is reduced (Figure 11.1(a)). When the values of a unit's G are randomly chosen (i.e. stochastic G manipulation; Li *et al.* 2000) from a set of values with a lower average (i.e. mean G reduction, but keeping the range of the distribution constant), the unit's response to a given external signal fluctuates more across discrete time steps. This implies decreased signal transmission fidelity (Figure 1B). In other words, a given amount of random variations in G—simulating random fluctuations in dopamine transmitter substance due to probabilistic transmitter release or stochasticity in receptor binding efficacy (Hessler *et al.* 1993)—generates more haphazard activation during signal processing if the average of the processing units' Gs is reduced. This functional interaction between fluctuation and level depicts a potential neurochemical mechanism for a common hypothesis of an ageing-related increase in neural noise introduced by Welford (1965): As ageing attenuates neuromodulation, the impact of transmitter fluctuations due to probabilistic transmitter release and other sources of neuronal noise (e.g. background spiking activity) on the overall level of haphazard neuronal activity is being amplified.

Reduced representational distinctiveness

With respect to the efficiency of conjunctive coding, of particular interest here is that the simulations also show that, as reduced responsivity leads to increased intra-network random activation variability, another subsequent effect is a decrease in the **distinctiveness** of the network's internal representations. Low representational distinctiveness means that the activation profiles formed across the network's hidden units for different stimuli are less readily

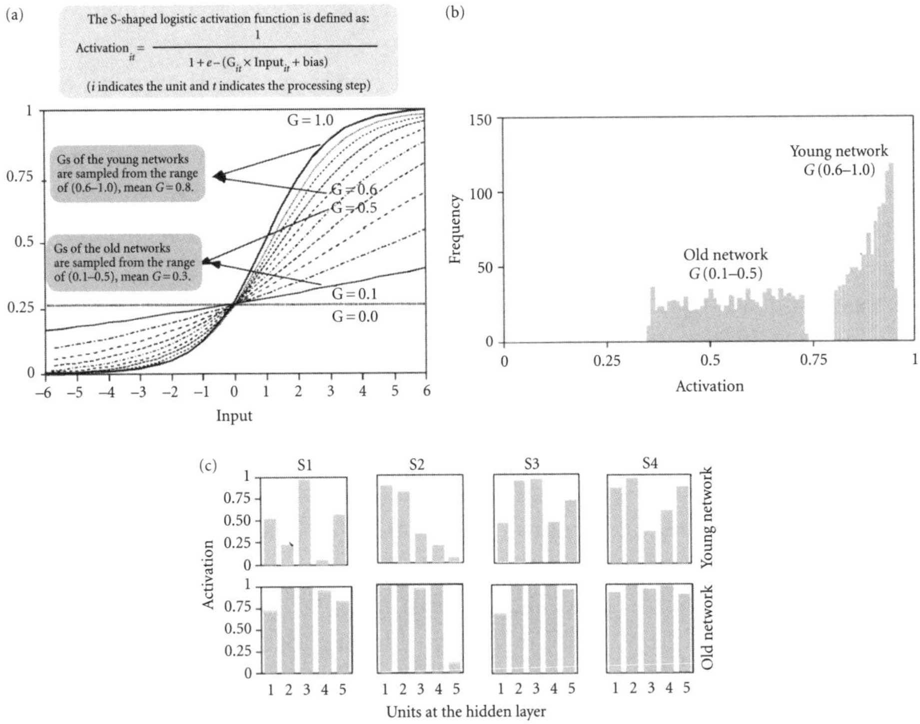

Figure 11.1 Simulations of gain modulation, neuromodulation, and ageing. (a) The S-shaped logistic activation function at different values of *G*. Physiological evidence suggests that the logistic function with a negative bias captures the function relating the strength of an input signal to a neuron's firing rate, with its steepest slope around the baseline firing rate. Reducing mean *G* flattens the activation function such that a unit becomes less responsive. Ageing-related decline of dopaminergic modulation can be simulated by sampling values of *G* from a distribution with a lower mean. (b) *G* and the variability of activation across processing steps. Reducing mean *G* (0.8 and 0.3 for the 'young' and 'old' networks, respectively) increases the temporal variability of a unit's response to an identical input signal (set to 4.0) across 1000 trials. (c) Internal activation patterns across five hidden units of one 'young' and one 'old' network in response to four different stimuli (S1–S4). The internal representations of the four stimuli are much less differentiable in the 'old' network than in the 'young' network. (Adapted with permission from S.-C. Li *et al. Neurocomputing*, **32–33**, 879–890, 2000.)

differentiable from each other. Figure 11.1(c) shows the internal activation patterns across units at the hidden layer of a 'young' (higher mean *G* in the top row) and an 'old' (lower mean *G* in the bottom row) network in response to four input stimuli. Because more units are required to distributively code the feature combinations of the different stimuli, the internal stimulus representations are less distinctive (patterns representing different memory events are less differentiable from each other) in the 'old' than in the 'young' network.

Taken together, a potential biological implication of these theoretical effects could be that, as people age, declining dopaminergic modulation reduces cortical neuron responsivity and increases neural noise in the ageing brain. Consequently, the efficiency of distributed coding of neuronal activity is reduced, such that the internal representations elicited by different stimuli and contexts become less differentiated. This theoretical sequence of potential effects has been tested in a series of simulations that captured a range of cognitive ageing phenomena, such as adult age differences in learning rate, asymptotic performance, interference susceptibility, working memory, complexity cost, intra- and inter-individual variability, ability dedifferentiation, and the coactivation of different neurocognitive processes (Li *et al.* 2001; Li and Sikström 2002).

Neurocognitive representations of concurrent exogenous and endogenous events (e.g. perception and sensation) and later reinstatements of these events (e.g. memory and action) are the primitives of subsequent information processing carried out by various neural circuits. It has been argued that perceptual, motor, and memory processes all involve the binding together of multiple representations of stimulus features, task goals, and contexts (Johnson 1992; Treisman 1998; Wolpert *et al.* 2001; Nadel *et al.* 2000). Thus deficient neuromodulation resulting in less efficient distributed conjunctive coding may have implications for ageing-related deficits in memory binding.

Relating reduced representational distinctiveness with deficits in conjunctive binding

Neurocomputational models aid the search for mechanisms that bind diverse features into coherent representations through formal analysis and hypothesis testing. Thus far, associative network theories emphasize distributed dynamical processes that tune each processing unit to subsets rather than to all relevant features (O'Reilly and Busby 2002; cf. Singer 1998). As reviewed above, earlier simulation work has shown that deficits in neuromodulation can result in less distinctive stimulus representations and, by implication, less efficient distributed conjunctive coding. Less distinctive representation can lead to erroneous conjunctions, which is deleterious in distributed and context dependent coding (Singer 1998) and thus may affect the efficacy of memory binding. We extend this principle to model ageing-related deficits in two aspects of memory binding.

A feature–association conjunctive binding model of ageing-related associative deficits

Deficits in associative conjunction binding in older adults has been systematically investigated in a series of recent experiments that examined both inter-item associations and intra-item feature conjunctions (Naveh-Benjamin 2000; Naveh-Benjamin *et al.* 2003). Of particular interest, one of the experiments clearly demonstrated that ageing differentially affects the encoding and storage of associative memory more than item memory (Naveh-Benjamin 2000, Experiment 2). Participants in this experiment were presented with word pairs during the study phase, but were instructed to study the word pairs either as two single words (the study words instruction) or as pairs (the study pairs instruction). During the testing phase, the participants were tested with both an associative test and an item test. The associative test required correct recognition of studied word pairs (targets) from rearranged word pairs (lures), whereas the item test required correct recognition of studied words (targets) from non-studied words (lures). The results showed that, when the associations between word pairs were learned intentionally (i.e. under the study pair instruction), older adults exhibited differentially poorer performance in the associative test than younger adults.

A feature–association conjunctive binding model (Li *et al.* 2005) was constructed to simulate the ageing-related deficit of associative binding observed in Naveh-Benjamin's (2000) experiment. The model (Fig. 11.2) involves parallel processing paths for feature conjunctive binding of item information and for

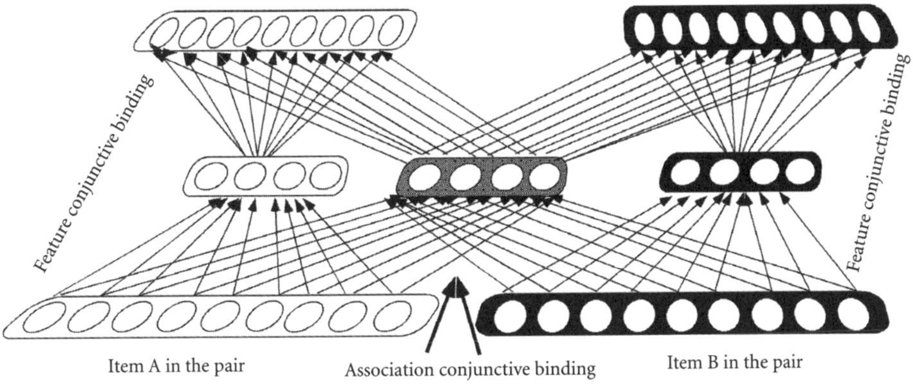

Figure 11.2 Schematic diagram of the network structure for the feature–association conjunctive binding model. (Adapted with permission from S.-C. Li *et al. Psychological Science*, **16**, 445–450, 2005.)

association conjunctive binding of inter-item associations. The multiple features of the two items in a given study pair are distributedly processed within each of the corresponding feature conjunctive binding paths, with converging connections from the input item-feature layer to the internal item-representation layer and divergent connections from the internal layer to the output item-response layer. The association conjunctive binding path in the middle processes inter-item association. The features of both items are distributedly processed through the input connections that converge on the internal association-representation layer and the divergent connections to the output item-response layer.

Network architecture

The networks had 18 inputs, 12 hidden units, and 18 output units that were separately connected by feedforward connections between layers within the feature conjunctive binding and the association conjunctive binding path. The first half of nine input and output units are dedicated to feature information for the study item on the left side of a given study pair (e.g. item A from the A–B pair). The second half of the remaining nine input and output units are dedicated to feature information for the item on the right side of the pair (e.g. item B from the A–B pair). The first four hidden units code distributed representation of feature conjunction of item A in the pair. The middle four hidden units are dedicated to the distributed representation of the association between the two items. Finally, the last four hidden units code the distributed representation of feature conjunction of item B. The specific network architecture of presenting item–item associations as intra-layer associations is designed specifically to stimulate Naveh-Benjamin's (2000) experimental paradigm closely. The effect of reducing the gain parameter in simulating the ageing deficit of paired associate memory using the more traditional way of representing item–item associations as input–output associations has been demonstrated elsewhere (Li *et al.* 2000). Although the model is currently set up to account for associative binding at the inter-item level, conceivably a similar architecture could also be used to simulate specific feature binding effects if within-item feature specificities are systematically present in the stimulus patterns.

Parameter values

Learning rate, momentum, and bias were fixed parameters and were set to 0.1, 0.8, and –4.0, respectively. The networks were initialized with random weights in the range $[-1,1]$. The stochastic gain manipulation (Li *et al.* 2000) affected all hidden and output units of the networks. Two groups of 10 networks were identical in all respects except for the mean values of their gain (G) parameters.

The two network groups can be considered as the yoked control for each other, as identical sets of 10 random seeds were used to define the initial weight configurations for both groups. The mean G of each of the 10 old networks was 0.9, whereas the mean G of each of the 10 young networks was 1.2. The range of the uniform distribution from which the values of G were sampled was fixed at 0.4 for both groups of networks.

Study and test phases

Before providing the networks with the study pairs for learning, both groups of networks were trained to reach the same performance level with a sample of single-item patterns to establish initial item knowledge. During the study phase, the networks were trained to learn item pairs for 10 trials. Connection weights were trained with back-propagation learning. Analogous to Naveh-Benjamin's (2000) experimental manipulation of study instructions, the emphasis on studying the presented pairs as either single items or intact pairs was implemented by either presenting only the item pairs (the study pair instruction) or presenting the item pairs as well as individual items of the pair to the network during the study phase (the study item instruction). At the test phase, both groups of networks were tested under two conditions. In the associative test condition, the networks were presented with intact target pairs and rearranged lure pairs. In the item test condition, the networks were presented with single target items and single lures. A standard indicator of the match between the expected outputs and the actual network outputs (the cosine between target and actual outputs (Goebel and Lewandowsky 1991)) was computed. If a test pair (or item) was a target test pair (or target item) and the cosine was greater than a fixed threshold, a hit was scored. If a test pair (or item) was a lure pair (or lure item) and the cosine was greater than the threshold, a false alarm was scored. The response threshold was fixed at a cosine of 0.99 for the study pair introduction and a cosine of 0.975 for the study word introduction.

Results

With only two assumptions—ageing-related deficit in dopaminergic modulation can be simulated by reducing the mean G of the network activation function and the response criterion is slightly lower in the incidental learning condition (the study word instruction)—the model was able to capture the age effects observed in Naveh-Benjamin's (2000) four experimental conditions (Fig. 11.3). The simulation accounts for differential ageing effects on item and associative memory. The performance of old networks was relatively spared in the item test and more impaired in the associative test. In particular, details of the three-way age $\times$ instruction $\times$ test type interaction, indicating that older adults had

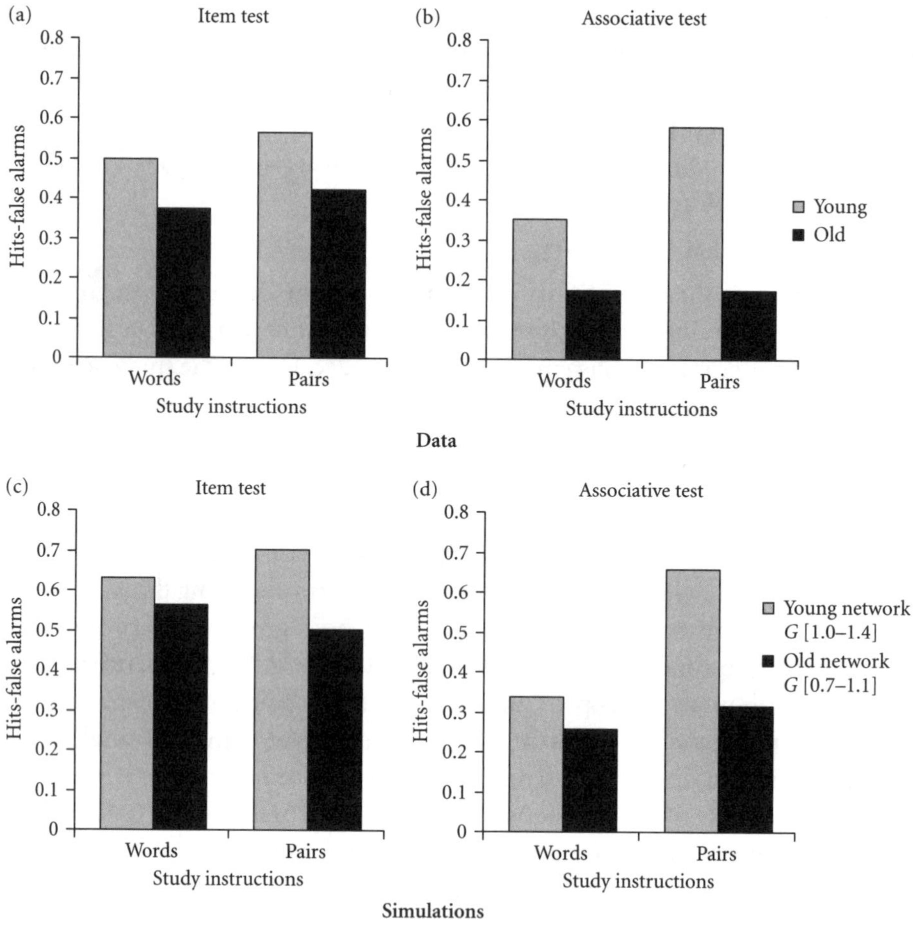

Figure 11.3 Empirical data (replotted from Naveh-Benjamin 2000, Experiment 2) and simulation results of adult age differences in associative binding. (Adapted with permission from S.-C. Li *et al. Psychological Science*, **16**, 445–450, 2005.)

disproportionately greater difficulty in encoding and storing associative information when the associations were learned intentionally, (i.e. comparing young and old associate test performance across study instructions Figs 11.3(b) and 11.3(d)), were captured well by the simulation results (Li *et al.* 2005).

Internal activation patterns

Examining the internal feature conjunctive representations of the items and the internal association conjunctive representations at the hidden layer revealed that the disproportionately poor associative memory of the old networks was indeed caused by less efficient coding of associative information owing to inferior *G* modulation. Figure 11.4 shows summary activation maps of individual networks with a range of mean G values from 1.6 to 0.6. On the vertical axis, the first 18 patterns correspond to activations in response to the associative test, whereas the remaining 12 patterns correspond to activations in response to the item test. On the horizontal axis, the first four units correspond to the distributed representation of feature conjunction of item A in the pair, the middle four units correspond to the distributed representation of association conjunction of the

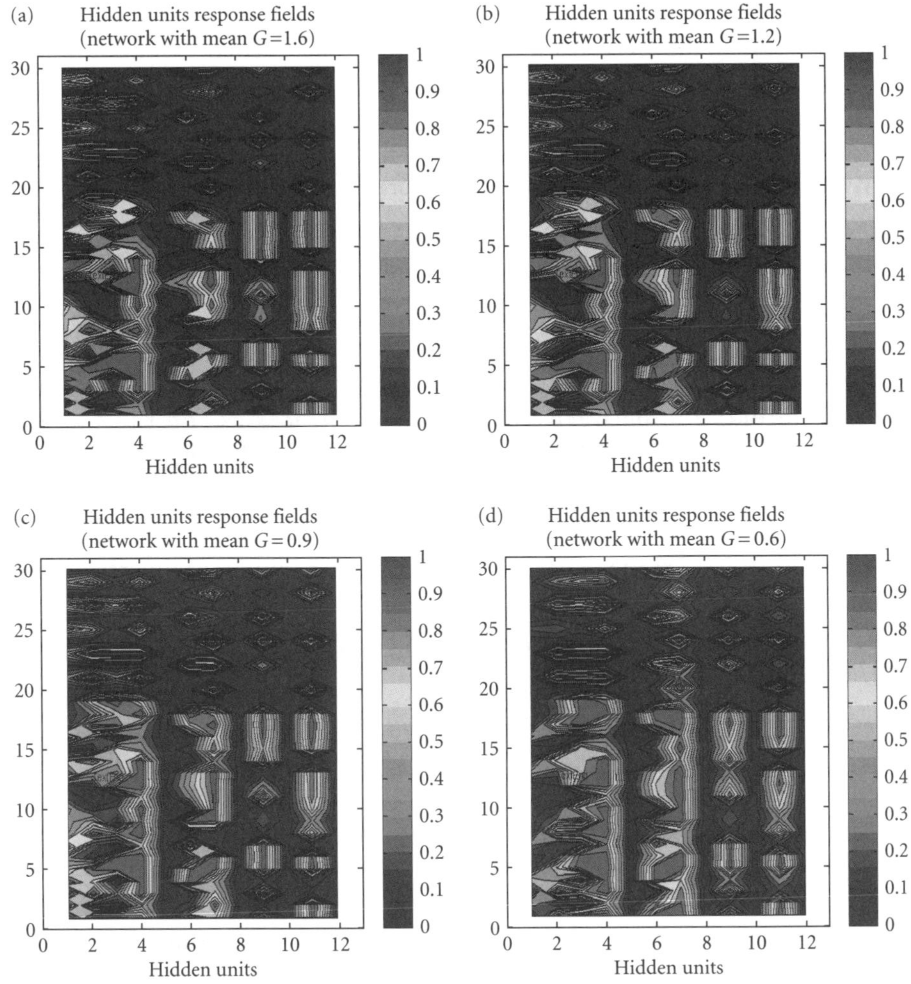

Figure 11.4 Summary hidden-unit activation maps of four networks illustrating the effects of reducing mean G on the distinctiveness of distributed coding of associative information. Red coloration indicates that the units are highly activated, whereas blue coloration indicates low activation (see text for explanation). See also colour plate section.

pair, and the last four units correspond to the representation of the feature conjunction of item B in the pair. Overall, far fewer units were involved in coding item than associative information (comparing the top and bottom portions of the activation maps). Most relevantly, the effect of the *G* manipulation is clearest in the activation patterns represented by the middle four units when responding to the associative test (i.e. activation patterns corresponding to the first 18 stimulus patterns across hidden units 5–8). Going from high mean *G* (Fig. 11.4(a)) to low mean *G* (Fig. 11.4(d)), the distributed coding of associative conjunction goes from highly distinctive with only a few highly activated units to less distinctive with the majority of units being highly active. These internal activation patterns show that reducing mean *G* to simulate ageing-related deficit in neuromodulation leads to less efficient distributed coding of associations between items, which, in turn, contributes to the poor associative memory of the old networks.

Contextual support and representational distinctiveness

As reviewed above, in addition to the deficit of associative binding between items, old adults also have difficulty in remembering contextual details of memory events. Comparing across a wide range of studies, Spencer and Raz (1995) showed that context memory is more sensitive to ageing than content memory. In line with more recent conceptions of situated cognition that stress the dynamic interaction between neurocognitive processes and the contexts (reviewed by Clark 1999), Craik (1983) suggested that the overall behaviour reflects compensation of some interactive mix of self-initiated processing by enhanced environmental contextual support. On the one hand, older adults show deficits in context memory; on the other hand, cognitive ageing researchers have suggested that, in comparison with themselves, the memory performance of older adults can be enhanced by providing contextual support (Craik and Anderson 1999).

In an earlier study (Li 2005), we explored the trade-offs between ageing-related decline in the neuromodulation of representational distinctiveness and the influence of contextual support in enhancing representational distinctiveness to counteract the effect of deficient neuromodulation in a different network architecture. The earlier model examined the effects of contextual support in a fully connected network without separated feature and associative conjunctive binding pathways. Simulation results from that study showed that reducing mean *G* (simulating ageing-related deficiency in dopaminergic modulation) gave rise to less distinctive representations of study items, which led to the poor memory performance. However, providing external contextual cues improved the memory performance of the old networks, relative to themselves, through context-dependent enhancement of efficiency in distributed conjunctive coding.

Discussion

Thus far, results from the neurocomputional simulations reviewed and presented in this chapter show that deficient neuromodulation may play a role in ageing-related deficits of memory binding. Specifically, the simulations explicate a sequence of effects from reduced responsivity of a single unit due to non-optimal *G* modulation, through less efficient distributed conjunctive coding of stimulus patterns across assemblies of units, to behavioural manifestations of an associative binding deficit. Clearly, this cross-level theoretical link is a conjecture awaiting further vigorous empirical testing. At the same time, our proposal can serve as a vantage point for discussing relations between various binding mechanisms that have been proposed so far.

Relations to other theories of binding

Among the various views on perceptual and memory binding, it has been suggested that the brain may use two general coding principles to represent relations between currently perceived object features or the regenerated representations of stored experiences. One principle involves coarse population codes of percepts or stored representations that are bound together through conjunction units (Barlow 1972), and the other involves dynamic context-dependent temporal binding of cell assembly codes (von der Malsburg 1985; Singer and Gray 1995). Obviously, these two principles differ: The first achieves binding by convergence (conjunction binding) and the second through temporal synchrony. However, both principles operate on distributed coding. Moreover, the two principles may complement each other. It has been suggested that stereotyped, frequently occurring, and particularly relevant conjunctions should be represented by specific binding units, because this strategy is faster and less susceptible to binding errors; whereas unanticipated conjunctions should be recruited by dynamically configured population codes that represent meta-conjunctions for which there are no pre-existing binding units (Singer 1999). Therefore mechanisms that may affect the representational distinctiveness of the distributed coding of neuronal activities related to stimulus and response, such as neuromodulation simulated in our model, would have implications for both binding principles.

Thus far, the effect of neuromodulation on temporal binding has rarely been investigated. However, two computational models suggest that neuromodulation may affect synchronization (e.g. the stability of synchronization and degrees of synchrony) by either influencing the intrinsic complexity of single-cell dynamics or the effective structure of whole networks (Harris-Warrick and Marder 1991; Wennekers and Pasemann 2001; Breakspear *et al.* 2003). For instance, increasing a parameter that corresponds to increasing the population of transmitter receptors decreases the coupling strength required to achieve stable synchronization (Breakspear *et al.* 2003). In other words, with deficient neuromodulation the ageing brain may require greater coupling strength between cortical columns to achieve synchronization-based binding. The details of how neurochemically modulated representation distinctiveness may affect the coupling strength between local networks and the overall stability of synchronization are open questions for future investigation.

It has also been proposed recently that the neocortex and the hippocampus may engage in two types of conjunctive learning (O'Reilly and Rudy 2001). The neocortex uses distributed overlapping representations for intentional effortful conjunctive learning, whereas the hippocampus uses relatively sparse coding for relatively more automatic incidental conjunction. Although our simulations did not explicitly model both anatomical regions and focused only on the neocortex, our results did show a clear effect of neuromodulation of representational distinctiveness on internally learned conjunctive binding (i.e. with the study pair instruction). There is recent evidence showing ageing-related differences in the functional connectivity between the PFC and hippocampus. In old adults, a stronger connectivity between dorsal lateral PFC and regions involved in attention regulation and the hippocampus is related to better memory performance (Grady *et al.* 2003). Considering our simulation results together with the empirical finding, we conjecture that dopaminergic modulation of representational distinctiveness in regions of the neocortex, such as the PFC, may affect the functional connectivity of the frontal-hippocampal circuitry (Grady *et al.* 2003). If the representations of neural activities elicited by different stimuli are less distinct in the neocortex because of suboptimal neuromodulation, processes requiring dynamic interactions between these representations and neural activities in other brain regions, such as the hippocampus, are likely to be affected. Other researchers (Mitchell *et al.* 2000) have suggested that the dynamics of the frontal-hippocampal circuitry may be implicated in ageing-related deficit of memory binding.

Finally, feature integration theory (Treisman and Gelade 1980) suggests that attention plays an important role in solving the binding problem, but at the same time attention limits may be set by the number of distinctly firing neuronal assemblies to code separate objects (Treisman 1996). Our simulations suggest that neuromodulation affects the distinctiveness of distributed conjunctive coding and may have implications for the relation between attention and basic binding mechanisms. With respect to ageing research, these theoretical observations imply that ageing-related conjunctive binding deficits should not be restricted to mechanisms of episodic memory binding, but should generalize to other binding mechanisms, such as the relations between attention, working memory, and perceptual binding.

Relation to other memory models

Regarding comparisons with other memory models, the feature–association conjunctive binding model (Li *et al.* 2005) is conceptually similar to global memory models which assume combination of multiple memory cues, distributed storage, and separate representations of item and associative information, such as the TODAM model (Murdock 1993). Not all classical memory models can account for the distinctions between item and associative memory (reviewed by Clark and Gronlund 1996). As shown, our model accounts for the finding that item memory is less sensitive to instruction manipulation (intentional versus incidental) than associative memory (Hockley and Cristi 1996).

In addition, the feature–association conjunctive binding model accounts for the differential ageing of item and associative memory. However, a limitation of the model is that it does not directly address the issue of retrieval time course. One possibility of extending the model is by augmenting it with an attractor network involving recurrent connections between the representation and output layers. Nevertheless, assuming that processing times are monotonically related to lack of match between target and actual outputs (Seidenberger and McClelland 1989), the performance advantage of item over associative test in our current implementation suggests that the retrieval time course is faster for item than for associative information, and that this effect is stronger in old networks. However, the model's ability to account simultaneously for the effects of stimulus repetition and response deadline on memory ageing (Jacoby 1999; Light *et al.* 2004) needs to be investigated in future modifications of the model that directly incorporate temporal dynamics.

Conclusion

The neurocognitive system may require multiple mechanisms across different levels to store and dynamically represent relations between multiple objects and complex memory events. Research on adult lifespan differences in associative and context memory is helpful for identifying basic factors contributing to binding mechanisms. Neurocomputational simulations of ageing-related decline in representational distinctiveness suggest that neuromodulatory processes may play a basic role in binding by affecting the efficiency of distributed conjunctive coding across cells within an assembly. The neurocognitive system's task to bind together multiple less distinctive assembly codes is harder for individuals, such as older adults, whose neuromodulatory processes function suboptimally.

References

Arnsten, A.F.T. and Goldman-Rakic, P.S. (1985). Alpha 2-adrenergic mechanisms in prefrontal cortex associated with cognitive declines in aged non-human primates. *Science*, **230**, 1273–1276.

Arnsten, A.F.T., Cai, J.X., Murphy, B.L., and Goldman-Rakic, P.S. (1994). Dopamine D_1 receptor mechanisms in the cognitive performance of young adult and aged monkeys. *Psychopharmacology*, **116**, 143–151.

Bäckman. L. and Farde, L. (2005) The role of dopamine functions in cognitive ageing. In *Cognitive Neuroscience of Aging: Linking Cognitive and Cerebral Aging* (ed R.Cabeza, L.Nyberg, and D.C. Park). New York: Oxford University Press, pp. 58–84.

Bäckman, L., Ginovart, N., Dixon, R.A., *et al.* (2000). Age-related cognitive deficits mediated by changes in the striatal dopamine system. *American Journal of Psychiatry*, **157**, 635–637.

Barlow, H.B. (1972). Single units and cognition: a neurone doctrine for perceptual psychology. *Perception*, **1**, 371–394.

Braver, T.S., Barch, D.M., Keys, D.A., *et al.* (2001). Context processing in older adults: evidence for a theory relating cognitive control to neurobiology in healthy ageing. *Journal of Experimental Psychology: General*, **130**, 746–763.

Breakspear, M., Terry, J.R., and Friston, K.J. (2003). Modulation of excitatory synaptic coupling facilitates synchronization and complex dynamics in a nonlinear model of neuronal dynamics. *Neurocomputing*, **52–54**, 151–158.

Camperi, M. and Wang, X.J. (1998). A model of visuospatial working memory in prefrontal cortex: recurrent network and cellular bistability. *Journal of Computational Neuroscience*, **5**, 383–405.

Chalfonte, B.L. and Johnson, M.K. (1996). Feature memory and binding in young and older adults. *Memory and Cognition*, **24**, 403–416.

Churchland, P.S. and Sejnowski, T.J. (1988). Perspectives on cognitive neuroscience. *Science*, **242**, 741–745.

Clark, A. (1999). An embedded cognitive science? *Trends in Cognitive Sciences*, **3**, 345–351.

Clark, S.E. and Gronlund, S.D. (1996). Global matching models of recognition memory: how the models match the data. *Psychological Bulletin and Review*, **3**, 37–60.

Craik, F.I.M. (1983). On the transfer of information from temporary to permanent memory. *Philosophical Transactions of the Royal Society London, Series B, Biological Sciences*, **302**, 341–359.

Craik, F.I.M. and Anderson, N.D (1999). Applying cognitive approach to problems of ageing. In *Attention and Performance XVII* (ed D. Gopher and A. Koriat). Cambridge, MA: MIT Press, pp. 583–615.

de Keyser, J., De Backer, J.P., Vauquelin, G., and Ebinger G. (1990). The effect of ageing on the D1 dopamine receptors in human cortex. *Brain Research*, **528**, 308–310.

Durstewitz, D., Kelc, M., and Güntürkün, O. (1999). A neurocomputational theory of the dopaminergic modulation of working memory functions, *Journal of Neuroscience*, **19**, 2807–2822.

Giorgi, O., Calderini, G., Toffano, G., and Biggio, G. (1987). D_1 dopamine receptors labeled with ^{3}H-SCH 23390:decrease in the striatum of aged rats. *Neurobiology of Aging*, **8**, 51–54.

Goebel, R.P. and Lewandowsky, S. (1991). Retrieval measures in distributed memory models. In *Relating Theory and Data: Essay on Human Memory in Honor of Bennet B. Murdock* (ed W.E. Hockley and S. Lewandowsky). Hillsdale, NJ: Erlbaum.

Goldman-Rakic, P.S., Muly, E.C., 3rd, and Williams, G.V. (2000). D1 recoptors in prefrontal cells and circuits. *Brain Research Reviews*, **31**, 295–301.

Grady, C.L., McIntosh, A.R., and Craik, F.I.M. (2003). Age-related differences in the functional connectivity of the hippocampus during memory encoding. *Hippocampus*, **13**, 572–586.

Harris-Warrick, R.M. and Marder, E. (1991). Modulation of neural networks for behavior. *Annual Review of Neuroscience*, **14**, 39–57.

Hasselmo, M.E. (1995). Neuromodulation and cortical function: modeling the physiological basis of behavior. *Behavioural Brain Research*, **67**, 1–27.

Head, D., Raz, N., Gunnin-Dixon, F., Williamson, A., and Acker, J. D. (2002). Age-related differences in the course of cognitive skill acquisition: the role of regional cortical shrinkage and cognitive resources. *Psychology and Aging*, **17**, 72–84.

Hessler, N.A., Shirke, A.M., and Malinow, R. (1993). The probability of transmitter release at a mammalian central synapse. *Nature*, **366**, 569–572.

Hockley, W.E. and Cristi, C. (1996). Tests of separate retrieval of item and associative information using a frequency-judgment task. *Memory and Cognition*, **24**, 796–811.

Johnson, M.K. (1992). MEM: mechanisms of recollection. *Journal of Cognitive Neuroscience*, **4**, 268–280.

Johnson, M.K., Hashtroudi, S., and Lindsay, D.S. (1993). Source monitoring. *Psychological Bulletin*, **114**, 3–28.

Kaasinen V., Vilkman, H., Hietala, J., *et al.* (2000). Age-related dopamine D_2/D_3 receptor loss in extrastriatal regions of the human brain. *Neurobiology of Aging*, **21**, 683–688.

Kausler, D. H. (1994). *Learning and Memory in Normal Aging*. New York: Academic Press.

Kliegl, R. and Lindenberger, U. (1993). Modeling intrusions and correct recall in episodic memory: adult age differences in encoding of list context. *Journal of Experimental Psychology: Learning, Memory, and Cognition*, **19**, 617–637.

Köning, P., Engel, A.K., Roelfsema, P.R., and Singer, W. (1995). How precise is neuronal synchronization? *Neural Computation*, **7**, 469–485.

Li, S.-C. (2002). Connecting the many levels and facets of cognitive ageing. *Current Directions in Psychological Science*, **11**, 38–43.

Li, S.-C. (2005). Neurocomputational perspectives linking neuromodulation, processing noise, representational distinctiveness, and cognitive ageing. In *Cognitive Neuroscience of*

Aging: Linking Cognitive and Cerebral Aging (ed R. Cabeza, L. Nyberg, and D.C. Park). New York: Oxford University Press, pp. 354–380.

Li, S.-C. and Sikström, S. (2002). Integrative neurocomputational perspectives on cognitive ageing, neuromodulation, and representation. *Neuroscience and Biobehavioral Reviews*, **26**, 795–808.

Li, S.-C., Lindenberger, U., and Frensch, P. A. (2000). Unifying cognitive ageing: from neuromodulation to representation to cognition. *Neurocomputing*, **32–33**, 879–890.

Li, S.-C., Lindenberger, U., and Sikström, S. (2001). Aging cognition: from neuromodulation to representation. *Trends in Cognitive Sciences*, **5**, 479–486.

Li, S.-C., Lindenberger, U., Hommel, B., Aschersleben, G., Prinz, W., and Baltes, P.B. (2004). Lifespan transformations in the couplings among intellectual abilities and constituent cognitive processes. *Psychological Science*, **15**, 155–163.

Li, S.-C., Naveh-Benjamin, M., and Lindenberger, U. (2005). Aging neuromodulation impairs associative binding. *Psychological Science*, **16**, 445–450.

Light, L.L. (1991). Memory and aging: four hypotheses in search of data. *Annual Review of Psychology*, **42**, 333–376.

Light, L.L., Patterson, M.M., Chung, C., and Healy, M.R. (2004). Effects of repetition and response deadline on associative recognition in young and older adults. *Memory and Cognition*, **32**, 1182–1193.

McIntyre, J.S. and Craik, F.I.M. (1987). Age differences in memory for item and source information. *Canadian Journal of Psychology*, **41**, 175–192.

MacKay, D.G. and Burke, D.M. (1990). Cognition and aging: a theory of new learning and the use of old connections. In *Aging and Cognition: New Knowledge Organization and Utilization* (ed T.M. Hess). Amsterdam: Elsevier, pp. 213–263.

MacRae, P.G., Spirduso, W.W., and Wilcox, R.E. (1988). Reaction time and nigrostriatal dopamine function: the effect of age and practice. *Brain Research*, **451**, 139–146.

Mitchell, K.J., Johnson, M.K., Raye, C.L., and D'Esposito, M. (2000). FMRI evidence of age-related hippocampal dysfunction in feature biding in working memory. *Cognitive Brain Research*, **10**, 197–206.

Morrison, J.H. and Hof, P.R. (1997). Life and death of neurons in the ageing brain. *Science*, **278**, 412–429.

Murdock, B.B., Jr (1993). TODAM 2: a model for the storage and retrieval of item, associative, and serial-order information. *Psychological Review*, **100**, 183–203.

Nadel, L., Samsonovich, A., Ryan, L., and Moscovitch, M. (2000). Multiple trace theory of human memory: Computational, neuroimaging, and neuropsychological results. *Hippocampus*, **10**, 352–368.

Naveh-Benjamin, M. (2000). Adult age differences in memory performance: tests of an associative deficit hypothesis. *Journal of Experimental Psychology: Learning, Memory, and Cognition*, **26**, 1170–1187.

Naveh-Benjamin, M., Hussain, Z., Guez, J., and Bar-On, M. (2003). Adult age differences in episodic memory: further support for an associative-deficit hypothesis. *Journal of Experimental Psychology: Learning, Memory, and Cognition*, **29**, 826–837.

Nieuwenhuis, S., Ridderinkhof, K.R., Talsma, D., *et al.* (2002). A computational account of altered error processing in older age: dopamine and error-related processing. *Cognitive, Affective, and Behavioral Neuroscience*, **2**, 19–36.

O'Reilly, R.C. and Busby, R.S. (2002). Generalizable relational binding from coarse-coded distributed representations. In *Advances in Neural Information Processing Systems (NIPS) 14* (ed T.G. Dietterich, S. Becker, and Z. Gahramani). Cambridge, MA: MIT Press.

O'Reilly, R.C. and Rudy, J.W. (2001). Conjunctive representations in learning and memory: Principles of cortical and hippocampal function. *Psychological Review*, **108**, 311–345.

Raz, N. (2000). Aging of the brain and its impact on cognitive performance: integration of structural and functional findings. In *The Handbook of Aging and Cognition* (2nd edn) (ed F.I.M. Craik and T.A. Salthouse). Mahwah, NJ: Erlbaum, pp. 1–90.

Rizzuto, D.S. and Kahana, M.J. (2001). An auto-associative neural network model f paired-associate learning. *Neural Computation*, **13**, 2075–2092.

Schillen, T.B. and König, P. (1994). Binding by temporal structure in multiple feature domains of an oscillatory neuronal network. *Biological Cybernetics*, **70**, 397–405.

Schneider, E.L., Rowe, J.W., Johnson, T.E., Holbrook, N., and Morrison, J. (ed) (1996). *Handbook of the Biology of Aging*. New York: Academic Press.

Segovia G., Porras, A., Del Arco, A., and Mora, F. (2001). Glutamatergic neurotransmission in ageing: A critical perspective. *Mechanisms of Ageing and Development*, **122**, 1–29.

Seidenberger, M.S. and McClelland, J.L. (1989). A distributed, developmental model of word recognition and naming. *Psychological Review*, **96**, 523–568.

Servan-Schreiber, D., Printz, H., and Cohen, J.D. (1990). A network model of catecholamine effects: gain, signal-to-noise ratio, and behavior. *Science*, **249**, 892–895.

Singer, W. (1998). Consciousness and the structure of neuronal representations. *Philosophical Transactions of the Royal Society London, Series B, Biological Sciences*, **353**, 1829–1840.

Singer, W. (1999). Neuronal synchrony: a versatile code for the definition of relations? *Neuron*, **24**, 49–65.

Singer, W. and Gray, C.M. (1995). Visual feature integration and the temporal correlation hypothesis. *Annual Review of Neuroscience*, **18**, 555–586.

Sowell, E.R., Peterson, B.S., Thompson, P.M., Welcome, S.E., Henkenius, A.C., and Toga, A.W. (2003). Mapping cortical change across the human life span. *Nature Neuroscience*, **6**, 308–315.

Spencer, W.D. and Raz, N. (1995). Differential effects of ageing on memory for content and context: a meta-analysis. *Psychology and Aging*, **10**, 527–539.

Treisman, A. (1996). The binding problem. *Current Opinion in Neurobiology*, **6**, 171–178.

Treisman, A. (1998). Feature binding, attention and object perception. *Philosophical Transactions of Royal Society London, Series B, Biological Sciences*, **353**, 1295–1306.

Treisman, A. (1999). Solutions to the binding problem: progress through controversy and convergence. *Neuron*, **24**, 105–110.

Treisman, A. and Gelade, G. (1980). A feature integration theory of attention. *Cognitive Psychology*, **12**, 97–136.

von der Malsburg, C. (1985). Nervous structures with dynamical links. *Berichte der Bunsen-gesellschaft physikalische Chemie*, **89**, 703–710.

Welford, A.T. (1965). Performance, biological mechanisms and age: a theoretical sketch. In *Behavior, Aging, and the Nervous System* (ed A.T. Welford and J.E. Birren). Springfield, IL: Thomas, pp. 3–20.

Wennekers, T. and Pasemann, F. (2001). Generalized types of synchronization in networks of spiking neurons. *Neurocomputing*, **38–40**, 1037–1042.

Wolpert, D.M., Ghahramani, Z., and Flanagan, J. R. (2001). Perspectives and problems in motor learning. *Trends in Cognitive Sciences*, **5**, 487–494.

Wong, D.F., Young, D., Wilson, P.D., Meltzer, C.C., and Gjedde, A. (1997). Quantification of neuroreceptors in the living brain. III: D2-like dopamine receptors: theory, validation and changes during normal ageing. *Journal of Cerebral Blood Flow and Metabolism*, **17**, 316–330.

Zacks, R.T., Hasher, L., and Li, K.Z.H. (2000). Human memory. In *The Handbook of Aging and Cognition* (2nd edn) (ed F.I.M. Craik and T.A. Salthouse). Mahwah, NJ: Erlbaum, pp. 293–357.

Zahrt, J., Taylor, J.R., Mathew, R.G., and Arnsten, A.F. (1997). Supranormal stimulation of dopamine D1 receptors in the rodent prefrontal cortex impairs spatial working memory performance. *Journal of Neuroscience*, **17**, 8528–8535.

Section 3

Binding in perception and knowledge representation

Chapter 12

Object tokens, binding, and visual memory

Anne Treisman

Introduction

At any moment of time the scene around us is filled with multifeatured objects, which we see from particular angles, distances, and illuminations, and which may themselves move and change. We must recognize their identities in order to retrieve semantic information relevant to our behaviour. However, we also need to represent their current state in order to interact with them, and store an episodic memory of the particular events in which they play a role. Kahneman, Gibbs, and I developed the object file metaphor to help capture this type-token distinction in the perceptual domain and collected data showing object-specific priming to support the idea (Kahneman *et al.* 1992). I also applied it to feature binding (Treisman 1992), to visual working memory (Wheeler and Treisman 2002), to negative priming (Treisman and DeSchepper 1996), and to long-term learning in visual search (Treisman 1992).

Object files in perception

I will start by outlining the perceptual framework. We drew a distinction between the activation of stored types, which mediates identification, and the creation of temporary episodic tokens, which mediates seeing (Kahneman and Treisman 1984). We called the episodic representations 'object files', and suggested that they hold the current description, location, orientation, and distance of the objects around us. Object files are temporary structures, addressed through their spatial locations, in which information accrues over time, just as information about a particular crime might be collected in a specific police file. If the object moves or changes, the object file is updated, creating a perceptually continuous entity

Object files are assumed to play a number of different roles in perception and in memory.

1. Object files are the perceptual units into which a scene is parsed, becoming the potential objects of attention. It is much easier to attend to a whole object than to single out one of its properties. It is also much easier to divide attention between two properties of the same object than between the same two properties when they are seen as belonging to separate objects (Treisman *et al.* 1983; Duncan 1984).
2. Object files allow us to represent novel objects for which we have no prior representations, no object type to reactivate. If an object file matches a known type in semantic memory, its identity is accessed. However, object files can also represent unknown objects.
3. Object files allow us to represent multiple identical objects—to differentiate a flock of sheep from a single very large or sheepish sheep. This might be difficult if all we could vary was the degree of activation of the type node for sheep.
4. Object files serve as vehicles to bind features. Feature integration theory (Treisman and Gelade 1980) proposed that the correct selection of features is achieved through spatial attention. Features that share the same location usually belong to the same object, and so the correct binding can be determined by serial attention to different locations, temporarily excluding features from unattended locations. Evidence for this view includes the facts that search for conjunctions of features is usually serial, and that when focused attention is diverted or overloaded, illusory conjunctions are often formed (Treisman and Schmidt 1982). For example, a red S and a blue O might generate an illusory blue S or red O.
5. Object files also bind successive states of an object over time, updating their representations as the objects move and change. The visual system assumes the continuity of objects in the real world. Kahneman *et al.* (1992) suggested that each object that appears in the scene 'looks for' its immediate past history. When a spatiotemporally compatible match is found, the contents of the earlier object file are compared with the currently present features. If there is a mismatch, we update the file, or, if the change is too great, we open a new one and see a new object. Evidence for this came from the object-specific priming that we found when participants were asked to name letters presented successively, either in the same or in a different moving frame.
6. Object files provide an interface between early vision, top-down knowledge, and conscious experience. The hypothesis is that without an object file, the object is not consciously seen. However, the reverse may not be the case: not all object files become conscious (see the section below on negative priming).

The main theme of this chapter concerns what happens to object files once the objects are no longer visible. How do we store bindings in memory and recognize them over short intervals of time. Wolfe *et al.* (2002) recently gave a short and simple answer: 'We don't'. The conclusion stemmed mostly from the marked 'change blindness' shown when we try to detect a difference between two alternating versions of the same scene (Rensink *et al.* 1997; Simons and Levin 1997). Large changes like the disappearance of an engine on an aeroplane may take many seconds to detect. Instead of the teeming colourful world of detail we think that we have in memory, it seems instead to be a sparse abstracted schematic world, inhabited at most by three or four more detailed objects. We retain the illusion of a rich and detailed memory because in everyday life we are seldom tested. As O'Regan (1992) points out, the real world normally provides an external memory to supply details as we need them.

Within the framework of feature integration theory, there are several forms in which information is encoded and a number of levels at which it could be stored.

1. Features and locations are encoded in separate parallel maps before attention binds them to form integrated objects. They may also leave temporary unbound traces in those separate maps.
2. The object tokens that are formed in object files through focused attention can be transferred to visual working memory for early explicit recall and recognition.
3. They can also be stored in episodic long-term memory as consciously retrievable traces of particular incidents.
4. The object files may remain as implicit traces of perceptual experiences that prime or interfere with later re-perceptions.
5. Finally, they can contribute to the formation of learned associations in semantic memory between features that have been repeatedly perceptually bound.

I will outline some research on each of these kinds of memory and some tentative suggestions about how they may be related over short and longer intervals, in both explicit and implicit memory.

Visual working memory: features and objects

Luck and Vogel (1997) presented displays of coloured squares and tested recognition 900 ms later. The second display either matched the first exactly or had one feature changed. The maximum number of objects that participants could remember accurately was only three or four. However, the number was the same whether the objects had one relevant feature (colour), or two, or even four (colour, length, orientation, and a break in the line). Luck and Vogel suggested that what is encoded and stored in visual working memory (VWM) is a small set of bound objects, to which any number of features can be added for free if they characterize one of the original objects. However, there is an alternative explanation which should be considered. Performance in Luck and Vogel's experiment might also reflect a set of separate feature stores, holding a set of four colours in one, a set of four shapes in another, and so on. Luck and Vogel claimed to have ruled out this alternative by showing that objects that were each characterized by two features within a single dimension (colour) rather than a colour and a shape, for example, also functioned as single memory units. In this case, memory could not recruit new storage space for the additional features, since only one dimension (colour) was varied.

Wheeler and Treisman (2002) were unable to replicate this result. We found that three bicoloured objects were remembered no better than six unicoloured objects. There was no benefit at all from combining colours within fewer objects (Fig. 12.1). This was true whatever patterns we used to integrate the colours, including checkerboards, centre squares with surrounds, and so on. This result is consistent with a similar finding testing parts of shapes. Lee and Chun (2001) compared the capacity of visual memory in change detection for what they called locations and objects. They used either superimposed or separated presentation of three pairs of boxes and lines (cf. Duncan 1984) and found no difference in memory. If we think of the component shapes as equivalent to the colours in our experiment, the inference is the same—integrating two shapes into a single compound unit produces no increase at all in the capacity of VWM. These failures revive the possibility of parallel independent feature stores, each with its own limited capacity, as an explanation of memory for multidimensional stimuli.

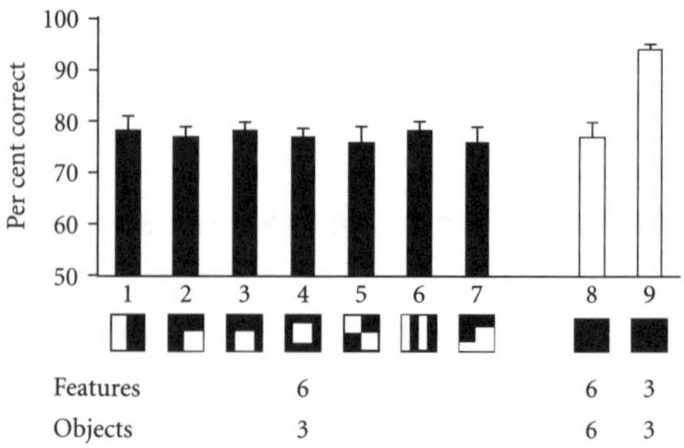

Figure 12.1 Results of the experiment by Wheeler and Treisman (2002) on VWM for combinations of colours. There are no significant differences between these various patterns and the sets of six separate squares, suggesting that integrality has no effect on VWM for colour combinations.

A similar conclusion was reached by Magnussen (2000) from very different data—the psychophysics of delayed discrimination with sine wave gratings varying in spatial frequency, orientation, colour, or motion. He describes a 'low-level perceptual memory mechanism located early in the visual processing stream . . . composed of a series of parallel special-purpose perceptual mechanisms with independent but limited processing resources. Each mechanism is devoted to the analysis of a single dimension and is coupled to a memory store'. Magnussen suggests that even higher-level memory may reflect the same feature traces. 'It remains a distinct possibility that our visual memories, like on-line perceptions, are based on the resurrection of a pattern of precisely-stored single attributes'. The data described in the remainder of this chapter suggest instead that higher-level or longer-term recall depends on a separate memory for object tokens, which incorporates the particular binding in which the features are presented. Working memory can draw on both these object tokens and the traces of separate features lingering in separate sensory feature maps.

My students and I have run a number of further experiments using the change detection paradigm to explore the parameters of explicit voluntary memory over brief intervals of time. We used two different ways of testing the idea that VWM holds bound objects. In the first, we made it impossible to rely on feature stores by specifically asking for recognition of the binding. In the second, we tested how far participants could avoid remembering the binding when they were asked to ignore it and to remember only the features.

In the first two experiments, Wheeler and Treisman (2002) compared memory for features (colour and location in one experiment, colour and shape in the other) with memory for their binding (Fig. 12.2). In the first experiment, we presented participants with an array of three or six coloured squares for 150 ms, followed by a delay of 900 ms, and then a second array which was identical on 50 per cent of trials or could contain either a new feature (colour or location) or unchanged features but a change in their binding (the colours switched between two locations) (Fig. 12.3). The conditions were blocked so that participants knew whether they would be tested on colour, location, either of the two features, or the bindings. In another version of the experiment, different shapes were used and changes of locations were replaced by changes of shapes. Figures 12.3(a) and 12.4(a) show the results. In both experiments, the changes of binding were less likely to be detected than new features. Thus the features seem to be stored at least partly independently of the bound object tokens.

However, the story changed when we used a single probe rather than a whole display. In this condition, the changes of binding were detected as accurately as changes in the least good single feature (Figs 12.3(b) and 12.4(b)). This was true

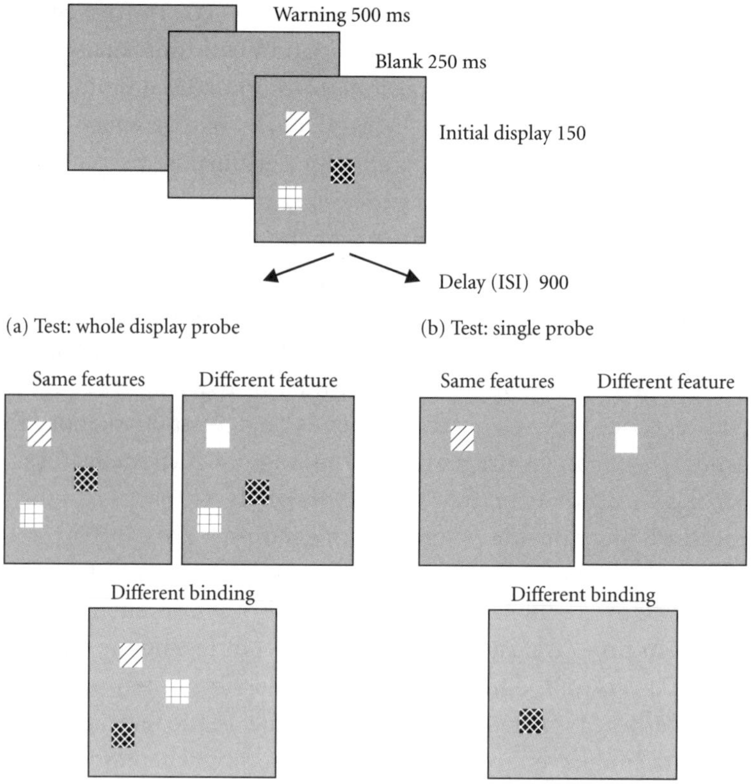

Figure 12.2 Schematic description of the experiment by Wheeler and Treisman (2002) on memory for colours and locations.

for both colour–location and colour–shape binding. One possibility is that there was simply a greater decision load with the whole display. There were several items to be checked in a whole display probe and only one in the single probe condition, giving more chance for error. This did not seem to be the reason. When we presented the whole display at test and then cued one relevant item to be checked, performance was equally bad. The binding must be stored, since it was available with the single probe, but it may be especially vulnerable to the visual interference created by the whole display at test.

We tried to distinguish two forms that this interference might take.

1. Focused attention may be needed, not only to bind the features during the initial encoding of the display, but also to maintain the bindings in VWM. The new visual stimuli in the whole display probe may draw attention away from the stored items in VWM and destroy their binding. The whole display competes for attention more than the single item.

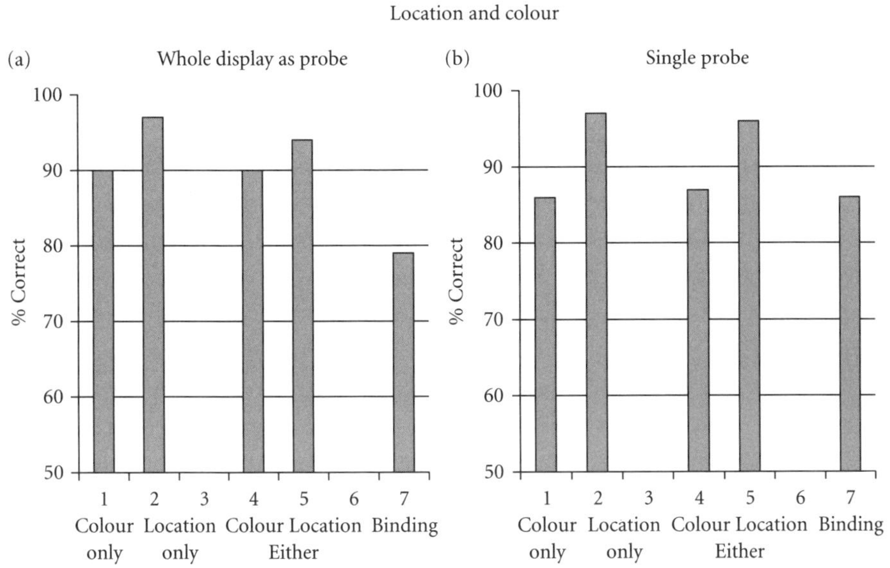

Figure 12.3 Results of the experiment by Wheeler and Treisman (2002) on VWM for colour and location. With the whole display probe, accuracy of detection of changes of binding is significantly lower than detection of changes of either feature separately. The difference disappears with the single probe.

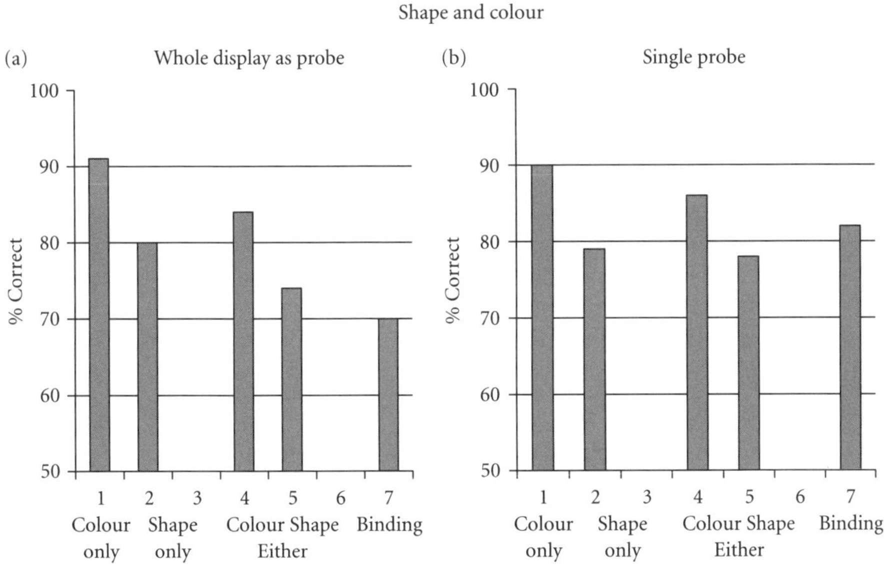

Figure 12.4 Results of the experiment by Wheeler and Treisman (2002) on VWM for colour and shape. Again, with the whole display probe, memory for binding is worse than memory for the separate features, whereas with the single probe there is no difference.

2. Feature bindings may be especially vulnerable to new visual stimuli overwriting previously registered visual information. This would be consistent with the object file model. When Kahneman, Gibbs, and I were exploring the object-specific priming effects that prompted the theory, we asked how far back the priming could originate: just one change back or more? We tried showing two prime letters successively in the same object frame and checked whether there was any object-specific priming from the letter before last as well as from the last letter. The answer was 'no'. Each new state of an object apparently erases the one that precedes it in the same object file. In the present paradigm, the whole display probes appeared in the same locations as the original memory display. The visual system may simply have updated the preceding traces to represent the current state of the world. In the colour–shape experiment, the single probe was presented in the centre of the display rather than in one of the original locations. The colour–location probe was necessarily presented in one of the original locations, but, since it was the only item present, it could draw focused attention, which might allow participants to detect the change when it occurred.

Wheeler and I leaned towards the first account—that it takes attention to maintain bindings in VWM. Now I am not so sure, as I will explain below. Whichever is correct, the fact that the features survive even when the binding is lost suggests that they may be stored at the feature level as well as forming part of the stored object files.

So far I have described experiments looking at explicit memory for binding. In the next experiment, Treisman and Zhang (2006) turned the question around to ask: When items are attended, is binding automatic, so that object files are the only memory traces available? Or can we choose to store features separately and unbound when this is what the task requires? If VWM holds only object files, and the bindings are changed in the probe, this should disrupt memory for the features as well.

We presented three coloured shapes for 150 ms, followed after 900 ms by a probe display (Fig. 12.5). Participants looked for a change in one feature: shape or colour. The bindings could be the same as in the original display or they could be switched around. Participants were told that they should respond 'New' only if a new shape or colour was present, ignoring possible changes of binding. Feature recognition was significantly worse when the binding changed: 62 per cent with changed binding versus 69 per cent when the binding matched. It appears that when participants attend to the display, they automatically store the binding and hold it in VWM, even when it is irrelevant and may interfere with recognition.

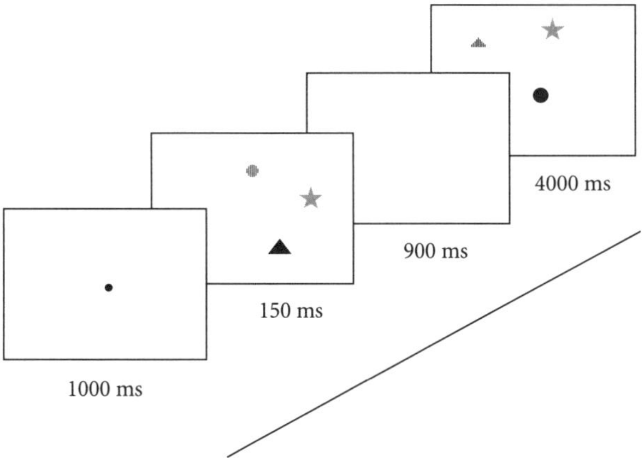

Figure 12.5 Design of experiment by Treisman and Zhang on memory for features with the same or different binding and location.

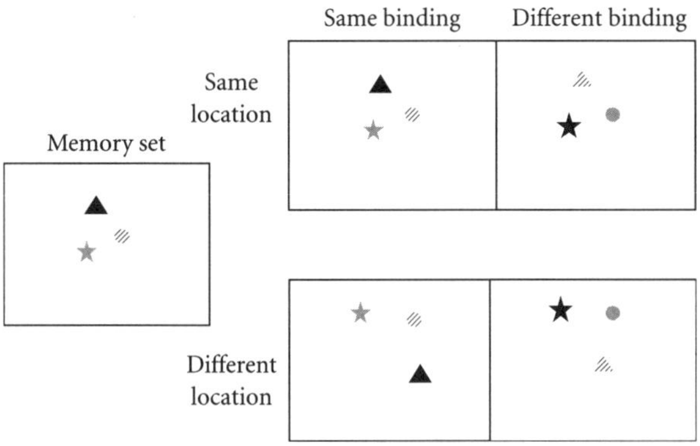

Figure 12.6 Different conditions in the feature recognition experiment by Treisman and Zhang.

We had claimed that attention is necessary for binding. We now find that it may also be sufficient.

Can we say any more about how the features are stored? Are they bound to each other, independently of location, or is each of the features bound to its location and only indirectly to the other features in the same location? In half the blocks we tested recognition in the same locations and in half the blocks we presented the recognition probes in new locations, which had previously been empty (Fig. 12.6). Surprisingly, we found that changing the locations had no overall effect on feature recognition. It is not that the locations were forgotten, because we found large interactions of location with binding (Fig. 12.7). People were better with the same location when the binding was the same and worse when it was different, but there was no overall advantage to using the original locations.

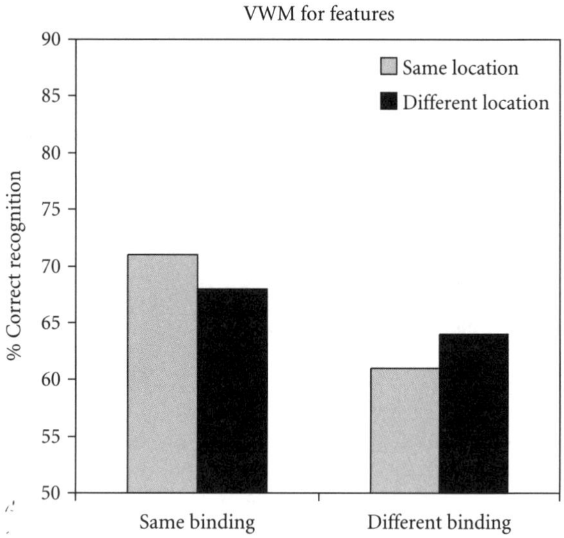

Figure 12.7 Accuracy of detection of feature changes in the experiment by Treisman and Zhang as a function of whether or not the binding and locations were changed. Changing the binding is disruptive. Changing the location has no overall effect, but there is an interaction with changed binding, suggesting that locations are stored only with the bound form of feature memory.

A related experiment was reported by Prabhakaran *et al.* (2000). Memory for letters was tested with probes that were presented either in the same location or in the location previously occupied by a different letter. Unlike our results, recognition in their experiment was more accurate (88.5 compared with 85.7 per cent) and faster (1139 compared with 1261 ms) when the location was the same, suggesting that 'verbal and spatial information in the bound displays were maintained in an integrated fashion in VWM'. However, the advantage of keeping the same locations was not large. It seems that features are stored in object files, but that memory can also be supplemented by information from separate feature stores when binding is not directly tested. Prabhakaran *et al.* also looked at the brain areas activated selectively in the bound condition and found that right prefrontal areas were involved. They suggested that there might be a specialized memory in this brain area for integrated information, perhaps analogous to Baddeley's episodic buffer (Baddeley 2000).

While feature information can be retrieved from either integrated representations or independent feature stores, feature integration theory suggests that locations are critical for the encoding of conjunctions. Are they equally critical for their storage and retrieval, or is it the case that, once the features are bound, the location information can be dropped without losing the conjunctions? Zhang and I used the same stimuli to test VWM for binding. In this experiment, the same features always appeared in the initial display and in the recognition probe (Fig. 12.6). The task was to detect a change of binding rather than the presence of a new feature. In half the trials the binding between two of the objects was changed and in half it remained the same. Participants now performed considerably worse when the objects were presented in new locations, with an average drop of 9 per cent ($F(1,23) = 57.5, P < 0.001$). Unlike the previous tests of memory for features, memory for the bindings was sharply impaired when the locations were new, as though the binding is maintained, as well as initially established, through attention to the locations. Again, this fits well with the object file model. A crucial claim was that object files are addressed by their spatio-temporal coordinates. When these allow a plausible continuity in the object (as when the locations are the same, or when the object is seen in real or apparent motion between the original and new location), the contents of the object file are compared automatically and updated if necessary to match the features currently present. When continuity is not established, as when the objects are presented in arbitrary new locations, new object files are likely to be opened and the comparison with the old ones is less efficient.

We ran some further variants of this experiment, each with 12 participants. In one, the delay was reduced to 100 ms (in the range of iconic memory) to see whether the role of location in memory for binding is different immediately after presentation. In fact, the pattern was similar, but at 100 ms the effect of location was considerably stronger, averaging 18 per cent instead of 9 per cent (Fig. 12.8). The interaction of delay and location was significant ($F(1, 23) = 13.68, P < 0.01$) with errors on 40 per cent of trials when the locations were changed compared

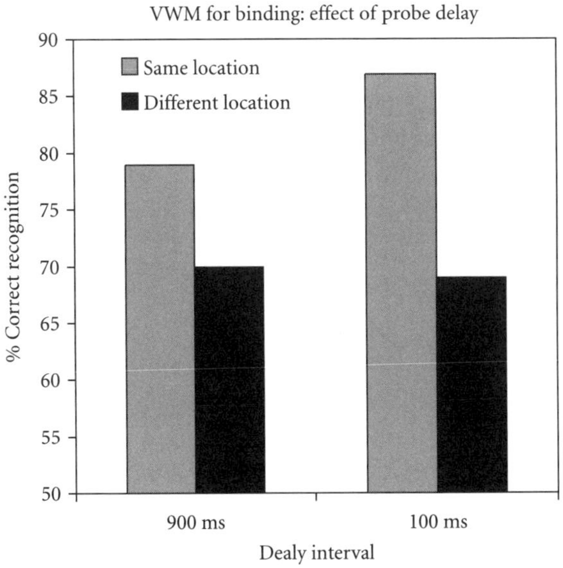

Figure 12.8 Accuracy of detection of changes of binding in experiment 2 by Treisman and Zhang as a function of location changes and probe delay. Changes of location are much more disruptive than they were for detection of feature changes, and the disruption is greater at the shorter delay interval.

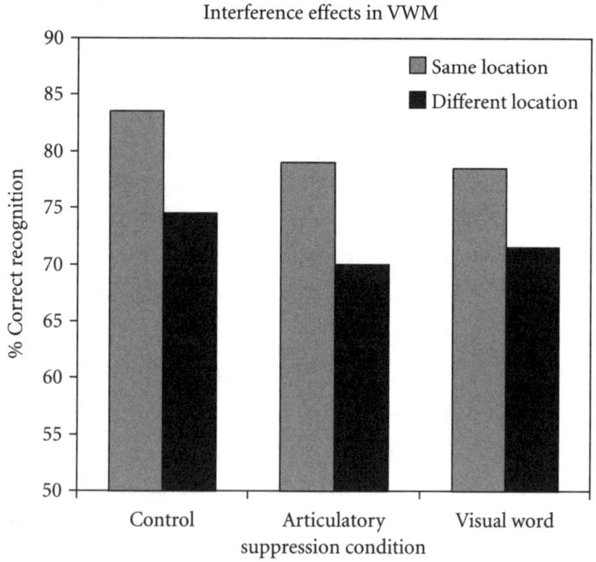

Figure 12.9 Accuracy of detection of changes of binding as a function of articulatory suppression and visual word interference.

with 14 per cent in the same location. The result suggests that the object files are initially closely dependent on location and that the direct link between the features is gradually consolidated over the first second of delay, reducing without eliminating the dependence on location.

Articulatory suppression, which is presumed to reduce or eliminate verbal coding, had little effect. Performance was slightly worse after a 900-ms delay of repeating 'Coca-Cola' relative to an unfilled delay in which naming was possible, but the difference was not significant ($F(1, 23) = 2.37$, $P = 0.137$) (Figs 12.9(a) and 12.9(b)), suggesting that verbal coding is little used, at least with these brief delays. What about visual interference? Presenting a visual word in the centre of the display during the interval between display and test had no effect at all (Fig. 12.9(c)), although reading is automatic and participants almost certainly read the word. The word may be sufficiently different from the coloured shapes not to be taken as an update on the same object files.

What conclusions on VWM can we draw so far? They seem to fit well with the ideas that came out of the earlier work and also add to them. We can set up at most two or three object files which contain bound features and which can survive for at least 900 ms, and probably longer. Adding features on more different dimensions within the same number of object files comes free, or at low cost. The binding is vulnerable to overwriting when a new display of objects is presented, although the features may survive intact. Recognizing features is harder when their binding is changed, suggesting that when we attend to objects, we bind their features automatically whether the binding is relevant or not. Moving the objects to new locations leaves feature recognition unimpaired but damages recognition of the bindings quite severely, especially immediately after presentation. Features are stored in two different forms: as entries in an object file, and also as separate traces, independent of their locations, as predicted by the hypothesis that features and locations are registered initially in separate maps. The object files integrate information across the two sets of representations, binding the features to their locations. Initially the locations are strongly integrated with the object file, but this dependence diminishes as the memory delay increases and direct bindings between features within object files are consolidated.

Relation between visual working memory and long-term memory

Another question concerns the relation between VWM and long-term memory (LTM). There have been a number of hypotheses (Fig. 12.10). In an early account by Atkinson and Shiffrin (1971), short-term memory was a gateway or way-station to LTM. The representations were presumably transformed into a different format to gain admission, since they were vulnerable to different forms of interference. A second account, proposed by Anderson (1983) and also adopted by Cowan (1995, 1999), makes VWM a temporarily activated subset of LTM, presumably implying that it shares both the format and the information encoded in that subset. In a third account, VWM is seen as a separate system with its own properties, accessed in parallel with LTM rather than necessarily preceding it, although information can be transferred in either direction between the two. Baddeley's multistore model of VWM is the best-known elaboration of this view (Baddeley 1986). It is also supported by neuropsychological evidence of dissociations resulting from brain lesions in different brain systems (Della Sala and Logie

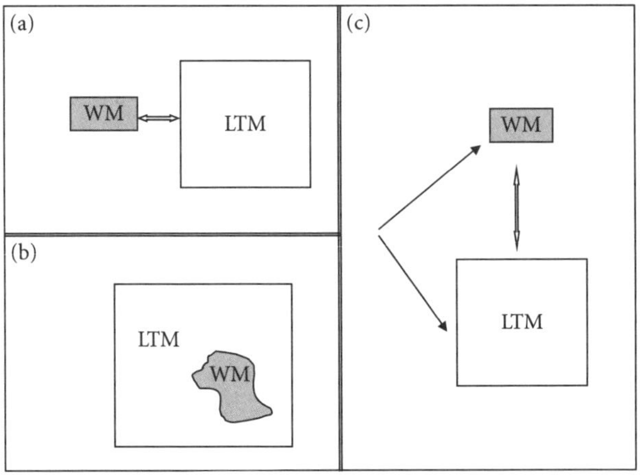

Figure 12.10 Three possible relationships between VWM and LTM: (a) the traditional sequential model; (b) VWM as a temporarily activated subset of LTM; (c) separate and independent stores with the possibility of parallel access.

1993). There could be an evolutionary advantage for a separate VWM, since the properties it needs are quite different from those needed in LTM. They include instant or rapid access, literal recall, quick erasure, and the ability to carry out various online operations or transformations of the material. Baddeley (2000) has more recently added a bridging store that he calls the episodic buffer. It has many of the characteristics of LTM, including semantic and syntactic chunking and multimodal binding, but it retains other characteristics of VWM, such as limited capacity, temporary availability, and immunity to the forms of amnesia that devastate LTM.

Recently, a number of authors (e.g. Crowder 1993; Cowan 1999; Ranganath *et al.* 2003; Ruchkin and Grafman 2003) have argued against any separation between VWM and LTM on the grounds that similar brain areas are activated in imaging studies of both. However, differences in brain activation between short- and long-term memory tasks can also be found (e.g. Braver *et al.* 2001; Cabeza *et al.* 2002). The assumption that items can enter either or both VWM and LTM in parallel, directly from perceptual encoding, makes it difficult to test whether they are distinct systems or a single unitary store activated in different ways. The more similar the information in VWM is to that stored in LTM, the more plausible the single-store view becomes.

Conditions that increase the likelihood of testing VWM rather than the early stages of LTM (assuming that they are separate systems) include repeatedly reusing the same items in different contexts, so that the information from each trial must be deleted and replaced to minimize inter-trial interference. Using trial-unique items increases the probability of automatic long-term storage and retrieval, since novelty gives an advantage in retention, thus blurring the distinction between VWM and LTM when recall is tested at short intervals.

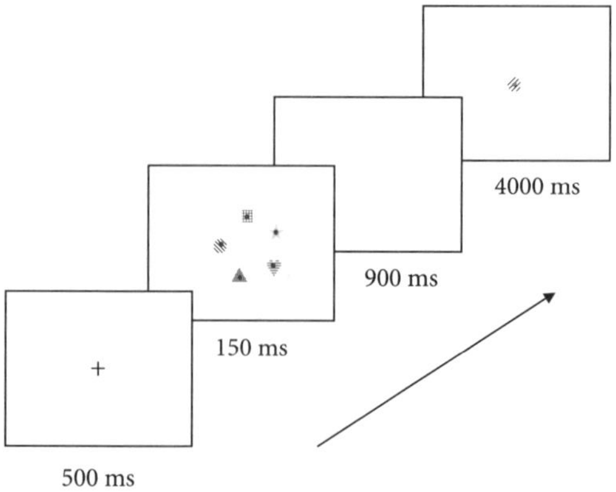

Figure 12.11 Design of the experiment by Treisman and Dishon-Berkovits. Participants attended to either colour or shape, and the experiment explored the effect of consistent pairings of the two features on both LTM and VWM.

Dishon-Berkovits and I ran a preliminary experiment to test possible interactions between VWM and LTM. If VWM is an activated subset of LTM, one might expect any relevant learning to show up in both. We explored the possibility that VWM would benefit from long-term learning of contingencies between properties, so that consistent property bindings would also provide facilitation when tested in VWM paradigms. We presented a circular array of five coloured shapes in a change detection paradigm similar to those described earlier (Fig. 12.11). This time the task was to attend to one dimension of the stimuli (either their colour or their shape) and state whether the probe matched on the attended dimension. Participants always knew which dimension was relevant.

The new factor in this experiment was the introduction of long-term consistencies between the two dimensions, colour and shape. Some combinations of colour and shape were much more frequent than others. For example, for one subject red might be paired with triangle, blue with circle, green with square, and so on in 80 per cent of the trials. In a surprise test after the experiment, we asked whether these contingencies had been learned, measuring explicit recall of the high-frequency pairings. That was the long-term learning component, recording the trial-to-trial accumulation of frequencies.

We tested a VWM expression of this long-term binding by looking for dependencies between colour and shape in the within-trial responses. If the predictable pairings were represented in VWM as well as LTM, performance should be better for a group exposed to the frequent colour–shape conjunctions than it was for a control group in which there were no contingencies—shape and colour varied orthogonally.

We also looked at the effects of short-term within-trial colour–shape binding. The irrelevant dimension could either agree with the relevant dimension in being old or new or it could disagree (old when the relevant dimension was new or new when it was old). Thus each test item could either match or mismatch in terms of the response that the two features would evoke on any given trial. If the shape and colour are automatically bound in VWM, a mismatch should interfere with the response and a match should facilitate it.

Thus we used three different measures of memory for colour–shape bindings: recall of the high-frequency colour–shape pairings in the surprise test at the end of the experiment (LTM), better VWM performance with associated pairs than with random pairings (LTM effect on VWM), and within-trial binding in VWM, shown in the effects of consistency in the responses evoked by the relevant and irrelevant dimensions.

Finally, for each of these three measures of associative memory, we also asked if it matters whether the colours and shapes are presented in an integrated form

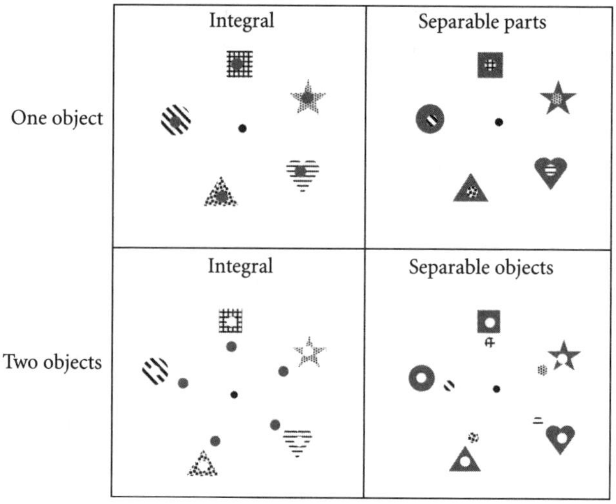

Figure 12.12 Different forms of integrality or separability of shape and colour in two versions of the experiment by Treisman and Dishon-Berkowitz.

or are spatially separated, either as parts within an object or as different objects (Fig. 12.12). Xu (2002) found a large benefit in change detection in either of two different features (colour and orientation) when the features characterized different parts of the same object (mushroom stem and cap) relative to separate stems and caps. In contrast, Walker and Hinkley (2003) found that recognition memory for colours cued by their associated shapes was at chance when naming was prevented and the colours were presented as a non-integral background to the white shapes with which they were associated. On the other hand, we found no significant effect overall of integrality (68.6 per cent integral and 68.2 per cent separable). Surprisingly, accuracy was closely matched for recognition of a grey shape with a coloured central dot, a coloured shape with a grey central dot, a separate coloured shape adjacent to a grey dot, and a separate grey shape adjacent to a coloured dot. The difference from Walker and Hinkley's results may be due to the fact that both our integral and separable stimuli were presented as figures, whereas their separable colours were presented as backgrounds to the figural shapes and therefore may have been subject to some attentional suppression. Xu's results may differ from ours because memory was tested explicitly for both colours and shapes, whereas our participants responded explicitly to only one of the two features. Implicit processing, shown in indirect measures of consistency, may be less constrained by perceptual organization than explicit processing. Another difference is that the components of our separate pairs were still spatially grouped, whereas those in Xu's experiment were independently located. Since we found no effects of integrality, the remaining discussion will refer to results pooled across the integrality–separability factor.

To see if there was any long-term learning of the colour–shape contingencies, we looked at the post-experiment questionnaire. Participants did far better than chance when asked to report the pairings at the end of the experiment. In the shape-relevant condition participants had a mean accuracy of 65 per cent, and in the colour-relevant condition they had a mean accuracy of 36 per cent, where the chance probability of obtaining a correct pairing was about 15 per cent. Thus participants did learn at least some of the consistencies across trials. However, we found absolutely no benefit from these long-term contingencies in VWM recognition. Compared with control groups for whom the colours and shapes were orthogonally combined, there was a small and insignificant benefit of correlation in the experiment with integral or separable parts and an almost significant cost of correlation in the experiment with integral or separable objects ($P = 0.059$). We have no explanation for the apparent reversal, but we can conclude that there is no evidence for any consistent use of long-term contingencies in the VWM task. There was also no within-trial difference between the correlated items and the one randomly paired item within the correlated condition. Finally, there was no correlation between long-term learning and VWM performance. The Pearson correlation between the number of correct pairings reported by each participant and his or her overall mean accuracy in the VWM task was -0.19. Thus, although participants did learn some of the pairings between the relevant and irrelevant dimensions in the correlated conditions, that 'knowledge' did nothing to improve their recognition performance in VWM.

What about binding within VWM? Perhaps we found no benefit from the correlated colours and shapes simply because the task did not require any binding. Recognition was tested only for one of the two features (shape or colour). Our earlier experiment suggests that binding is automatic when the objects are attended to, and we also have evidence here that the colours and shapes were bound, even though recall of the bindings was not required. We compared performance when the irrelevant feature evoked the same response as the relevant feature or the opposite response (match versus mismatch to the initial display). We did find an effect of consistency, suggesting again that binding occurs automatically in VWM. However, it was present only when shape was relevant, giving a significant interaction between match/mismatch and colour versus shape. The findings suggest an asymmetry in the processing of colour and shape in VWM: Shapes retrieve colours more readily than the reverse. In sum, we seem to have some binding in VWM and in LTM, but no interaction between the two sets of associations. The results fit better with separate differently specialized stores than with the activated subset view. Of course, it is possible that both forms of short-term storage are used: persisting passive activation in LTM, and voluntary active rehearsal in VWM. The question would then become which form is responsible for performance in particular specific conditions. In the next section we discuss a passive form of memory revealed through priming that can affect immediate as well as long-delayed responses.

Implicit memory for bound object tokens

One of the surprising findings in this research has been how little we store of what we have just seen. Three or four bound objects is not much. The change blindness phenomenon is another dramatic demonstration of this limit (Rensink *et al.* 1997; Simons and Levin 1997). Does the brain really not have the capacity to lay down more information about the world around us?

Perhaps the limit is more on conscious access than on storage. Some implicit measures of memory offer quite dramatic evidence of long-term storage of a large number of novel objects to which participants had not even paid attention. Tipper (1985) found that responses are slower to a currently attended object when it has previously been ignored, a phenomenon he called 'negative priming'. He used a small set of familiar objects, and so his results could perhaps be explained with the notion of object types; for example, the representation of a trumpet in the mental dictionary of objects could be made temporarily less accessible, so that it is harder to respond with its name. DeSchepper and I ruled out this possibility by using novel nonsense shapes that participants had never seen before, similar to those used earlier by Rock and Gutman (1981). Participants had to decide whether the green shape in overlapped red and green pairs matched a white shape to the right of it (Fig. 12.13). We found clear negative priming from the previously unattended red shapes after a single exposure to a novel shape (DeSchepper and Treisman 1996).

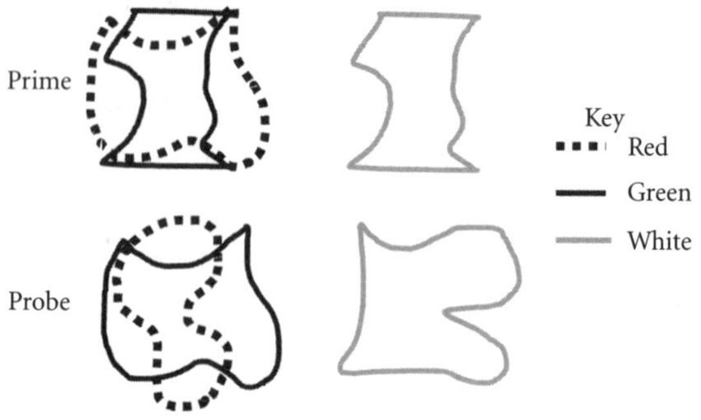

Figure 12.13 Example of displays in the negative priming experiment by DeSchepper and Treisman (1996). Participants decided whether the green shape in the overlapped pair matched the white shape to the right. The ignored red shape on one trial could become the attended green shape on a subsequent trial, giving slightly longer mean response latencies.

Our results cannot be explained in terms of activation or inhibition of stored representations of familiar types. We used 270 nonsense shapes, each seen only once before being tested. In our original experiment, the representation of the previously ignored red shape must have been held in memory for at least 1–2 s to affect the next trial. We tested whether it lasted longer than that and found that the negative priming effect was undiminished after 3, 10, 100, and 200 intervening trials. Growing more and more surprised, we asked new groups of participants to come back after a day, a week, and a month, and we still saw effects of the initial exposure. There were substantial individual differences, and so we divided the participants according to whether they showed negative priming after one trial, and then tested them on a different set of shapes after the various delays shown in Fig. 12.14. Both groups showed significant effects, but they took the form of inhibition for the group who showed negative priming and facilitation for the others. What seems to happen with the passage of time is that the inhibition decreases and the positive facilitation increases, as if the response tags saying 'ignore me' and creating the inhibitory effect are lost earlier than the traces of the shapes. These survive independently of the response tags and prime perception of the shapes when they are presented again.

Are these memory traces available to the participants when we ask for explicit recognition of the unattended shapes? It seems not. Participants were at chance in both immediate and delayed tests in deciding which shapes they had seen but ignored and which had not been presented. Apparently attention is needed to

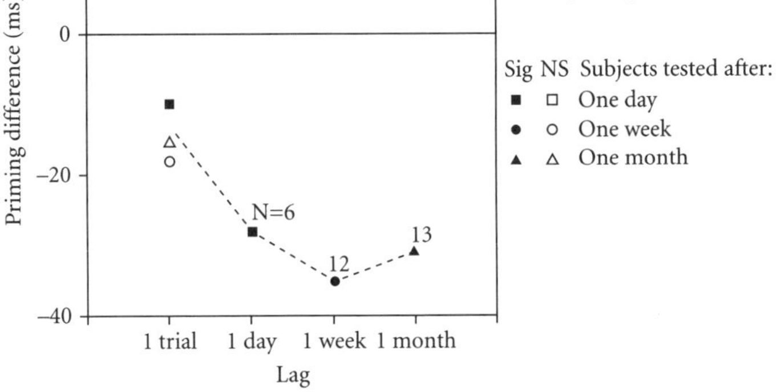

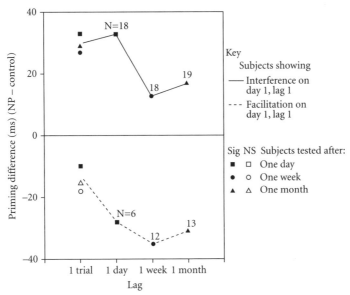

Figure 12.14 Negative and positive priming results at different delays for participants divided according to whether or not they had shown negative priming in an initial test with a different set of shapes.

make memories explicitly available. This may help to account for the apparent discrepancy between the negative priming results, implying persistent detailed traces of a large set of novel shapes after a single unattended exposure, and the very limited storage suggested by the change blindness results. The memory traces that mediate priming are usually thought to be changes in the perceptual system that initially registered them—a kind of 'greasing of pathways'. This may be plausible in some cases of positive priming, but in our negative priming experiments the implicit traces seem to be individuated tokens. They involve some binding of colour to shape and they must be labelled as relevant or irrelevant to the action, to be attended or to be ignored. Whether these are the same tokens that, if attended, would become available to conscious voluntary retrieval, or different tokens with different properties is not yet clear. However, the fact that the traces in negative priming last a long time and are not simply increases in the fluency of processing, as could be the case in positive or repetition priming, does suggest distinct object representations which can in some way be tagged as relevant or irrelevant.

Search, priming, and long-term contingencies

Another form of conjunction priming can be seen across trials in visual search tasks. Treisman *et al.* (1992) introduced long-term contingencies here also. We showed that conjunction targets are detected faster when they frequently occur in a particular location than when they can appear anywhere in the display (Fig. 12.15). For example if the pink Q target usually appears at 3 o'clock in a circular array whereas the green R target can appear anywhere, the pink Q in its habitual location is detected up to 300 ms faster—a large effect. This was true, even when participants were quite unaware of the contingencies. It seems to reflect implicit learning.

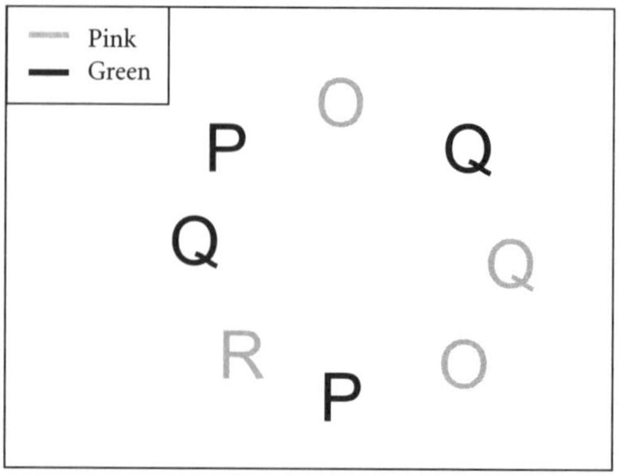

Figure 12.15 Example of display in search for conjunction targets (e.g. pink Q and green R) with two targets appearing mostly in consistent locations and two others in randomly varying locations.

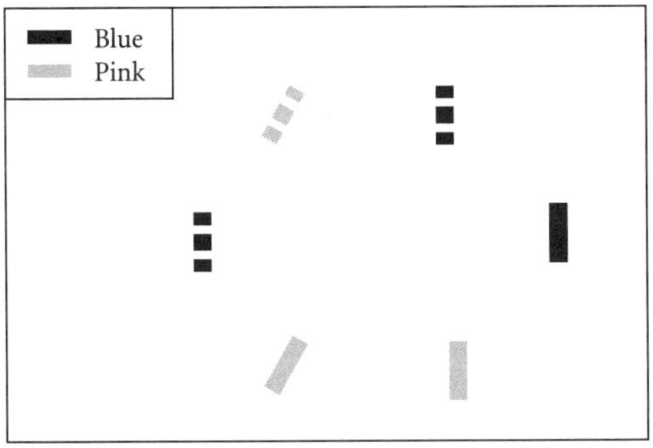

Figure 12.16 Example of display in search for conjunction targets (e.g. solid vertical bar) with irrelevant feature (e.g. blue) consistently paired on most trials.

In another experiment we introduced contingencies in other irrelevant properties in addition to location (Fig. 12.16). We found that detection was also faster for the frequent pairings when, for example, a solid blue bar target was usually vertical, or when a tilted broken target was usually pink, even though the targets were defined only by the first two features listed. This reflects some long-term but implicit learning of object tokens with all their features bound together, even those irrelevant to the task.

In an experiment that is so far unpublished we tried setting up contingencies in the distractor items rather than the targets. Chun and Jiang (1998) found implicit priming from a consistent spatial layout of distractor items in a visual search task. We found the same. Participants apparently learned associations between particular distractors and the locations in which they typically appeared. They showed faster responses when the display conformed to those associations. However, we observed a further surprising effect, suggesting very specific memorial matching. We analysed the results according to the degree of contrast between a current target and the distractor that had in the past most often occupied the same location, and found a substantial effect on detection times. For example, if a particular location normally contained a green P, participants were quicker to detect the very different pink Q target in that location than a more similar green R. It was as if they were matching the new display against an expected spatial layout of object tokens and detecting mismatches faster when they were more salient. I believe that this fits well with the object file framework. It lends some reality to the notion that new objects are matched to the traces of past object tokens that occupied the same locations earlier in time. All these conjunction priming effects suggest that implicit traces of many bound object tokens can survive in memory for long periods, despite interference from multiple intervening displays, even when explicit access to them has apparently been lost or was never established.

Conclusions

1. For explicit VWM, object tokens are stored in a limited-capacity vulnerable store that maintains the bindings of features for just two to four objects. Attention is required to sustain the memories. They are matched to new stimuli on the basis of their locations, and the object files are updated, erasing memory for their earlier states. In addition, we retain some traces of unbound features, which allow better recognition of feature changes than of binding changes.
2. Although the data do not yet rule out a unitary store, our evidence is consistent with the idea that VWM is a separate system from LTM, specialized for different tasks and storing information in different forms, In the task we used, in which the bindings were not explicitly relevant, we found little effect of feature integrality. However, it is possible that there would be more effect of the presentation format if the features had not been perceptually grouped in both cases, or if participants were asked to recall the bindings explicitly, as in the experiment by Xu (2000).
3. Perception also leaves implicit traces that can speed or slow performance when the tokens are presented again. Capacity here is much larger and the duration of the traces much longer. These implicit traces do meet some of the criteria for tokens. They bind features and can be tagged for their relevance to action. It appears unlikely that simply changing the ease of activating previously used perceptual pathways could mediate these effects.

The story that tentatively begins to emerge can be summarized as follows. In perceiving the world, we first form representations of the separate features that are present. We then bind the features through their locations to form integrated object tokens. Memory traces remain of both the separate features and the object tokens. The former are independent of their locations, while the tokens are at least initially accessed through the locations in which the bindings were formed. Only a few bound tokens (two to four) can be explicitly maintained in VWM and subsequently accessed in recognition memory tasks. This requires continued attention. Without attention, or with new intervening presentations, the bindings are quickly lost., at least to explicit conscious awareness. However, many additional object tokens may remain implicitly available to prime their later re-perception or to inhibit it if they were previously ignored. Thus there seems to be a dissociation between, on the one hand, forming multiple bound object tokens that persist over time and may prime future perception and, on the other hand, storing the tokens explicitly in a voluntarily accessible form. The main costs in human memory appear to relate to voluntary retrieval. Why the latter should pose such a severe memory bottleneck if the former is possible is an intriguing topic for future research.

Acknowledgements

The research was supported by grants from the National Institutes of Health Conte Center (P50 MH62196), from the Israeli Binational Science Foundation (1000274), and from the National Institutes of Health (RO1 MH 58383).

References

Anderson, J.A. (1983). *The Architecture of Cognition*. Cambridge, MA: Harvard University Press.

Atkinson, R.C. and Shiffrin, R.M. (1971). The control of short term memory. *Scientific American*, **225**, 82–90.

Baddeley, A. (1986). *Working Memory*. Oxford: Oxford University Press.

Baddeley, A.D. (2000). The episodic buffer: a new component of working memory? *Trends in Cognitive Sciences*, **4**, 417–423

Braver, T., Barch, D., Kelley, W.M., *et al.* (2001). Direct comparison of prefrontal cortex regions engaged by working and long-term memory tasks. *NeuroImage*, **14**, 48–59.

Cabeza, R., Dolcos, F., Graham, R., and Nyberg, L. (2002). Similarities and differences in the neural correlates of episodic memory retrieval and working memory. *NeuroImage*, **16**, 317–330.

Chun, M.M. and Jiang, Y. (1998). Contextual cueing: implicit learning and memory of visual context guides spatial attention. *Cognitive Psychology*, **36**, 28–71.

Cowan, N. (1995). *Attention and Memory: An Integrated Framework*. Oxford: Oxford University Press.

Cowan, N. (1999). An embedded-processes model of working memory. In *Models of Working Memory* (ed A. Miyake and P. Shah). New York: Cambridge University Press, pp. 62–101.

Crowder, R. G. (1993). Short-term memory: where do we stand? *Memory and Cognition*, **21**, 142–145.

Della Sala, S. and Logie, R.H. (1993). When working memory does not work: the role of working memory in neurospychology. *Handbook of Neuropsychology*, Vol. 8. (ed H. Spinnler and F. Boller). Amsterdam: Elsevier, pp. 1–62.

DeSchepper, B. and Treisman, A. (1996). Visual memory for novel shapes: implicit coding without attention. *Journal of Experimental Psychology: Learning, Memory, and Cognition*, **22**, 27–47.

Duncan, J. (1984). Selective attention and the organization of visual information. *Journal of Experimental Psychology: General*, **113**, 501–517.

Kahneman, D. and Treisman, A. (1984). Changing views of attention and automaticity. In *Varieties of Attention* (ed. R. Parasuraman and R. Davies). New York: Academic Press, pp. 29–61.

Kahneman, D., Treisman, A., and Gibbs, B. (1992). The reviewing of object files: object-specific integration of information. *Cognitive Psychology*, **24**, 175–219.

Lee, D. and Chun, M.M. (2001). What are the units of visual short-term memory: objects or spatial locations? *Perception and Psychophysics*, **63**, 253–257.

Luck, S.J. and Vogel, E.K. (1997). The capacity of visual working memory for features and conjunctions. *Nature*, **390**, 279–281.

Magnussen, S. (2000). Low level memory processes in vision. *Trends in Neuroscience*, **23**, 247–251.

O'Regan, K. (1992). Solving the 'real' mysteries of visual perception: the world as an outside memory. *Canadian Journal of Psychology*, **46**, 461–488.

Prabhakaran, V., Narayanan, K., Zhao, Z., and Gabrieli, J.D. (2000). Integration of diverse information in working memory within the frontal lobes. *Nature Neuroscience*, **3**, 85–90.

Ranganath, C., Johnson, M.K., and D'Esposito, M. (2003). Prefrontal activity associated with working memory and episodic long-term memory, *Neuropsychogia*, **41**, 378–389.

Rensink, R.A., O'Regan, J.K. and Clark, J. (1997). To see or not to see: the need for attention to perceive changes in scenes. *Psychological Science*, **8**, 368–373.

Rock, I. and Gutman, D. (1981). The effect of inattention and form perception. *Journal of Experimental Psychology: Human Perception and Performance*, **7**, 275–285.

Ruchkin, D.S., Grafman, J., Cameron, K., and Berndt, R.S. (2003). Working memory retention systems: a state of activated long-term memory. *Behavioral and Brain Science*, **26**, 709–728.

Simons, D.J. and Levin, D.T. (1997). Change blindness. *Trends in Cognitive Sciences*, **1**, 261–267.

Tipper, S.P. (1985). The negative priming effect: inhibitory effects of ignored primes. *Quarterly Journal of Experimental Psychology*, **37A**, 571–590.

Treisman, A. (1992). Perceiving and re-perceiving objects. *American Psychologist*, **47**, 862–875.

Treisman, A. and DeSchepper, B. (1996). Object tokens, attention, and visual memory. In *Attention and Performance XVI: Information Integration in Perception and Communication* (ed T. Inui and J. McClelland). Cambridge, MA: MIT Press, pp. 15–46.

Treisman, A. and Gelade, G. (1980). A feature integration theory of attention. *Cognitive Psychology*, **12**, 97–136.

Treisman, A. and Schmidt, H. (1982). Illusory conjunctions in the perception of objects. *Cognitive Psychology*, **14**, 107–141.

Treisman, A., Kahneman, D., and Burkell, J. (1983). Perceptual objects and the cost of filtering. *Perception and Psychophysics*, **33**, 527–532.

Treisman, A., Vieira, A. and Hayes, A. (1992). Automaticity and preattentive processing. *American Journal of Psychology*, **105**, 341–362.

Treisman, A. and Zhang, W. (in press). Location and binding in visual working memory. *Memory and Cognition.*

Walker, P. and Hinkley, L. (2003). Visual memory for shape-color conjunctions utilizes structural descriptions of letter shape. *Visual Cognition*, **10**, 987–1000.

Wheeler, M.E. and Treisman, A.M. (2002). Binding in short-term visual memory. *Journal of Experimental Psychology: General*, **131**, 48–64.

Wolfe, J.M., Oliva, A., Butcher, S.J., and Arsenio, H.C. (2002). An unbinding problem? The disintegration of visible, previously attended objects does not attract attention. *Journal of Vision*, **2**, 256–271.

Xu, Y. (2002). Limitations in object-based feature encoding in visual short-term memory. *Journal of Experimental Psychology: Human Perception and Performance*, **28**, 458–468.

Chapter 13

Psychophysiological evidence for binding and unbinding arithmetic knowledge representations

Frank Rösler, Kerstin Jost, and Michael Niedeggen

Introduction

Mental calculation is a complex cognitive skill requiring the interplay of several distinct processing components. Ad hoc, one can conceive at least three processes which may be invoked by a particular mental calculation problem: **retrieval of well-established facts** from declarative memory (e.g. $3 \times 4 = 12$), **retrieval of calculation rules** (e.g. any number multiplied by zero will be zero), and, if a result is not immediately available from memory, the **application of production rules** to compute the correct solution (e.g. 36×8: first calculate 30×8, then calculate 6×8, and then add the two partial results) (McCloskey 1992). More complex arithmetic problems, such as multidigit operations, require the partitioning of the problem into several simpler problems (Hitch 1978). The sequence of steps has to be planned and controlled, and intermediate results must be maintained in working memory (Dehaene and Cohen 1995). Moreover, conceptual knowledge (e.g. understanding the arithmetic operations and laws pertaining to these operations) is crucial in solving such complex problems (Sokol and McCloskey 1991). It is evident from these examples that mental arithmetic involves well-learned procedures, problem-solving skills, and a reliance on working memory. It is also evident that executive functions which bind representations in working memory, start and stop production rules, guide access to stored facts, or maintain representations of partial results and of production rules in an active state must also be involved.

Binding and unbinding of arithmetic knowledge

Transient binding and unbinding of associations seems to be of particular importance for mental calculation. Hearing or seeing a multiplication problem such as $3 \times 8 = ?$ will trigger the correct result 24. But how is this achieved? The correct result 24 must also be linked in long-term memory to other operand combinations, such as 4×6, and, vice versa, each of the two operands 3 and 8 must have links to other multiples of the three or eight times tables. Even this cannot be the whole story, as exactly the same operands must also have links to possible sums such as $3 + 8 = 11$ and $4 + 6 = 10$. These few examples show immediately that mental calculation knowledge must be stored in a highly interconnected network of numerical representations whose links are transiently activated by the particular operand combination and the particular operation sign. Moreover, the activation of the relevant link must be 'protected' against competing activations which are triggered by the same operands. The complexity of the task to be solved by the system becomes even more obvious if one considers that these transient bindings, which are relevant for one problem, might be irrelevant and even a hindrance in the next problem in a computation sequence or the next step in a multidigit problem. For example, consider the problem sequence $(3 + 4) \times 4 = ?$. Here the operand 4 must first be transiently bound to the intermediate result of the sum $3 + 4 = 7$ and in the next step the same numerical representation 4 must be bound to the multiplication result $7 \times 4 = 28$. Most likely, the first binding must be suppressed or inhibited in order to activate the second binding. This needs continuous and well-tuned control of the activation levels of number representations. If we replace the numbers by words and the operation signs by grammatical rules, the scenario looks similar to language processing episodes. There also, exactly the same elements (morphemes, function words, and content words) must be transiently bound and unbound in order to compute the correct meaning of a sentence (e.g. 'That man that had been attacked by the robber sat on a bank in front of the bank which was located at the bank of the river').

The existence of such interactions between competing associations of number representations can easily be demonstrated by carry-over effects from one problem to the next in longer sequences of problems. For example, Campbell and colleagues (Campbell and Clark 1989; Campbell 1991) studied errors in sequences of multiplication problems and found that preceding results and operands had a substantial impact on how fast and how accurately a current problem was solved in a speeded production task. There were both negative and positive priming effects, i.e. inhibition and facilitation of results by related answers retrieved on previous trials.

Such interactions can also be observed between representations which belong to different knowledge domains as addition and multiplication facts (Miller *et al.* 1984). We investigated how addition and multiplication might interfere by presenting both types of problems in either a 'blocked' or a 'mixed' condition in a verification task (Jost and Rösler 2003). In the blocked condition participants performed one operation for 32 trials and then switched to the other operation in the next block. In the mixed condition, participants had to switch between addition (A) and multiplication (M) every second trial (AAMMAAMM). The problems were presented in a verification task with 50 per cent incorrect solutions. Half of the incorrect solutions were correct for the alternative competing operation, i.e. it was the product if an addition was required (e.g. $3 + 5 = 15$), or the sum if a multiplication was required (e.g. $4 \times 5 = 9$). These interfering results were contrasted with non-interfering results which were completely unrelated to the problems, i.e. incorrect with respect to both operations (e.g. $4 \times 5 = 21, 3 + 6 = 10$).

For multiplication problems the sum of the two operands proved to be more difficult to reject in the mixed than in the blocked condition (Fig. 13.1(a), black bars) and this rejection time was significantly longer than the time for accepting the correct result (for similar findings see Winkelmann and Schmidt 1974; Zbrodoff and Logan 1986). The interference effect was most prominent in trials in the mixed condition which involves a switch from the addition to the multiplication operation. Thus non-relevant representations of addition results appear to remain partially bound to the operands when they define a multiplication problem. No comparable intrusion effect was found for addition problems: Response times (RTs) for interfering products and correct sums were almost the same (Fig. 13.1(b), black bars). However, another effect can be seen for addition; the a priori unrelated solution (Result ± 1) caused the greatest RT delay in both mixed and blocked conditions.

The asymmetric effect of related solutions suggests that if both task sets are relevant the operands of a problem automatically activate addition facts but not necessarily multiplication facts. However, the particularly long RT in addition

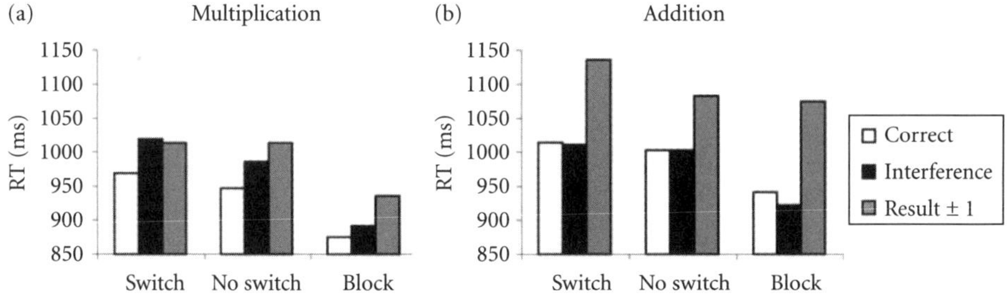

Figure 13.1 Evidence for transient bindings of arithmetic facts. Response time (RT) for (a) multiplication and (b) addition trials in mixed and blocked conditions. In the mixed condition, trials were analysed separately for switch trials (sequences AM or MA) and no-switch trials (sequences AA or MM). The RTs show different transfer effects for the two operations and the two conditions.

problems in which the solution deviates only slightly from the correct sum suggests that the system not only tests the correctness of an offered solution but also evaluates its magnitude (and plausibility). If the magnitude lies within the range of the correct result, a careful time-consuming rechecking procedure seems to take place before a verification response is committed. This suggests that control functions other than pure fact retrieval seem to be invoked if highly overlearned single-digit addition problems have to be verified.

Event-related potentials reflect binding phenomena during mental calculation

Although such behavioural studies can reveal features of the hidden processes which are triggered by mental calculation problems, they have a major limitation. All the conclusions about hypothetical processes mediating between a particular stimulus pattern (a problem) and a response (production or verification of a result) are indirect and retrospective. They are derived from RTs or error patterns, i.e. behavioural data which are collected at the very end of the processing sequence. To obtain more direct insight into the processes which are triggered by a mental calculation problem and the hypothesized effects of binding and unbinding of numerical representations, we measured event-related potentials (ERPs) while participants verified or produced the results of simple single-digit problems.

ERPs can be extracted from the EEG by signal extraction methods of averaging and filtering. They reflect systematic activation changes within circumscribed cortical cell assemblies which follow or precede critical events: the presentation of a stimulus or the execution of a response. Research has convincingly shown that the components of the ERP have systematic relationships with information processing steps which mediate between stimulus and response (Rugg and Coles 1995a). In particular, processes which are related to language comprehension and memory activation leave prominent and function-specific signatures in the ERP (Brown and Hagoort 1999; Rösler and Heil 2003). Therefore this method also appears promising for investigating the intricacies of mental calculation processes.

The arithmetic N400 effect

ERP research has identified one phenomenon which appears to reflect activation states of representations in semantic memory. Words which do not fit into a semantic context, such as semantically incongruous sentence endings (e.g. 'He spread his warm bread with *socks*' versus '. . . with *butter*'), evoke a prominent negativity over the parietal cortex. The amplitude difference between ERPs elicited by incongruous and congruous endings is known as the N400 effect (Kutas and Hillyard 1980). The interesting observation is that this phenomenon is not just a correlate of surprise. Rather, its amplitude covaries systematically with the semantic relationship between preceding context and the target word which evokes the phenomenon. Completing a sentence fragment such as 'He liked lemon and sugar in his . . .' with 'tea' (best fit, close association), 'coffee' (no fit, related association), or 'butter' (no fit, unrelated) reveals that words which perfectly fit into the established context evoke hardly any negativity at all, those which do not fit at all evoke a strong negativity, and those which are partially associated with the previous context evoke a negativity somewhere in between. Modality of stimulus presentation (visual, auditory) or the type of language (German, English, American sign language) does not affect the phenomenon; it can be observed equally well in all these stimulus situations (Holcomb 1985; Neville 1985; Van Petten *et al.* 1991). The semantic context, i.e. a word which does not optimally fit into the context because of semantic restrictions, is decisive.

The effect is not linked to sentence contexts; it can also be observed in a typical priming paradigm with a lexical decision. There the target evokes an N400 whose amplitude depends on how closely the target is associated with the preceding prime (Fig. 13.2(a)) (Rösler *et al.* 2001). The amplitude is the stronger the less the target is primed. Therefore it is not the sentence context in a narrow sense, but rather the semantic context which triggers the N400 effect. Moreover, these findings suggest that the N400 effect reflects aspects of how the semantic lexicon is organized—it reflects associative relations. The amplitude is sensitive to all kinds of semantic associations: relationships which exist due to categorical associations (tool–hammer), frequency of usage (United–States), etc. In each case the amplitude increases with a larger associative distance of priming context and target (Van Berkum *et al.* 1999). One hypothesis for integrating these findings suggests that the N400 amplitude reflects additional 'search' or activation processes in semantic memory to integrate a currently processed piece of information into the activation pattern already established by the previous context (Rösler and Hahne 1992). The more the memory representation of a target is activated by the prime, the smaller the amplitude will be. Reversing the argument suggests that the amplitude reduction of the N400 effect, measured in relation to the maximum amplitude triggered by a completely unprimed target, can reveal the amount of context-related preactivation which a representation has already received from a priming context (Fig. 13.2(b)).

We investigated whether there is a similar effect if arithmetic facts have to be activated in memory (Niedeggen *et al.* 1999). Subjects saw a multiplication

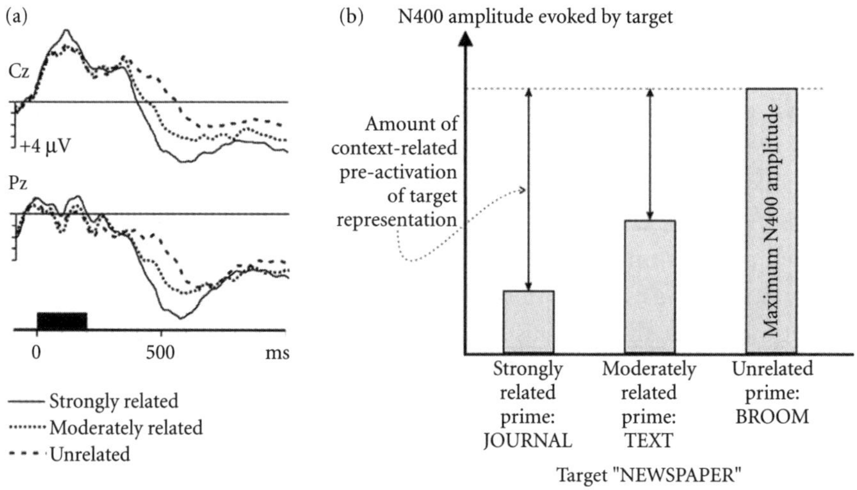

Figure 13.2 Strength of associations and the semantic N400 effect. (a) ERPs from a lexical decision task in which the semantic relationship between prime and target was varied systematically. The amplitude between 300 and 700 ms increased monotonically with decreasing strength of the semantic relationship (data from Rösler *et al.* 2001). (b) Model to explain the amplitude modulation of the N400 effect. It is assumed that the N400 reflects activation processes in semantic memory: the smaller the N400 amplitude, the stronger are target representations activated by the priming context.

problem which was followed by either a correct or an incorrect solution, and they had to verify the equation. As can be seen in Figure 13.3, an arithmetic incongruency (right) evokes a very similar ERP signature to a semantic incongruency (left). Thus there is an arithmetic N400 effect which might reflect associative relations of arithmetic knowledge.

The characteristic features, especially the topography, of the incongruency N400 effect in the arithmetic and semantic conditions are very similar. This was further corroborated in a recent study in our laboratory in which we directly compared factors affecting N400 amplitude in both the arithmetic and the linguistic condition (Jost *et al.* 2004). Onset latency was almost the same for both conditions; the only difference was that the maximum amplitude was generally smaller and was reached slightly earlier in the arithmetic condition. However, differences in latency and amplitude remained within the limits observed for linguistic N400 effects in other studies.

Thus it can be concluded that the same functional mechanism appears to be triggered by the incongruency manipulation in the one or the other domain. 'Additional semantic integration' is the broadest theoretical construct that has been suggested to explain N400 effects such as those evoked by unexpected

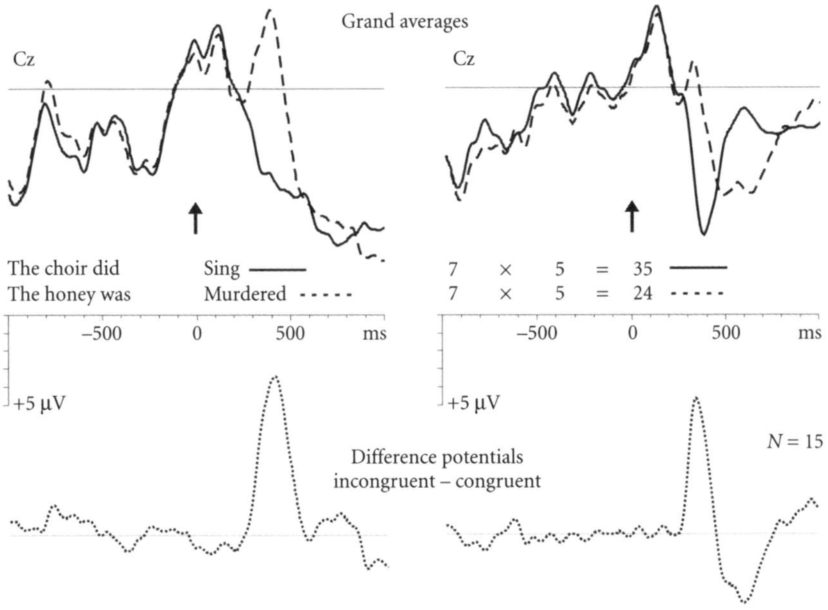

Figure 13.3 The semantic (left) and arithmetic (right) N400 effect. In each condition the incongruent completion of the sentence or the equation, respectively, evokes a pronounced negativity between 300 and 500 ms at central-parietal scalp locations. The difference potentials show the N400 effect with an amplitude maximum at about 400 ms in the semantic condition and 350 ms in the arithmetic condition. (Data from Niedeggen *et al.* 1999).

words in sentences, unprimed words in lexical decision tasks, or incorrect solutions of multiplication problems. In each case unexpected semantic elements, which do not fit with the preceding context of meaning, can be assumed to need extra effort in order to stabilize the system with a coherent semantic meaning. Since the amplitude of the incongruency N400 seems to be inversely proportional to the level of pre-activation which an item has received from the previous context (Niedeggen and Rösler 1999; Rösler *et al.* 2001; Khader *et al.* 2003), we believe that the N400 amplitude is functionally related to activation in memory networks. N400 amplitude appears to reflect the amount of additional activation in the knowledge network that is necessary to push a memory representation of a perceptually triggered concept above threshold. The more such a concept is pre-activated by the preceding context, the less additional activation is necessary and thus the smaller is the N400 amplitude. This functional relationship appears to hold for each type of semantic knowledge: linguistic entities in the narrow sense (words primed by other words, sentences, or longer texts), declarative knowledge entities (e.g. exemplars primed by categories), or, as shown here, arithmetic facts.

Amplitude of the N400 effect and strength of bindings

Reaction time studies in numerical decision tasks produced several systematic effects which, as in semantic priming studies, disclose the pattern of bindings which exist permanently in memory or which are activated transiently by a particular problem. For example, solutions of a multiplication problem which are incorrect but are multiples of one of the operands (e.g. $3 \times 6 = 24$) are harder to reject in a verification task than incorrect solutions which are completely unrelated to each operand (e.g. $3 \times 6 = 14$) (Campbell 1987). Moreover, incorrect solutions which are numerically close to the correct result are harder to reject than incorrect solutions which are numerically distant (e.g. $3 \times 6 = 24$ versus $3 \times 6 = 48$) (Stazyk *et al.* 1982). Thus the response time in a numerical decision task is directly proportional to the table-relatedness of the solution to one of the operands and inversely proportional to the numerical distance between the correct and incorrect solution. The effect of table-relatedness suggests that not only does the combination of operands activate the correct result, but that each operand alone activates other results which belong to the same multiplication table (Campbell 1991, 1995). On the other hand, the numerical distance effect suggests that solutions which are numerically close to the correct result receive more activation than solutions whose magnitude is clearly out of range (Ashcraft and Stazyk 1981).

Do these factors of table-relatedness and numerical distance become manifest in the arithmetic N400? If so, do they tell us anything about how arithmetic facts are stored or which bindings exist between operands, problems, and results?

To find an answer to these questions we performed a study in which the two factors were systematically manipulated (Niedeggen and Rösler 1999). Table-relatedness was varied on two levels (the incorrect result could be either related or unrelated to the multiplication table of one of the operands) and numerical distance was varied on three levels (the incorrect result could have a numerically close, medium, or large distance from the correct result). For the multiplication problem 3×6, the three related incorrect results were 24, 30, and 36, and the three unrelated incorrect results were 26, 32, and 38. In total, subjects saw 600 multiplication problems with single-digit operands (2×3 to 8×9). Ties (2×2) and operations with 1 or 0 were excluded because these may have a different status in memory. Half of the trials had correct solutions and half had incorrect solutions, and the incorrect solutions varied with respect to the two factors 'table-relatedness' and 'numerical distance'. Each of the six incorrect conditions had 50 trials. The two operands and the solution were presented one after the other, and the participant had a maximum of 1500 ms to signal the decision by a finger lift. The EEG was recorded from 61 Ag–Ag–Cl electrodes, with a bandpass from DC to 50 Hz and a sampling rate of 250 Hz.

The RTs replicate the well-known effects (Fig. 13.4(b)): RT decreases with increasing numerical distance, and the RT to table-related incorrect solutions is always longer than to table-unrelated solutions. The ERPs revealed a well-developed arithmetic N400 effect. Figure 13.4(a) shows the difference potentials separately for the three numerical distance conditions and the related versus unrelated incorrect results. The most interesting aspect of these data is the amplitude modulation of the N400 effect depending on the relatedness and the numerical distance of the incorrect solution. A related incorrect solution evokes the N400 effect with a smaller amplitude than a completely unrelated incorrect solution, but this only holds if the numerical distance is either small or medium. If the related solution is numerically very distant from the correct result, the amplitude of the N400 effect is as large as for an unrelated solution.

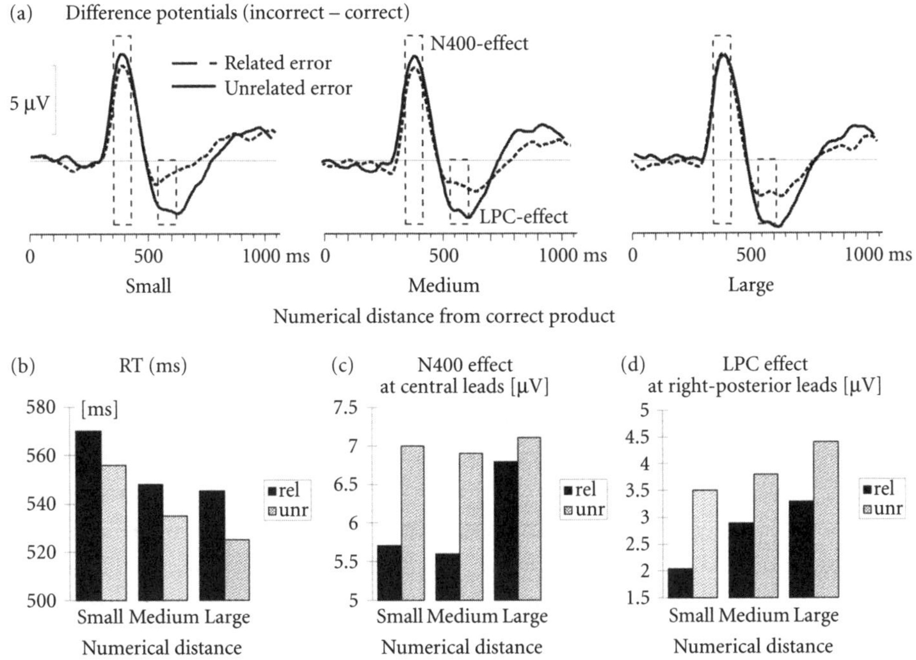

Figure 13.4 Effects of table-relatedness and numerical distance of an incorrect solution on the RTs and ERPs in an arithmetic verification task. (a) Difference potentials between incorrect and correct solutions at electrode Cz separately for table-related and table-unrelated errors and an increasing numerical distance of the incorrect solution from the correct solution. (b) Average RTs, (c) average amplitude of the N400 effect, and (d) average amplitude of the late positive component for the six conditions. The windows in which the amplitudes were measured are shown in (a) (Data from Niedeggen and Rösler 1999.)

The pattern of results is similar to that observed with linguistic material, where the target-evoked N400 effect reflects the associative strength between prime and target or between sentence context and final word. Here, the arithmetic N400 effect seems to be sensitive to the associations that exist between multiplication problems, their operands, and a table of solutions.

However, this is only part of the story. There is another component in the ERP which is also affected by the experimental manipulations. This amplitude modulation concerns the late positive component (LPC) which can also be seen in the difference potential 'incorrect–correct solution' between 500 and 600 ms. This positive component always has a larger amplitude for unrelated than for related errors and it increases with the numerical distance of the incorrect solutions from the correct solution.

Seeing the three dependent variables together (RT, N400 amplitude, and LPC amplitude) reveals the following story. First, the RT and the amplitude of the N400 effect dissociate, and, secondly, the RT and the LPC amplitude show reciprocal effect patterns. From the perspective of the independent variables which were manipulated in this experiment, we found the following.

Relatedness and numerical distance act additively on decision time. This is in line with the hypothesis (Ashcraft 1992) that RT reflects the difficulty of rejecting results which have an associative relationship with the correct results: the more it is associated, the more difficult it will be to reject it, i.e. the longer it will take to get the situation straight.

Exactly the same pattern is revealed by the LPC amplitude, where again both table-relatedness and numerical distance act additively. We could argue that this effect reflects something like 'surprise' which is associated with implausible results. The surprise increases with numerical distance and unrelatedness.

However, the situation is different with the N400 effect; both factors act non-additively on the amplitude of the N400 effect. As mentioned above, we assume that the N400 amplitude reflects problem-related spread of activation. The amplitude is smaller the more a numerical representation is already pre-activated by the preceding context, i.e. the two operands and their combination. The non-additive effect suggests that the activation which originates from a problem is limited to those results which are numerically close to the correct result. However, this is a tricky finding: The effect can hardly be due to a simple passive spread of activation which decreases with increasing associative distance. In that case the coactivation of incorrect and table-related results should decrease monotonically with numerical distance. Rather, it looks as if the particular operand combination restricts the spread of activation to numerically plausible results. Although all table-related results must somehow be bound to each operand, the problem as such seems to transiently restrict the set of activated bindings (see also Campbell 1995).

The result is also of particular interest from a methodological point of view. The N400 effect appears to reflect something different from the behavioural effect, i.e. the RTs. While the RT is an omnibus measure which integrates the timing of all processing steps intervening between stimulus and response, the N400 effect appears to be a manifestation of a single process or of a subset of these mediating processes only. Thus ERPs can be used to monitor processes which take place within behaviourally mute epochs. On the other hand, the LPC effect has a much closer link to RT; the two variables behave almost as mirror images of each other—the shorter is RT, the larger is the LPC amplitude.

Returning to the questions raised at the beginning of this section, the experiment described here provides the following answers. Table-relatedness and numerical distance both have an influence on the amplitude of the arithmetic N400 effect. This influence is interactive. The amplitude does not monotonously decrease with increasing numerical distance of an offered result from the correct solution, as one would predict if the spread of activation were just a passive process. Rather, the N400 amplitude was found to be reduced only for offered solutions which have a table-relatedness to the operands (i.e. which are other multiples of one or other of the operands) and which are numerically not too distant from the correct result (i.e. which are numerically plausible). This gives some clue as to how arithmetic facts are stored and which transient bindings exist between operands, problems, and results. On the one hand, the results suggest that two operands of a multiplication problem activate more than just the correct result. Owing to overlearned associations, they also activate other multiples of the same multiplication table. However, on the other hand, this spread of activation seems to be limited by the problem, i.e. the combination of the two operands. Thus the problem appears to activate an estimate of the expected problem size, and this expected size seems to restrict the spread of activation to acceptable table-related problems only.

Small and large single-digit multiplication problems

There is another variable, in addition to table-relatedness and numerical distance, which also affects processing times of simple single-digit multiplication problems. Responses are in general slower and more error prone if the operands, and hence the correct solutions, become numerically larger (e.g. 7×8 compared with 2×3) (Stazyk *et al.* 1982; Miller *et al.* 1984; Campbell and Graham 1985). This so-called problem size effect, or more generally difficulty effect, holds for both production and verification tasks (Parkman 1972; Campbell 1987; Zbrodoff and Logan 1990; Campbell and Fugelsang 2001).

Within the theoretical framework of activation spread, the problem size effect is attributed to differences in the strength of associative bindings. It is argued that larger problems are less frequently encountered at school and later in life, and therefore the respective solutions are less tightly bound to the operands. Consequently, it takes longer to accumulate enough activation to retrieve the result. However, it has also been argued that the prolonged reaction times for large problems are not caused by differences in retrieval speed but by a shift to non-retrieval procedures such as a decomposition of the problem into a set of smaller problems (e.g. $7 \times 8 = \{[(7 \times 2) \times 2] \times 2\}$) (LeFevre *et al.* 1996a). Another possible factor was mentioned by Campbell (1995), who suggested that problems also activate a magnitude representation which reflects the approximate numerical size of the solution. As is known from psychophysics, numerical magnitudes are related to the objective size by a log linear function, i.e. the internal scale is more compressed for large than for small numbers. Thus larger magnitudes will be less well discriminated from each other than smaller magnitudes (Dehaene 1989; Brysbaert 1995). Therefore, in the case of large problems, correct and incorrect table-related solutions are psychologically more similar and this could cause more interference between the activated nodes. Such an effect could either slow down the activation accumulation at the correct node or prolong the decision process between the evidence for correct and incorrect solutions (Atkinson and Juola 1974).

The hypotheses about the cause of the problem size effect should find different expressions in the ERPs. If the difference between large and small problems is only a question of different binding strength which affects the speed of activation, then only the amplitude of the arithmetic N400 should be affected. The activation spreading from the operands to the correct solution should be less for large than for small problems and therefore the difference potential between large and small problems should show an N400 effect. This effect should have the same topographical features as the typical incongruency N400 effect, i.e. the difference between incorrect and correct solutions.

In contrast, if the problem size effect is not caused by differences in activation strength alone but also by distinct solution strategies or additional rechecking processes, then these processes should not become manifest in an amplitude modulation of the N400 effect. Instead, large problems should evoke an additional ERP phenomenon which is distinct from a typical N400. This expectation rests on the assumption that functionally distinct mechanisms express themselves in distinct ERP components which, among other things, differ in scalp topography (Rugg and Coles 1995b).

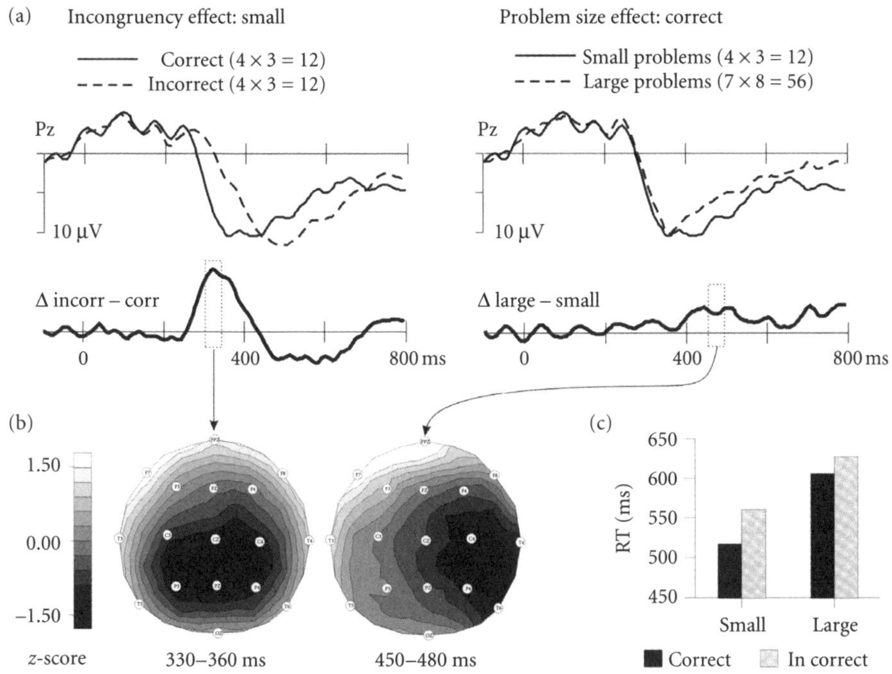

Figure 13.5 Effects of incongruency and problem size in an arithmetic verification task. (a) ERPs evoked by correct and incorrect solutions (left panel) and by solutions of small and large multiplication problems (right panel). The top tracings show the grand average ERPs and the tracings below are the difference potentials which visualize the arithmetic incongruency effect and the arithmetic problem size effect in the ERP. (b) Standardized topographies of the incongruency and the problem size effects. (c) Average verification times. (Data from Jost *et al.* 2004.)

To test this we performed the following experiment (Jost *et al.* 2004): We used 56 different single-digit multiplication problems (without ties or 0 and 1 problems) and presented these in a verification task with 50 per cent incorrect trials. Problems with both operands < 5 were classified as small, and problems with both operands > 5 as large (Zbrodoff and Logan 1990; Kiefer and Dehaene 1997). Problems with one operand < 5 and one operand > 5 (e.g. 3×8) were defined as small if they contained a 2 or a 5, and otherwise as large (see Campbell and Tarling (1996) for a similar classification). Both levels of problem size comprised 28 operand combinations. All problems were presented twice in random order. The experiment was performed with 16 participants.

The RTs (Fig. 13.5(c)) again show an incongruency effect for both small and large problems, i.e. it always took more time to reject an incorrect solution than to accept a correct solution. In addition, there is a reliable problem size effect, i.e. decisions took longer for large than for small problems and this held for both correct and incorrect solutions.

The ERPs evoked by correct and incorrect solutions confirmed the incongruency effect described above which shows up as an arithmetic N400 effect in the difference potential 'incorrect–correct' (Fig. 13.5(a), left panel). This N400 effect was found for both large and small problems (Jost *et al.* 2004). A careful analysis of the scalp topography (Fig. 13.5(b), left panel) and its direct comparison with linguistic incongruency conditions revealed that the arithmetic and the semantic or linguistic N400 effects have approximately the same topography. The maximum is located over the parietal-central scalp. This suggests that the two phenomena are probably due to comparable functional mechanisms.

In contrast, the problem size effect shows a completely different picture. A difference between small and large problems is also present but this amplitude difference appears much later and has a completely distinct topography (Figs 13.5(a) and 13.5(b), left panels). The effect maximum is located over the right hemisphere extending towards postero-temporal regions. The observed pattern of results clearly suggests that the arithmetic problem size effect and the arithmetic incongruency effect cannot be attributed to the same functional mechanism. Both manipulations prolong the decision, as found in other studies (Campbell 1987; Zbrodoff and Logan 1990; Campbell and Fugelsang 2001), but they become manifest in ERP components with a distinct topography.

The most interesting finding of this study is the late effect with a maximum over the right cortex. Siegler (1988) suggested that arithmetic problems may trigger additional solution strategies if an associated result is not immediately available (see also LeFevre *et al.* 1996a,b). The negativity observed over the right hemisphere might reflect different strategies, such as decomposition, but there is another explanation which seems equally plausible. Both neuropsychological case reports and brain imaging studies have shown that number comparison tasks and magnitude estimations recruit cell assemblies in the right hemisphere (Dehaene 2000). Although the surface topography of an ERP effect gives only limited information about the location of its generator(s), nevertheless it is striking that the problem size effect observed in the present study had its maximum amplitude over the right hemisphere, exactly over those brain areas which have been found to be essential for magnitude estimation in production tasks (Kiefer and Dehaene 1997). Thus it is possible that the negativity observed for large problems is a manifestation of such magnitude estimation processes.

With respect to the possible cause of the problem size effect in a verification task, the ERPs in this study suggest that the RT increase with increasing problem size is not primarily due to a slower spread of activation. Rather, compared with smaller problems, larger problems seem to invoke additional processes (e.g. additional size estimation or rechecking processes) in order to make the correct verification decision. Again, this shows that verifying a single-digit multiplication problem appears to involve more than just fact retrieval and response selection. Problems which, from a phenomenological perspective, would be categorized as equivalent (e.g. single-digit multiplications) appear to be different on a psycho(physiological)logical level of analysis.

Beyond fact retrieval

The previously reported study suggests that other strategies will be employed if fact retrieval is unreliable or fails completely. Apart from this, there are by definition multiplication problems which are not necessarily solved by direct fact retrieval, but rather by retrieving and applying a general rule. For example, multiplication by 0 or 1 appears to be such an exception ($N \times 0 = 0$; $N \times 1 = N$) (Parkman 1972; Stazyk *et al.* 1982). Studies of patients with circumscribed brain lesions suggest a double dissociation between retrieval-based and rule-based multiplication (Sokol *et al.* 1991; Pesenti *et al.* 2000). Although there is little doubt that multiplication problems can trigger fact retrieval and rule application, it is not entirely clear which problems invoke which strategy. Some researchers found particularly long RTs and high error rates for zero problems, possibly an indication of rule application (Parkman 1972; Stazyk *et al.* 1982), while others found the reverse pattern, faster responses for zero than for non-zero problems (Miller *et al.* 1984; LeFevre *et al.* 1996a).

To test differences between fact retrieval and rule application in single-digit multiplication problems we designed an experiment in which participants had to produce the result (Jost *et al.* 2004). This production was embedded in a chain calculation problem, i.e. a sequence of simple calculations had to be performed and the final result had to be verified at the very end of the sequence (e.g. $3 \times 5+2 = 17$). Thus, participants were forced to produce the interim result of the multiplication problem before they could go on with the next calculation step. Moreover, the multiplication result had to be produced without any overt response. This procedure enabled movement artefacts to be avoided in the EEG recording.

Three types of multiplications (problems with small or large non-zero operands and problems with one zero operand) were compared with a control condition not involving any type of multiplication within the critical epoch. In this condition only the operands of the first problem had to be stored and one of the operands had to be used for the subsequent addition or subtraction. For example, the subject saw 3 ! 4 (in contrast to '×', '!' indicated the store condition);

if the next operand (e.g. +1) was shown on the left-hand side of the display the subject had to add 1 to the stored 3, but if it appeared on the right-hand side 1 had to be added to the stored 4. Thus, while the subject had to retrieve a multiplication result contingent on the two operands in multiplication trials, they had just to store the first two digits in this control condition. This provides an 'active' or 'high-level' baseline, because the operands must be perceived and stored in each multiplication condition as well. Therefore computing the differences between multiplication conditions and the storage condition should reveal the net effects due to different solution strategies.

Among others, we analysed a slow negative wave evoked by the second operand, i.e. an ERP phenomenon which accompanied the silent production of the result. Slow negative waves accompany almost any cognitive processing and they have two interesting features. Their topographic maximum is determined by the modality and the type of task (e.g. linguistic tasks evoke a left anterior and spatial tasks a parietal maximum), and their amplitude reflects processing effort, i.e. larger negativities are evoked by more difficult tasks (Rösler *et al.* 1997). There is also strong evidence that slow negative waves reflect a relative increase of excitatory post-synaptic potentials within cortical cell assemblies (Birbaumer *et al.* 1990). Thus slow negative waves indicate to what extent identical or distinct neural cell assemblies are recruited during a particular processing episode.

The experimental conditions significantly affected the slow negative wave whose timing coincides with the production phase proper. It was most pronounced for large multiplications, intermediate for small and zero problems, and smallest for the storage condition. This suggests that different problems recruit neural resources to a different extent. However, the most important finding was that the negativity revealed clear topographic differences between the conditions (Fig. 13.6). These indicate activation of distinct generator ensembles (Urbach and Kutas 2002) and therefore support the hypothesis that even highly overlearned single-digit multiplication problems are solved by means of different solution strategies. Compared with small problems, larger problems evoked a stronger negativity over fronto-central and right temporal sites, and zero problems evoked a left anterior negativity. These topographic differences indicate not only that zero and small non-zero problems are solved by means of distinct strategies (rule application and fact retrieval, respectively) but also that larger less overlearned problems invoke additional processes as well as pure knowledge activation. To our knowledge this is the first study which shows clear-cut biological correlates of distinct 'microprocesses' invoked by single-digit multiplication problems.

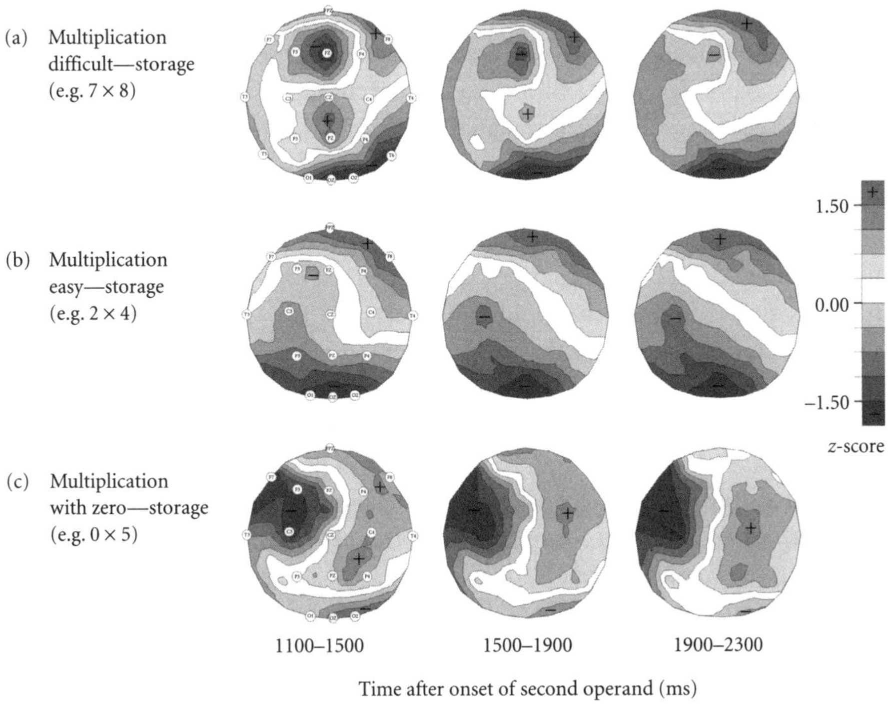

Figure 13.6 Topography of slow negative waves in an arithmetic production task with different types of single-digit multiplication problems. *Z*-standardized maps for three time epochs after presenting the second operand of a multiplication problem in a longer sequence of computations are shown. The maps were computed from difference potentials which contrasted the three multiplication conditions ((a) difficult, large operands; (b) easy, small operands; (c) one zero operand) with a non-multiplication condition in which single-digit numbers only had to be stored. The net effect (difference between multiplication and storage) reveals a significantly distinct topography for the three types of problem. (Data from Jost *et al.* 2004.) See also colour plate section.

The two studies summarized above and in the previous section showed ERP correlates of the arithmetic problem size effect. In the first study, with a verification task, larger problems evoked a stronger relative negativity between 400 and 600 ms with a maximum around 475 ms over the right central to temporal cortex (at CP6–T46 according to the extended 10–20 system). In the second study, with an implicit production task, larger multiplication problems compared with the control condition evoked a relative stronger negativity 1000–2300 ms after problem onset with two maxima, one peaking around 1300 ms after problem onset over fronto-central scalp sites (at Fz) and a second one which appeared at the same time over occipital to right temporal sites (extending between Oz and T46). It prevailed longer than the frontal negativity (for >1 s) and shrank towards Oz with increasing time. These substantial differences must be attributed to the different tasks: verfication versus production. On the micropsychological level these two tasks seem to involve very distinct sets of processes and it can only be speculated how the observed phenomena might be related to each other. Nevertheless, there is at least some convergence, i.e. the right central to temporal negativity which, although having a different timing, has at least some overlapping topography in both studies (around T46). Therefore one could argue that it is at least in part a manifestation of similar processes—as argued, rechecking or size estimation. On the other hand, the fronto-central negativity in the production situation must be attributed to a completely different functional origin. We might speculate that this negativity is related to executive control which initiates the fact retrieval and the additional size estimation and rechecking processes. That it becomes manifest in the production task only could be due to the fact that this task furnished longer processing times; thus distinct processes had a better chance of being separated over time. The different amount of temporal overlap of subprocesses in the two tasks could also contribute to the different topographies, because a measured topography reflects the net effect of all generated potentials at a particular time. In any case, speculation about the similarity and dissimilarity of the processes involved in the two task situations must be substantiated by further studies which directly manipulate the postulated processes and monitor the three-dimensional location of the cortical generators involved by means of functional MRI.

Summary and conclusions

Priming and switching paradigms, in combination with ERP measures, has proved a useful approach to the study of distinct memory activation and control processes in mental calculation tasks. In particular, microprocesses, such as activation and inhibition of representations that are triggered by the problem itself, by immediately preceding problems, or by the larger context of task-relevant problems presented in one experiment, appear to leave distinct signatures in the ERP.

The range of experimental manipulations realized in the reported studies is still very limited. Therefore generalizations may be problematic and we should be cautious in prematurely relating the observed ERP effects to narrowly defined cognitive functions. Nevertheless, the following tentative conclusions about functional relations between arithmetic ERP-effects and cognitive processes may be feasible.

The arithmetic N400 effect with a central-parietal maximum triggered by incongruent solutions in verification tasks seems to reflect activation spread within the network of fact associations (see our comments above on the similarity between arithmetic and linguistic N400 effects). The amplitude of this effect was found to be inversely proportional to the amount of activation spread triggered by a prime. Therefore the amplitude of this effect can be used to monitor the associative network structure between numbers, arithmetic problems, and results.

Another relative negativity with a later latency than the typical N400 effect and a clearly right parietal to right temporal topography seems to reflect additional processes of magnitude estimation and/or rechecking, if less overlearned facts (such as larger problems) have to be verified. A similar effect was observed in an implicit production task but the latency was further delayed, a finding which is probably due to fundamental task differences between verification and production.

Further task-accompanying relative negativities were observed in the production task. Of particular interest are a fronto-central and a left anterior negativity. The first was tentatively related to executive functions when less overlearned facts have to be produced (control of fact retrieval and rechecking strategies), and the second was specifically associated with problems which can be solved by applying a general rule rather than by individual fact retrieval.

Finally, the effects of an LPC were also observed in the arithmetic verification and production experiments. The amplitude shifts in this component observed by Niedeggen and Rösler (1999) are compatible with the idea that more unexpected, surprising, and implausible results in a verification task evoke a stronger LPC. This is in line with the rich literature on the functional significance of the LPC or P300 which suggests that the LPC indicates the invocation of context-updating processes if the system has to readjust its expectations (Donchin and Coles 1988). On the other hand, an amplitude modulation of the LPC in the production design of Jost *et al.* (2004) was interpreted as indicating the automatic evaluation of the expected difficulty of a problem, an idea which can also be subsumed under the broader concept of 'context-updating' processes (see Neumann *et al.* 1986).

The reported findings show that even very simple single-digit production and verification problems are not exclusively solved by pure fact retrieval. Rather, other solution strategies have to be employed if direct fact retrieval is not sufficient or inappropriate. Among others, we could provide evidence that, compared with smaller problems (e.g. 2×3) larger single-digit multiplications (e.g. 7×8) appear to involve additional processing steps, such as plausibility checks and magnitude estimations. The ERP topography also suggests that problems which can be solved by means of rule knowledge (such as multiplication by zero, e.g. 3 × 0) invoke different processes than those which can be solved by direct fact retrieval. Moreover, if the system has to switch between distinct knowledge domains, such as addition and multiplication facts, additional processes are invoked which control the intrusion effects of competing memory representations.

Transient activations and inhibitions, i.e. transient bindings and unbindings of associations, can be understood as the 'basic elements' of executive functions (Rösler 2004). Thus this work with simple arithmetic problems (single-digit multiplications and additions) has a close relationship with more complex multidigit problems. With the latter, distinct representations must also be transiently activated and inhibited, and likewise, as in our more controlled priming and switching paradigms, it has to be assumed that the processing of a particular calculation step will be influenced by the immediately preceding steps. Therefore the present work is intended to provide further insight into elementary processes of mental calculation which are relevant for both simple and more complex problems.

References

Ashcraft, M.H. (1992). Cognitive arithmetic: a review of data and theory. *Cognition*, **44**, 75–106.

Ashcraft, M.H. and Stazyk, E.H. (1981). Mental addition: a test of three verification models. *Memory and Cognition*, **9**, 185–196.

Atkinson, R.C. and Juola, J.F. (1974). Search and decision processes in recognition memory. In *Learning, Memory, and Thinking* (ed D.H. Krantz, R.C. Atkinson, R.D. Luce, and P. Suppes). San Francisco, CA: W.H. Freeman, pp. 243–293.

Birbaumer, N., Elbert, T., Canavan, A.G.M., and Rockstroh, B. (1990). Slow potentials of the cerebral cortex and behaviour. *Physiological Reviews*, **70**, 1–41.

Brown, C.M. and Hagoort, P. (1999). *The Neurocognition of Language*. Oxford: Oxford University Press.

Brysbaert, M. (1995). Arabic number reading: on the nature of the numerical scale and the origin of phonological recoding. *Journal of Experimental Psychology: General*, **124**, 434–452.

Campbell, J.I.D. (1987). Production, verification, and priming of multiplication facts. *Memory and Cognition*, **15**, 349–364.

Campbell, J.I.D. (1991). Conditions of error priming in number-fact retrieval. *Memory and Cognition*, **19**, 197–209.

Campbell, J.I.D. (1995). Mechanisms of simple addition and multiplication: a modified network-interference theory and simulation. *Mathematical Cognition*, **1**, 121–165.

Campbell, J.I.D. and Clark, J.M. (1989). Time course of error priming in number-fact retrieval: Evidence for excitatory and inhibitory mechanisms. *Journal of Experimental Psychology: Learning, Memory, and Cognition*, **15**, 920–929.

Campbell, J.I.D. and Fugelsang, J. (2001). Strategy choice for arithmetic verification: effects of numerical surface form. *Cognition*, **80**, B21–B30.

Campbell, J.I.D. and Graham, D.J. (1985). Mental multiplication skill: structure, process and acquisition. *Canadian Journal of Psychology*, **39**, 338–366.

Campbell, J.I.D. and Tarling, D.P.M. (1996). Retrieval processes in arithmetic production and verification. *Memory and Cognition*, **24**, 156–172.

Dehaene, S. (1989). The psychophysics of numerical comparison: a re-examination of apparently incompatible data. *Perception and Psychophysics*, **45**, 557–566.

Dehaene, S. (2000). Cerebral bases of number processing and calculation. In *The New Cognitive Neurosciences* (ed M. Gazzaniga). Cambridge, MA: MIT Press, pp. 987–998.

Dehaene, S. and Cohen, L. (1995). Towards an anatomical and functional model of number processing. *Mathematical Cognition*, **1**, 83–120.

Donchin, E. and Coles, M.G. (1988). Is the P300 component a manifestation of context updating? *Behavioral and Brain Sciences*, **11**, 357–427.

Hitch, G.J. (1978). The role of short-term working memory in mental arithmetic. *Cognitive Psychology*, **10**, 302–323.

Holcomb, P.J. (1985). Unimodal and multimodal models of lexical memory: an ERP analysis. *Psychophysiology*, **22**, 576.

Jost, K. and Rösler, F. (2003). Interference effects of addition and multiplication knowledge. Manuscript, Department of Psychology, Philipps University, Marburg.

Jost, K., Beinhoff, U., Hennighausen, E., and Rösler, F. (2004). Facts, rules, and strategies in single-digit multiplication: evidence from event-related brain potentials. *Cognitive Brain Research*, **20**, 183–193.

Jost, K., Hennighausen, E., and Rösler, F. (2004). Comparing arithmetic and semantic fact retrieval: effects of problem size and sentence constraint on event-related brain potentials. *Psychophysiology*, **41**, 46–59.

Khader, P., Scherag, A., Streb, J., and Rösler, F. (2003). Differences between noun and verb processing in a minimal phrase context: a semantic priming study using event-related brain potentials. *Cognitive Brain Research*, **17**, 293–313.

Kiefer, M. and Dehaene, S. (1997). The time course of parietal activation in single-digit multiplication: evidence from event-related potentials. *Mathematical Cognition*, **3**, 1–30.

Kutas, M. and Hillyard, S.A. (1980). Reading senseless sentences: brain potentials reflect semantic incongruity. *Science*, **207**, 203–205.

LeFevre, J.A., Bisanz, J., Daley, K.E., Buffone, L., Greenham, S.L., and Sadesky, G.S. (1996a). Multiple routes to solution of single-digit multiplication problems. *Journal of Experimental Psychology: General*, **125**, 284–306.

LeFevre, J.A., Sadesky, G.S., and Bisanz, J. (1996b). Selection of procedures in mental addition: reaqssessing the problem size effect in adults. *Journal of Experimental Psychology: Learning, Memory, and Cognition*, **22**, 216–230.

McCloskey, M. (1992). Cognitive mechanisms in numerical processing: evidence from acquired dyscalculia. *Cognition*, **44**, 107–157.

Miller, K., Perlmutter, M., and Keating, D. (1984). Cognitive arithmetic: comparison of operations. *Journal of Experimental Psychology: Learning, Memory, and Cognition*, **10**, 46–60.

Neumann, U., Ullsperger, P., Gille, H.G., Pietschmann, M., and Erdmann, U. (1986). Effects of graduated processing difficulty on P300 component of the event-related brain potential. *Zeitschrift für Psychologie*, **194**, 25–37.

Neville, H.J. (1985). Biological constraints on semantic processing: a comparison of spoken and signed languages. *Psychophysiology*, **22**, 576.

Niedeggen, M. and Rösler, F. (1999). N400-effects reflect activation spread during arithmetic fact retrieval. *Psychological Science*, **10**, 271–276.

Niedeggen, M., Rösler, F., and Jost, K. (1999). Processing of incongruous mental calculation problems: evidence for an arithmetic N400-effect. *Psychophysiology*, **36**, 307–324.

Parkman, J.M. (1972). Temporal aspects of simple multiplication and comparison. *Journal of Experimental Psychology*, **95**, 437–444.

Pesenti, M., Depoorter, N., and Seron, X. (2000). Noncommutability of the $N + 0$ arithmetical rule: a case study of dissociated impairment. *Cortex*, **36**, 445–454.

Rösler, F. (2004). Einige Gedanken zum Problem der 'Entscheidungsfindung' in Nervensystemen. In *Zur Freiheit des Willens* (ed Berlin: Brandenburgische Akademie der Wissenschaften). Berlin: Akademie Verlag, pp. 23–34.

Rösler, F. and Hahne, A. (1992). Hirnelektrische Korrelate des Sprachverstehens: zur psycholinguistischen Bedeutung der N400-Komponente im EEG. *Sprache und Kognition*, **11**, 149–161.

Rösler, F. and Heil, M. (2003). The principle of code-specific memory representations. In *Principles of Learning and Memory* (ed R.H. Kluwe, G. Lüer, and F. Rösler). Basel: Birkhäuser, pp. 71–92.

Rösler, F., Heil, M. and Röder, B. (1997). Slow negative brain potentials as reflections of specific modular resources of cognition. *Biological Psychology*, **45**, 109–141.

Rösler, F., Streb, J., and Haan, H. (2001). Event-related brain potentials evoked by verbs and nouns in a primed lexical decision task. *Psychophysiology*, **38**, 694–703.

Rugg, M.D. and Coles, M.G.H. (ed) (1995a). *Electrophysiology of Mind*. Oxford: Oxford University Press.

Rugg, M.D. and Coles, M.G.H. (1995b). The ERP and cognitive psychology: conceptual issues. In *Electrophysiology of Mind* (ed M.D. Rugg and M.G.H. Coles). Oxford: Oxford University Press, pp. 27–39.

Siegler, R.S. (1988). Strategy choice procedures and the development of multiplication skill. *Journal of Experimental Psychology: General*, **117**, 258–275.

Sokol, S.M. and McCloskey, M. (1991). Cognitive mechanisms in calculation. In *Complex Problem Solving: Principles and Mechanisms* (ed R.J. Sternberg and P.A. Frensch). Hillsdale, NJ: Erlbaum.

Sokol, S.M., McCloskey, M., Cohen, N.J., and Aliminosa, D. (1991). Cognitive representations and processes in arithmetic: inferences from the performance of brain-damaged subjects. *Journal of Experimental Psychology: Learning, Memory, and Cognition*, **17**, 355–376.

Stazyk, E.H., Ashcraft, M.H., and Hamann, M.S. (1982). A network approach to simple multiplication. *Journal of Experimental Psychology: Learning, Memory, and Cognition*, **8**, 320–335.

Urbach, T.P. and Kutas, M. (2002). The intractability of scaling scalp distributions to infer neuroelectric sources. *Psychophysiology*, **39**, 791–808.

Van Berkum, J.J.A., Hagoort, P., and Brown, C.M. (1999). Semantic integration in sentences and discourse: evidence from the N400. *Journal of Cognitive Neuroscience*, **11**, 657–671.

Van Petten, C., Kutas, M., Kluender, R., Mitchiner, M., and McIsaak, H. (1991). Fractionating the word repetition effect with event-related potentials. *Journal of Cognitive Neuroscience*, **3**, 131–150.

Winkelmann, J.H. and Schmidt, J. (1974). Associative confusions in mental arithmetic. *Journal of Experimental Psychology*, **102**, 734–736.

Zbrodoff, N.J. and Logan, G.D. (1986). On the autonomy of mental processes: a case study of arithmetic. *Journal of Experimental Psychology: General*, **115**, 118–130.

Zbrodoff, N.J. and Logan, G.D. (1990). On the relation between production and verification tasks in the psychology of simple arithmetic. *Journal of Experimental Psychology: Learning, Memory, and Cognition*, **16**, 83–97.

Chapter 14

Motivated binding: top-down influences in the encoding of compound objects

Andreas Voss, Klaus Rothermund, and
Jochen Brandtstädter

Introduction

Beliefs, expectations, motives, and emotions often involve changes in cognitive processing. Such top-down influences are particularly strong when the stimulus information is ambiguous, i.e. when bottom-up factors are comparatively weak, and they involve all stages of processing (Yantis 2000). Action-theoretical approaches in particular have stressed the functional links between motivation and cognition; different action phases have been shown to engage particular 'mind sets' that support an ongoing course of action (Gollwitzer 1995). However, with respect to the conditions that guide attentional processes, different positions exist that imply partly divergent predictions. For example, it has been argued that 'negative' stimuli tend to grab attention (Pratto and John 1991), whereas notions of 'perceptual defence' implicate a tendency to blot out or reject threatening stimuli (Erdelyi 1974). The two arguments overlap, and to some extent also converge, with a third line of argument that focuses on stimulus relevance as a modulating factor (Lazarus *et al.* 1953; Averill and Rosenn 1972; Miller 1979; Folk *et al.* 1992; Bacon and Egeth 1994, 1997). Of course, attentional asymmetries will affect not only perception, but also processes of encoding and recall.

A consideration of the different stages of cognitive processing may help to improve our understanding of how and when top-down factors come into play (Fig. 14.1). In the initial stage of a (visual) perceptual process, all objects in the visual field are stored in the iconic memory, which has a high capacity but stores objects only briefly. Therefore, as long as it is available, critical information has to be extracted from a large set of objects that are perceived simultaneously. Up to this point of processing, single features in the visual field are received 'free floating', i.e. without being bound together as compound objects (Treisman 1986,

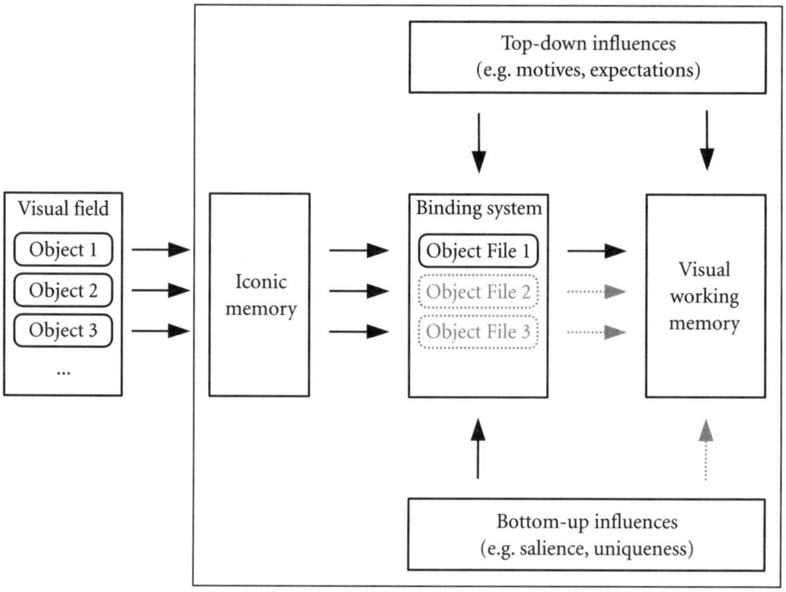

Figure 14.1 A model of visual encoding. All objects in the visual field are stored simultaneously in the iconic memory. For further processing, the different features of each object are integrated to object files which are subsequently stored in the visual working memory (VWM). Top-down factors may enhance or decrease the priority of certain objects in the binding system and may also guide further processing in the VWM. Bottom-up influences mainly affect the priority of the initial binding process. In the model they are separated from incoming objects to emphasize that bottom-up influences (e.g. uniqueness) are not attributes of single objects but reflect relations between objects in the visual field.

1993, 1999). The features are perceived in parallel mode. Consequently, feature perception is relatively independent of set size. However, to transfer objects into visual working memory (VWM), it is necessary to integrate the features to separate objects (see Chapter 12). This binding process is a time-consuming operation. To bind the perceived features to integrated percepts, objects have to be analysed **serially**. Consequently, in a conjunction search task, response times are a function of set size (Treisman and Sato 1990; Wolfe 1996). Additional evidence for the cognitive effort required by binding comes from the phenomenon of 'illusory conjunctions' (Treisman 1999; Wheeler and Treisman 2002). If stimuli that involve particular conjunctions of features are shown for short exposition times, the observer may form wrong or 'illusory' conjunctions. For example, if a yellow O and a red X are shown, the conjunctions red–O and yellow–X may be reported. A 'spotlight of attention' metaphor has been suggested to account for this phenomenon (Treisman and Sato 1990; Wheeler and Treisman 2002). According to this idea, correct binding requires that each single object in the visual field is focused for a period of time, with other objects being inhibited in this phase (see also Oberauer 2005. The features that are linked to a particular visual object are simultaneously focused and tend to form an integrated percept. When the features of one object are bound, the 'spotlight' will shift to the next object. However, if such a serial focusing of the presented objects is prevented, the binding process will be deficient and illusory conjunctions will occur.

The integrated information for each object resulting from the binding process forms an object file (Kahneman *et al.* 1992; see also Chapter 12). The object files are subsequently stored in VWM and thus are available for further processing. As mentioned above, feature integration is a serial process which involves a kind of bottleneck allowing no more than about 25 objects per second to be processed (Wolfe 1996). Therefore, selection is necessary in order to separate important and unimportant stimuli rapidly. The attentional system controls which information is 'read' from the iconic memory first. Attentional capture is typically driven by phenomenal attributes such as uniqueness or abrupt onset (Yantis 1996), as well as by the meanings and implications associated with a stimulus. Of particular interest here is the latter case, in which top-down influences are salient. However, at this juncture the question arises as to how top-down factors can operate in early selection. Is it possible to 'prefer' certain objects in a phase in which features are still stored unbound in the iconic memory? We argue that this is possible. Early selection requires that information gathered from parallel processing is used to infer (possible) meanings of objects. Because no binding has yet occurred in this phase of perception, single features have to be used to assess whether an object may be important or not. A theoretical approach that converges with this account is the guided search (GS) model (Wolfe 1994, 1996). GS assumes that the visual field is represented by different (spatially organized) internal feature maps (Treisman 1986). Further processing is controlled by an activation map which integrates bottom-up information from the feature map as well as top-down selective tendencies. For example, expectation of a particular object, such as a red X, should enhance sensitivity for object-related features by strengthening the linkage between the corresponding feature maps and the activation map. The joint activation effect from bottom-up and top-down processes then determines the priorities for serial analyses, which in turn is a precondition of feature binding.

If we assume top-down control of the binding system, another aspect of binding has to be considered. It is possible that object files store not only perceptual features, but also additional information from long-term memory. Most important, evaluative information associated with a certain stimulus may be bound together with the perceptual information (see Chapter 23 for a discussion of memory associations as binding phenomena). The assumption of early binding of evaluative information to perceptual objects also helps to explain the findings of automatic stimulus evaluation (see Fazio *et al.* (1986) for the automatic activation of attitudes; see also Murphy and Zajonc (1993)).

Figure 14.1 shows a schematic representation of the encoding process described above. Our focus here is on top-down influences. We posit that top-down factors may affect early phases of encoding before feature integration is completed. As can be seen in Figure 14.1, top-down influences may also guide later processing; for example, top-down controlled attention will determine storage of objects in long-term memory. In the following, we will briefly discuss top-down influences in the encoding of danger stimuli before presenting some experimental findings.

Attention to danger signals: the role of control

We apply the encoding model to stimuli signalling an impending danger. Danger signals are linked to aversive consequences and therefore should adopt a negative valence. However, the valence aspect as such does not warrant conclusions concerning the sensitivity for danger signals; as intimated above, sensitizing as well as inhibiting effects might be expected (Erdelyi 1974; Pratto and John 1991). While it appears uncontroversial that stimulus relevance is an important moderating condition (Folk *et al.* 1992; Bacon and Egeth 1994, 1997), the definition of relevance seems crucial in this case. We assume that a factor of key importance is the degree to which people have control over an impending danger. Consider, for example, a symptom indicating a particular disease. If the disease can be prevented or successfully treated at an early stage, much depends on early detection, and one would perhaps even be willing to accept false positives in order not to miss the chance of successful intervention. Of course, things are different when the disease is neither preventable nor curable. Generally, attending to a problem seems to have less adaptive value when problem-oriented action is not possible, and might even bind resources that would be better invested for more tractable problems.

Although we have couched this argument in somewhat intentionalist terms, there are reasons to assume that it also applies to mechanisms of selective attention. A theoretical rationale for this assumption is provided by the theory of assimilative and accommodative coping (Brandtstädter and Renner 1990; Brandtstädter and Rothermund 2002a,b). The model distinguishes two different modes of dealing with aversive situations (dangers, losses, etc.). In the assimilative mode, the person actively tries to change the situation (counteract the danger, avoid the loss, etc.); attention is focused on information that relates to this goal. In the accommodative mode, the aversive discrepancy is neutralized by adjusting preferences and ambitions. Which of these modes dominates in a given situation crucially depends on action resources and perceived control; when efficient action is blocked, the person gradually disengages from the goal of preventing or avoiding the problem, and the system shifts towards accommodation. With regard to cognitive processing, the accommodative mode involves a withdrawal of attention from the problem and a reduced sensitivity for cues related to it (Rothermund 1998; Brandtstädter and Rothermund 2002a). Thus, in the present context, the dual-process model predicts a sensitizing effect for danger signals that can be linked to efficient action, whereas sensitivity should be reduced when the person has, or believes that he or she has, no control over the danger.

We have tested theses assumptions in an experimental arrangement that draws on the paradigm of 'illusory conjunctions'. Danger signals were defined by particular letter–colour combinations that signalled a loss of points in a game-like task; the loss was controllable (i.e. it could be averted by adequate action) for one group of participants and uncontrollable for the rest. Although binding is necessary to identify the danger stimulus, we assume that the attentional asymmetries would emerge at early levels of analysis by sensitizing the perceptual process for critical features in the case of controllable dangers and lowering sensitivity for these features in the uncontrollable case. Corresponding effects are expected for the encoding, and consequently for the recall, of the 'bound' signals.

We tested these hypotheses using a task in which selected conjunctions of features were presented tachistoscopically. The stimulus material comprised three optically distinct letters (E, O, and V), of dimensions 4 × 6 mm, that were presented on a screen in three different colours (red, green, and blue) against a black background. Three of the nine possible letter–colour conjunctions were presented in each trial. Then a probe stimulus (PS) was shown, and participants had to indicate whether this probe had been part of the previous stimulus set (PS was notified only after the presentation of the stimulus set). The experimental procedure was arranged as a game-like task; to enhance accuracy motivation, 10 points were credited for a correct response (cinema tickets were offered for the best performance). For each participant, one particular letter–colour conjunction, the danger stimulus (DS), signalled a potential loss (subtraction of 20 points); the negative consequence followed presentation of the DS, independent of whether it was given as the PS or whether it was detected or not. Both features of the DS (shape and colour) were counterbalanced across participants. The factor 'control' was varied between subjects in the following way: in the 'controllable' condition, participants had an opportunity to avoid the loss by solving an additional task; in the 'uncontrollable' condition, neutralization of the loss depended on the 'response' of a random generator on which participants had no influence.

Study I

In the first study, data were obtained from 108 students (psychology undergraduates). The experimental sessions comprised 324 trials each; the DS was presented in a third of these trials. The single trials comprised the following steps. First, a fixation point was presented on the screen. After 800 ms the stimulus set appeared and remained on the screen for 100 ms before it was replaced by a backward mask. Participants were then asked whether a given PS had been shown, which in one out of nine trials was the DS. Feedback was given immediately after the response. Trials in which the DS was present were followed by an additional task; in the 'controllable' condition, participants had to indicate the position of the DS in the stimulus set presented previously. If the correct position was chosen, the loss was averted. In the 'uncontrollable' condition, a random generator 'selected' the position. Pay-off conditions for the two groups were matched (for details see Brandtstädter *et al.* 2004). In both conditions, participants received immediate feedback whether or not a loss occurred.

The nine letter–colour conjunctions can be classified into four sets of stimuli: (1) the 'dangerous' conjunction (DS; one conjunction); (2) stimuli sharing the colour feature with the DS (D–colour; two conjunctions); (3) stimuli sharing the letter feature with the DS (D–shape; two conjunctions); (4) stimuli differing in shape and colour from the DS (neutral; four conjunctions). Response distributions under these conditions were analysed drawing on procedures from signal detection theory (Macmillan and Creelman 1991). Sensitivity parameters (d') were calculated from hit rates and false alarm rates. Individual sensitivity scores were used as dependent variables in a 2 × 4 (Group: Control versus No Control × Stimulus Type: DS, D–colour, D–shape, neutral) analysis of variance (ANOVA).

Significant main effects obtained for Stimulus Type ($F(3, 104) = 16.54$, $P < 0.001$) and Control ($F(1, 106) = 6.11$, $P = 0.01$). The main effects were qualified by a Control × Stimulus Type interaction ($F(3, 104) = 25.42$, $P < 0.001$). This pattern suggests that recall of the DS depends on the Control factor in the theoretically predicted way (Fig. 14.2). The danger sign was recalled more accurately when the DS was instrumental in averting impending loss and less accurately when this was not the case.

As shown in Figure 14.2, the effect of control tends to spill over to some extent to stimuli sharing the colour feature with the DS. However, this does not imply that the pattern is uniform over individuals. To gauge individual differences,

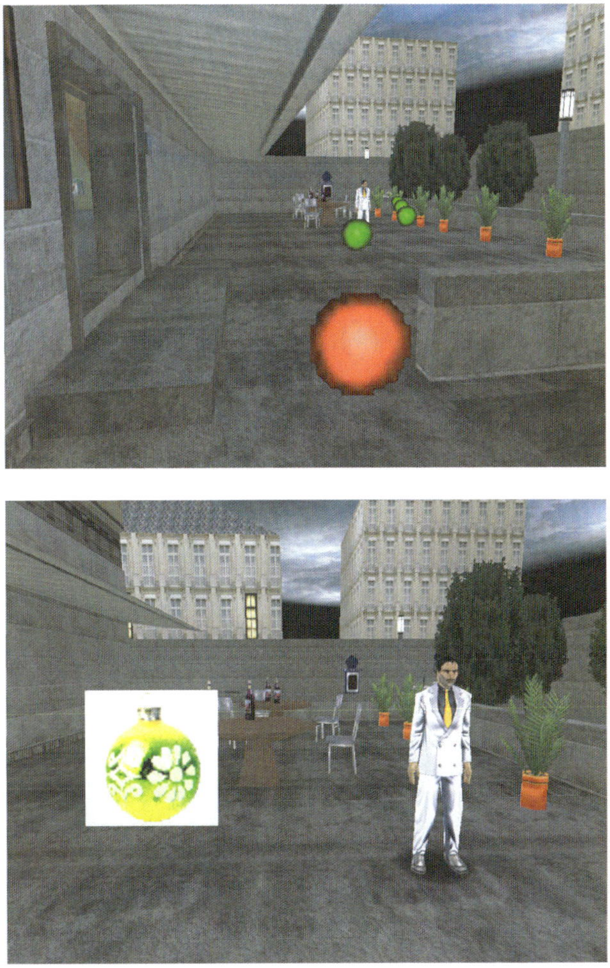

Figure 3.2 Snapshot of the encoding phase of Experiment 2. (a) The participant follows a trail of green dots (the next dot to move over is coloured red), and (b) encounters a distinct person in a distinct location and is presented with the image of a distinct object.

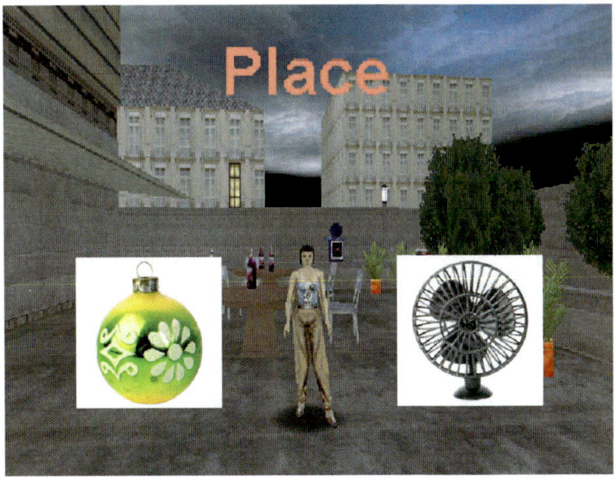

Figure 3.3 An example of a context-dependent paired forced choice question from Experiment 2, showing a Place question: 'Which object did you see in this place?'

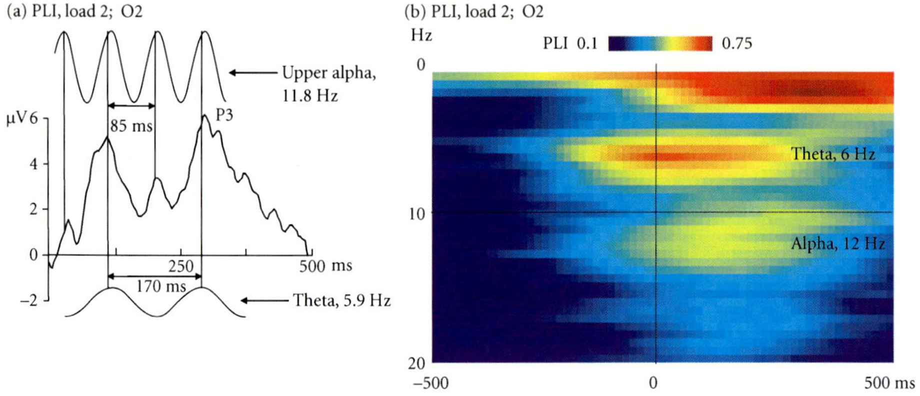

Figure 5.4 (a) ERP and (b) phase locking during successful retrieval (following the presentation of a probe item) in a Sternberg memory scanning task with number-words as items. See p. 131 for detailed caption.

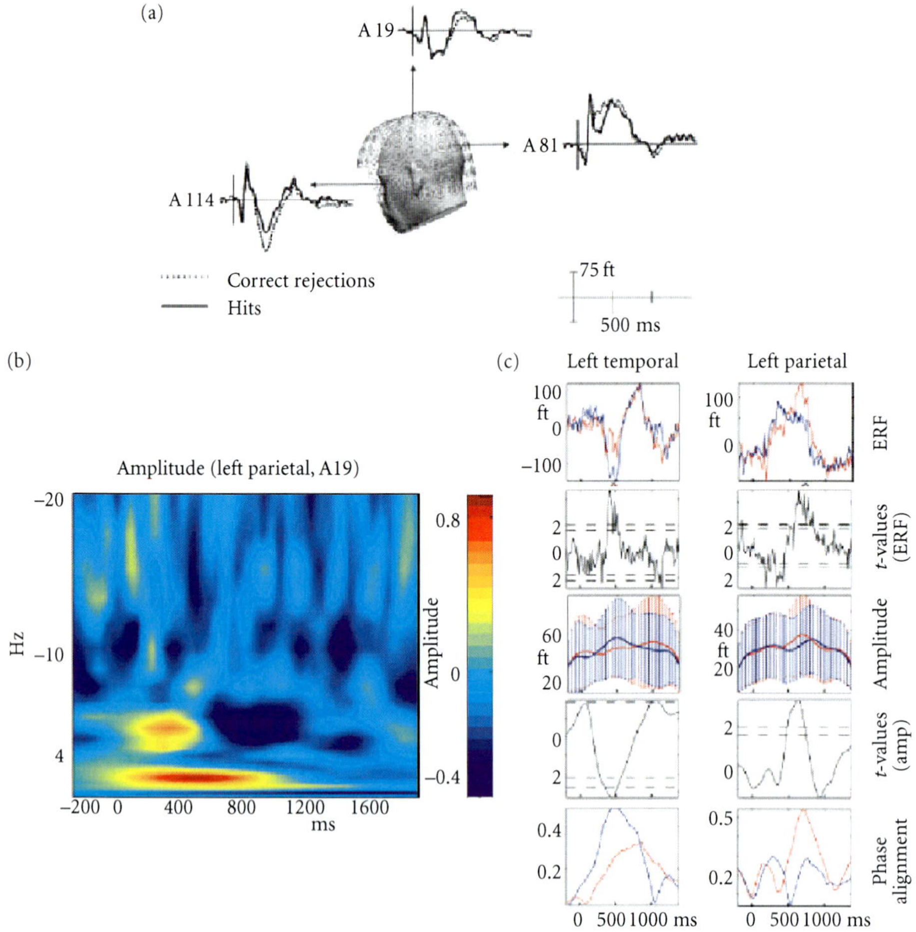

Figure 6.1 (a) Grand average (11 subjects) ERFs elicited by correctly recognized studied (old) words (hits, solid lines) and correctly rejected unstudied (new) words (dotted lines). (b) Time–frequency spectra of the ERF difference between old and new words at sensor A19 obtained by wavelet transformation of the ERF (hence after averaging of single trials). (c) Evidence for evoked responses from single-subject data at a left temporal and a left parietal sensor: comparisons of ERFs, phase alignment, and amplitudes. See p. 150 for detailed caption.

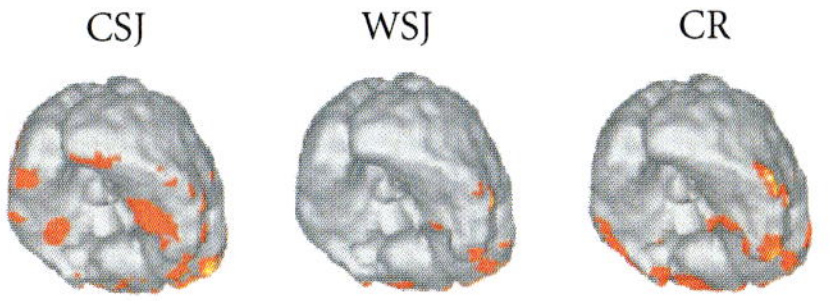

Figure 6.2 Current density distributions of induced theta oscillations for correct source judgements (CSJ), wrong source judgements (WSJ), and correct rejections (CR).

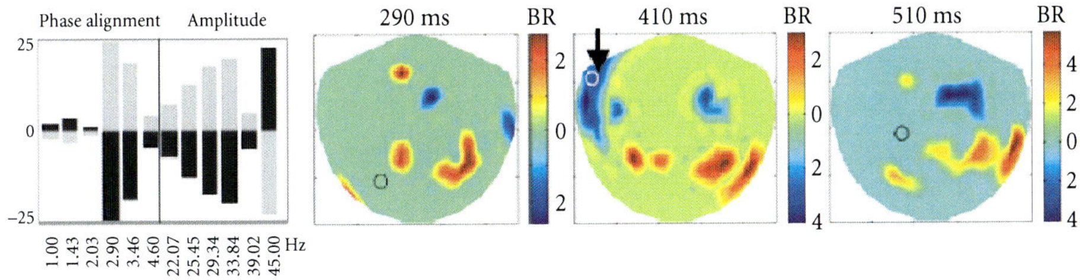

Figure 6.3 Partial least-squares analysis of the covariance between phase alignment in the delta and theta range and amplitude in the beta and gamma range. The left panel illustrates how phase alignment of frequencies ranging from 1 to 4.6 Hz and amplitude of frequencies ranging from 22 to 45 Hz jointly distinguish hits (grey bars) and correct rejections (black bars). The topographic maps on the right display the topography of the corresponding frequency patterns at early, N400, and LPC time windows. See p. 156 for detailed caption.

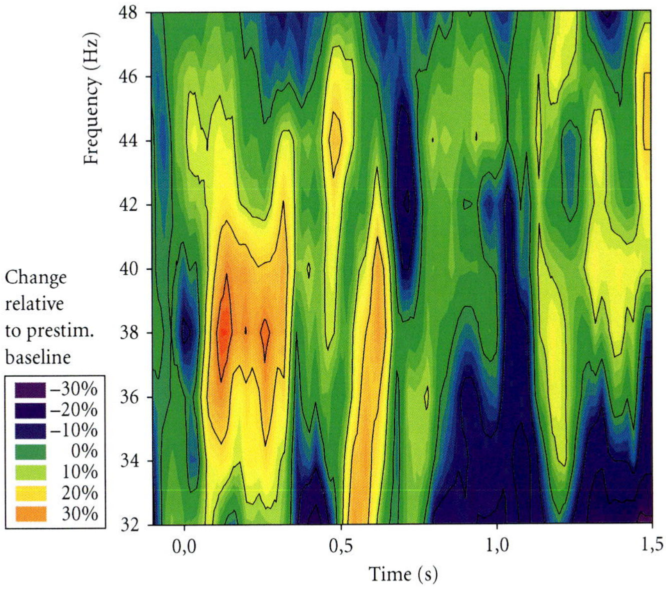

Figure 7.3 Differences of phase synchronization between rhinal cortex and hippocampus (per cent) relative to prestimulus baseline for subsequently recalled versus unrecalled words. See p. 182 for detailed caption.

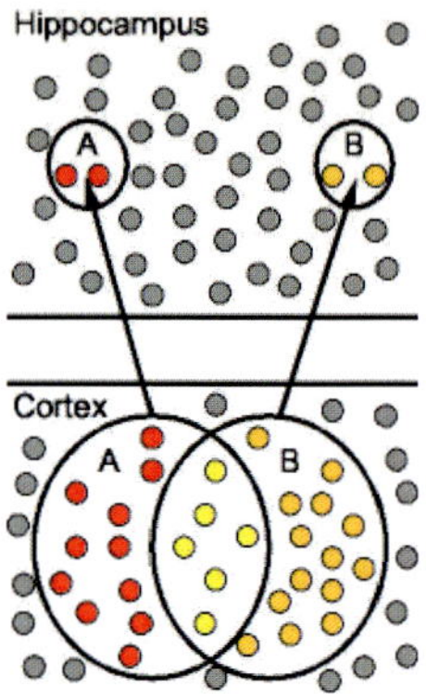

Figure 8.9 Sparse representations in the hippocampus relative to the cortex leads to pattern separation (less probability of activation patterns overlapping, as is evident in the figure), and to units in hippocampus representing larger conjunctions of features in the cortex. See p. 214 for detailed caption.

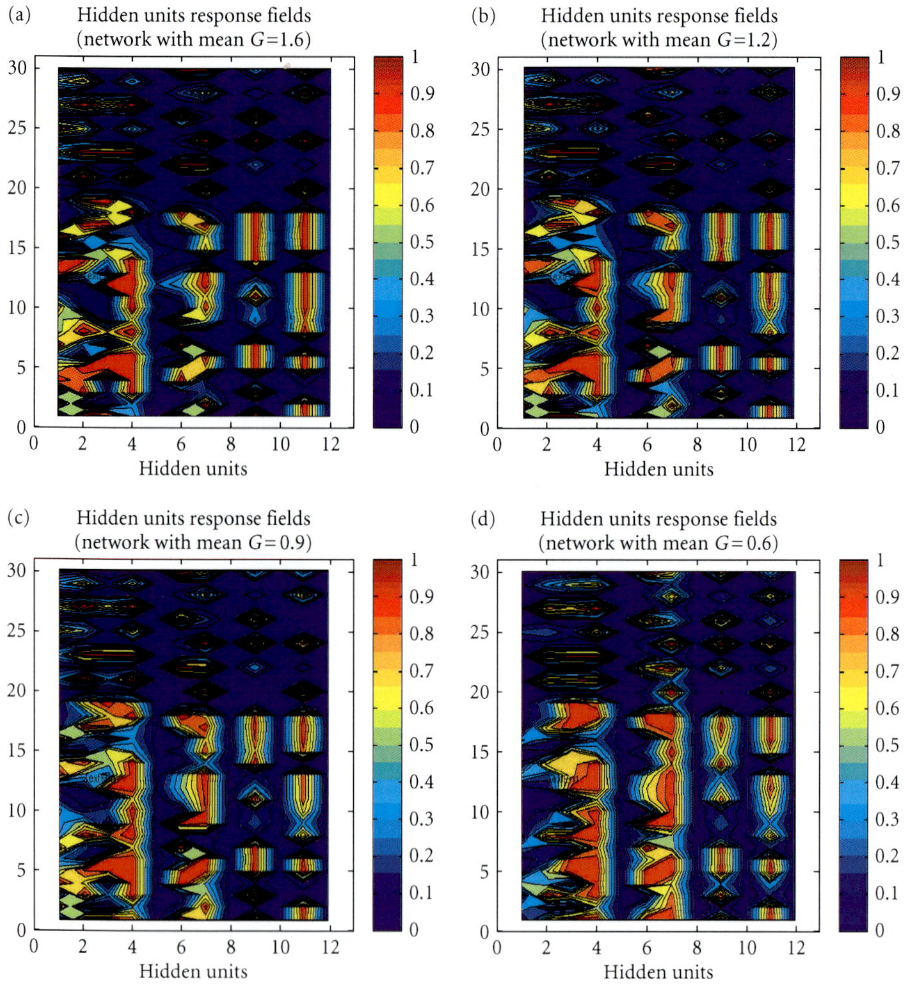

Figure 11.4 Summary hidden-unit activation maps of four networks illustrating the effects of reducing mean G on the distinctiveness of distributed coding of associative information. Red coloration indicates that the units are highly activated, whereas blue coloration indicates low activation (see text for explanation).

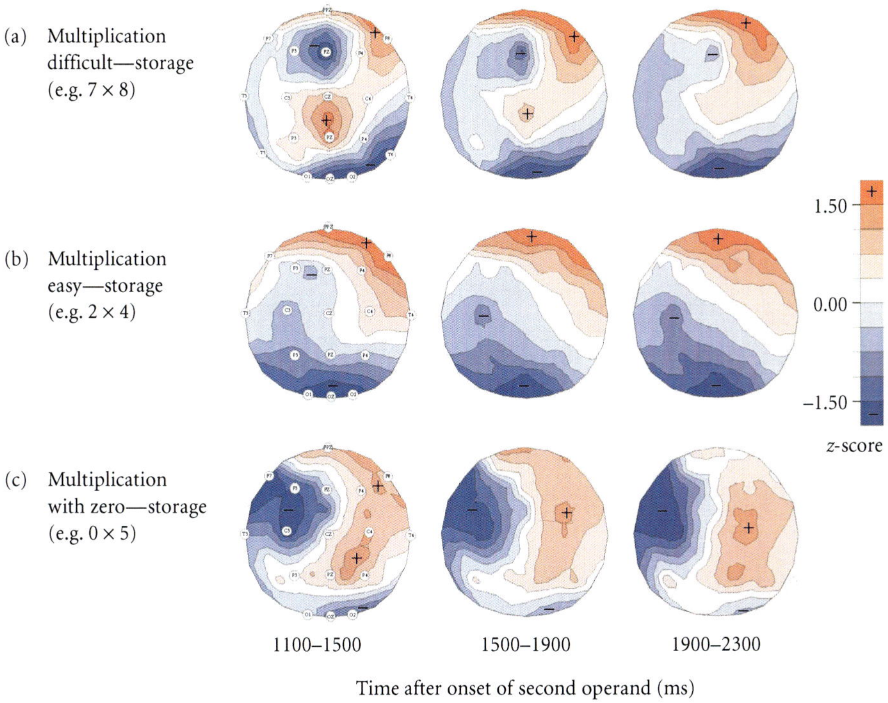

Figure 13.6 Topography of slow negative waves in an arithmetic production task with different types of single-digit multiplication problems. *Z*-standardized maps for three time epochs after presenting the second operand of a multiplication problem in a longer sequence of computations are shown. The maps were computed from difference potentials which contrasted the three multiplication conditions ((a) difficult, large operands; (b) easy, small operands; (c) one zero operand) with a non-multiplication condition in which single-digit numbers only had to be stored. See p. 355 for detailed caption.

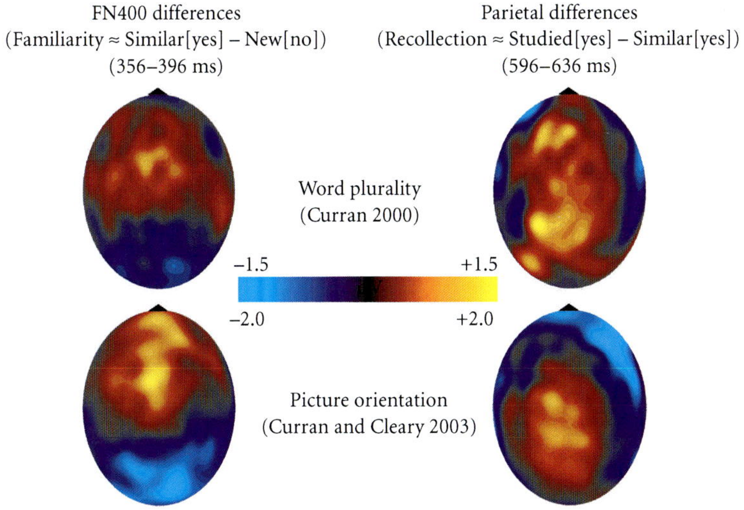

Figure 18.2. Topographical comparison of the FN400 familiarity effect with the parietal recollection effect. (a) Figures from the plurality recognition experiment; (b) figures from the picture orientation recognition experiment (subjects with good studied–similar discrimination only). See p. 472 for detailed caption.

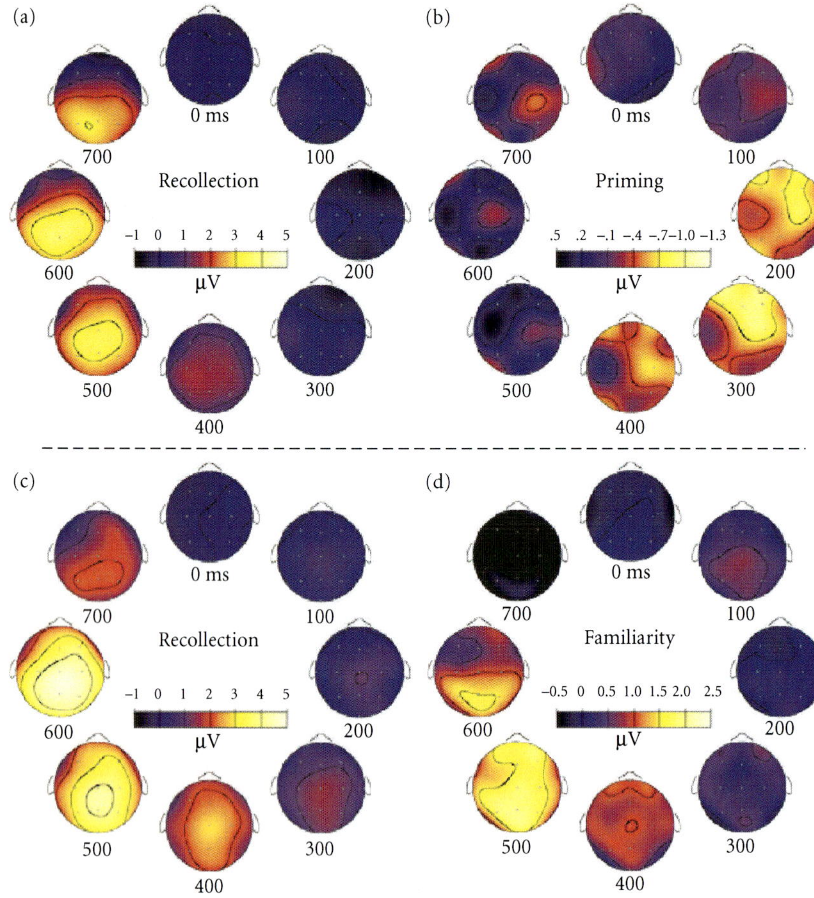

Figure 21.3 Topographic maps of brain potentials associated with different memory phenomena: (a) recollection and (b) perceptual priming in one experiment (Paller 2003a); (c) recollection and (d) pure familiarity in another experiment (Yovel and Paller *et al.* 2004). See p. 537 for detailed caption.

Figure 24.1 Hemispheric asymmetry in PFC activity between two RM tasks: word-pair cued recall and context recognition. Left PFC activity was greater for cued recall than for context recognition, possibly reflecting greater production demands, whereas right PFC activity was greater for context recognition than for cued recall, possibly reflecting greater monitoring demands. (Reproduced from R. Cabeza *et al., Journal of Cognitive Neuroscience*, **15**, 249–259, 2003.)

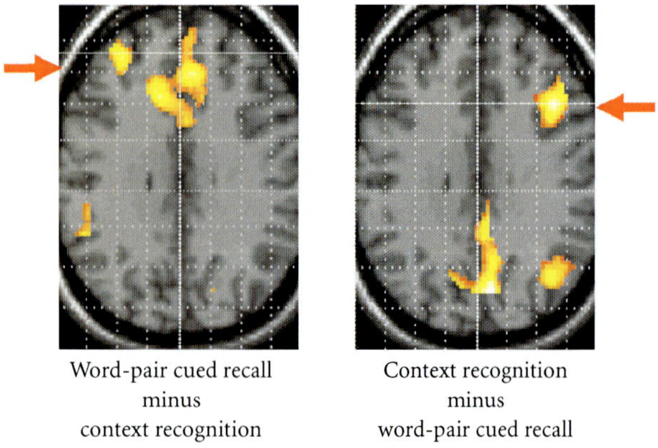

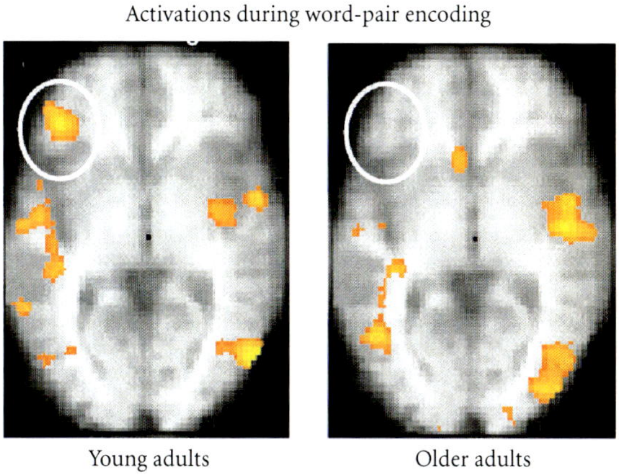

Figure 24.2 During word-pair learning, left ventrolateral PFC was significantly activated in young adults but not in older adults, possibly reflecting age-related deficits in memory encoding processes. (Based on results originally reported in R. Cabeza, *Psychology and Aging*, **17**, 85–100, 2002.)

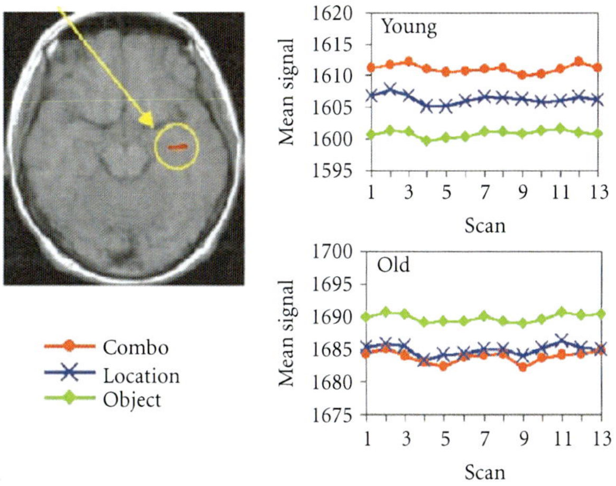

Figure 24.3 During a working memory task, young adults showed greater hippocampal activity when maintaining information about objects in different screen locations (combo trials), than when maintaining the objects or the locations alone (object and location trials). In contrast, older adults did not show greater hippocampal activity for combo trials. (Reproduced from K.J. Mitchell *et al.*, *Cognitive Brain Research*, **10**, 197–206, 2000.)

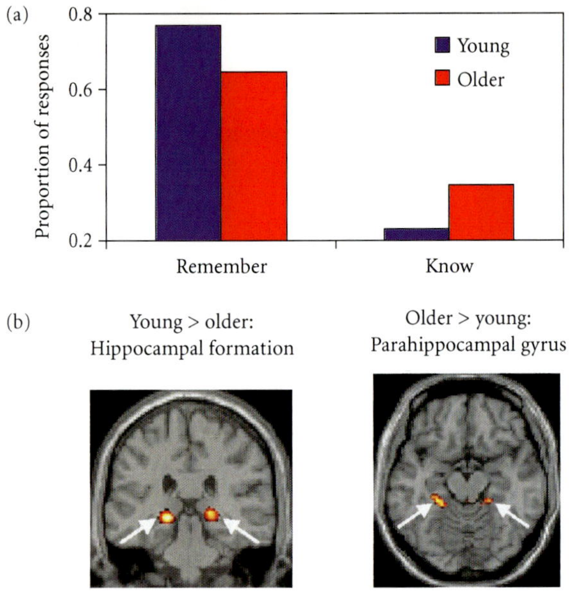

Figure 24.4 (a) During episodic retrieval, older adults produced fewer 'remember' responses (recollection), but more 'know' responses (familiarity), than young adults. (b) During the same episodic retrieval task, the hippocampus was more activated in young adults than in older adults, whereas the parahippocampal gyrus was more activated in older adults than in young adults. See p. 605 for detailed caption. (Reproduced from R. Cabeza *et al.*, *Cerebral Cortex*, **14**, 364–375, 2004.)

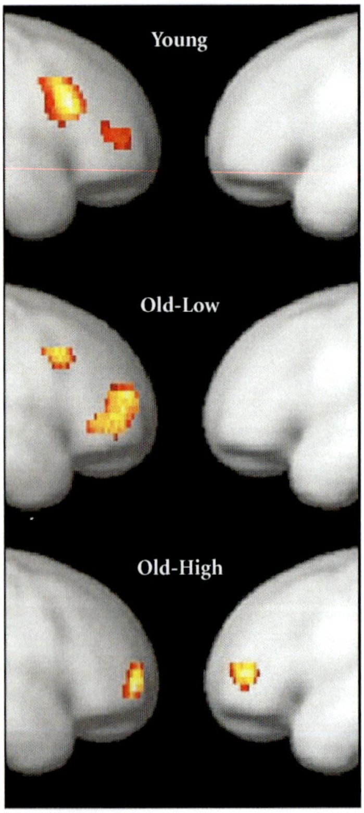

Figure 24.5 Consistent with the compensatory interpretation of bilateral PFC recruitment in older adults, high-performing but not low-performing older adults showed bilateral PFC activation during context memory (Reproduced from R. Cabeza *et al.*, *NeuroImage*, **17**, 1394–1402, 2002).

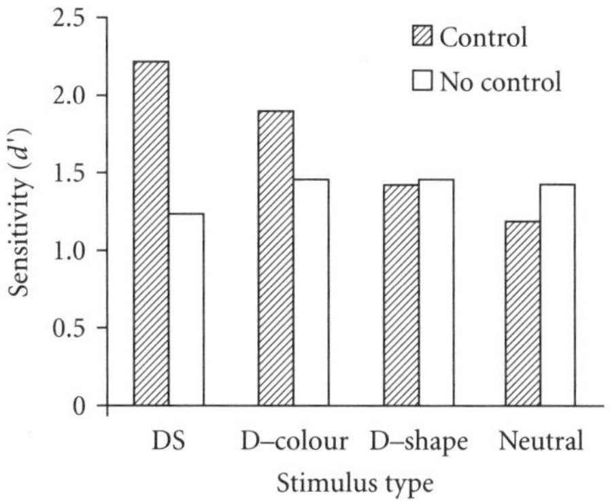

Figure 14.2 Sensitivity *d'* for different stimulus types as a function of control (Study I). DS, danger stimulus, conjunction of colour and letter; D–colour, stimuli sharing the colour of the danger stimulus but not its shape; D–shape, stimuli sharing letter of the *DS* but not its colour; Neutral, stimuli sharing neither shape nor colour with DS.

Table 14.1 Results of the cluster analysis for participants from the 'controllable danger' condition (Study I)

Cluster number	N	Mean relative sensitivity d'			Focus of attention
		Danger stimulus	Danger–colour only	Danger–shape only	
I	23	1.65**	1.41**	0.25*	Strong focus on danger–colour
II	25	0.31*	0.18*	−0.06	Weak focus on danger–colour
III	6	1.66**	0.14	1.39**	Strong focus on danger–shape

$^*P < 0.05$; $^{**} P < 0.01$.

relative sensitivities for the DS, D–shape and D–colour conjunctions were calculated by subtracting sensitivity for the neutral stimuli. The new values were entered into a cluster analysis (SPSS QUICK CLUSTER procedure). For participants with control over danger, a three-cluster solution emerged. Cluster means are shown in Table 14.1. Obviously, the degree to which stimulus type affects relative achievement in the recall task differs between clusters. In cluster I, heightened sensitivity for the DS goes with enhanced sensitivity for the colour feature (D–colour); this also holds for cluster II, but here the effects are less strong. In contrast, visual search appears to be primarily driven by the shape feature (D–shape) in cluster III, which, however, comprises only six participants. A 3 × 3 (Stimulus Type × Cluster) ANOVA reveals significant main effects for Stimulus Type ($F(2, 50) = 18.69$; $P < 0.001$) and Cluster ($F(2, 51) = 48.44$; $P < 0.001$), as well as an interaction ($F(4, 102) = 16.20$; $P < 0.001$). No clear pattern emerged for participants in the No Control Group.

The findings from this exploratory study conform to our predictions. When subjects have control over the aversive consequences, sensitivity to the danger signal is enhanced and the binding system appears to be tuned to features of the danger stimulus. Consequently, danger signals are encoded (and recalled) correctly more often than other stimuli. Although performance was best for probes including both danger features, this does not imply that the conjunction as such is addressed in early selection. Instead, the cluster-analytic results indicate that, for most participants, the colour feature guided the selection process. For participants who did not have active control over the negative consequences, the pattern was completely reversed. In this group, binding accuracy was worst for the danger stimulus. It should be noted that this pattern cannot be attributed to response tendencies. In terms of GS theory (Wolfe 1994, 1996), the features of the danger stimulus appear to be suppressed in the activation map and therefore, in relation to other stimuli, disadvantaged in the binding system as well as in VWM.

We could be be criticized for using a game-like situation where not much is at stake; however, it is all the more noticeable that the predicted asymmetry appears even under such conditions. A more serious limitation of the experimental arrangement may consist in the particular demands of the additional task used in the 'Controllable Danger' condition. Successful performance in this task was dependent on the detection of the DS in the preceding trial, and this in turn may have facilitated the search for danger signals in the detection task. Study II addresses this point.

Study II

In a supplementary experiment, the 'Control' condition of Study I was replicated with a particular modification. The additional task used to avert the danger was designed differently so that successful performance no longer depended on the detection of the DS in the preceding trial. Again, we expect an increased binding accuracy for the DS and for conjunctions sharing a feature with the DS compared with neutral conjunctions.

Eighteen psychology undergraduates participated in this supplementary experiment. The procedure for the additional task was altered as follows: 800 ms after the feedback for the detection task, the word 'Danger' was displayed on the screen whenever the critical letter–colour conjunction of the DS had been present in the stimulus set; 300 ms later, the original stimulus set was presented again, and participants had to rapidly indicate the position of the DS in the triangular display by pronouncing a corresponding number (1 indicated the upper

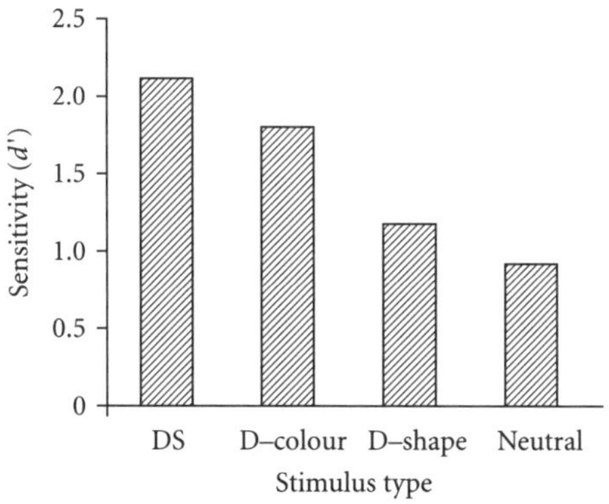

Figure 14.3 Sensitivity *d*′ for different stimulus types (Study II). DS, danger stimulus, conjunction of colour and letter; D–colour, stimuli sharing the colour of the danger stimulus but not its shape; D–shape, stimuli sharing letter of the *DS* but not its colour; Neutral, stimuli sharing neither shape nor colour with DS.

position, 2 the lower right position, and 3 the lower left position). Response latencies were recorded by a microphone that was connected to the computer. The 'defence' (averting a loss of points) was successful if a correct response was given within a latency of 500 ms. In this approach, detection of the DS may be helpful for solving the additional task, but it is not a necessary condition for success as in the previous paradigm.

Figure 14.3 shows the mean sensitivity scores (d' values; see above) for the four levels of Stimulus Type (DS, D–colour, D–shape, neutral) that were calculated from hit rates and false alarm rates in the recall task. The pattern replicates the results for the 'Controllable Danger' condition in Study I. Again, a strong effect of stimulus category emerges ($F(3, 15) = 12.56$, $P < 0.001$); planned contrasts with the neutral stimuli show that sensitivity was significantly increased for all stimuli involving a danger feature. To compare the two different additional tasks (Study I, controllable condition, versus Study II), a 2×4 (Task Type $\times$ Stimulus Type ANOVA was conducted. No significant main effects or interactions involving Task Type emerged (all $F < 1$), indicating that the two tasks have an equivalent effect.

Discussion

The present chapter addresses top-down influences on the encoding of objects. More specifically, we expected top-down influences to moderate perceptual sensitivity. If top-down processes direct attention to a particular class of stimuli, examples from this class will not just be reported more readily, but will be more easily identified and remembered. The difference between perceptual and response system effects is captured by the distinction between response bias and sensitivity in signal detection theory (Snodgrass and Corwin 1988). As outlined in the Introduction, features are not yet integrated to compound percepts in early visual processing. At this early level, top-down influences should operate on the basis of features and not on the basis of conjunction information; for example, attention could be directed to all red objects but not specifically to red circles only. A binding of features of separate dimensions (e.g. colour and shape) to integrated percepts (object files) requires focused attention, which is a limited resource. The 'spotlight of attention' (Treisman 1993) focuses on only a small segment of the visual field at a time. Inhibition of objects outside the attentional focus may also play an important role in this process (Oberauer 2005). The 'spotlight of attention' metaphor shows that binding is a time-consuming process; consequently, a conjunction search proceeds serially. In our studies, we used this fact to infer the attentional capture of different types of stimuli from binding accuracy. The tachistoscopic presentation of stimuli did not afford enough time to process all stimuli serially, so that correct binding indicates that a given object had a high priority in the search process.

Following this rationale, two studies were conducted. Top-down influences were expected to guide the allocation of attentional resources to different types of stimuli. Binding accuracy was compared between a danger signal (defined as a conjunction of colour and shape), stimuli sharing a single feature with this danger signal, and neutral stimuli. Personal control over aversive consequences in case of danger was varied between participants. Proceeding from the account of assimilative and accommodative coping (Brandtstädter and Rothermund 2002 a,b), we argued that danger signals should attract attention if a potential loss can be actively averted; in contrast, we expected an inhibition of danger signals if no control was possible. Here, the notion of control does not imply perfect control, but a probabilistic link between action and outcome (see also Maier 1989). As predicted, we found that sensitivity for stimuli signalling a negative consequence was enhanced when participants had a chance to actively avert this consequence, and suppressed when they had no control over the impending danger.

This finding fits well with the GS model (Wolfe 1994, 1996). According to this model, the amount of activation in an internal activation map representing locations in the visual field is determined not only by bottom-up but also by top-down processes. Top-down influences moderate the transmission of activation from initial feature maps to the activation map. For example, activation for all locations where a certain feature is represented (e.g. the feature 'red') is enhanced because of the high relevance of this feature in the current situation. The distribution of activation in the activation map then guides a serial process of feature integration that starts at the location that has the largest activation and proceeds downwards.

The enhanced sensitivity for stimuli signalling controllable dangers can be explained by assuming that locations where the critical features are present enter the binding process with high priority. However, an additional cluster analysis revealed the limits of such top-down influences. For each participant in the controllable condition, only one of the two features the critical conjunction that had an influence on the serial feature integration process. Apparently, top-down influences on the activation map are restricted to a single feature, which explains why there is no efficient conjunction search (if the stimulation on the activation map could be enhanced for more than one feature simultaneously, this would imply that objects sharing both of two critical features would always be the first to attract attention). Although sensitivity was highest for stimuli sharing both features of the (controllable) danger stimulus, the results suggest that this is due to a summation of effects of a guided search for different features across participants. This result stands in contrast with postulates of the GS model which allow for a simultaneous pre-activation of multiple features (Wolfe *et al.* 1989).

Thus privileged processing of controllable dangers seems to be located at an early selection stage that is based on a pre-activation of single features. Although these influences cannot bypass the binding process, they can guide the priorities with which objects sharing certain features enter into the feature integration process. However, it is less clear whether such a pre-activation of features can also account for the reduced sensitivity that emerged for the uncontrollable danger stimuli in Study I. This finding suggests that top-down influences may affect perception not only through an increase in the activation of certain features, but also through inhibitory processes. Contrary to the findings for the controllable danger condition, the pattern of results for the uncontrollable condition indicates that this effect is not based on an inhibition of single features because a reduced sensitivity was found only for the feature conjunction that made up the danger stimulus. This suggests an active suppression of perceptual objects that are irrelevant for the regulation of action, such as negative priming (Tipper 2001). By definition, object-based influences are located at a post-binding stage of perception. Thus the reduced sensitivity for stimuli signalling uncontrollable dangers that was found in our data appears to reflect a fast decay (e.g. in VWM) of object representations that are irrelevant for the regulation of action. In line with the assumption of a 'perceptual defence' against negative or threatening information, uncontrollable dangers become actively suppressed after having been identified in the feature integration process. However, our findings do not support the assumption that dangerous or negative information is generally suppressed (McGinnies and Sherman 1952; Erdelyi 1974, 1993). Whether such information is preferred or suppressed in the perceptual process seems to depend on whether the danger can be averted by active efforts. Thus this assumption, which is consistent with the dual-process model of action regulation (Rothermund 1998; Brandtstädter and Rothermund 2002a), accounts for at least some of the inconsistencies in research findings concerning the perception of valent information.

These considerations converge with observations from other lines of research. For example, Rothermund *et al.* (2002) found reduced pain sensitivity for heat stimuli after a prolonged exposition to uncontrollable painful pressure stimuli, indicating that the perceptual information (i.e. the pain) was inhibited in the helplessness condition. More direct evidence for a deeper processing of action relevant stimuli comes from experimental findings pointing to an increased sensitivity for perceptual cues that are relevant for tendencies of approach or avoidance (Wentura *et al* 2000; Wentura and Rothermund 2003). Similarly, research on the self-ascription of negative and positive attributes has revealed that self-assessments for uncontrollable attributes are subject to a self-enhancement bias, whereas self-evaluation for controllable attributes is characterized by a problem focus (Dunning 1995; Rothermund *et al.* 2005).

Summary and conclusions

Top-down influences on the encoding of valent stimuli appear to be mediated by processes of selective attention that can bias perceptual processes at the pre- and post-binding stages. A pre-activation of features guides attention so that relevant objects have privileged access to the feature integration process. A second type of influence operating at the post-binding stage appears to influence the duration with which object representations remain active in VWM. Inhibitory effects help to suppress the access of irrelevant information to further information processing. The core assumption of the present research was that attentional processes and motivated binding depend on and are integrated in processes of action regulation (Brandtstädter and Rothermund 2002a,b). Our findings suggest that perceived personal control over outcomes triggers a problem focus that enhances sensitivity for danger signals. In contrast, experiences of helplessness or low control appear to activate an accommodative mindset in which negative or threatening information is actively suppressed so that processing resources can be reallocated to more promising domains.

Acknowledgements

The research reported in this chapter was supported by a grant to JB from the Deutsche Forschungsgemeinschaft (DFG).

References

Averill, J.R., and Rosenn, M. (1972). Vigilant and nonvigilant coping strategies and psychophysiological stress reactions during the anticipation of electric shock. *Journal of Personality and Social Psychology*, **23**, 128–141.

Bacon, W.F. and Egeth, H.E. (1994). Overriding stimulus-driven attentional capture. *Perception and Psychophysics*, **55**, 485–496.

Bacon, W.F. and Egeth, H.E. (1997). Goal-directed guidance of attention: evidence from conjunctive visual search. *Journal of Experimental Psychology: Human Perception and Performance*, **23**, 948–961.

Brandtstädter, J. and Renner, G. (1990). Tenacious goal pursuit and flexible goal adjustment: explication and age-related analysis of assimilative and accommodative strategies of coping. *Psychology and Aging*, **5**, 58–67.

Brandtstädter, J. and Rothermund, K. (2002a). Intentional self development: exploring the interfaces between development, intentionality, and the self. In *Motivation, Agency, and the Life Course. Nebraska Symposium on Motivation*, Vol. 47 (ed L.J. Crockett). Lincoln, NE: University of Nebraska Press, pp. 31–75.

Brandtstädter, J. and Rothermund, K. (2002b). The life-course dynamics of goal pursuit and goal adjustment: a two-process framework. *Developmental Review*, **22**, 117–150.

Brandtstädter, J., Voss, A., and Rothermund, K. (2004). Perception of danger signals: the role of control. *Experimental Psychology*, **51**, 1–9.

Dunning, D. (1995). Trait importance and modifiability as factors influencing self-assessment and self-enhancement motives. *Personality and Social Psychology Bulletin*, **21**, 1297–1306.

Erdelyi, M.H. (1974). A new look at the new look: perceptual defense and vigilance. *Psychological Review*, **81**, 1–25.

Erdelyi, M.H. (1993). Repression: the mechanism and the defense. In *Handbook of Mental Control* (ed D.M. Wegner and J.W. Pennebaker). Englewood Cliffs, NJ: Prentice-Hall, pp. 126–148.

Fazio, R.H., Sanbonmatsu, D.M., Powell, M.C., and Kardes, F.R. (1986). On the automatic activation of attitudes. *Journal of Personality and Social Psychology*, **50**, 229–238.

Folk, C.L., Remington, R.W., and Johnston, J.C. (1992). Involuntary covert orienting is contingent on attentional control settings. *Journal of Experimental Psychology: Human Perception and Performance*, **18**, 1030–1044.

Gollwitzer, P.M. (1995). The volitional benefits of planning. In *The Psychology of Action: Linking Cognition and Motivation to Behavior* (ed P.M. Gollwitzer and J.A. Bargh). New York: Guilford Press, pp. 287–312.

Kahneman, D., Treisman, A., and Gibbs, B. (1992). The reviewing of object files: object-specific integration of information. *Cognitive Psychology*, **24**, 175–219.

Lazarus, R.S., Yousem, H., and Arenberg, D. (1953). Hunger and perception. *Journal of Personality*, **21**, 312–328.

McGinnies, E. and Sherman, H. (1952). Generalization of perceptual defense. *Journal of Abnormal and Social Psychology*, **47**, 81–85.

Macmillan, N.A. and Creelman, C.D. (1991). *Detection Theory: A User's Guide*. New York: Cambridge University Press.

Maier S. F. (1989). Learned helplessness: Event Covariation and Cognitive Changes. In *Contemporary learning theories: Instrumental conditioning theory and the impact of biological constraints on learning* (eds B. Klein and R. R. Mowrer). Hillsdale, NJ: Erlbaum, pp. 51–86.

Miller, S.M. (1979). Coping with impending stress: psychophysiological and cognitive correlates of choice. *Psychophysiology*, **16**, 572–581.

Murphy, S.T., and Zajonc, R.B. (1993). Affect, cognition, and awareness: affective priming with optimal and suboptimal stimulus exposures. *Journal of Personality and Social Psychology*, **64**, 723–739.

Oberauer, K. (2005). Binding and inhibition in working memory: individual and age differences in short-term recognition. *Journal of Experimental Psychology: General*, **134**, 368–387.

Pratto, F. and John, O.P. (1991). Automatic vigilance: the attention-grabbing power of negative social information. *Journal of Personality and Social Psychology*, **61**, 380–391.

Rothermund, K. (1998). Persistenz und Neuorientierung: Mechanismen der Aufrechterhaltung und Auflösung zielbezogener kognitiver Einstellungen [Persistence and reorientation: maintaining and dissolving goal-related cognitive sets]. University of Trier Internet document. Available online at: http://ub-dok.uni-trier.de/diss/diss11/19990701/19990701.htm

Rothermund, K., Brandtstädter, J., Meiniger, C., and Anton, F. (2002). Nociceptive sensitivity and control: hypo- and hyperalgesia under two different modes of coping. *Experimental Psychology*, **49**, 57–66.

Rothermund, K., Bak, P.M., and Brandtstädter, J. (2005). Biases in self-evaluation: effects of attribute controllability. *European Journal of Social Psychology*, **35**, 281–290.

Snodgrass, J.G., and Corwin, J. (1988). Pragmatics of measuring recognition memory: applications to dementia and amnesia. *Journal of Experimental Psychology: General*, **117**, 34–50.

Tipper, S. P. (2001). Does negative priming reflect inhibitory mechanisms? A review and integration of conflicting views. *Quarterly Journal of Experimental Psychology: Comparative and Physiological Psychology*, **54a**, 321–343.

Treisman, A. (1986). Features and objects in visual processing. *Scientific American*, **255**, 114–125.

Treisman, A. (1993). The perception of features and objects. In *Attention: Selection, Awareness, and Control. A Tribute to Donald Broadbent* (ed A.D. Baddeley and L. Weiskrantz). Oxford: Clarendon Press, pp. 5–35.

Treisman, A. (1999). Feature binding, attention and object perception. In *Attention, Space, and Action. Studies in Cognitive Neuroscience* (ed G.W. Humphreys, J. Duncan, and A. Treisman). New York: Oxford University Press, pp. 91–111.

Treisman, A. and Sato, S. (1990). Conjunction search revisited. *Journal of Experimental Psychology: Human Perception and Performance*, **16**, 459–478.

Wentura, D. and Rothermund, K. (2003). The 'meddling-in' of affective information: a general model of automatic evaluation effects. In *The Psychology of Evaluation: Affective Processes in Cognition and Emotion* (ed J. Musch and K.C. Klauer). Mahwah, NJ: Erlbaum, pp. 51–86.

Wentura, D., Rothermund, K., and Bak, P. (2000). Automatic vigilance: the attention-grabbing power of approach and avoidance-related social information. *Journal of Personality and Social Psychology*, **78**, 1024–1037.

Wheeler, M.E. and Treisman, A.M. (2002). Binding in short-term visual memory. *Journal of Experimental Psychology: General*, **131**, 48–64.

Wolfe, J.M. (1994). Guided search 2.0: a revised model of visual search. *Psychonomic Bulletin and Review*, **1**, 202–238.

Wolfe, J.M. (1996). Extending Guided Search. Why Guided Search needs a preattentive 'item map'. In *Converging Operations in the Study of Visual Selective Attention* (ed A.F. Kramer and M.G.H. Coles). Washington, DC: American Psychological Association, pp. 247–270.

Wolfe, J.M., Cave, K.R., and Franzel, S.L. (1989). Guided search: an alternative to the feature integration model for visual search. *Journal of Experimental Psychology: Human Perception and Performance*, **15**, 419–433.

Yantis, S. (1996). Attentional capture in vision. In *Converging Operations in the Study of Visual Selective Attention* (ed A.F. Kramer and M.G.H. Coles). Washington, DC: American Psychological Association, pp. 45–76.

Yantis, S. (2000). Goal-directed and stimulus driven determinants of attentional control. In *Control of Cognitive Processes: Attention and Performance XVIII* (ed S. Monsell and J. Driver). Cambridge, MA: MIT Press, pp. 73–103.

Chapter 15

Brain correlates of binding processes of emotion and memory

Esther Fujiwara and Hans J. Markowitsch

Introduction

Although global and severe memory disorders primarily result from organic brain damage, it has long been known that intra-psychic processes, such as emotional disturbances or stress, can influence cognitive functions and therefore memory. Autobiographical episodic memory is the memory system most vulnerable to disturbances resulting from organic diseases or functional disorders. We assume that its vulnerability originates from obligatory complex interactions between memory and processing of one's self and emotions. In this chapter, following a brief overview of contemporary memory systems and their brain correlates, we elucidate binding mechanisms within autobiographical episodic memory with respect to emotion and processing of the self. These mechanisms may be disrupted, and we suggest that emotional or self-related disturbances can result in autobiographical memory loss. Behavioural and neuroimaging results from psychiatric patients are presented to exemplify this relationship. The chapter closes with a model describing possible mechanisms of autobiographical episodic memory interruptions resulting from emotional or self-related disturbances.

Memory processes and memory systems

Memory can be divided according to processes, aspects of time, and contents. In long-term memory formation, different steps of information processing are traversed. Prior to permanent storage, information first has to be registered at the sensory organs (**registration**) and initially pre-processed (**encoding**). The pre-processed information is then embedded into information networks which already exist and associated with previous contents (**consolidation**). Once information is successfully consolidated, memory engrams are stored permanently (**storage**) and, in principle, can be retrieved later (**retrieval**). Every time stored information is retrieved, it will be re-encoded. Thus the initial memory trace undergoes considerable changes (Tulving 2001). The traditional classification along the dimension of time corresponds to the concepts of short- and long-term memory as well as working memory (Baddeley *et al.* 2001). A further time-based categorization relates to the onset of amnesia in patients. Here, one can distinguish memories acquired before a critical incident from information to be learned subsequently. In the case of organic amnesia, these incidents refer to brain injury (e.g. resulting from head trauma, hypoxia, or encephalitis), whereas in psychological or non-organic forms of amnesia they may consist of the experience of a psychological trauma or stressful event (Kopelman 2002). In either case, if patients are unable to access information that happened before the critical incident they are said to be suffering from retrograde amnesia, whereas the inability to acquire new information after the incident is called anterograde amnesia.

It has long been known that memory in amnesic patients is not evenly affected by deteriorations. Contents-based classifications of memory may be the best way to describe the pattern of memory loss seen in amnesia. According to Tulving (2002), long-term memory can be divided into separate but interdependent and hierarchically organized subdivisions. From the lowest level of complexity to the highest, these systems are termed procedural memory, priming, perceptual memory, semantic memory, and episodic memory (Markowitsch 2003b). The two most elaborate memory systems, episodic and semantic memory, and the differences between them are of particular interest in the current context. Whereas semantic memory is believed to be present-oriented and covers context-free facts and general knowledge such as names of cities and countries, episodic memory requires 'mental time travel' to the past and contains context-embedded specific and distinctive events from one's own past.

The terms 'episodic memory' and 'autobiographical memory' are often used interchangeably. This may partly result from the fact that Tulving himself never drew a definite distinction between episodic autobiographical memory and episodic recall and recognition of items such as words or pictures to be remembered in experimental settings (Tulving 2001). However, both forms of episodic memory are clearly differentiable in several aspects (e.g. emotional connotation, personal significance, complexity of the information, temporal distance of the 'time travel'). Although Tulving eventually referred to episodic memories for single items from experimental settings as 'mini-events' (e.g. Tulving 1983), their contents are unlikely to match episodes from one's own autobiography. However, rather than referring to the different contents of autobiographical episodic memories versus non-autobiographical episodic memories, Tulving emphasized the similarities of retrieval consciousness associated with both types of episodic memories. In this vein, Tulving (2001) claims that the contents of all memory systems are associated with different levels of awareness. Episodic information is thought to be **autonoetic** in that it requires an awareness of one's own self (Markowitsch 2003a). This is the case even if the content of an episodic memory only comprises single items from experimental settings, since one has mentally to go back to the learning episode ('mini-event') when the item was encountered. Reconsidering the difference between autobiographical and non-autobiographical episodic memory, it may be obvious that retrieval of both requires autonoetic consciousness and that this holds even if their contents undoubtedly differ. Thus one has to be aware that a certain event has happened with regard to its temporo-spatial context and to oneself experiencing it in the past, regardless of whether or not its contents are autobiographically relevant. The contents of the semantic memory system are believed to be **noetic**. This includes the possibility of consciously retrieving semantic information but excludes the obligatory involvement of the self. In other words, one can know semantic facts without remembering where and when one has acquired this knowledge. Note that some autobiographical information has a context-free character (e.g. names of former friends or previous telephone numbers) and is also known as 'personal semantic memory' (Kopelman and Kapur 2001). However, also within impersonal semantic memory, clear context independence is not always given. While world knowledge, such as that obtained from the news media, basically possesses semantic qualities, it can involve additional autobiographical–episodic components. For instance, in remembering the terror attack on the World Trade Center one might recapitulate the fact that this event has happened (semantic memory), but one might also remember more specific circumstances such as one's own reactions or feelings at that time (episodic information). Conway (2001) further developed how to distinguish between episodic autobiographical memory and semantic autobiographical knowledge, which will be discussed below.

The hierarchical organization of the memory systems implies that lower systems can operate without higher systems. In ontogenetic and phylogenetic development, episodic memory evolves latest and may be restricted to humans (Tulving 2001; Suddendorf and Busby 2003). Accordingly, it is possible that other species exhibit only lower memory systems such as perceptual memory, which can be tested by visual or auditory recognition paradigms (Aggleton and Pearce 2001). Further support of the hierarchy described relates to human ontogenesis. By the age of about 4 years or less, children are capable of acquiring semantic knowledge about the world without, however, displaying episodic memory abilities. They are not yet able to retrieve temporally and contextually specific events from their personal past (Reese 2002; Uehara 2000). Moreover, patients with acquired brain lesions or neurodegenerative diseases (Hamann and Squire 1995; Vargha-Khadem *et al.* 2001) usually show deficits when acquiring new episodic memory information but their ability to learn semantic or perceptual information is spared. Selective lesions or initial damage to the hippocampal formation (e.g. in Alzheimer's disease (Garrido *et al.* 2002)) is believed to be responsible for these deficits, whereas damage extending to broader areas of the medial and lateral temporal lobes can also compromise semantic memory (Grossman *et al.* 2003).

Memory and the brain

Amnesic patients normally show impairment in conscious forms of memory, whereas unconscious systems are mostly preserved. As mentioned above, this discrepancy can usually be seen in patients with organic amnesias, resulting from bilateral medial temporal lobe lesions (Corkin *et al.* 1997) or medial diencephalic pathology (alcoholic Korsakoff syndrome (Phaf *et al.* 2000)) for example. Similar dissociations are apparent in psychiatric patients (Kazes *et al.* 1999; Ellwart *et al.* 2003). Correspondingly, in functional neuroimaging studies with healthy subjects, memory systems and processes have been associated with clearly differentiable brain regions (see *Neuropsychologia*, **41** (3), Special Issue on Functional Neuroimaging of Memory).

Starting with the lower memory systems, encoding and consolidation of procedural memory require structures of the basal ganglia and cerebellum (Mandolesi *et al.* 2001); acquisition of priming and perceptual memory are organized in uni- and polymodal cortical areas (Buckner and Koutstaal 1998). The medial temporal lobe, medial diencephalon, and, more loosely, the basal forebrain act as bottleneck structures for the episodic and semantic memory systems (Markowitsch 2000). Even small lesions to these structures can lead to massive impairment of the storage of new materials (Markowitsch *et al.* 1993; von Cramon *et al.* 1993). It is believed that episodic and semantic encoding and consolidation depend on two separable but interrelated circuits within the limbic system: the Papez circuit and the amygdaloid circuit. The Papez circuit comprises mammillary bodies, anterior nuclei of the thalamus, the hippocampal formation, and their connecting fibres (e.g. cingulum, fornix). Whereas Papez himself considered this circuit to be specifically involved in processing of emotional material (Papez 1937), it is now believed to be responsible for transfer of all short-term memory information into long-term stores. Instead, the amygdaloid circuit, comprising the amygdala, the mediodorsal nucleus of the thalamus, the subcallosal area of the basal forebrain, and their connecting fibres, is now considered to be particularly involved in encoding and consolidation of emotional memories (Markowitsch 1998). Patients with highly circumscribed lesions within the Papez circuit can exhibit extensive anterograde memory problems (Calabrese *et al.* 1995), whereas memory deficits that result from damage to the amygdaloid circuit are more subtle and possibly restricted to emotional contents. A few single and multiple case studies of patients with selective bilateral amygdala calcification resulting from Urbach–Wiethe disease (Siebert *et al.* 2003) point to this particular deficit in perception and acquisition of emotional information in these patients. As will be outlined in more detail below, there is a large body of evidence about autobiographical memory disturbances in affective disorders, implicating abnormal functioning of the amygdala (e.g. in depression (Van Vreeswijk and De Wilde 2004)). Therefore lesions to the amygdaloid circuit may also compromise autobiographical memory. Although there is no direct evidence from brain-damaged subjects (i.e. Urbach–Wiethe patients), amygdala lesions may correspond to autobiographical memory disturbances, at least with regard to retrieval specificity. Beyond medial temporal and medial diencephalic regions, there is growing evidence for the importance of (pre-)frontal brain areas in episodic memory formation (Fletcher and Henson 2001).

Retrieval of perceptual, priming, and procedural memory contents relies on similar structures to those involved during their acquisition. Depending on the nature of the task, different polymodal association areas are implicated in priming and perceptual memory. Once procedural and priming memory contents are successfully consolidated, retrieval requires less activity in the brain regions initially involved (Schacter and Buckner 1998). Concerning episodic and semantic memory, Tulving *et al.* (1994) have proposed and recently revised (Habib *et al.* 2003) a hemispheric encoding–retrieval asymmetry (HERA) model. They suggested that, being stimulus independent, the right hemisphere is specialized for episodic retrieval, whereas the left hemisphere is more involved in retrieval of semantic information (and encoding of both episodic and semantic information). The brain region most critically involved in retrieval from both memory systems is the prefrontal cortex. Reanalysing previous neuroimaging results with healthy subjects, Fletcher and Henson (2001) differentiated retrieval control processes such as specification of search parameters, monitoring of retrieval results, and maintenance of information, and assigned them to different regions within the prefrontal cortex. The right temporo-frontal junction is a further critical component of episodic memory retrieval in healthy subjects (Fink *et al.* 1996; Markowitsch *et al.* 2000b) as well as in patients with structural brain damage (Levine *et al.* 1998) or functional disturbance in this area (Markowitsch *et al.* 1997a). Summarizing previous results from patients and normal subjects, we list

Table 15.1 Brain regions associated with memory systems and processes

	Procedural memory	Priming	Perceptual memory	Semantic memory	Episodic memory
Encoding and consolidation	Basal ganglia Cerebellar regions	Primary and association cortex	Posterior sensory cortex	Cerebral cortex Limbic structures	Limbic system Prefrontal cortex
Storage	Basal ganglia Cerebellar regions	Primary and association cortex	Posterior sensory cortex	Cerebral cortex (mainly association areas)	Cerebral cortex (mainly association areas) Limbic regions
Retrieval	Basal ganglia Cerebellar regions	Primary and association cortex	Posterior sensory cortex	Fronto-temporal cortex (left)	Fronto-temporal cortex (right) Limbic regions

Reproduced from M. Brand and H.J. Markowitsch, in *Principles of Learning and Memory* (ed R.H. Kluwe, G. Lüer, and F. Rösler). Basel: Birkhäuser, 2003, pp. 172–84.

brain structures and circuits associated with the memory systems and processes discussed above in Table 15.1 (Brand and Markowitsch 2003).

Emotional modulation of memory processes

Emotional characteristics of information are of particular importance for their encoding and consolidation as well as for storage and retrieval. Brain areas associated with emotional processing and emotional memory comprise the amygdala, the prefrontal cortex (especially the ventromedial prefrontal and orbitofrontal cortex), the anterior cingulate gyrus, the ventral striatum, and the insula (Davidson and Irwin 1999). Of these, the amygdala is most intensively studied and amygdaloid involvement has been observed in numerous emotion-processing and emotional memory studies of animals and healthy human subjects (LeDoux 2000). Selective structural damage to the amygdala can lead to deterioration of emotional processing and memory, as in patients with Urbach–Wiethe disease (Siebert *et al.* 2003). Furthermore, in patients with affective disorders of psychiatric origin, enduring amygdaloid metabolic hyper- or hypoactivity critically contributes to memory deficits (von Gunten *et al.* 2000). The basolateral nucleus of the amygdala is considered a crucial brain structure for the modulation of memory through emotional arousal (Cahill and McGaugh 1998). It possesses various systemic hormonal afferents whose input is combined and distributed via efferents to subcortical and cortical memory-relevant brain structures (e.g. the hippocampal formation) (Aggleton 2000). It has been suggested that this modulation is mediated by the effects of stress hormones, including glucocorticoids, interacting with noradrenergic receptors in the basolateral amygdala (McGaugh and Roozendaal 2002) and other neurotransmitter systems (Vallée *et al.* 2001). In animal experiments glucocorticoids were found to enhance amygdala-dependent processes (emotional learning) while simultaneously inhibiting hippocampus-dependent processes (non-emotional learning) (Roozendaal *et al.* 1999; McGaugh 2002). It is important to note that modulation of memory formation via glucocorticoids is dose dependent. Generally, memory-enhancing effects are obtained with low to moderate doses over short periods of time, whereas memory-deteriorating effects are observed after longer-lasting exposure to glucocorticoids at higher doses (Kim and Yoon 1998; de Kloet *et al.* 1999; Lupien *et al.* 2002). Although this interaction has been primarily studied in the context of memory formation, there is growing evidence for the importance of glucocorticoid modulation of memory retrieval (Roozendaal 2002; de Quervain *et al.* 2003). Outside the amygdala, glucocorticoid receptors are located in various memory-relevant structures, such as the anterior temporal lobes and the hippocampal formation, making them particularly vulnerable to stress effects (McEwen 1999; Bremner and Vermetten 2001). Given that autobiographical episodic memory is mostly characterized by its emotional nature, its particular vulnerability to stress-related deteriorations is not surprising. In the following sections we will first focus on neural correlates of autobiographical memory in healthy subjects and then turn to their deterioration mediated by emotional and/or self-related disturbances in patients.

Autobiographical memory: emotions and the self

Remembering autobiographical events requires retrieval of episodic memory contents and related emotions, and a sense of one's own self and past life history (Tulving 2001). The vivid recollection of personal episodes is, at least partly, related to the evocation of the formerly experienced emotional states (Dolan *et al.* 2000; Markowitsch 2000). To assign events to autobiographical memory, episodic memory contents have to be integrated and bound with a sense of self-coherence and self-continuity across the individual time axis reaching into the past as well as the future (Larsen *et al.* 1996). Thus, autobiographical episodic memory comprises the emotional evaluation of personal life experiences with respect to ourselves.

The relationship between autobiographical memory and the self is powerful if not inseparable. As was pointed out by Conway and Pleydell-Pearce (2000), autobiographical knowledge may define the range of goals of the self, which in turn modulate the construction of new autobiographical memories. In their view, emotional autobiographical memories derive from experiences of goal attainment or failure, and retrieval of or forgetting emotional personal events may serve to reduce perceived discrepancies in the self. Wilson and Ross (2003) proposed similar interdependencies. Their temporal self-appraisal theory proposes a bidirectional relation between autobiographical memory and current identity. It suggests that autobiographical memory serves to enhance feelings of personal identity and consistency through time. These authors provide evidence of self- and time-dependent memory biases and demonstrate how perceived self-improvement over a lifetime can distort autobiographical recall (e.g. Karney and Frye 2002). On the other hand, current self-views can be changed by the emotional connotation and temporal remoteness of retrieved autobiographical memories (Ross and Wilson 2002).

How do we consciously experience previous emotional states ourselves and relate them to our autobiography? According to Damasio (1994, 1999), metaphysical ideas about these entities as being conscious thoughts separate from one's own body and any physical reality should be doubted. In this vein, Churchland (2002) pointed out that conscious thinking results from activities of the physical brain, aspects of self-regulation and self-cognition can be non-conscious, and any introspective experience of the self is inseparable from the body. To begin with emotions, Damasio (1994, 1999) suggested that they were complex expressions of homeostatic regulatory systems of organisms. In his terminology, the core of an emotion is the collection of changes in the body and mind mediated by several body organs and a limited number of brain circuits. This collection takes place under control of a brain system binding momentary thoughts with the current situation or event. On the one hand, reactions resulting from this collection involve bodily changes through a so-called body-loop; on the other hand, changes within the brain can be induced by minimally engaging the body via simulation through as-if-body-loops. An advantage of the latter mechanism is that, on the basis of former experiences, organisms can internally simulate internal and external events, which then can be used in a generalized and therefore energetically economic way (see also Churchland (2002) who proposed that a system's efficiency is linked to increasing abilities to emulate events and states internally). Damasio proposed four stages of life regulatory mechanisms: basic reflexes, emotions, feelings, and knowing of one's own feelings. In his model, these mechanisms are associated with different levels of consciousness. On top of basic life regulation (e.g. reflexes), emotions are triggered if an object or situation occurs and is associated with specific somatic and mental changes. Furthermore, if an organism is capable of forming mental representations or images of the changes induced by emotions, a feeling is experienced. On the highest level, some organisms can consciously experience themselves as being the owners of their feelings. Reflexes, emotions, and feelings do not necessarily require consciousness, whereas knowing of feelings is a conscious process. Damasio (1999) suggests that emotions and feelings, as well as increasing levels of consciousness, provide the basis for survival-oriented behaviours. If organisms are capable of experiencing themselves as being the owners of emotions and feelings, as-if-body loops are necessarily involved. Therefore increasing levels of consciousness are associated with higher degrees of simulation capacity and therefore generalization and adaptivity. Higher levels of consciousness are associated with increasingly complex forms of self-representation. Along with this idea, Churchland (2002) claims that neuroscientific exploration of the self and its brain correlates requires a reformulation of the idea of the self from a singular entity into a concept allowing for plurality of self-representing functions. Damasio (1999) gives a possible classification of a plurality of selves (see also Gallagher 2000; O'Brien and Opie 2003). On the most basic level, he suggests a non-conscious proto-self, which is an ongoing collection of representations of the multiple dimensions of the state of the current organism. On a higher level, he places a core self as a transient but conscious reference or feedback to the organism in which events are happening. The level of consciousness associated with the core self is labelled core consciousness. Core consciousness results from confrontation with an external or internal object or event automatically inducing mental representations experienced with a sense of ownership of these images. Therefore core consciousness is normally associated with a feeling of knowing that oneself is the owner of an experience. Because of its transient nature, the core self does not require embedding in a personal history or past experiences. However, organisms without the ability to form autobiographical memories can be conscious of their moment-to-moment core selves. Finally, at the top of the hierarchy, extended consciousness enables organisms to experience autobiographical selves. Extended consciousness is understood as the capacity to generate a sense of individual perspective and ownership over a larger range of knowledge than that surveyed in core consciousness. A substantial part of this knowledge is autobiographical memory. A summary of Damasio's model is given in Figure 15.1.

Because of the inseparable interaction of brain and body in Damasio's theories, neural substrates and representations of the body form the basis of emotion and proto-self (e.g. representation of the bodily internal milieu in the brainstem, hypothalamus, and basal forebrain; representation of body posture and location in relation to the outside world in the somatosensory system). However, core and autobiographical self and associated core and extended consciousness require

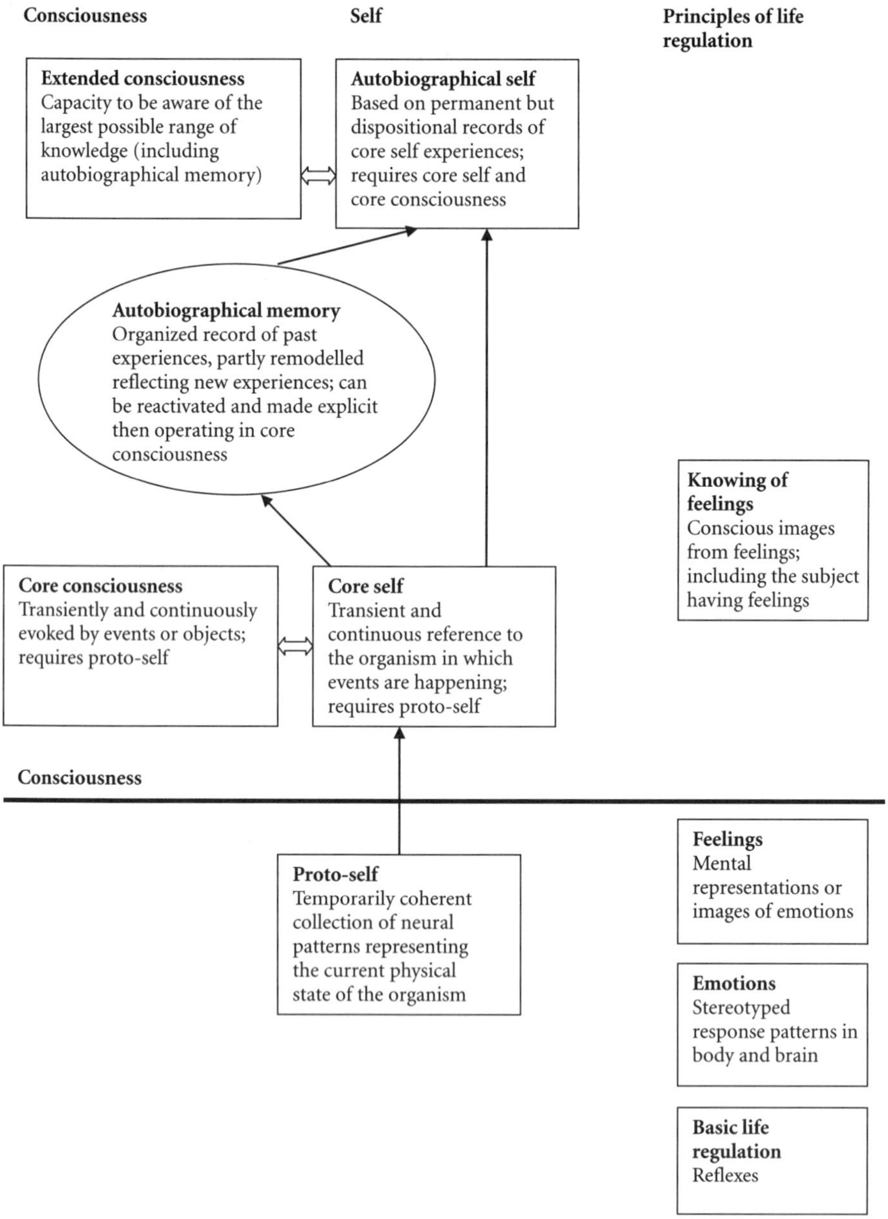

Figure 15.1 Classifications of consciousness, self, and life regulatory systems according to Damasio (1999).

brain structures receiving converging signals from various sources capable of processing signals from the whole organism as well as from objects of the outside world. The convergence zones, a network comprising the prefrontal cortex, cingulate cortex, thalamus, and superior colliculi, are assumed to serve this purpose

(Damasio 1999). Similarly, according to Mesulam (2000, p. 93), 'from a strictly behavioral point of view, the existence of consciousness might be inferred when a living organism responds to environmental events in an adaptive way that is not entirely automatic'. Mesulam argues that species with more complex nervous systems will also have more complex forms of consciousness. His argument implies that, because of the large-scale networks in the human nervous system, the possibilities for an asynchronous action are also increased, especially under conditions of brain damage or dysfunction. Indeed, neurological and psychiatric patients suffering from disturbances of autobiographical memory, emotion, and self may be the best and most concrete indicators of the existence of the classifications discussed above. These will be described in the last section of this chapter. First, we turn to brain correlates of autobiographical memory associated with emotion and self in healthy subjects.

Autobiographical memory and self: processing in the brain

Let us return to autobiographical memory, which in Damasio's terminology is a major part of the knowledge used in extended consciousness. Conway (2001) suggests that a distinction be drawn between autobiographical knowledge and episodic memory. He takes episodic memory to be more time-restricted and largely sensory–perceptual in nature. During episodic memory retrieval, these sensory characteristics trigger 'recollective experience', which he describes as the sense or experience of one's own self in the past. In contrast, retrieval of temporally extended autobiographical knowledge, which also contains personal semantics, evokes feelings of familiarity. Only then may it lead to a recollective experience, if its retrieval additionally activates interconnected episodic memories. For integration into autobiographical knowledge, these single episodes have to possess sensory–perceptual features and they have to be experienced in relation to the self and pre-existing autobiographical knowledge. Therefore Conway assumes that sensory–perceptual episodic memory is associated with posterior sensory cortices, while the more comprehensive autobiographical knowledge is suggested to involve broader networks of cortical and subcortical structures. The assumption that episodic memory retrieval reactivates posterior sensory brain regions was supported by an EEG study (Conway *et al.* 2003) in which participants had to retrieve truly experienced versus imagined events. Retrieval of the experienced events was associated with higher activity shifts over occipito-temporal regions than retrieval of imagined events. However, Markowitsch *et al.* (2000b) revealed a somewhat contrary result in their positron-emission tomography (PET) study. Here, activation of the precuneus region in the occipito-temporal junction area was observed during processing of imagined and fictitious events but not during processing of true autobiographical events. Although the difference between real and fictive autobiographical episodes may reside in remembered sensory–perceptual characteristics of real episodes, it is unclear from these results whether this is the most crucial differentiating variable. Re-experiencing of former self and emotions may play a far more important role, as was indicated by the results obtained by Markowitsch *et al.* (2000b). Generally, neuroimaging studies on autobiographical episodic memory employ stimuli which are episodic in nature but, as a matter of definition, belong to the personal past of the subjects and thus to their general autobiographical knowledge. Therefore, while Conway's model (Conway 2001) is intriguing, no definitive neuroimaging evidence yet exists to confirm or refute it.

Alternatively, emotional and self-related information processing could also be a crucial link to autobiographical episodic memory. A more or less consistent network of implicated brain regions is reported in previous neuroimaging studies comprising, bilaterally, the ventrolateral, dorsolateral, and ventromedial prefrontal cortex, the temporal pole, the lateral and medial temporal cortex including the hippocampal and parahippocampal complex, the temporo-parietal junction area, and the posterior cingulate/retrosplenial cortex and cerebellar regions (Maguire 2001). Assuming that self-related processing is crucial for autobiographical episodic memory retrieval, bilateral medial and right prefrontal cortices appear to be prominent regions in which consistent overlap in activation has been observed in both autobiographical episodic retrieval and self-processing tasks (Markowitsch 2003a). Keenan *et al.* (2000) found a general right-hemispheric preponderance during processing of one's own compared with other people's faces in laterality tasks, and this was localized within the right prefrontal cortex in event-related potential (ERP) and functional MRI (fMRI) experiments (Keenan *et al.* 2001). Similarly, in a PET study during which participants encoded trait adjectives with reference to either one's self or other people, the bilateral medial and right prefrontal cortex was involved only in the self-referential condition, as revealed by partial least-squares analysis (Craik *et al.* 1999). Bilateral medial prefrontal engagement was also seen in fMRI experiments during self-referential cognition (Johnson *et al.* 2002; Kelley *et al.* 2002; Zysset *et al.* 2002), with a possible differentiation of more ventral parts associated with emotional aspects and dorsal parts mediating attentional demands of the task (Gusnard *et al.* 2001). It has been argued that the medial prefrontal cortex is involved in a network of medial brain regions that are, by default or during rest, more active than inactive. Conversely, these regions showed a decrease rather than an increase in activity if task-related processing was compared with resting states of the brain (Raichle *et al.* 2001). Furthermore, this default mode of the brain may be associated with (unintentional) self-related thinking, which will be attenuated during task-related processing, especially in attention-demanding tasks (Gusnard *et al.* 2001). In this vein, Kelley *et al.* (2002) investigated self- and other-related processing. Across conditions they revealed an attenuation of medial prefrontal activity compared with a baseline. Contrasting self-related with other-related processing was associated with higher activity in the self-related than in the other-related condition, but lower than the baseline. In fact, in this study the explicit self-related processing was associated with smaller decreases from a low-level baseline than an actual increase in activity. Kelley *et al.* (2002) argued that their result mimics the normal mode of operation of the medial prefrontal cortex, i.e. it is more active in resting states (unintentional self-related cognition) and explicit self-referential thoughts than during attention-demanding tasks. It may be inferred that cognitive–attentional processes associated with an experimental setting and task have led to a general attenuation of the (naturally high) medial prefrontal cortex activity. In turn, the self-referential aspect of the task condition raised its activity back towards its default level. However, the picture is complicated by other studies of self-referential cognition that point to actual increases in medial prefrontal cortex activity compared with control tasks (Johnson *et al.* 2002; Schmitz *et al.*, 2004).

In non-autobiographical episodic retrieval, medial and right ventral parts of the prefrontal cortex corresponded to active retrieval in contrast with automatic recollection (Petrides 2002). In a series of PET studies, Lepage *et al.* (2000) found the right ventral prefrontal region activated when participants were in an episodic retrieval mode, a state in which one consciously focuses on the act of episodic memory retrieval (e.g. focusing attention on a specific past experience, treating incoming and online information as retrieval cues, becoming aware of retrieval products). How can one reconcile the apparently conflicting findings of right-hemispheric activation in some studies, medial and left prefrontal findings in others, and both in still others? Fink *et al.* (1996) provide one important clue. Healthy subjects showed that to-be-retrieved materials with explicit emotional connotation engaged the right hemisphere in particular (but see Piefke *et al.* 2003). Further evidence shows that studies that revealed right-hemispheric engagement (Fink *et al.* 1996, Ryan *et al.* 2001) may all involve enhanced emotional engagement compared with the majority of studies showing medial or left prefrontal activation (Andreasen *et al.* 1999; Conway *et al.* 1999; Maguire *et al.* 2000; Maguire and Frith 2003; Piefke *et al.* 2003). Following this line of reasoning, it is noteworthy that participants were relatively naive before scanning, since they were unaware of the purpose of previously conducted autobiographical interviews for stimulus acquisition (Fink *et al.* 1996), or stimuli were partly acquired by interviews of spouses rather than participants themselves (Ryan *et al.* 2001). Considering the effect that this would have had on the participants, in all the latter studies confrontation with autobiographical stimuli most probably invoked a higher degree of emotional involvement (e.g. feelings of surprise, ambiguity, emotional re-experiencing) as well as heightened visual attention to the stimuli during the scanning, which may both correspond to right-hemispheric activity (Davidson 2002; Cabeza *et al.* 2003).

In summary, we conclude that medial prefrontal areas are specifically engaged in the processing of one's own self. The more emotional the information, the more these activations extend ventrally and to the right prefrontal cortex. This may be the case in autobiographical episodic memory studies, in which subjects are naive to the stimuli and therefore re-experience cues of autobiographical episodes with a higher degree of emotional and visual attentional involvement during the scanning. These latter results may be most appropriate for explaining findings of autobiographical memory deficits in neurological and psychiatric patients with right-hemispheric frontal lesions or functional disturbances. In the next section we will focus on autobiographical memory deficits and their parallels in self-related and emotional disturbances in psychiatric patients. Neuroimaging results are reported to elucidate possible corresponding functional brain correlates.

Dissociation of self, emotion, and memory: autobiographical memory and its disturbances in psychiatric disorders

Schizophrenia

Among psychiatric disorders affecting a sense of integrated self and consciousness, schizophrenia first comes to mind. Following Gallagher (2000), particular psychotic experiences such as hallucinations, thought insertion, or delusions of self-control elucidate distortions in the access to one's own self being an immediate and pre-reflective point of origin for action, experience, and thought. This form of self, comparable with the core self of Damasio (1999), is normally immune to errors of misidentification. Its processes and contents are experienced with a sense of self-ownership ('I am undergoing a certain experience') and self-agency ('It is me causing an action or thought'), a condition that is also referred to as the immunity principle. Following Frith's (1992) model, Gallagher (2000) suggests that defective monitoring can account for these phenomena, leaving the sense of self-ownership intact while the sense of agency is disrupted. If delusions of control or thought insertion occur, schizophrenic patients may still have the sense that it is their body that is moving or their thoughts appearing in consciousness. However, the actions or thoughts would not evoke the sense of being self-generated but rather of being outside their control, which can be understood as disruptions of self-agency. Frith (1992) suggests that these monitoring errors occur because of dysfunctional comparisons between internally predicted outcomes of actions or thoughts and the sensory or cognitive feedback caused by the actions or thoughts (see also Damasio 1999).

Schizophrenia is associated with structural abnormalities or dysfunctions in the prefrontal cortex (Byne and Davis 1999; Broadbelt *et al.* 2002) which can account for the behavioural aberrances described. In particular, cognitive functions mostly relying on the prefrontal cortex are often disturbed in schizophrenia (Velligan and Bow-Thomas 1999), including complex memory functions such as autonoetic remembering versus noetic knowing (Sonntag *et al.* 2003) and autobiographical memory (Feinstein *et al.* 1998; Elvevåg *et al.* 2003). The results obtained by Feinstein *et al.* (1998) suggest that remote memory deficits in schizophrenia depend not only on dysfunctional retrieval but also on additional encoding deficits in the storage of long-term memory contents probably related to temporo-parietal dysfunctions. Schizophrenic patients may further show reduced recall of specific temporal and contextual details of personal events (Riutort *et al.* 2003), a condition known as over-generalized autobiographical memory and frequently observed in depression (see below). Interestingly, in a study by Corcoran and Frith (2003), the autobiographical event memory performance of schizophrenic patients was impaired, and this impairment correlated with their deficient theory of mind abilities. Theory of mind or 'mind reading' refers to the capacity to infer one's own or other people's mental states, intentions, and attitudes, and is considered an essential basis for social skills (Baron-Cohen 1995). From their results, Corcoran and Frith (2003) hypothesized that schizophrenic patients are unable to apply the necessary context for retrieval of specific social information, be it explicitly autobiographical, as in personal events, or not, as in ToM situations. Thus, in schizophrenia with its decoupling of certain aspects of the self from ongoing and former experiences, autobiographical episodic memory may lack the contextual and emotional details of healthy subjects' memories. Reduced levels of (self-)awareness in general may correspond to these impairments and may be evident on the brain level. In this regard, Andreasen (2000) suggests that functional disturbances in schizophrenia occur within a network of cortical–cerebellar–thalamic–cortical loops in which the prefrontal cortex plays the most crucial role.

Depression and stress-related disorders

Emotional disturbances can also be a major cause of deterioration in remembering autobiographical episodes, as is evident in major depression. A frequently reported finding is that the autobiographical event memory of depressive patients lacks specificity, indicating that, compared with healthy subjects, depressive patients tend to recall more over-generalized events. Instead of reporting temporally and contextually distinctive episodes, they give categoric descriptions of summarized repeated occasions (Williams 1996; Barnhofer *et al.* 2002; de Decker *et al.* 2003). This retrieval style is further associated with poor recovery from the disease (Brittlebank *et al.* 1993). A possible underlying mechanism is described by Williams (1996) and referred to as 'mnemonic interlock'. He suggests that over-general autobiographical retrieval is encouraged by a ruminative self-focus which in turn fosters over-general retrieval. Although over-general autobiographical retrieval also serves to avoid memories of negative emotional aspects of events in healthy subjects (Raes *et al.* 2003), in depressive patients this behaviour is assumed to develop early in life so that avoidance of conscious recollection becomes an automatized habit. Furthermore, according to Williams, depressive patients show a tendency to retrieve negative self-referential categoric descriptions (e.g. 'I have always failed'). If potentially negative retrieval cues are encountered, these categoric descriptions are triggered in an automatized way. Activation of related and frequently used self-descriptions is elicited only within this level of description stage (e.g. 'I used to fail at school', 'I never had friends', etc.), meaning that retrieval moves across the hierarchy rather than down to more specific levels. Thus, over-general memory emerges from a blockade or truncation ('mnemonic interlock') of the search for specific events and instead results in an over-elaboration of self-related general categories. Williams further assumes that mnemonic interlocks can only be overridden at high costs of effort. Individuals with working memory or attentional impairments, resulting from either structural brain damage to the frontal lobes or functional metabolic disturbances in frontal brain regions, as seen in depression (Drevets 2001), may show particular problems in inhibiting the automated categoric search and therefore be barely able to access specific memories. Thus, in major depression, emotionally motivated over-stable self-views may prevent autonoetic remembering of autobiographical episodes and instead foster noetic retrieval of categoric events. It is not known how this tendency develops in childhood and later on, but one of the most likely triggers is the experience of trauma.

A large body of evidence emphasizes the close relationship between stress and depression (Di Chiara *et al.* 1999; Holsboer 2001), and patients with post-traumatic stress disorder (PTSD) show a heightened prevalence of comorbid depression (Franklin and Zimmerman 2001). On the brain level, the mediating factor between the two diseases can be seen in a dysregulation of glucocorticoid signalling. As glucocorticoids are required for reliable memory formation and retrieval, especially if the memory contents are of an emotional nature (see above), hypersecretion of glucocorticoids and reduced responsiveness to glucocorticoids, as seen in depression, or hypocortisolism, as in PTSD (Raison and Miller 2003), may correspond to deficits in retrieving specific autobiographical events. On a structural level, Schore (2002) found a heightened vulnerability of basal right-hemispheric brain regions (e.g. brainstem, limbic system) to childhood trauma and stressful attachments during upbringing. Resulting impairments of primarily right-hemispheric functions, such as attachment and relationship behaviour, affect regulation and stress modulation as well as autobiographical episodic retrieval, and may therefore further promote subsequent dysfunctional coping strategies and later development of PTSD and depression. The results of direct comparisons of the impacts of traumatic experiences with depressive symptoms on over-general autobiographical retrieval are controversial. Some studies have suggested a major influence of trauma (Harvey *et al.* 1998; de Decker *et al.* 2003), whereas others have found depression to be more relevant (Wessel *et al.* 2001; Arntz *et al.* 2002). Likewise, both factors have been identified as possible precursors in the most dramatic case of autobiographical memory disturbance, i.e. dissociative or functional retrograde amnesia (Markowitsch 1999).

Dissociative disorders and functional retrograde amnesia

Dissociative disorders, also known as conversion disorders, provide one of the most impressive examples for outlining the sensitivity to emotionally motivated autobiographical memory loss. Although domains other than memory can be affected (e.g. motor symptoms in conversion paralysis), three dissociative disorders centre on memory pathology: dissociative amnesia, dissociative fugue, and dissociative identity disorder (American Psychiatric Association 1994, World Health Organization 1994). Dissociative amnesia and dissociative fugue most often occur after the experience of psychological trauma or extremely stressful situations and time periods. Both syndromes involve the inability to retrieve all or part of the personal past. In dissociative fugue this retrieval failure is accompanied by suddenly and unexpectedly leaving one's usual environment for days, weeks, or even months, and can include assuming a new identity. Awareness of basic life regulation is usually preserved (e.g. feeding, communication, use of common devices and transportation), so that patients do not give the clinical impression of disorganized thought as seen in schizophrenia. In dissociative identity disorder, patients have the subjective and stable experience of at least two separable identities or personalities within their body. These are symmetrically or asymmetrically amnesic for each other. Each identity has its own perceptual, cognitive, and communicative pattern relating to self and environment, and at least two of the personalities repeatedly assume control of the behaviour. Symptoms of fugue and amnesia can co-occur in dissociative identity disorder, and it usually results from experience of extremely traumatic (childhood) events. Following van der Kolk (1994), the mechanism of dissociation enables the individual to fragment, de-realize, and depersonalize traumatic experiences, but this pattern of unbinding experiences from the experiencing self remains stable in everyday life. Acute dissociative reactions to a trauma, as may be experienced in acute stress disorder, are predictive of later development of PTSD (Marshall and Schell 2002; Birmes *et al.* 2003). This indicates that dissociation, although a powerful psychological protection in the acute situation, is disadvantageous as a long-term stress-coping mechanism. In this regard, Harvey *et al.* (1998) investigated a sample of motor vehicle accident survivors and found that inaccessibility of episodic memories for the trauma in the acute post-traumatic time accounted for PTSD severity at a 6-months follow up.

Decoupling of emotion, self, and autobiographical memory can be assumed in all forms of selective but extensive remote memory loss. The term functional retrograde amnesia (RA) (Markowitsch 1999) is commonly used as a cumulative category for cases in which the amnesia can certainly be traced back to psychological aetiology, such as dissociative amnesia, (Schacter *et al.* 1982; Glisky *et al.* 2004), as well as those in which organic versus psychogenic causation remains obscure (De Renzi *et al.* 1995; Mackenzie Ross 2000). The amnesic symptoms always comprise autobiographical remote memory, sometimes also extending to semantic and procedural memory. If domains other than the autobiographical episodic domain are affected, it can nevertheless be reasoned that emotional connotation and self-relevance of personal semantics and even procedural knowledge might lead to their deterioration (e.g. as in conversion paralysis, in which, by emotional-motivational processes, patients are unable to perform certain or most actions). However, autobiographical episodic memory is, although not exclusively, most sensitive to emotional and self-related disturbances. In functional RA, retrieval deficits may extend to the entire previous life or may comprise specific, often trauma-related, information and time periods. Many functional RA patients improve over days or weeks, whereas others exhibit apparent permanent memory loss (Markowitsch 1999).

The unequivocal distinction between organic and psychogenic aetiology in functional RA breaks down for several reasons. As was pointed out by Kopelman

(2002) and Markowitsch (1996), somatic and psychiatric problems commonly co-occur in selective retrograde amnesia. For instance, some previous cases had detectable brain pathology which was insufficient to account for the severity of the retrieval deficits (Costello *et al.* 1998, Kapur 2000). Thus, even in the presence of brain pathology, psychological processes may influence the onset, severity, and recovery of amnesic symptoms. Secondly, in the absence of structural brain damage, functional metabolic disturbances were seen in several functional RA patients. Implicated brain regions comprised temporal regions of the right (Sellal *et al.* 2002) and left (Papagno 1998) hemispheres, the bilateral temporal regions (De Renzi and Lucchelli 1993; Nakamura *et al.* 2002), the right temporo-frontal junction area (Markowitsch *et al.* 1997a), the frontal or parietal areas of the left (Stracciari *et al.* 1994) or right (Starkstein *et al.* 1997) hemispheres, and the posterior cingulate gyrus (Lucchelli *et al.* 1995). As outlined above, autobiographical episodic memory retrieval involves distributed networks within the brain. Thus it is not surprising that functional resting state irregularities of functional RA are not restricted to a specific area. However, considering brain regions relevant for autonoetic or extended consciousness, self-processing, emotion processing, and autobiographical episodic memory retrieval, it appears that dysfunctions in the right hemisphere, presumably within the frontal and temporal lobes, probably account for retrieval deficits in functional RA. This is most apparent in previous functional neuroimaging studies of functional RA patients during active states, i.e. during attempts to retrieve the forgotten past.

In this regard, the brain activation of patient NN (Markowitsch *et al.* 1997b), who suffered from autobiographical episodic functional RA following a fugue, was studied with ^{15}O-PET while he attempted to retrieve remote autobiographical episodes. NN showed a largely left-lateralized activation pattern of the temporo-frontal regions compared with the right-lateralized activity seen in healthy control subjects (Fink *et al.* 1996). In the healthy subjects, a lateralization to the left hemisphere was detected during retrieval of semantic information. Thus, NN's brain activity was supposed to reflect processing of one's own autobiography as if it was personally irrelevant, semantic information. This may correspond to an emotional detachment from personal memories, as was obvious on the behavioural level (Markowitsch *et al.* 1997b). On the other hand, an overly emotional processing of remote memories was hypothesized for the functional RA patient of Yasuno *et al.* (2000). Studies with ^{15}O-PET showed that their patient processed semantic remote information (famous faces) with enhanced activation in the right prefrontal cortex and right anterior medial temporal regions, including the amygdala, as well as decreased activity in the right anterior cingulate. In contrast, healthy control subjects showed bilateral hippocampal activity and, corresponding to the semantic nature of the stimuli, more left-lateralized prefrontal activation. Because of the enhanced amygdala activity, the authors assumed an overly emotional and particularly negatively valenced processing of semantic remote information in their patient. Moreover, after recovery from functional RA, the patient's right-hemispheric limbic and cortical hyperactivity during this task had resolved to normal at a 1-year follow-up examination (see also case AMN in Markowitsch *et al.* (1998, 2000a)).

One further patient, studied by Costello *et al.* (1998), is also relevant. This case is somewhat different from those discussed above because the onset of his amnesia was clearly an organic disease (stroke) and he sustained haemorrhage to the left dorsolateral prefrontal cortex. However, the patient also presented with signs of psychogenic rather than organic RA. $H_2{}^{15}O$-PET measurement during attempts to retrieve remote versus newly acquired autobiographical episodes or impersonal information revealed increased activity in the precuneus and decreased activity in the right posterior ventrolateral frontal cortex and the left superior frontal cortex in the region of the structural damage. It was suggested that the retrieval deficit had been caused by a lack of activation in the right ventral frontal cortex, corresponding to deficient recursive self-cueing during autobiographical retrieval. In this regard, patient ML (Levine *et al.* 1998) is of particular interest. ML sustained severe head trauma with brain lesion restricted to the right ventral prefrontal cortex and underlying white matter, and extending to the uncinate fascicle that connects the frontal inferior frontal cortex and the anterior temporal pole. Behaviourally, he correspondingly showed selective impairment of self-monitoring functions and autonoetic memory retrieval.

Only intact functional and structural connectivity of brain regions processing emotions, self, and memory enables conscious retrieval of one's own autobiographical episodes. If one or more of these components undergo change, the entire or parts of the ability to remember personal past experiences autonoetically is affected. We consider that the prefrontal brain regions of the right hemisphere are the most critical for this function.

Conclusion

In the following model, developed following Oakley (1999), we illustrate theoretical mechanisms of interruptions of autonoetic memory retrieval (Fig. 15.2).

In the normal processing stream, single features (F) of external sensory input as well as internal states like feelings and thoughts are perceived. These single features or objects are further bound to more complex representations (R) in that they become embedded in larger contexts. For example, they are related to features of other currently or previously perceived information. Contextual embedding or build-up of representations is accomplished by a control system, such as the supervisory attentional system of Shallice (1988). This system provides access to formerly stored contextual information and mediates associations between single features. We suggest that proper functioning of the control system depends on current demands and expectations, originating from the individual (emotions, motives, goals, beliefs), from other individuals (emotions, expectations, relationship demands), and external conditions (task requirements). The control system receives ongoing updates from all sources, and compares and adjusts them. In the normal case (1), it is able to bind perceived features to complex

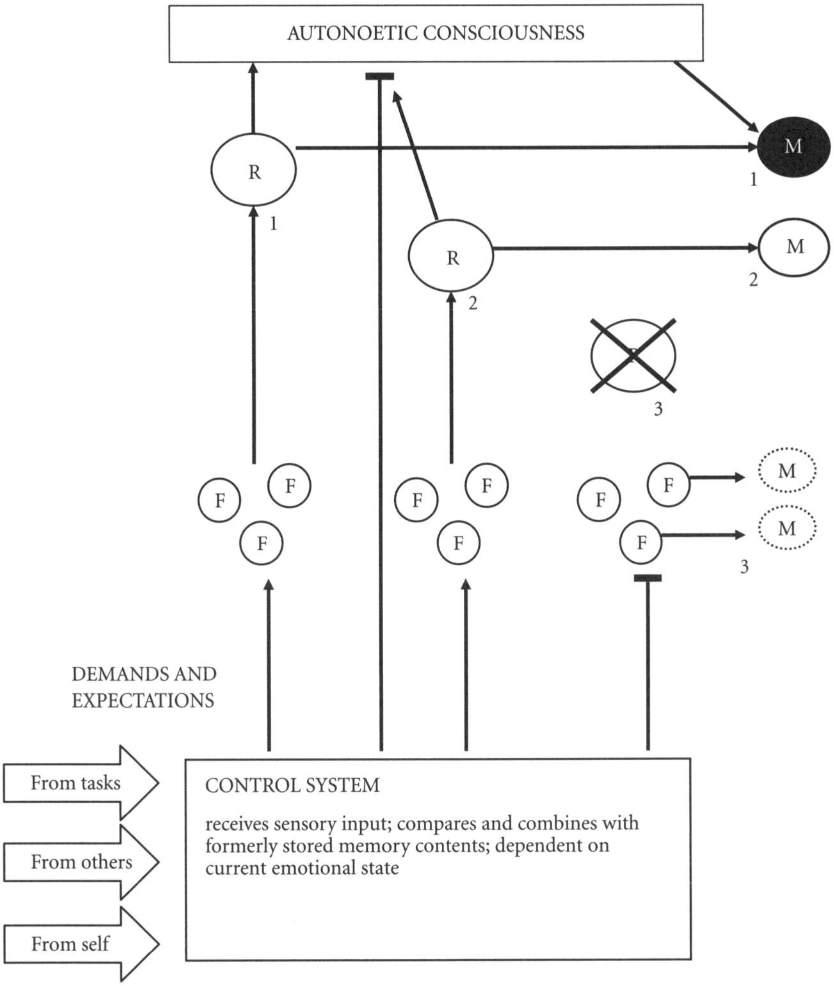

Figure 15.2 Model illustrating possible mechanisms for interruptions of autonoetic memory developed following to Oakley (1999): R, representation; F, feature of internal or external information; M, memory. For explanation see text.

representations and transfer them to autonoetic consciousness. Thus representations are perceived with a sense of one's own self. This in turn triggers memories related to the current representation which are accordingly remembered autonoetically. The model covers two possible cases of autonoetic memory disturbance.

In case (2), if demands and expectations conflict emotionally with the built representations, the emotionally motivated or biased control system actively withholds representations from autonoetic consciousness. Thus memories related to the representations are not experienced autonoetically. Although single features of information can still be bound to representations, they are actively withheld from autonoetic consciousness. Corresponding memories are still retrievable but experienced without a sense of self. An example of this mechanism can be seen in the dissociation between impaired explicit and intact implicit memories in patients with functional RA (Kopelman *et al.* 1994; Markowitsch *et al.* 1997a). Furthermore, the problems with autonoetic retrieval experienced by depressive patients may originate from conflicts between emotionally biased self-views and task demands (e.g. processing a positively valenced cue). The built representation of the retrieval cue is not transferred to autonoetic consciousness and related former memories (e.g. joyful situations) are not autonoetically retrieved. Another example refers to the phenomenon of repressive coping style in healthy individuals (Weinberger 1990). Repressive individuals act in socially desirable ways and generally self-report low levels of (negative) affect. In turn, their actual physiological reactivity points to elevated arousal patterns such as those in anxiety disorders (Pauls and Stemmler 2003). A repressive personality style is often observed in social situations where repressive individuals expect social judgement about their overt emotional state (cf. conflicts between demands from others, self, task in our model). A few studies have compared brain activity in repressive and non-repressive subjects (Kline *et al.* 1998; Tomarken and Davidson 1998). Revealing higher involvement of left compared with right frontal brain regions in repressive subjects, these studies suggested that cognitive processes of the left frontal lobe exert control over right-hemispheric emotional processes. Furthermore, in a study by Blagov and Singer (2004) repressive individuals displayed lower autobiographical memory specificity than non-repressive subjects, a finding directly corresponding to our assumption that self- and emotion-related disturbances, or even slight alterations as in repressive personality style, can influence autobiographical retrieval.

In case (3) the binding of single features to complex representations may already be in conflict with current demands and expectations. Features are not embedded in contexts and either corresponding memories are not accessible (consciously and unconsciously) or only fragmentary memories are retrieved. This may result if either the control system is itself disturbed, as in brain-damaged patients, or if single features of the information highly exceed current expectations such as in extremely stressful situations. The latter mechanism can be seen in symptoms of memory fragmentation and inability to verbalize memories in PTSD (Nadel and Jacobs 1998). Furthermore, in almost all patients suffering from autobiographical episodic retrieval deficits, either structural or functional disturbances, if detectable, include frontal/prefrontal cortex (see above). Even in cases in which no such disturbances are seen, executive dysfunctions eventually accompany the retrieval failure point to frontal lobe involvement.

Our model centres on a control system based on frontal brain regions. It depends on sensory–perceptual input from sensory cortices, and it accomplishes adjustment between current and formerly stored information and therefore contents from long-term memory stores in the temporal lobes. It is necessary for emotional evaluation and thus is modulated by input from the limbic system. Whereas its mechanisms can be interrupted by disturbances in all its components, it can itself actively disturb its components. Inhibition of episodic memory retrieval was found to rely on control functions in a series of behavioural experiments by Anderson and Green (2001). Here, healthy subjects were capable of selectively suppressing memories by executive inhibitory control and the number of inhibition trials was related to lower later memory performance. Furthermore, Anderson *et al.* (2004) showed that experimentally induced voluntary suppression of memory for certain words was associated with reduced right hippocampal and increased bihemispheric dorsolateral prefrontal brain activity. As suggested by our model, in this study inhibitory control mediated by prefrontal brain areas was related to decreases in memory-relevant regions of the medial temporal lobe system. It can be argued whether motivated forgetting of personally irrelevant information, as in Anderson and Green (2001), parallels the presumably unconscious inhibition of autobiographical memories as in functional RA (Kihlstrom 2002). However, the results obtained by Anderson and colleagues (Anderson and Green 2001; Anderson *et al.* 2004) point to mechanisms that may underlie self-motivated failures of autonoetic remembering of one's own past.

In summary, we conclude that binding of emotions and self to memory is necessary for autonoetic remembering of autobiographical episodes. Disturbances in emotion and self-processing can contribute to distortions in autobiographical memory retrieval, as was illustrated in the examples of schizophrenia and depression. Finally, the most comprehensive decoupling of emotions and self from memory may result in complete loss of one's own autobiography, as is obvious in dissociative or functional amnesia.

References

Aggleton, J.P. (2000). *The Amygdala: A Functional Analysis.* Oxford University Press, Oxford.

Aggleton, J.P. and Pearce, J.M. (2001). Neural systems underlying episodic memory: insights from animal research. *Philosophical Transactions of the Royal Society of London, Series B: Biological Sciences*, **356**, 1467–1482.

American Psychiatric Association (1994). *Diagnostic and Statistical Manual of Mental Disorders* (4th edn). Washington, DC: American Psychiatric Association.

Anderson, M.C. and Green, C. (2001). Suppressing unwanted memories by executive control. *Nature*, **310**, 366–369.

Anderson, M.C., Ochsner, K.N., Kuhl, B., *et al.* (2004). Neural systems underlying the suppression of unwanted memories. *Science*, **303**, 232–235.

Andreasen, N.C. (2000). Is schizophrenia a disorder of memory or consciousness? In *Memory, Consciousness, and the Brain* (ed E. Tulving). Philadelphia, PA: Psychology Press, pp. 243–261.

Andreasen, N.C., O'Leary, D.S., Paradiso, S., *et al.* (1999). The cerebellum plays a role in conscious episodic memory retrieval. *Human Brain Mapping*, **8**, 226–234.

Arntz, A., Meeren, M., and Wessel, I. (2002). No evidence for overgeneral memories in borderline personality disorder. *Behaviour Research and Therapy*, **40**, 1063–1068.

Baddeley, A., Chincotta, D., and Adlam, A. (2001). Working memory and the control of action: evidence from task switching. *Journal of Experimental Psychology: General*, **130**, 641–657.

Barnhofer, T., de Jong-Meyer, R., Kleinpass, A., and Nikesch, S. (2002). Specificity of autobiographical memories in depression: an analysis of retrieval processes in a think-aloud task. *British Journal of Clinical Psychology*, **41**, 411–416.

Baron-Cohen, S. (1995). *Mindblindness.* Cambridge, MA: MIT Press.

Birmes, P., Brunet, A., Carreras, D., *et al.* (2003). The predictive power of peritraumatic dissociation and acute stress symptoms for posttraumatic stress symptoms: a three-month prospective study. *American Journal of Psychiatry*, **160**, 1337–1339.

Blagov, P.S. and Singer, J.A. (2004). Four dimensions of self-defining memories (specificity, meaning, content, and affect) and their relationships to self-restraint, distress, and repressive defensiveness. *Journal of Personality*, **72**, 481–511.

Brand, M. and Markowitsch, H.J. (2003). The principle of bottleneck structures. In *Principles of Learning and Memory* (ed R.H. Kluwe, G. Lüer, and F. Rösler). Basel: Birkhäuser, 2003, pp. 172–84.

Bremner, J.D. and Vermetten, E. (2001). Stress and development: behavioral and biological consequences. *Development and Psychopathology*, **13**, 473–489.

Brittlebank, A.D., Scott, J., Williams, J.M., and Ferrier, I.N. (1993). Autobiographical memory in depression: state or trait marker? *British Journal of Psychiatry*, **162**, 118–121.

Broadbelt, K., Byne, W., and Jones, L.B. (2002). Evidence for a decrease in basilar dendrites of pyramidal cells in schizophrenic medial prefrontal cortex. *Schizophrenia Research*, **58**, 75–81.

Buckner, R.L. and Koutstaal, W. (1998). Functional neuroimaging studies of encoding, priming, and explicit memory retrieval. *Proceedings of the National Academy of Sciences of the United States of America*, **95**, 891–898.

Byne, W. and Davis, K.L. (1999). The role of prefrontal cortex in the dopaminergic dysregulation of schizophrenia. *Biological Psychiatry*, **45**, 657–659.

Cabeza, R., Dolcos, F., Prince, S.E., Rice, H.J., Weissman, D.H., and Nyberg, L. (2003). Attention-related activity during episodic memory retrieval: a cross-function fMRI study. *Neuropsychologia*, **41**, 390–399.

Cahill, L. and McGaugh, J.L. (1998). Mechanisms of emotional arousal and lasting declarative memory. *Trends in Neurosciences*, **21**, 294–299.

Calabrese P., Markowitsch, H. Z., Harders, A. G., Scholz, M., and Gehlen, W. (1995). Fornix damage and memory. A case report. *Cortex*, **31**, 555–564.

Churchland, P.S. (2002). Self-representation in nervous systems. *Science*, **296**, 308–310.

Conway, M.A. (2001). Sensory–perceptual episodic memory and its context: autobiographical memory. *Philosophical Transactions of the Royal Society of London, Series B, Biological Sciences*, **356**, 1375–1384.

Conway, M.A. and Pleydell-Pearce, C.W. (2000). The construction of autobiographical memories in the self-memory system. *Psychological Review*, **107**, 261–288.

Conway, M.A., Turk, D.J., Miller, S.L., *et al.* (1999). A positron emission tomography (PET) study of autobiographical memory retrieval. *Memory*, **7**, 679–702.

Conway, M.A., Pleydell-Pearce, C.W., Whitecross, S.E., and Sharpe, H. (2003). Neurophysiological correlates of memory for experienced and imagined events. *Neuropsychologia*, **41**, 334–340.

Corcoran, R. and Frith, C.D. (2003). Autobiographical memory and theory of mind: evidence of a relationship in schizophrenia. *Psychological Medicine*, **33**, 897–905.

Corkin, S., Amaral, D.G., Gonzalez, R.G., Johnson, K.A., and Hyman, B.T. (1997). HM's medial temporal lobe lesion: findings from magnetic resonance imaging. *Journal of Neuroscience*, **17**, 3964–3979.

Costello, A., Fletcher, P.C., Dolan, R.J., Frith, C.D., and Shallice, T. (1998). The origins of forgetting in a case of isolated retrograde amnesia following a hemorrhage: evidence from functional imaging. *Neurocase*, **4**, 437–446.

Craik, F.I.M., Moroz, T.M., Moscovitch, M., *et al.* (1999). In search of the self: a positron emission tomography study. *Psychological Science*, **10**, 26–34.

Damasio, A.R. (1994). *Descartes' Error: Emotion, Reason, and the Human Brain*. New York: Grosset–Putnam.

Damasio, A.R. (1999). *The Feeling of What Happens: Body and Emotion in the Making of Consciousness*. New York: Harcourt Brace.

Davidson, R.J. (2002). Anxiety and affective style: role of prefrontal cortex and amygdala. *Biological Psychiatry*, **51**, 68–80.

Davidson, R.J. and Irwin, W. (1999). The functional neuroanatomy of emotion and affective style. *Trends in Cognitive Sciences*, **3**, 11–21.

de Decker, A., Hermans, D., Raes, F., and Eelen, P. (2003). Autobiographical memory specificity and trauma in inpatient adolescents. *Journal of Clinical Child and Adolescent Psychology*, **32**, 22–31.

de Kloet, E.R., Oitzl, M.S., and Joëls, M. (1999). Stress and cognition: are corticosteroids good or bad guys? *Trends in Neurosciences*, **10**, 422–426.

de Quervain, D.J., Henke, K., Aerni, A., *et al.* (2003). Glucocorticoid-induced impairment of declarative memory retrieval is associated with reduced blood flow in the medial temporal lobe. *European Journal of Neuroscience*, **17**, 1296–1302.

De Renzi, E. and Lucchelli, F. (1993). Dense retrograde amnesia, intact learning capability and abnormal forgetting rate: a consolidation deficit? *Cortex*, **29**, 449–466.

De Renzi, E., Lucchelli, F., Muggia, S., and Spinnler, H. (1995). Persistent retrograde amnesia following a minor trauma. *Cortex*, **31**, 531–542.

Di Chiara, G., Loddo, P., and Tanda, G. (1999). Reciprocal changes in prefrontal and limbic dopamine responsiveness to aversive and rewarding stimuli after chronic mild stress: implications for the psychobiology of depression. *Biological Psychiatry*, **46**, 1624–1633.

Dolan, R.J., Lane, R., Chua, P., and Fletcher, P. (2000). Dissociable temporal lobe activations during emotional episodic memory retrieval. *NeuroImage*, **11**, 203–209.

Drevets, W.C. (2001). Neuroimaging and neuropathological studies of depression: implications for the cognitive-emotional features of mood disorders. *Current Opinion in Neurobiology*, **11**, 240–249.

Ellwart, T., Rinck, M., and Becker, E.S. (2003). Selective memory and memory deficits in depressed inpatients. *Depression and Anxiety*, **17**, 197–206.

Elvevåg, B., Kerbs, K.M., Malley, J.D., Seeley, E., and Goldberg, T.E. (2003). Autobiographical memory in schizophrenia: an examination of the distribution of memories. *Neuropsychology*, **17**, 402–409.

Feinstein, A., Goldberg, T.E., Nowlin, B., and Weinberger, D.R. (1998). Types and characteristics of remote memory impairment in schizophrenia. *Schizophrenia Research*, **30**, 155–163.

Fink, G.R., Markowitsch, H.J., Reinkemeier, M., Bruckbauer, T., Kessler, J., and Heiss, W.-D. (1996). Cerebral representation of one's own past: neural networks involved in autobiographical memory. *Journal of Neuroscience*, **16**, 4275–4282.

Fletcher, P.C. and Henson, R.N.A. (2001). Frontal lobes and human memory: insights from functional imaging. *Brain*, **124**, 849–881.

Franklin, C.L. and Zimmerman, M. (2001). Posttraumatic stress disorder and major depressive disorder: investigating the role of overlapping symptoms in diagnostic comorbidity. *Journal of Nervous and Mental Disease*, **189**, 548–551.

Frith, C.D. (1992). *The Cognitive Neuropsychology of Schizophrenia*. Hove: Erlbaum.

Gallagher, I.I. (2000). Philosophical conceptions of the self: implications for cognitive science. *Trends in Cognitive Sciences*, **4**, 14–21.

Garrido, G.E., Furuie, S.S., Buchpiguel, C.A., *et al.* (2002). Relation between medial temporal atrophy and functional brain activity during memory processing in Alzheimer's disease: a combined MRI and SPECT study. *Journal of Neurology, Neurosurgery, and Psychiatry*, **73**, 508–516.

Glisky, E.L., Ryan, L., Reminger, S., and Hardt, O. (2004). A case of psychogenic fugue. I understand, aber ich verstehe nichts. *Neuropsychologia*, **42**, 1132–1147.

Grossman, M., Koenig, P., Glosser, G., *et al.* (2003). Neural basis for semantic memory difficulty in Alzheimer's disease: an fMRI study. *Brain*, **126**, 292–311.

Gusnard, D.A., Akbudak, E., Shulman, G.L., and Raichle, M.E. (2001). Medial prefrontal cortex and self-referential mental activity: relation to a default mode of brain function.

Proceedings of the National Academy of Sciences of the United States of America, **98**, 4259–4264.

Habib, R., Nyberg, L., and Tulving, E. (2003). Hemispheric asymmetries of memory: the HERA model revisited. *Trends in Cognitive Sciences*, **7**, 241–245.

Hamann, S.B. and Squire, L.R. (1995). On the acquisition of new declarative knowledge in amnesia. *Behavioral Neuroscience*, **109**, 1027–1044.

Harvey, A.G., Bryant, R.A., and Dang, S.T. (1998). Autobiographical memory in acute stress disorder. *Journal of Consulting and Clinical Psychology*, **66**, 500–506.

Holsboer, F. (2001). Stress, hypercortisolism and corticosteroid receptors in depression: implications for therapy. *Journal of Affective Disorders*, **62**, 77–91.

Johnson, S.C., Baxter, L.C., Wilder, L.S., Pipe, J.G., Heiserman, J.E., and Prigatano, G.P. (2002). Neural correlates of self-reflection. *Brain*, **125**, 1808–1814.

Kapur, N. (2000). Focal retrograde amnesia and the attribution of causality: an exceptionally benign commentary. *Cognitive Neuropsychology*, **17**, 623–637.

Karney, B.R. and Frye, N.E. (2002). 'But we've been getting better lately': comparing prospective and retrospective views of relationship development. *Journal of Personality and Social Psychology*, **82**, 222–238.

Kazes, M., Berthet, L., Danion, J.M., *et al.* (1999). Impairment of consciously controlled use of memory in schizophrenia. *Neuropsychology*, **13**, 54–61.

Keenan, J.P., Freund, S., Hamilton, R.H., Ganis, G., and Pascual-Leone, A. (2000). Hand response differences in a self-face identification task. *Neuropsychologia*, **38**, 1047–1053.

Keenan, J.P., McCutcheon, N.B., and Pascual-Leone, A. (2001). Functional magnetic resonance imaging and event related potentials suggest right prefrontal activation for self-related processing. *Brain and Cognition*, **47**, 87–91.

Kelley, W.M., Macrae, C.N., Wyland, C.L., Caglar, S., Inati, S., and Heatherton, T.F. (2002). Finding the self? An event-related fMRI study. *Journal of Cognitive Neuroscience*, **14**, 85–94.

Kihlstrom, J.F. (2002). No need for repression. *Trends in Cognitive Sciences*, **6**, 502.

Kim, J.J. and Yoon, K.S. (1998). Stress: metaplastic effects in the hippocampus. *Trends in Neurosciences*, **21**, 505–509.

Kline, J.P., Allen, J.J., and Schwartz, G.E. (1998). Is left frontal brain activation in defensiveness gender specific? *Journal of Abnormal Psychology*, **103**, 149–153.

Kopelman, M.D. (2002). Disorders of memory. *Brain*, **125**, 2152–2190.

Kopelman, M.D. and Kapur, N. (2001). The loss of episodic memories in retrograde amnesia: single-case and group studies. *Philosophical Transactions of the Royal Society of London, Series B, Biological Sciences*, **356**, 1409–1421.

Kopelman, M.D., Christensen, H., Puffett, A., and Stanhope, N. (1994). The great escape: a neuropsychological study of psychogenic amnesia. *Neuropsychologia*, **32**, 675–691.

Larsen, S.F., Thompson, C.P., and Hansen, T. (1996). Time in autobiographical memory. In *Remembering Our Past* (ed D.C. Rubin). New York: Cambridge University Press, pp. 129–156.

LeDoux, J. (2000). Cognitive–emotional interactions: listen to the brain. In *Cognitive Neuroscience of Emotion. Series in Affective Science* (ed R. Lane and L. Nadel). New York: Oxford University Press, pp. 129–155.

Lepage, M., Ghaffar, O., Nyberg, L., and Tulving, E. (2000). Prefrontal cortex and episodic memory retrieval mode. *Proceedings of the National Academy of Sciences of the United States of America*, **97**, 506–511.

Levine, B., Black, S.E., Cabeza, R., *et al.* (1998). Episodic memory and the self in a case of isolated retrograde amnesia. *Brain*, **121**, 1951–1973.

Lucchelli, F., Muggia, S., and Spinnler, H. (1995). The 'petites madeleines' phenomenon in two amnesic patients: sudden recovery of forgotten memories. *Brain*, **118**, 167–183.

Lupien, S.J., Wilkinson, C.W., Briere, S., Menard, C., Ng Ying Kin, N.M., and Nair, N.P. (2002). The modulatory effects of corticosteroids on cognition: studies in young human populations. *Psychoneuroendocrinology*, **27**, 401–416.

McEwen, B.S. (1999). Stress and hippocampal plasticity. *Annual Review of Neuroscience*, **22**, 105–122.

McGaugh, J.L. (2002). Memory consolidation and the amygdala: a systems perspective. *Trends in Neurosciences*, **25**, 456–461.

McGaugh, J.L. and Roozendaal, B. (2002). Role of adrenal stress hormones in forming lasting memories in the brain. *Current Opinion in Neurobiology*, **12**, 205–210.

Mackenzie Ross, S. (2000). Profound retrograde amnesia following mild head injury: organic or functional? *Cortex*, **36**, 521–537.

Maguire, E.A. (2001). Neuroimaging studies of autobiographical event memory. *Philosophical Transactions of the Royal Society of London, Series B, Biological Sciences*, **356**, 1441–1451.

Maguire, E.A. and Frith, C.D. (2003). Lateral asymmetry in the hippocampal response to the remoteness of autobiographical memories. *Journal of Neuroscience*, **23**, 5302–5307.

Maguire, E.A., Mummery, C.J., and Büchel, C. (2000). Patterns of hippocampal-cortical interaction dissociate temporal lobe memory subsystems. *Hippocampus*, **10**, 475–482.

Mandolesi, L., Leggio, M.G., Graziano, A., Neri, P., and Petrosini, L. (2001). Cerebellar contribution to spatial event processing: involvement in procedural and working memory components. *European Journal of Neuroscience*, **14**, 2011–2022.

Markowitsch, H.J. (1996). Organic and psychogenic retrograde amnesia: two sides of the same coin? *Neurocase*, **2**, 357–371.

Markowitsch, H.J. (1998). The biological basis of memory. In *Memory in Neurodegenerative Disease: Biological, Cognitive, and Clinical Perspective* (ed A.I. Tröster). New york: Cambridge University Press, pp. 140–153.

Markowitsch, H.J. (1999). Functional neuroimaging correlates of functional amnesia. *Memory*, **5/6**, 561–583.

Markowitsch, H.J. (2000). Memory and amnesia. In *Principles of Behavioral and Cognitive Neurology* (ed M.M. Mesulam). Oxford: Oxford University Press, pp. 257–293.

Markowitsch, H.J. (2003a). Autonoetic consciousness. In *The Self in Neuroscience and Psychiatry* (ed T. Kircher and A. David). Cambridge: Cambridge University Press, pp. 180–196.

Markowitsch, H.J. (2003b). Psychogenic amnesia. *NeuroImage*, **20**, S132–S138.

Markowitsch, H.J., von Cramon, D.Y., and Schuri, U. (1993). Mnestic performance profile of a bilateral diencephalic infarct patient with preserved intelligence and severe amnesic disturbances. *Journal of Clinical and Experimental Neuropsychology*, **15**, 27–52.

Markowitsch, H.J., Calabrese, P., Fink, G.R., *et al.* (1997a). Impaired episodic memory retrieval in a case of probable psychogenic amnesia. *Psychiatry Research: Neuroimaging*, **74**, 119–126.

Markowitsch, H.J., Fink, G.R., Thöne, A., Kessler, J., and Heiss, W.-D. (1997b). A PET study of persistent psychogenic amnesia covering the whole life span. *Cognitive Neuropsychiatry*, **2**, 135–158.

Markowitsch, H.J., Kessler, J., Van der Ven, C., Weber-Luxenburger, G., Albers, M., and Heiss, W.D. (1998). Psychic trauma causing grossly reduced brain metabolism and cognitive deterioration. *Neuropsychologia*, **36**, 77–82.

Markowitsch, H.J., Kessler, J., Weber-Luxenburger, G., Van der Ven, C., Albers, M., and Heiss, W.D. (2000a). Neuroimaging and behavioral correlates of recovery from mnestic block syndrome and other cognitive deteriorations. *Neuropsychiatry, Neuropsychology and Behavioral Neurology*, **13**, 60–66.

Markowitsch, H.J., Thiel, A., Reinkemeier, M., Kessler, J., Koyuncu, A., and Heiss, W.-D. (2000b). Right amygdalar and temporofrontal activation during autobiographic, but not during fictitious memory retrieval. *Behavioural Neurology*, **12**, 181–190.

Marshall, G.N. and Schell, T.L. (2002). Reappraising the link between peritraumatic dissociation and PTSD symptom severity: evidence from a longitudinal study of community violence survivors. *Journal of Abnormal Psychology*, **111**, 626–636.

Mesulam, M.-M. (2000). Behavioral neuroanatomy: large-scale networks, association cortex, frontal syndromes, the limbic system, and hemispheric specializations. In *Principles of Behavioral and Cognitive Neurology* (ed M.M. Mesulam). Oxford: Oxford University Press, pp. 1–120.

Nadel, L. and Jacobs, W.J. (1998). Traumatic memory is special. *Current Directions in Psychological Science*, **7**, 156–157.

Nakamura, H., Kunori, Y., Mori, K., Nakaaki, S., Yoshida, S., and Hamanaka, T. (2002). Two cases of functional focal retrograde amnesia with impairment of object use. *Cortex*, **38**, 613–622.

Oakley, D.A. (1999). Hypnosis and conversion hysteria: a unifying model. *Cognitive Neuropsychiatry*, **4**, 243–265.

O'Brien, G. and Opie, J. (2003). The multiplicity of consciousness and the emergence of the self. In *The Self in Neuroscience and Psychiatry* (ed T. Kircher and A. David). Cambridge: Cambridge University Press, pp. 107–120.

Papagno, C. (1998). Transient retrograde amnesia associated with impaired naming of living categories. *Cortex*, **34**, 111–121.

Papez, J.W. (1937). A proposed mechanism of emotion. *Archives of Neurology and Psychiatry*, **38**, 725–743.

Park, R.J., Goodyer, I.M., and Teasdale, J.D. (2002). Categoric overgeneral autobiographical memory in adolescents with major depressive disorder. *Psychological Medicine*, **32**, 267–276.

Pauls, C.A. and Stemmler, G. (2003). Repressive and defensive coping during fear and anger. *Emotion*, **3**, 284–303.

Petrides, M. (2002). The mid-ventrolateral prefrontal cortex and active mnemonic retrieval. *Neurobiology of Learning and Memory*, **78**, 528–538.

Phaf, H.R., Geurts, H., and Eling, P.A. (2000). Word frequency and word stem completion in Korsakoff patients. *Journal of Clinical and Experimental Neuropsychology*, **22**, 817–829.

Piefke, M., Weiss, P.H., Zilles, K., Markowitsch, H.J., and Fink, G.R. (2003). Differential remoteness and emotional tone modulate the neural correlates of autobiographical memory. *Brain*, **126**, 650–668.

Raes, F., Hermans, D., de Decker, A., Eelen, P., and Williams, J.M.G. (2003). Autobiographical memory specificity and affect regulation: an experimental approach. *Emotion*, **3**, 201–206.

Raichle, M.E., MacLeod, A.M., Snyder, A.Z., Powers, W.J., Gusnard, D.A., and Shulman, G.L. (2001). A default mode of brain function. *Proceedings of the National Academy of Sciences of the United States of America*, **98**, 676–682.

Raison, C.L. and Miller, A.H. (2003). When not enough is too much: the role of insufficient glucocorticoid signaling in the pathophysiology of stress-related disorders. *American Journal of Psychiatry*, **160**, 1554–1565.

Reese, E. (2002). Social factors in the development of autobiographical memory: the state of the art. *Social Development*, **11**, 124–142.

Riutort, M., Cuervo, C., Danion, J.M., Peretti, C.S., and Salame, P. (2003). Reduced levels of specific autobiographical memories in schizophrenia. *Psychiatry Research*, **117**, 35–45.

Roozendaal, B. (2002). Stress and memory: opposing effects of glucocorticoids on memory consolidation and memory retrieval. *Neurobiology of Learning and Memory*, **78**, 578–595.

Roozendaal, B., Nguyen, B.T., Power, A.E., and McGaugh, J.L. (1999). Basolateral amygdala noradrenergic influence enables enhancement of memory consolidation induced by hippocampal glucocorticoid receptor activation. *Proceedings of the National Academy of Sciences of the United States of America*, **96**, 11642–11647.

Ross, M. and Wilson, A.E. (2002). It feels like yesterday: self-esteem, valence of personal past experiences, and judgments of subjective distance. *Journal of Personality and Social Psychology*, **82**, 792–803.

Ryan, L., Nadel, L., Keil, K., *et al.* (2001). Hippocampal complex and retrieval of recent and very remote autobiographical memories: evidence from functional magnetic resonance imaging in neurologically intact people. *Hippocampus*, **11**, 707–714.

Schacter, D.L. and Buckner, R.L. (1998). On the relations among priming, conscious recollection, and intentional retrieval: evidence from neuroimaging research. *Neurobiology of Learning and Memory*, **70**, 284–303.

Schacter, D.L., Wang, P.L., Tulving, E., and Freedman, M. (1982). Functional retrograde amnesia: a quantitative case study. *Neuropsychologia*, **20**, 523–532.

Schmitz, T.W., Kawahara-Baccus, T.N., and Johnson, S.C. (2004). Metacognitive evaluation, self-relevance, and the right prefrontal cortex. *NeuroImage*, **22**, 941–947.

Schore, A.N. (2002). Dysregulation of the right brain: a fundamental mechanism of traumatic attachment and the psychopathogenesis of posttraumatic stress disorder. *Australian and New Zealand Journal of Psychiatry*, **36**, 9–30.

Sellal, F., Manning, L., Seegmuller, C., Scheiber, C., and Schoenfelder, F. (2002). Pure retrograde amnesia following mild head trauma: a neuropsychological and metabolic study. *Cortex*, **38**, 499–509.

Shallice T (1988). *From Neuropsychology to Mental Structure*. Cambridge: Cambridge University Press.

Siebert, M., Markowitsch, H.J., and Bartel, P. (2003). Amygdala, affect and cognition: evidence from 10 patients with Urbach–Wiethe disease. *Brain*, **126**, 2627–2637.

Sonntag, P., Gokalsing, E., Olivier, C., *et al.* (2003). Impaired strategic regulation of contents of conscious awareness in schizophrenia. *Consciousness and Cognition*, **12**, 190–200.

Starkstein, S.E., Sabe, L., and Dorrego, M.F. (1997). Severe retrograde amnesia after a mild closed head injury. *Neurocase*, **3**, 105–109.

Stracciari, A., Ghidoni, E., Guarino, M., Poletti, M., and Pazzaglia, P. (1994). Post-traumatic retrograde amnesia with selective impairment of autobiographical memory. *Cortex*, **30**, 459–468.

Suddendorf, T. and Busby, J. (2003). Mental time travel in animals? *Trends in Cognitive Science*, **7**, 391–396.

Tomarken, A. J. and Davidson R. J. (1998) Frontal brain activation in repressors and non repressors. *Journal of Abnormal Psychology*, **103**, 339–349.

Tulving, E. (1983). *Elements of Episodic Memory*. Oxford: Clarendon Press.

Tulving, E. (2001). Episodic memory and common sense: how far apart? *Philosophical Transactions of the Royal Society of London, Series B, Biological Sciences*, **356**, 1505–1515.

Tulving, E. (2002). Episodic memory: from mind to brain. *Annual Review of Psychology*, **53**, 1–25.

Tulving, E., Kapur, S., Craik, F.I., Moscovitch, M., and Houle, S. (1994). Hemispheric encoding/retrieval asymmetry in episodic memory: positron emission tomography findings. *Proceedings of the National Academy of Sciences of the United States of America*, **9**, 2016–2020.

Uehara, I. (2000). Differences in episodic memory between four- and five-year-olds: false information versus real experiences. *Psychological Reports*, **86**, 745–755.

Vallée, M., Mayo, W., Koob, G.F., and Le Moal, M. (2001). Neurosteroids in learning and memory processes. *International Review of Neurobiology*, **46**, 273–320.

van der Kolk, B.A. (1994). The body keeps the score: memory and the evolving psychobiology of posttraumatic stress. *Harvard Review of Psychiatry*, **1**, 253–265.

Van Vreeswijk, M.F. and De Wilde, E.J. (2004). Autobiographical memory specificity, psychopathology, depressed mood and the use of the Autobiographical Memory Test: a meta-analysis. *Behaviour Research and Therapy*, **42**, 731–743.

Vargha-Khadem, F., Gadian, D.G., and Mishkin, M. (2001). Dissociations in cognitive memory: the syndrome of developmental amnesia. *Philosophical Transactions of the Royal Society of London, Series B, Biological Sciences*, **356**, 1435–1440.

Velligan, D.I. and Bow-Thomas, C.C. (1999). Executive function in schizophrenia. *Seminars in Clinical Neuropsychiatry*, **4**, 24–33.

von Cramon, D.Y., Markowitsch, H.J., and Schuri, U. (1993). The possible contribution of the septal region to memory. *Neuropsychologia*, **31**, 159–180.

von Gunten, A., Fox, N.C., Cipolotti, L., and Ron, M.A. (2000). A volumetric study of hippocampus and amygdala in depressed patients with subjective memory problems. *Journal of Neuropsychiatry and Clinical Neurosciences*, **12**, 493–498.

Wessel, I., Meeren, M., Peeters, F., Arntz, A., and Merckelbach, H. (2001). Correlates of autobiographical memory specificity: the role of depression, anxiety and childhood trauma. *Behaviour Research and Therapy*, **39**, 409–21.

Weinberger, D. A. (1990). The construct validity of the repressive coping style. In *Repression and Dissociation* (ed J. L. Singer). Chicago: The Chicago University Press, pp. 337–386.

Williams, J.M.G. (1996). Depression and the specificity of autobiographical memory. In *Remembering Our Past* (ed D.C. Rubin). New York: Cambridge University Press, pp. 244–67.

Wilson, A.E. and Ross, M. (2003). The identity function of autobiographical memory: time is on our side. *Memory*, **11**, 137–149.

World Health Organization (1994). *International Statistical Classification of Diseases and Health Related Problems, Tenth Version (ICD-10)*. Geneva: World Health Organization.

Yasuno, F., Nishikawa, T., Nakagawa, Y., *et al.* (2000). Functional anatomical study of psychogenic amnesia. *Psychiatry Research: Neuroimaging*, **99**, 43–57.

Zysset, S., Huber, O., Ferstl, E., and von Cramon, D.Y. (2002). The anterior frontomedial cortex and evaluative judgment: an fMRI study. *NeuroImage*, **15**, 983–991.

Section 4

Binding processes during retrieval

Chapter 16

Associations and dissociations in recognition memory systems

M. W. Brown and E. C. Warburton

Introduction

Medial temporal lobe amnesia is characterized by a loss of episodic memory: patients fail to remember new events that can be set in an autobiographical context (an episode). An important typical feature of such amnesia is a loss of recognition memory. In recent years, the relationship between episodic memory and recognition memory has become contentious. The source of contention centres on an uncertainty over the relative contributions of the hippocampus and the perirhinal cortex to recognition memory. Resolving this issue is critical to understanding the processes disrupted in medial temporal lobe amnesia. It also has major implications for interpreting the findings from animal models of such amnesia.

Since the influential article by Scoville and Milner (1957), clinical findings have centred on the hippocampus as the critical locus of damage responsible for medial temporal lobe amnesia. A standard feature of this classical anterograde amnesic syndrome is a loss of recognition memory. These facts raise a potential anomaly as recent results from animal work have repeatedly highlighted a major role in recognition memory for a region close to the hippocampus, the perirhinal cortex, rather than the hippocampus itself. Thus groups working with animals all agree that the severity of impairment in standard tests of recognition memory in rats and monkeys is greater after perirhinal lesions than after hippocampal lesions, even though controversy remains concerning the extent of impairment following hippocampal lesions (Gaffan and Murray 1992; Suzuki *et al.* 1993; Meunier *et al.* 1993, 1996; Mumby and Pinel 1994; Alvarez *et al.* 1995; Ennaceur *et al.* 1996; Murray and Mishkin 1998; Aggleton and Brown 1999; Beason-Held *et al.* 1999; Zola *et al.* 2000). In this chapter we review some of the evidence that indicates that this apparent conflict can be resolved by considering potentially different roles in recognition memory for the hippocampus and the perirhinal cortex.

Anyone who has known a friend or relative in the early stages of Alzheimer's disease will be aware that one of the distressing manifestations of the condition is the constant repetition of questions and stories by the sufferer. In registering these repetitions, the normal observer is using a mechanism that has been impaired in the disease sufferer. In the normal person, the ability to judge what is novel and what is familiar, what has occurred recently, and what has never been encountered before is commonplace and usually effortless. Thus recognition memory is a central part of our ability to remember. It requires a capacity for both identification and judgement concerning the prior occurrence of what has been identified (Mandler 1980). The most parsimonious model regards recognition memory as a unitary process directly linked to other forms of explicit memory and hence dependent on the same systems (Haist and Shimamura 1992; Hirshman and Master 1997; Donaldson 1999). In this way, recognition memory is viewed as an integral component of the class of memory lost in amnesia. An alternative view is that there are different component processes within recognition memory (Mandler 1980; Jacoby and Dallas 1981; Gardiner and Parkin 1990), and that only one of these maps directly onto the class of memory always lost in anterograde amnesia (Aggleton and Brown 1999).

When you meet someone, you may recollect information such as where you met previously or the person's name, and hence you are able to recognize the person as someone you have previously encountered. Contrastingly, you may immediately know that the person is familiar, but nothing more. Thus, subjectively, it is possible to consider recognition memory as subdivided into at least two processes, familiarity discrimination ('know') and recollective match ('remember'), which automatically imply a successful familiarity judgement. Single-process models of recognition memory assume that 'knowing' reflects a weaker trace strength than 'remembering', so that they only differ quantitatively. In contrast, dual-process models see these as qualitatively different modes of recognition memory.

In this chapter we will consider evidence from neuronal recording and immunohistochemical imaging studies for there being two different aspects to recognition memory, and the differential involvement of the perirhinal cortex and hippocampus in each of them. These two aspects of recognition memory, familiarity discrimination for individual stimulus items and recollection of potentially many items and their contextual associations, differ markedly in their reliance on associative information. Accordingly, these two aspects of recognition memory have markedly different requirements for the binding of information in memory.

The involvement of the perirhinal cortex in recognition memory

Recent research has identified what appears to be at least part of the neuronal mechanism underlying familiarity discrimination (Brown and Xiang 1998; Brown and Bashir 2002; Brown and Aggleton 2001). This research has indicated a central role in familiarity discrimination for changes in neuronal responses in the perirhinal cortex of the temporal lobe when visual stimuli are repeated. The perirhinal cortex (classically, Brodmann's area 35, but more recently redefined to include both area 35 and area 36 (Amaral *et al.* 1987; Burwell *et al.* 1995)) is found anteriorly and inferiorly in the medial temporal lobe of primates. It is lateral to the hippocampal formation, to which it provides many inputs (Burwell *et al.* 1995; Suzuki 1996a;b Burwell and Amaral 1998; Lavenex and Amaral 2000). In monkeys it lies medial and anterior to area TE, a high-order visual processing area. The perirhinal cortex receives information from widespread areas of the cerebral cortex, including areas involved in visual (notably area TE in monkeys), auditory, somatosensory, and olfactory processing, as well as return pathways from the hippocampal formation (Burwell *et al.* 1995; Suzuki 1996a,b; Burwell and Amaral 1998; Lavenex and Amaral 2000). It is similarly placed with broadly equivalent connections in the rodent (Witter *et al.* 1989; Burwell *et al.* 1995; Shi and Cassell 1997; Witter *et al.* 2000). Thus the perirhinal cortex is a multimodal area at the top of the hierarchy of sensory processing areas (Felleman and Van Essen 1991; Lavenex and Amaral 2000; Witter *et al.* 2000). Indeed, it has been suggested to be essential to the perception of objects as entities in themselves (Buckley and Gaffan 1998b; Murray and Bussey 1999). Such a region, where the sensory processing streams provide information concerning the identity of a stimulus, is well placed to be involved in processes concerning memory for the past history of the stimulus. Consistent with this view, there is evidence that the perirhinal cortex is involved in paired associate learning and aversive and appetitive conditioning, as well as in recognition memory (Murray *et al.* 1993, 1998; Corodimas and LeDoux 1995; Higuchi and Miyashita 1996; Suzuki 1996b; Buckley and Gaffan 1998a; Murray and Bussey 1999). It is with the functions of the perirhinal cortex in the familiarity discrimination component of recognition memory that the first section of this chapter is concerned. The potential contributions of the hippocampal system to spatial and recollective aspects of recognition memory are considered in the second section (Brown and Aggleton 2001).

The essential role of the perirhinal cortex in visual recognition memory has been established by ablation studies, chiefly in the monkey (Zola-Morgan *et al.* 1989; Gaffan and Murray 1992; Suzuki *et al.* 1993; Meunier *et al.* 1993, 1996), but also in the rat (Otto and Eichenbaum 1992; Mumby and Pinel 1994; Ennaceur *et al.* 1996). Thus there is major impairment of tasks, particularly visual delayed matching or non-matching to sample tasks, that depend for their successful performance upon judgement of the prior occurrence of infrequently repeated individual items (Murray 1996; Murray and Bussey 1999; Brown and Aggleton 2001). While the degree of impairment following hippocampal lesions is still disputed, all groups agree that impairment following perirhinal lesions is far greater than that following hippocampal, amygdalar, or prefrontal lesions (Aggleton *et al.* 1986; Mumby *et al.* 1992, 1995; Zola-Morgan and Squire 1993; Zola-Morgan *et al.* 1994; Alvarez *et al.* 1995; Murray 1996; Meunier *et al.* 1997; Murray and Mishkin 1998; Aggleton and Brown 1999; Beason-Held *et al.* 1999; Murray and Bussey 1999; Zola *et al.* 2000; Brown and Aggleton 2001; Baxter and Murray 2001). Thus evidence from primate and rat ablation studies strongly indicates that the perirhinal cortex is a nodal point of a system that is concerned with judgements concerning the prior occurrence of individual visual items.

Candidate neuronal substrates of familiarity discrimination

Given the central involvement of the perirhinal cortex in familiarity discrimination, what are the candidate neuronal substrates that could explain the behavioural results? Any substrate must be capable of explaining learning that occurs in a single exposure, is long lasting, and has high capacity, in particular the ability to remember the prior occurrence of very large numbers of complex stimuli. The substrate should be found in both trained and untrained situations because familiarity discrimination itself (and correspondingly its counterpart process, novelty detection) should be innate rather than needing to be learned. It must also adequately deal with a stimulus encountered by the subject for the first time ever, and not merely with stimuli that have been frequently encountered and hence are highly familiar. Evidence for potential substrates comes from studies of the response characteristics of perirhinal neurons. Several activity changes that might provide candidate potential substrates have been discovered by recording the responses of neurons during the performance of recognition memory tasks by monkeys (Gross *et al.* 1972; Fuster and Jervey 1981; Brown *et al.* 1987; Miller and Desimone 1994; Xiang and Brown 1997; Brown and Xiang 1998). These putative candidate substrates are response differences between match and mismatch trials, delay activity, response reductions or response increments on stimulus repetition, and synchronized neuronal firing (Fig. 16.1). However, of these substrates only one, response reductions on stimulus repetition, has so far been demonstrated to have the necessary properties and to occur in a variety of behavioural situations (Brown and Xiang 1998; Brown and Aggleton 2001).

The first reported memory-related difference in responsiveness of inferior temporal neurons in a recognition memory task was that between responses on

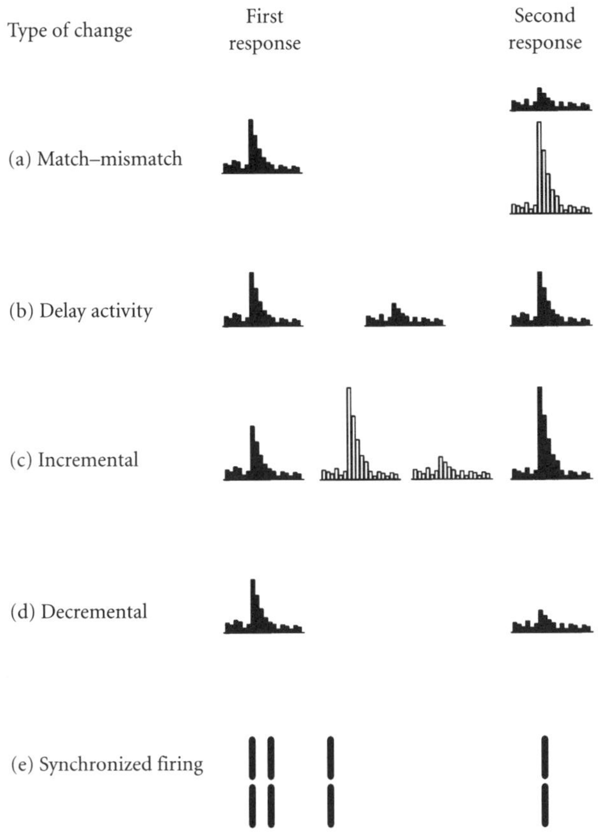

Figure 16.1 Types of neuronal activity change found in perirhinal cortex during performance of familiarity discrimination tasks. The size of the histogram represents the magnitude of the response to an individual stimulus. A change in size denotes a change in response on repetition. (a) Match–mismatch response differences. (b) Delay activity. (c) Response enhancement. (d) Response reductions. (e) Synchronized firing.

match and mismatch trials while monkeys performed a delayed matching task (Gross *et al.* 1972). There are many reports of such differences using tasks where a match–mismatch judgement must be made to a single target stimulus on each trial and the target stimuli are selected from a small number of frequently repeating items (Gross *et al.* 1972; Mikami and Kubota 1980; Brown 1982; Riches *et al.* 1991; Nakamura and Kubota 1995; Young *et al.* 1997). However, when a novel stimulus is introduced into such a delayed matching task, neurons with such responses typically continue to signal that the trial type is match or non-match and not whether a particular stimulus is novel or familiar (Riches *et al.* 1991). Thus the response changes between match and mismatch trials are the same for novel as for familiar stimuli and therefore do not differentially signal the novelty or familiarity of the stimulus. Accordingly, such differences cannot provide a substrate of general familiarity discrimination (Brown and Xiang 1998; Brown and Aggleton 2001).

The next potential mechanism to be discovered was delay activity. This is a persistent change in neuronal firing that occurs in the delay interval after the presentation of a stimulus in the acquisition phase of a memory task and lasts until the occurrence of the same or a different stimulus in the subsequent behavioural choice/decision phase (Fuster and Jervey 1981; Riches *et al.* 1991; Miller *et al.* 1993; Colombo and Gross 1994; Miller and Desimone 1994; Desimone 1996). Delay activity has not been demonstrated under conditions that require long-term rather than short-term memory (e.g. where more than one stimulus must be remembered at a time) nor when the eventual occurrence of the choice phase of a task is unpredictable (e.g. where it may not occur until after a delay of many minutes filled with other activities) (Desimone 1996; Brown and Xiang 1998; Brown and Aggleton 2001). Additionally, delay activity has not been shown to persist over long periods of time nor has it been shown to occur endogenously without an animal having being trained in a task where recurrence of stimuli is predictable. Thus delay activity may rather represent a substrate of an attentive or short-term memory mechanism, although one that could contribute to short-term recognition memory (Desimone 1996; Brown and Xiang 1998).

Similarly, responses that increment on repetition, i.e. are larger to a repeated stimulus than to one occurring for the first time, have only been observed when an animal has been trained to discriminate between a specific stimulus which, when repeated, signals the availability of reward and other stimuli which, when repeated, do not signal the availability of reward (Miller and Desimone 1994). Again, these response increments have only been demonstrated under conditions where only one stimulus had to be held in mind at a time. In such situations, as already suggested above, short-term memory and attentive mechanisms provide alternative means of solving the task (Brown and Xiang 1998; Brown and Aggleton 2001). Furthermore, response increments have not been shown to occur when time delays are long. Therefore such response increments provide an additional recognition memory mechanism with specific advantages under particular conditions, but do not provide an adequate substrate for general untrained familiarity discrimination.

In contrast, response reductions on stimulus repetition have been reported under a variety of conditions (Brown *et al.* 1987; Riches *et al.* 1991; Eskandar *et al.* 1992; Fahy *et al.* 1993; Li *et al.* 1993; Miller *et al.* 1993; Sobotka and Ringo 1993; Miller and Desimone 1994; Zhu *et al.* 1995a,b; Xiang and Brown 1998). An example is shown in Figure 16.2. The details of such neuronal response reductions on stimulus repetition have been extensively reviewed elsewhere (Brown 1996; Desimone 1996; Eichenbaum *et al.* 1996; Ringo 1996; Brown and

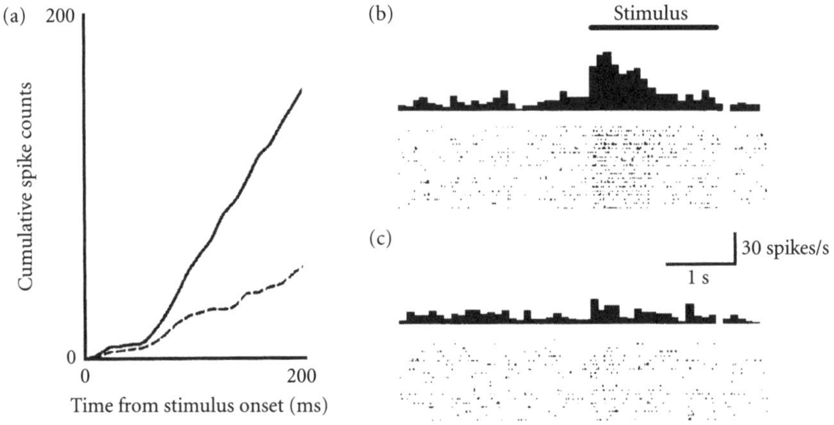

Figure 16.2 Speed of processing. (a) The cumulated action potential counts after stimulus onset (time = 0) for 20 novel (continuous line) and 20 familiar (dashed line) pictures of a neuron recorded in area TE. Peristimulus–time histograms and rasters for 20 novel (b) and 20 familiar (c) pictures for the neuron. (Copyright 2002 with permission from The Royal Society.)

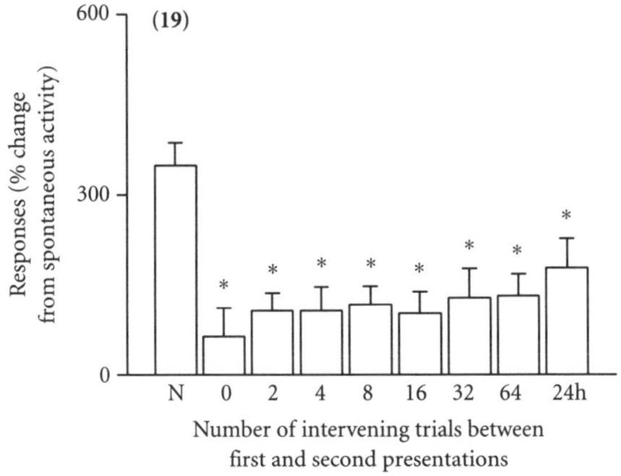

Figure 16.3 Mean population response across different intervals (number of intervening trials) for 19 recency neurons recorded in the perirhinal cortex. *Significant difference between mean response to first and subsequent presentation. (Reproduced with permission. Copyright (1998) Elsevier.)

Xiang 1998; Suzuki and Eichenbaum 2000; Brown and Aggleton 2001) and so will be given only briefly here. In monkeys such response reductions occur under closely controlled conditions and are not explicable by changes in alertness, attention, motivation, eye movements, or other behavioural changes (Brown and Xiang 1998). Critically, they occur after a single exposure to an initially novel stimulus even if the delay until the re-occurrence of the stimulus is 24 h or more (Fahy *et al.* 1993; Xiang and Brown 1998) (Fig. 16.3). Moreover, these reductions are found even when many stimuli must be remembered simultaneously and when intervals between repetitions are filled with presentations of other stimuli to which attention is being paid, so that long-term memory mechanisms are essential to task performance (Xiang and Brown 1998). Thus the response reductions evidence dependence on information held in long-term memory. No other type of response change capable of signalling information adequate to explain general long-term recognition memory has been reported in the perirhinal cortex. The high capacity of the system is evident because such reductions occur for repetitions of new stimuli even when an animal has already seen many hundreds of such items (Xiang and Brown 1998). Furthermore, neuronal response reductions are found whether or not an animal is using the stimulus repetitions to obtain reward (Riches *et al.* 1991; Fahy *et al.* 1993; Zhu *et al.* 1995a; Brown and Xiang 1998). The reductions are observable in rats as well as monkeys (Zhu *et al.* 1995a; Brown and Xiang 1998). As response reductions occur even in situations where an animal has received no specific training in a recognition memory task, they must be endogenous rather than induced by training. Any general familiarity discrimination mechanism needs to be able operate automatically and without direct or immediate feedback from reward systems.

A particular example of reduced neuronal activation produced by familiar compared with novel stimuli when animals have not been trained in a recognition memory task is provided by the results of rat immunohistochemical imaging studies. Such imaging is possible because the high proportion of perirhinal neurons whose responses diminish with stimulus repetition enables their distribution to be visualized by immunohistochemistry for the products (Fos) of the immediate early gene c-*fos* (Zhu *et al.* 1995b; Zhu *et al.* 1996; Wan *et al.* 1999). This immediate early gene is generally turned on when neurons are activated (Herdegen and Leah 1998), enabling relative differences in activation to be determined from differences in the immunohistochemical staining of the neurons. To control for any non-specific differences produced by the presentation of novel compared with familiar stimuli, both types of stimuli were presented under the same conditions of movement, arousal, and motivation, and with similar eye movements, by using the paired viewing procedure (Zhu *et al.* 1996). In this procedure, the stimuli are presented in such a way that one eye sees only a novel picture while, at the same time, the other eye sees only a familiar picture (as shown in Fig. 16.4). A rat is trained to hold its head in an observing hole while the pairs of stimuli are presented. On doing so the rat receives juice, but the delivery of the juice is not dependent on the animal discriminating between the novel and familiar stimuli, so that any differences in neuronal activity produced by the relative familiarity of the stimuli must be endogenous and not induced by training in a recognition memory task. By presenting a series of such paired stimuli, the amount of neuronal activation evoked by novel and familiar stimuli can be assessed in the same rat by comparing the levels of Fos expression in the two

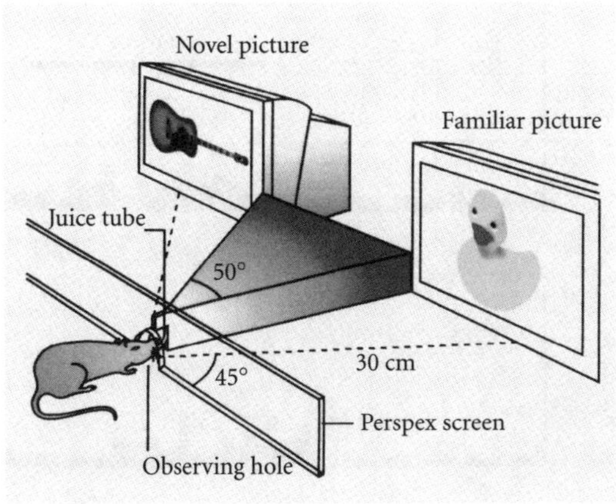

Figure 16.4 The paired viewing procedure for simultaneously presenting novel and familiar stimuli. (Reproduced with permission. Copyright (2001) Macmillan Magazine Ltd.)

hemispheres, one of which has chiefly processed the information from the familiar stimuli, while the other has chiefly processed the information from the novel stimuli. Under these conditions, more neurons are activated in the perirhinal cortex (and the adjacent temporal visual association cortex (area Te2)) by novel than by familiar stimuli, consistent with the results of electrophysiological studies (Zhu *et al.* 1996; Wan *et al.* 1999). It is important to note that these results rely on storage of information concerning the familiarity of the stimuli for at least 3 h, so that the differences are not dependent on short-term memory processes. Thus the results of Fos imaging studies are closely consistent with the recording studies in finding activity reductions for previously seen stimuli in perirhinal cortex.

The last potential substrate concerns the precise timing of action potentials within neuronal networks. Much less is known about the potential involvement of synchronized neuronal firing in familiarity discrimination. In relation to sensory processing it has been hypothesized that such coincident or near-coincident firing may carry important information (Singer and Gray 1995) and, in particular, that such temporally correlated firing may be important for binding together the different individual attributes of a stimulus into a unitary percept (Abeles 1982). Significant interactions between neurons have been revealed by cross-correlating the simultaneously recorded activity of pairs of neurons in monkeys (Gawne and Richmond 1993; Xiang and Brown 1997; Brown and Xiang 1998; Erickson *et al.* 2001). These interactions suggest that information of potential importance to recognition memory is being carried by relationships between the activity of perirhinal neurons. However, as far as has been determined to date, the incidence of simultaneous (within 6 ms) action potentials produced by simultaneously recorded pairs of neurons is very low. Moreover, more crucially, the timing of

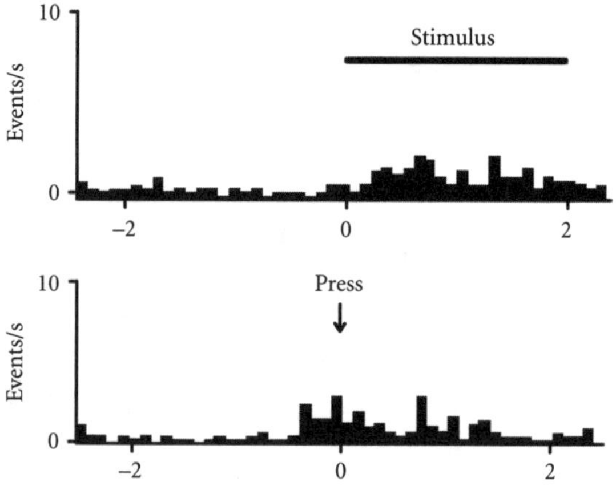

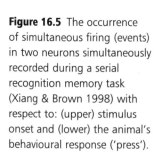

Figure 16.5 The occurrence of simultaneous firing (events) in two neurons simultaneously recorded during a serial recognition memory task (Xiang & Brown 1998) with respect to: (upper) stimulus onset and (lower) the animal's behavioural response ('press').

the occurrence of such simultaneous firing is typically late rather than early after stimulus onset, and is usually more closely related to the occurrence of an animal's behavioural response than to the stimulus onset itself (Brown 2000; J.-Z. Xiang and M.W. Brown, unpublished observations) (Fig. 16.5). Accordingly, the information carried by such firing provides a much slower signal than is provided by the change in firing rate of the individual neurons.

Do synaptic changes occur in the perirhinal cortex?

While ablation studies establish the importance of the perirhinal cortex for familiarity discrimination and recording studies establish that there are neurons within this cortex whose response reductions on stimulus repetition signal the type of information that is required to judge prior occurrence for individual stimuli, the evidence reviewed so far does not establish where the synaptic changes that underlie the neuronal response changes may first be generated. Important evidence concerning the location of such changes is provided by the speed and incidence of response reductions that survive over long delays between the first and subsequent occurrence of a stimulus. In monkeys it is possible to find neuronal response reductions more posteriorly, in regions concerned with the earlier stages of visual processing. However, these reductions do not survive more than some seconds or when more than a very few other stimuli are shown before a particular stimulus is repeated (Baylis and Rolls 1987; Maunsell *et al.* 1991; Miller *et al.* 1991; Vogels *et al.* 1995). Accordingly, such response reductions cannot explain those in anterior area TE and perirhinal cortex that survive many intervening stimulus presentations and delay intervals of many hours (Xiang and Brown 1998). Responses are reduced with stimulus repetition for approximately 25 per cent of all recorded neurons in the anterior TE, the perirhinal cortex, and the entorhinal cortex (Miller *et al.* 1993; Xiang and Brown 1998). For over 50 per cent of the neurons whose responses change on stimulus repetition, such reductions are found even after a 24-h delay. The incidence of such long memory spans is highest in the perirhinal cortex (Xiang and Brown 1998). Ablation of the entorhinal cortex in monkeys produces only a transient impairment of delayed non-matching to sample (Meunier *et al.* 1993; Leonard *et al.* 1995), so that the critical change cannot be dependent on the entorhinal cortex. Thus the critical response changes must either be first generated in the anterior TE and perirhinal cortex, or be fed back to these areas from later processing stages, such as the hippocampus or prefrontal cortex.

Response reductions signal prior occurrence with remarkable rapidity. Latency measures across all the neurons displaying response reductions in anterior area TE in the monkey indicate that within 90 ms of stimulus onset there is a significant difference in the population's activity dependent on whether the presented stimulus is novel or previously seen (Xiang and Brown 1998). In many neurons the latency of the response change is the same (to within the experimental error of 10–20 ms) as the latency of the neuron's visual response (Fahy *et al.* 1993; Miller *et al.* 1993; Xiang and Brown 1998) (Fig. 16.2). The speed of this change means that the initial change in response cannot be generated as a result of feedback from later processing stages such as the hippocampus or prefrontal cortex. Recordings in the monkey hippocampus and prefrontal cortex support this view (see further below). Thus the incidence of response changes on the repetition of infrequently encountered individual stimuli in the hippocampus is less than 1 per cent (Rolls *et al.* 1989, 1993; Riches *et al.* 1991; Xiang and Brown 1998). Moreover, the latencies of the changes in monkey hippocampal neuronal responses to infrequently repeated stimuli are long compared with those in the anterior TE and perirhinal cortex (Rolls *et al.* 1993; Xiang and Brown 1998). The incidence of response changes on stimulus repetition is much higher in certain parts of the monkey prefrontal cortex, but again the latencies of these changes are much longer than in the temporal cortex (Miller *et al.* 1996; Xiang and Brown 2004; Miller 1999). Furthermore, although changes in neuronal responses on stimulus repetition have been described in subcortical regions, such as the monkey basal forebrain nucleus (Rolls *et al.* 1982; Wilson and Rolls 1990), these changes occur with a longer latency than those in the anterior inferior temporal and perirhinal cortex (Brown and Xiang 1998). Additionally, it seems implausible that the relatively small number of neurons involved in such subcortical areas could have suficient information processing capacity to discriminate first themselves amongst hundreds of complex visual stimuli; such capacity is a prerequisite for the judgement of the prior occurrence of such stimuli. (It is important to note that there is evidence of such capacity for area TE and the perirhinal cortex.) Thus there is no evidence that the initial response reductions on stimulus repetition are fed back to the anterior TE and perirhinal cortex from other brain regions. Indeed, the rapidity of the discrimination makes such an explanation implausible.

Thus the available evidence indicates that the response reductions do not arise as a result of either feedforward signals from more posterior visual areas or feedback from other processing regions. Hence at least the initial reductions in response must be generated in the anterior TE and/or the perirhinal cortex. For visual processing, ablation experiments cannot easily distinguish between the contributions of the anterior TE and the perirhinal cortex, as ablating TE de-afferents the perirhinal cortex. Moreover, while the response changes occur at shorter latency in the anterior TE than in the perirhinal cortex, the memory spans of the response changes tend to be longer in the perirhinal cortex than in the anterior TE. Thus, in the monkey, the evidence indicates that response changes are generated within the region encompassing the anterior TE and the perirhinal cortex, and may involve both, but it does not clearly distinguish between them. However, in the rat there is evidence that critical changes are dependent on the perirhinal cortex. In rats familiarity discrimination can be measured by the preferential exploration of a novel compared with a familiar object (Ennaceur and Delacour 1988). Such discrimination is impaired by bilateral localized infusions of scopolamine into the perirhinal cortex via implanted cannulae when the drug is infused to be present at acquisition but not when it is present at retrieval (choice) (Warburton *et al.* 2003). Thus administration of scopolamine does not impair discrimination of the familiarity of an object encountered before the drug was given, i.e.if storage has occurred. Accordingly, if the critical information storage occurs outside the infused region (e.g. in area Te2, which is approximately the rat equivalent of monkey area TE) and independently of perirhinal involvement, performance should not be impaired when the drug is present in the perirhinal cortex during acquisition. However, there is impairment, so that storage must be within or dependent on the infused region, i.e. the perirhinal cortex.

Computational modelling and the feasibility of using neuronal response reductions as a basis for familiarity discrimination

Assuming that neuronal response reductions in the perirhinal cortex provide the substrate for familiarity discrimination, is it plausible that such a system could explain human capabilities? Human abilities are very impressive in the laboratory

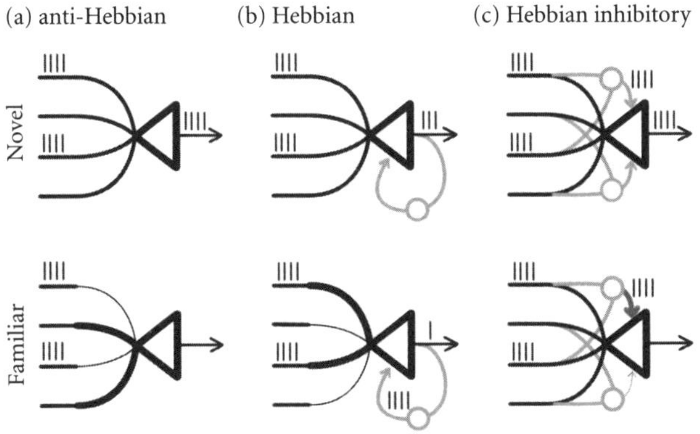

Figure 16.6 Synaptic and network mechanisms that may underlie the decrease of perirhinal neurons' response for familiar stimuli. Three mechanisms are shown (a) anti-Hebbian learning (synaptic weakening), (b) Hebbian learning (synaptic strengthening), and (c) Hebbian learning between inhibitory interneurons and novelty neurons.

as well as in everyday life, and include speed, accuracy, and huge capacity (Standing 1973; Seeck *et al.* 1997; Hintzman *et al.* 1998). However, the plausibility of perirhinal response reductions as a substrate for familiarity discrimination has been established by recent computational modelling (Bogacz *et al.* 1999, 2001; Bogacz and Brown 2003). The models are based on the response properties of perirhinal neurons. The basic premise is that individual synapses undergo a plastic use-dependent change upon their initial activation by a stimulus. This synaptic change stores the prior occurrence of the individual stimulus. In the models, the necessary synaptic changes could be effected by processes determined at individual synapses, such as those that are utilized by long-term potentiation or depression (Ito 1989; Bliss and Collingridge 1993; Kemp and Bashir 2001; Linden 1994; Abraham and Bear 1996; Brown and Xiang 1998; Brown and Bashir 2002.) (Fig. 16.6). Hence, such models can be made to operate using biologically plausible learning rules and connectivity.

Theoretical calculations and simulations indicate that under optimal conditions the capacity of such models to discriminate the familiarity of stimuli is potentially extremely large; the number of stimuli whose familiarity can be judged is proportional to the number of the modifiable synapses (Bogacz 2001; Bogacz *et al.* 2001; Bogacz and Brown 2003). Thus if it is assumed, based on data from Insausti *et al.* (1998) and Xiang and Brown (1998), that in the human perirhinal cortex there are approximately 10^7 neurons that judge familiarity and each has approximately10^4 synapses, it can be calculated that the model proposed by Bogacz *et al.* (2001) is able to discriminate the familiarity of approximately 10^9 stimuli with an error rate of 1 per cent. This capacity corresponds to that required to register and remember with high accuracy the occurrence of a new picture approximately every 3 s over a lifetime of 100 years. It is possible to achieve such a high capacity because the network is required to supply as its output only the relative familiarity of a stimulus. Correspondingly, the number of neurons required is less than 0.1 per cent of those in the whole cerebral cortex. As the output required is not complex, such a network can potentially arrive at a decision within milliseconds. Thus, for a relatively small outlay, the brain can have a system that signals the novelty or familiarity of a stimulus with great speed and accuracy.

Modelling has shown that several different network architectures might potentially enable familiarity discrimination to be performed rapidly and accurately for large numbers of stimuli. However, the particular architectures and learning rules have major influences on both the maximum capacity of the model and whether the types of responses simulated in the model mirror those observed in the real brain (Bogacz 2001; Bogacz *et al.* 2001; Bogacz and Brown 2003). Importantly, simulations of different models have revealed that the capacity of a model depends critically on the degree of correlation between the responses of the individual neurons to the incoming stimuli (Fig. 16.7). Clearly, if all the neurons responded in the same way to each different stimulus, the capacity of the whole model could be no more than the capacity of one of the individual component neurons and therefore would be very low. Thus it is essential that mechanisms within the network act to decorrelate responses so that individual neurons make independent calculations of the familiarity of a stimulus. Most computational networks for discriminating familiarity have used synaptic enhancement as the fundamental synaptic change (Bogacz *et al.* 1999; Sohal and Hasselmo 2000; Bogacz 2001; Bogacz *et al.* 2001; Norman and O'Reilly 2001). (The models also employ some form of synaptic weakening of relatively unstimulated synapses to maintain a constant overall level of network excitability.) Further, response increments are an essential feature of the models using synaptic enhancement that combine feature detection (learning to categorize or form a representation) with familiarity discrimination; the increased responses are designed to signal (represent) the presence of a particular stimulus (Sohal and Hasselmo 2000; Norman and O'Reilly 2001). Firstly, however, it should be noted that response increments on stimulus repetition are unusual and unimpressive in magnitude within the perirhinal cortex (Li *et al.* 1993; Xiang and Brown 1998). Secondly, if the representation has not yet been learnt and hence feature extraction is incomplete, the responses of the network's neurons are necessarily not independent (and hence are correlated). For this reason, simulations indicate that these models have a capacity that is greatly reduced compared with that theoretically possible when responses are uncorrelated (Bogacz and Brown 2003).

In the original model of Bogacz *et al* (2001) the fundamental synaptic change was one of enhancement on stimulus repetition, with response increments being

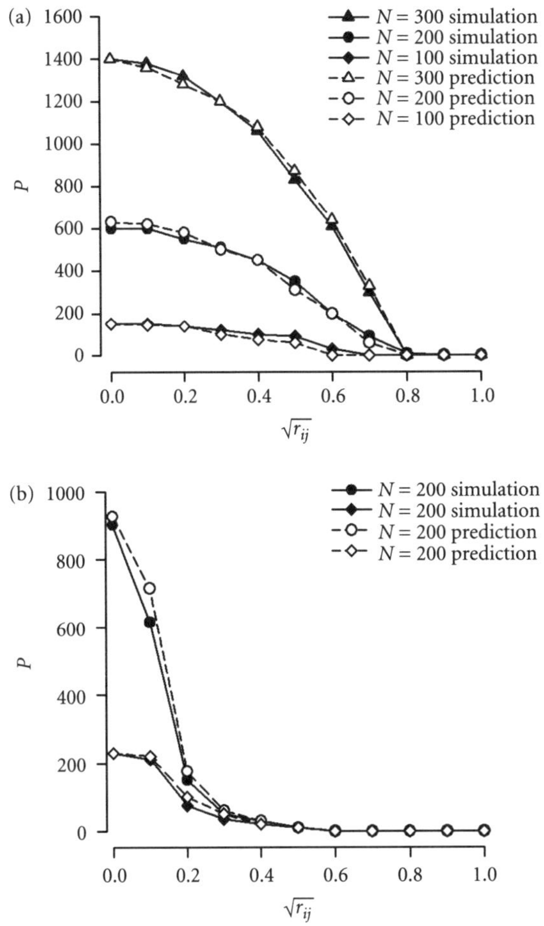

Figure 16.7 The capacities (number of stored patterns, *P*) of familiarity discrimination networks when the activity of the neurons in the network is correlated (square root of $|r_{ij}|$). (a) Simulations and mathematical calculations ('predictions') of the capacity of the anti-Hebbian model where synaptic weakening is the primary plastic change. (b) Capacity of the Hebbian model where synaptic strengthening is the primary plastic change. (Adapted with permission. Copyright (2003) Wiley.)

prevented by network connections that increased inhibition for repeated stimuli. Nevertheless, for a high capacity to be achieved by this model, it remains necessary for correlations between responses to be very low ($r_{ij} < 0.05$) (Bogacz and Brown 2003) (Fig. 16.7). In contrast, if the primary synaptic change is decremental rather than incremental, the neuronal responses tend to become less rather than more correlated as a result of the synaptic change that stores the occurrence. Correspondingly, the capacity of the network is far less affected by any initial correlations between the responses of its neurons (Bogacz and Brown 2003) (Fig. 16.7). The reason for this difference can be understood in principle from the following considerations. Fundamentally, if an incremental change is used, the network moves in the direction of feature extraction, i.e. neurons responsive to a particular stimulus feature tend to become more responsive to it when it recurs in the future while (through compensatory mechanisms) originally less responsive neurons become even less responsive. Such an outcome is favourable to building a representation by feature extraction. However, as shown by simulations, a familiarity discrimination network is far more efficient if feature extraction has already been completed and the responses of its component neurons are decorrelated, i.e. essentially the neurons of the network act to emphasize what is particular rather than what is commonplace in a stimulus (Bogacz and Brown 2003). Hence a network that uses synaptic enhancement as its primary plastic change tends to bind together stimulus features that occur together frequently. In contrast, a network that uses synaptic weakening as its primary plastic change tends to detect unbound features that have not co-occurred previously. Thus modelling provides an explanation for the observed direction of response change (reductions rather than increments) on stimulus repetition in perirhinal cortex. The counterpart of this direction of change is that, for a novel stimulus, the system generates a large signal which can potentially be used to allow further processing of this stimulus elsewhere (possibly including setting up a new representation outside the familiarity discrimination network).

In sum, computational modelling demonstrates that neuronal response reductions in the perirhinal cortex could potentially be used as a basis for familiarity discrimination; the necessary speed, accuracy, and capacity are theoretically achievable. The models rely on activity-dependent synapse-specific plasticity. Plastic mechanisms which do not produce changes that are localized to specific synapses would result in a catastrophic loss of capacity. Moreover, as measurements in the perirhinal cortex indicate that there are many more excitatory synapses than inhibitory synapses (Thompson *et al.* 2001), a high capacity can only be achieved by having modifiable excitatory synapses. Both long-term potentiation and long-term depression rely on activity-dependent synapse-specific plastic mechanisms. The arguments based on computational modelling presented above indicate that employing as the primary plastic mechanism one that reduces synaptic efficacy is likely to prove more efficient than employing one that enhances efficacy.

The involvement of the hippocampus in recognition memory

Evidence from lesion studies

The involvement of the hippocampal formation (defined as hippocampal fields CA1–4, the dentate gyrus, and the subiculum) in familiarity discrimination of infrequently encountered individual items in standard tests of monkey recognition memory is controversial. There is dispute concerning the effects of hippocampal lesions on recognition memory (Alvarez *et al.* 1995; Murray and Mishkin 1998; Beason-Held *et al.* 1999; Zola *et al.* 2000) although, as indicated above, any impairment is agreed to be less than that following perirhinal lesions. Importantly, a recent meta-analysis of such reports has established that memory impairment increases as perirhinal damage increases but, counter-intuitively, increases as hippocampal damage decreases (Baxter and Murray 2001). The latter finding is consistent with a malfunctioning hippocampus being more disruptive to familiarity discrimination than a non-existent one, as has been suggested by studies in the rat (Mumby *et al.* 1992). Similarly, the majority of rat ablation studies have failed to find consistent effects of hippocampal lesions on familiarity discrimination of individual stimuli (Mumby 2001)

These results for recognition memory tasks using infrequently repeating ('trial unique') stimuli can be contrasted for those using small stimulus sets. In such tasks the stimuli rapidly all become highly familiar so that recency rather than familiarity mechanisms are favoured. Moreover, typically, only one target stimulus must be remembered at a time in such tasks so that short-term or working-memory-based mechanisms provide the optimum strategy for task solution. Perirhinal lesions do not prevent performance of such tasks (Eacott *et al.* 1994).

In contrast with the still equivocal role in familiarity discrimination for individual items, if task complexity is increased, particularly if a judgement dependent on spatial memory is required, there is a very large body of evidence indicating that hippocampal lesions produce major impairments (O'Keefe and Nadel 1978; Morris *et al.* 1982; Aggleton *et al.* 1986; Eichenbaum *et al.* 1994; Eichenbaum *et al.* 1996; Gaffan 1994; Liu and Bilkey 1998a,b,c; Murray *et al.* 1998; Aggleton and Brown 1999; Brown and Aggleton 2001). Moreover, the importance of the hippocampal formation to allocentric spatial processing is well established (O'Keefe and Nadel 1978; Morris *et al.* 1982; Aggleton *et al.* 1986; Gaffan 1994). In contradistinction, lesion studies have shown that damage to the perirhinal cortex has relatively little or no effect on spatial memory tasks, and thus the perirhinal cortex is relatively unimportant in the processing of spatial stimuli (Gaffan 1994; Ennaceur *et al.* 1996; Bussey *et al.* 1999; but see Liu and Bilkey 1998a;b;c; Bilkey and Lui 2000).

Evidence from recording studies

The results of recording studies parallel those of ablation work. Thus, on the one hand, they indicate that the incidence of hippocampal neurons carrying information concerning the familiarity or recency of presentation of individual infrequently repeating stimuli is low (approximately 1 per cent) (Brown *et al.* 1987; Rolls *et al.* 1989,1993; Riches *et al.* 1991; Xiang and Brown 1998). This figure compares with 25 per cent found in the perirhinal cortex under the same conditions, as reported above. Moreover, for those hippocampal neurons that do change response on stimulus repetition, memory spans have not been demonstrated to be as long as those of many such neurons in the anterior inferior temporal, including the perirhinal, cortex (Rolls *et al.* 1993; Xiang and Brown 1998). Thus electrophysiological evidence of a major role for the hippocampus in long-term familiarity discrimination of individual items is weak.

As for the inferior temporal cortex, both delay activity and match–mismatch differences have been reported at high incidence in the hippocampus when small stimulus sets have been used in tasks where short-term or working-memory-based mechanisms may be used (Brown 1982; Riches *et al.* 1991, Colombo and Gross 1994; Hampson *et al.* 1999; Wiebe and Staubli 1999). Such activity changes have been found using odours as well as visual stimuli and in rats as well as monkeys (Eichenbaum *et al.* 1996; Otto and Eichenbaum 1992; Wood *et al.* 1999). As for the perirhinal cortex, it has been shown in monkeys that these activity changes do not reliably signal information about the novelty or familiarity of infrequently encountered individual stimuli (Riches *et al.* 1991). Rather, these activity changes signal information concerning the type of trial (match–mismatch) in which a stimulus occurs (Brown 1990; Riches *et al.* 1991; Otto and Eichenbaum 1992; Brown and Aggleton 2001). Hence, as in the perirhinal cortex, these match–mismatch activity changes, although probably important for solving repetitious recognition memory tasks, do not provide a possible substrate for general long-term familiarity discrimination.

Although the hippocampus has been shown to contain a much lower proportion of neurons that signal the prior presentation of infrequently occurring individual stimuli than the perirhinal cortex, there are many studies which show that the hippocampus contains many neurons which respond to the position or arrangement of stimuli in the environment (O' Keefe 1993; Eichenbaum *et al.* 1996; Muller 1996; Wiener 1996; O'Keefe *et al.* 1998). For example, individual neurons in the rat respond to particular spatial positions in the environment, described as place fields (O'Keefe and Nadel 1978; Muller 1996). In the monkey, increases in the firing of hippocampal neurons have been shown when the animal directs its gaze to a particular position in the environment, and these neurons have been described as spatial view cells (Rolls *et al.*,1998). The responses of perirhinal cortex neurons to the presentation of spatial stimuli have been little studied (Burwell *et al.* 1995).

Evidence from immediate early gene (c-*fos*) imaging

The rat Fos imaging studies which demonstrated that more neurons were activated in the perirhinal cortex (and the adjacent temporal visual association cortex (area Te2)) by novel than by familiar individual stimuli also revealed that very few neurons were activated in the hippocampus (Zhu *et al.* 1995b; Zhu *et al.* 1996; Wan *et al.* 1999). Thus, consistent with the results of recording studies, immunohistochemical imaging experiments indicate an important role for the perirhinal cortex and at most a minor role for the hippocampus in discriminating the relative familiarity of individual visual stimuli.

In contrast, Fos imaging reveals major hippocampal involvement when familiarity discrimination has a spatial or associational component, such as an encounter with a new environment or a new spatial arrangement of familiar individual items (Wan *et al.* 1999; Vann *et al.* 2000). Recognition memory encompasses discrimination of the novelty or familiarity of a spatial arrangement of equally familiar individual items (e.g. your reaction to someone else rearranging the familiar furniture in your own room). An environment can be regarded as a set of individual items in a particular spatial relation to each other. The percept and its recording in memory necessitate binding together in a complex associational matrix the particular positional interrelationships of the individual items (Brown 1990).

The experimental evidence comes from a series of Fos imaging studies. In an initial study, levels of neuronal activation were measured in rats presented with novel stimuli in a familiar environment compared with rats presented with novel objects in a novel environment (Zhu *et al.* 1997). Neuronal activation was significantly higher in the hippocampus when the environment was novel than when it was familiar. In contrast, neuronal activation in the perirhinal cortex did not differ in the novel and familiar environments. However, in this study differences in levels of attention and arousal between the rat groups may have accounted for, or contributed to, the different levels of hippocampal activation observed. Thus in a second experiment (Wan *et al.* 1999) the experimental design was modified so that two different stimuli, one novel and one familiar, could be were presented simultaneously using the paired viewing procedure. The stimuli were pictures, each containing three individual items, in which the particular arrangements of the individual items and not the items themselves were either novel or familiar. Indeed, all the individual items were equally familiar. The novel and familiar arrangements produced differences in neuronal activation in various parts of the hippocampus, although not all regions showed the same direction of change. In subfield CA1 of the hippocampus presentation of the novel arrangements produced greater neuronal activation than for the familiar arrangements. In contrast, there was significantly less neuronal activation for the novel compared with the familiar stimuli in the dentate gyrus and subiculum. The perirhinal cortex and area Te2 were not differentially affected by the presentation of the novel and familiar arrangements. This result is consistent with previous findings, as the individual items in the arrangements were equally familiar and it was the spatial configuration of the items which was either novel or familiar. These findings suggest that recognition memory for spatial arrangements of stimuli may depend on a neural system involving the hippocampus rather than the perirhinal cortex.

The observed increases in activation produced by the familiar stimuli in the dentate gyrus and subiculum were found primarily outside the principal cell layers and could reflect increased activity in inhibitory interneurons. The differential activity of inhibitory neurons could explain the reversed directions of the differences in activation for novel and familiar stimuli as the information passed from one region to the next through the hippocampal formation (Wan *et al.* 1999). Another possibility, that the changes in activation reflected differences in processing between the dorsal and ventral hippocampal formation, was excluded in further work (unpublished) in which samples of both subfield CA1 and the dentate gyrus were made at both dorsal and the ventral levels. However, these data indicated greater activation in the dorsal than the ventral hippocampus. This finding is consistent with lesion and electrophysiological studies indicating that the dorsal hippocampal formation is more important than the ventral for learning about the arrangements of spatial stimuli (E. Moser *et al.* 1993; M.B. Moser *et al.* 1995). Thus dorsal hippocampal lesions impair spatial memory performance in the water maze, while ventral hippocampal lesions have no effect (E. Moser *et al.* 1993; M.B. Moser *et al.* 1995), and the ventral hippocampus has fewer place cells with larger and less selective place fields than the dorsal hippocampus (Jung *et al.* 1994).

Further studies using Fos imaging in rats performing a spatial memory task have highlighted the importance of the hippocampus and post-rhinal cortex in processing novel arrangements of items (Vann *et al* 2000). In these experiments two groups of rats were trained in an eight-arm radial maze. One group was trained in one room and then subsequently tested in a different novel room containing new spatial cues. The second group was both trained and tested in the same room so that the room cues were highly familiar at test. A significant increase in the levels of neuronal activation in the hippocampus was found in both groups when compared with a control group which had been trained to run down only one arm of a radial arm maze, i.e. to run the same distance and obtain the same amount of reward but without the need to use spatial information. Furthermore, in the group of rats exposed to the novel room cues activation was greater in rhe dentate gyrus, CA3, CA1, and the subiculum. Additionally, all parts of the dorsal hippocampus showed significantly greater neuronal activation than the ventral hippocampus. There was a slight increase in the number of

Fos-stained neurons in the perirhinal cortex of the rats tested in the novel room compared with those tested in the familiar room. However, the difference did not reach significance, possibly because the number of novel stimuli was insufficient to produce a sufficiently great increase in neuronal activation.

These immunohistochemical findings indicate that the hippocampal formation is crucially involved in processing not only perceptual aspects of spatial information, but also its prior occurrence (Wan *et al.* 1999; Vann *et al.* 2000). Further, they confirm that the hippocampal formation is less important than the perirhinal cortex in familiarity discrimination for individual items. Thus hippocampal involvement mirrors that of the perirhinal cortex, which is critical to judging the prior occurrence of individual items but is less important than the hippocampal formation when the judgement concerns spatial information. Therefore Fos imaging demonstrates a double dissociation between the involvement of perirhinal cortex and the hippocampus in processes related to recognition memory (Wan *et al.* 1999; Vann *et al.* 2000). Many neurons of the perirhinal cortex, but not the hippocampus, are differentially activated by novel and familiar individual stimuli, whereas the hippocampus, but not the perirhinal cortex, is differentially activated by novel and familiar spatial arrangements of stimuli.

Hence the hippocampal formation seems to become involved when recognition memory involves spatial (and possibly other) relationships or associations between items (Brown 1990; Eichenbaum *et al.* 1994; Brown and Aggleton 2001). The inference is that the familiarity discrimination system centred on the perirhinal cortex is not sufficient to solve judgements concerning prior occurrence when the judgement cannot be made on the basis of individual items taken in isolation. When both the spatial position and the identity of an individual item is crucial to task performance, both the perirhinal cortex and the hippocampal formation appear to be crucial to its performance (Parker and Gaffan 1998). In such situations it is clear that there must be an interchange of information between the two structures. However, where the information is solely spatial or solely concerns individual items, it appears that the systems involving the two structures can operate independently. Accordingly, information concerning prior occurrence is not transferred between the perirhinal cortex and the hippocampus under all circumstances, and the contributions of the perirhinal cortex and the hippocampus to recognition memory processes are potentially separable (Brown and Xiang 1998; Aggleton and Brown 1999; Brown and Aggleton 2001).

It is important to note that the hippocampal involvement provides a potential link to the episodic memory impairment found in humans with hippocampal damage both because episodic memories normally include spatial information (the location of the episode) and because of the need to register the complex associational matrix of relationships between the individual items of the episode. Critically, in the general case the episode can be defined by these interrelationships rather than by the presence or absence of specific individual items (Brown 1990; Eichenbaum 1992; Eichenbaum *et al.* 1994). Therefore the information to be stored requires structural discrimination learning. Such learning is required when a task can only be solved by discriminating the relative positions of features of the environment rather than the location of a particular feature (Aggleton and Pearce 2001). Thus, for example, structural learning requires binding together not merely the occurrence of two different features or two different items but encoding the spatial relationship or ordering between the items, i.e. not merely 'Are A and B there?', but 'Is A to the left of B?'. It is hypothesized that such learning requires the hippocampal system and is beyond the capabilities of the perirhinal system operating on its own.

Is more than one recognition memory system necessary?

Studies of human visual recognition memory have demonstrated its speed, accuracy, and huge capacity (Standing 1973; Seeck *et al.* 1997). Moreover, familiarity ('know') decisions are made faster than recollect ('remember') decisions (Seeck *et al.* 1997) under a variety of controlled conditions where task instructions do not require decisions concerning recollection to be given first (Hintzman *et al.* 1998; McElree *et al.* 2000). Interestingly, this latency difference parallels the temporal ERP differences believed to reflect familiarity and recall (Curran 2000). Fast familiarity discrimination leading to rapid and accurate detection and hence potential reaction to novelty is likely to have evolutionary advantages.

The perirhinal neural network model described above establishes that it is indeed possible to construct a plausible system that achieves very fast and accurate familiarity discrimination (Bogacz *et al.* 1999, 2001). The theoretical network performs familiarity discrimination with great efficiency when compared with systems that rely on associative learning, in terms of both the relatively small number of neurons required and the speed of decision-making. Furthermore, the possession of a specific familiarity discrimination system has an additional advantage: it removes the necessity for perceptual categorization networks to register the prior occurrence of stimuli (Brown and Xiang 1998; Xiang and Brown 1998). Hence categorization networks are freed from the necessity of making long-term changes to their synaptic connections each time a novel stimulus is encountered. In such a case, the novel stimulus is perceived and classified by the unique pattern of activation it evokes within the categorization networks; however, its occurrence is registered and stored, and its novelty or familiarity judged by the familiarity discrimination network. Nevertheless, categorization networks will have to be modified if associations of the stimulus need to be remembered, or if a new category needs to be formed; the familiarity discrimination network as envisaged will not perform these functions. Indeed, an additional associative system is required to fulfil this function and so make possible associative or recollective aspects of recognition memory. Thus a minimum of two systems is necessary. The economical perirhinal system allows fast identification of novelty and familiarity discrimination of individual items but has limited capabilities. A second, hippocampal, system is necessary to deal with complicated aspects of recognition memory involving multiple items and their associations, including spatial aspects of recognition memory.

These two systems differ markedly in their requirements for the binding of features in memory. Familiarity discrimination is a non-associative form of learning. Correspondingly, the perirhinal system requires minimal binding capacity to register the occurrence of individual items that belong to an already established perceptual category. In contrast, spatial and episodic memories are essentially associative, so that in forming a memory the hippocampal system must be able to bind together in a complex matrix of interrelations many simultaneously perceived individual items. The anatomical connectivity of the hippocampal formation would appear to be ideally suited to such a role. For example, axons from CA3 pyramidal cells are each widely distributed to large numbers of CA1 pyramidal cells, thus forming a potential associational matrix of synaptic interconnections. Such an associational matrix provides a potential neuronal substrate for the multidimensional binding essential for spatial and episodic memories (Brown 1990).

References

Abeles, M. (1982). Role of cortical neuron: integrator or coincidence detector? *Israel Journal of Medical Sciences*, **8**, 83–92.

Abraham, W.C. and Bear, M.F. (1996). Metaplasticity: the plasticity of synaptic plasticity. *Trends in Neurosciences*, **19**, 126–130.

Aggleton, J.P. and Brown, M.W. (1999). Episodic memory, amnesia and the hippocampal-anterior thalamic axis. *Behavioral and Brain Sciences*, **22**, 425–489.

Aggleton, J.P. and Pearce, J.M. (2001). Neural systems underlying episodic memory: insights from animal research. *Philosophical Transactions of the Royal Society of London, Series B, Biological Sciences*, **356**, 1467–1482.

Aggleton, J.P., Hunt, P.R., and Rawlins, J.N.P. (1986) The effects of hippocampal lesions upon spatial and non-spatial tests of working memory. *Behavioural Brain Research*, **19**, 133–146.

Alvarez, P., Zola-Morgan, S., and Squire, L.R. (1995). Damage limited to the hippocampal region produces long-lasting memory impairment in monkeys. *Journal of Neuroscience*, **15**, 3796–3807.

Amaral, D.G., Insausti, R., and Cowan, W.M. (1987) The entorhinal cortex of the monkey: I. cytoarchitectonic organization. *Journal of Comparative Neurology*, **264**, 326–355.

Baxter, M.G. and Murray, E.A. (2001) Opposite relationship of hippocampal and rhinal cortex damage to delayed nonmatching-to-sample deficits in monkeys. *Hippocampus*, **11**, 61–71.

Baylis, G.C. and Rolls, E.T. (1987) Responses of neurons in the inferior temporal cortex in short term and serial recognition memory tasks. *Experimental Brain Research*, **65**, 614–622.

Beason-Held, L.L., Rosene, D.L., Killiany, R.J., and Moss, M.B. (1999) Hippocampal formation lesions produce memory impairment in the rhesus monkey. *Hippocampus*, **9**, 562–574.

Bilkey, D.K. and Liu, P. (2000) The effects of separate and combined perirhinal and prefrontal cortex lesions on spatial memory tasks in the rat. *Psychobiology* **28**, 12–20.

Bliss, T.V.P. and Collingridge, G.L. (1993) A synaptic model of memory: long-term potentiation in the hippocampus. *Nature* **361**, 31–39.

Bogacz, R. (2001). Computational models of familiarity discrimination in the perirhinal cortex. PhD Thesis, Department of Computer Science, University of Bristol.

Bogacz, R. and Brown, M.W. (2003). Comparison of computational models of familiarity discrimination in the perirhinal cortex. *Hippocampus*, **13**, 494–524.

Bogacz, R., Brown, M.W., and Giraud-Carrier, C. (1999). High capacity neural networks for familiarity discrimination. *Proceedings of the International Conference on Artificial Neural Networks*, pp. 773–776.

Bogacz, R., Brown, M.W., and Giraud-Carrier, C. (2001). Model of familiarity discrimination in the perirhinal cortex. *Journal of Computational Neuroscience*, **10**, 5–23.

Brown, M.W. (1982). Effect of context on the responses of single units recorded from the hippocampal region of behaviourally trained monkeys. In *Neuronal Plasticity and Memory Formation. IBRO Monograph Series.* Vol.9 (ed C. Ajmone-Marsan and H. Matthies). New York: Raven Press, pp. 557–573.

Brown, M.W. (1990). Why does the cortex have a hippocampus? In *Learning and Computational Neuroscience: Foundations of Adaptive Networks* (ed M. Gabriel and J. Moore). New York: MIT Press, pp. 233–282.

Brown, M.W. (1996). Neuronal responses and recognition memory. *Seminars in Neuroscience*, **8**, 23–32.

Brown, M.W. (2000). Temporally structured neuronal activity and recognition memory processes. *European Journal of Neuroscience*, **12**, 449.

Brown, M.W. and Aggleton, J.P. (2001). Recognition memory: What are the roles of the perirhinal cortex and hippocampus? *Nature Reviews Neuroscience*, **2**, 51–61.

Brown, M.W. and Bashir, Z.I. (2002). Evidence concerning how neurones of the perirhinal cortex may effect familiarity discrimination. *Philosophical Transactions of the Royal Society of London, Series B, Biological Sciences*, **357**, 1083–1095.

Brown, M.W. and Xiang, J.Z. (1998). Recognition memory: neuronal substrates of the judgement of prior occurrence. *Progress in Neurobiology*, **55**, 149–189.

Brown, M.W., Wilson, F.A.W., and Riches, I.P. (1987). Neuronal evidence that inferomedial temporal cortex is more important than hippocampus in certain processes underlying recognition memory. *Brain Research*, **409**, 158–162.

Buckley, M.J. and Gaffan, D. (1998a). Perirhinal cortex ablation impairs configural learning and paired-associate learning equally. *Neuropsychologia*, **36**, 535–546.

Buckley, M.J. and Gaffan, D. (1998b). Perirhinal cortex ablation impairs visual object identification. *Journal of Neuroscience*, **18**, 2268–2275.

Burwell, R.D. and Amaral, D.G. (1998). Cortical afferents of the perirhinal, postrhinal, and entorhinal cortices of the rat. *Journal of Comparative Neurology*, **398**, 179–205.

Burwell, R.D., Witter, M.P. and Amaral, D.G. (1995). Perirhinal and postrhinal cortices of the rat: a review of the neuroanatomical literature and comparison with findings from the monkey brain. *Hippocampus*, **5**, 390–408.

Bussey, T.J., Muir, J.L., and Aggleton, J.P. (1999). Functionally dissociating aspects of event memory: the effects of combined perirhinal and postrhinal cortex lesions on object and place memory in the rat. *Journal of Neuroscience*, **19**, 495–502.

Colombo, M. and Gross, C.G. (1994). Responses of inferior temporal cortex and hippocampal neurons during delayed matching to sample in monkeys (*Macaca fascicularis*). *Behavioral Neuroscience*, **108**, 443–455.

Corodimas, K.P. and LeDoux, J.E. (1995). Disruptive effects of posttraining perirhinal cortex lesions on conditioned fear: Contributions of contextual cues. *Behavioral Neuroscience*, **109**, 613–619.

Curran, T. (2000). Brain potentials of recollection and familiarity. *Memory and Cognition*, **28**, 923–938.

Desimone, R. (1996). Neural mechanisms for visual memory and their role in attention. *Proceedings of the National Academy of the United States of America*, **93**, 13494–13499.

Donaldson, W. (1999). The role of decision processes in remembering and knowing. *Memory and Cognition*, **26**, 523–533.

Eacott, M.J., Gaffan, D., and Murray, E.A. (1994). Preserved recognition memory for small sets, and impaired stimulus identification for large sets following rhinal cortex ablations in monkeys. *European Journal of Neuroscience*, **6**, 1466–1478.

Eichenbaum, H. (1992). The hippocampal system and declarative memory in animals. *Journal of Cognitive Neuroscience* **4**, 217–231.

Eichenbaum, H., Otto, T., and Cohen, N.J. (1994). Two functional components of the hippocampal memory system. *Behavioral and Brain Sciences*, **17**, 449–518.

Eichenbaum, H., Schoenbaum, G., Young, B., and Bunsey, M. (1996). Functional organization of the hippocampal memory system. *Proceedings of the National Academy of the United States of America*, **93**, 13500–13507.

Ennaceur, A. and Delacour, J. (1988). A new one-trial test for neurobiological studies of memory in rats. 1: Behavioral data. *Behavioural Brain Research*, **31**, 47–59.

Ennaceur, A., Neave, N., and Aggleton, J.P. (1996). Neurotoxic lesions of the perirhinal cortex do not mimic the behavioural effects of fornix transection in the rat. *Behavioural Brain Research*, **80**, 9–25.

Erickson, C.A., Jagadeesh, B., and Desimone, R. (2001). Clustering of perirhinal neurons with similar properties following visual experience in adult monkey. *Nature Neuroscience*, **3**, 1143–1148.

Eskandar, E.N., Richmond, B.J., and Optican, L.M. (1992). Role of inferior temporal neurons in visual memory. I: Temporal encoding of information about visual images, recalled images, and behavioral context. *Journal of Neurophysiology*, **68**, 1277–1295.

Fahy, F.L., Riches, I.P., and Brown, M.W. (1993). Neuronal activity related to visual recognition memory: long-term memory and the encoding of recency and familiarity information in the primate anterior and medial inferior temporal and rhinal cortex. *Experimental Brain Research*, **96**, 457–472.

Felleman, D.J. and Van Essen, D.C. (1991). Distributed hierarchical processing in the primate cerebral cortex. *Cerebral Cortex*, **1**, 1–47.

Fuster, J.M. and Jervey, J.P. (1981). Inferotemporal neurons distinguish and retain behaviorally relevant features of visual stimuli. *Science*, **212**, 952–955.

Gaffan, D. (1994). Scene-specific memory for objects: a model of episodic memory impairment in monkeys with fornix transection. *Journal of Cognitive Neuroscience*, **6**, 305–320.

Gaffan, D. and Murray, E.A. (1992). Monkeys (*Macaca fascicularis*) with rhinal cortex ablations succeed in object discrimination learning despite 24-hr intertrial intervals and fail at matching to sample despite double sample presentations. *Behavioral Neuroscience*, **106**, 30–38.

Gardiner, J.M. and Parkin, A.J. (1990). Attention and recollective experience in recognition memory . *Memory and Cognition*, **18**, 579–583.

Gawne, T.J. and Richmond, B.J. (1993). How independent are the messages carried by adjacent inferior temporal cortical-neurons? *Journal of Neuroscience*, **13**, 2758–2771.

Gross, C.G., Rochamiranda, C.E., and Bender, D.B. (1972). Visual properties of neurons in inferotemporal cortex of the macaque. *Journal of Neurophysiology*, **35**, 96–111.

Haist, F. and Shimamura, A.P. (1992). On the relationship between recall and recognition memory. *Journal of Experimental Psychology: Learning, Memory, and Cognition*, **18**, 691–702.

Hampson, R.E., Simeral, J.D., and Deadwyler, S.A. (1999). Distribution of spatial and nonspatial information in dorsal hippocampus. *Nature*, **402**, 610–614.

Herdegen, T. and Leah, J.D. (1998). Inducible and constitutive transcription factors in the mammalian nervous system: control of gene expression by Jun, Fos and Krox, and CREB/ATF proteins. *Brain Research: Brain Research Reviews*, **28**, 370–490.

Higuchi, S.I. and Miyashita, Y. (1996). Formation of mnemonic neuronal responses to visual paired associates in inferotemporal cortex is impaired by perirhinal and entorhinal lesions. *Proceedings of the National Academy of the United States of America*, **93**, 739–743.

Hintzman, D.L., Caulton, D.A., and Levitin, D.J. (1998). Retrieval dynamics in recognition and list discrimination: further evidence of separate processes of familiarity and recall. *Memory and Cognition*, **26**, 449–462.

Hirshman, E. and Master, S. (1997). Modeling the conscious correlates of recognition memory: reflections on the remember–know paradigm. *Memory and Cognition*, **25**, 345–351.

Insausti, R., Juottonen, K., Soininen, H., *et al.* (1998). MR volumetric analysis of the human entorhinal, perirhinal and temporopolar cortices. *American Journal of Neuroradiology*, **19**, 659–671.

Ito, M. (1989). Long-term depression. *Annual Review of Neuroscience*, **12**, 85–102.

Jacoby, L.L. and Dallas, M. (1981). On the relationship between autobiographical memory and perceptual learning. *Journal of Experimental Psychology: General*, **3**, 306–340.

Jung, M.W., Wiener, S.I., and McNaughton, B.L. (1994). Comparison of spatial firing characteristics of units in dorsal and ventral hippocampus of the rat. *Journal of Neuroscience*, **14**, 7347–7356.

Kemp, N. and Bashir, Z.I. (2001). Long-term depression: a cascade of induction and expression mechanisms. *Progress in Neurobiology*, **65**, 339–365.

Lavenex, P. and Amaral, D.G. (2000). Hippocampal–neocortical interactions: a hierarchy of associativity. *Hippocampus*, **10**, 420–430.

Leonard, B.W., Amaral, D.G., Squire, L.R., and Zola-Morgan, S. (1995). Transient memory impairment in monkeys with bilateral lesions of the entorhinal cortex. *Journal of Neuroscience*, **15**, 5637–5659.

Li, L., Miller, E.K., and Desimone, R. (1993). The representation of stimulus familiarity in anterior inferior temporal cortex. *Journal of Neurophysiology*, **69**, 1918–1929.

Linden, D.J. (1994). Long term synaptic depression in the mammalian brain. *Neuron*,**12**, 457–472

Liu, P., and Bilkey, D.K. (1998a). Excitotoxic lesions centered on perirhinal cortex produce delay-dependent deficits in a test of spatial memory. *Behavioral Neuroscience*, **112**, 512–524.

Liu, P. and Bilkey, D.K. (1998b). Lesions of perirhinal cortex produce spatial memory deficits in the radial maze. *Hippocampus*, **8**, 114–121.

Liu, P. and Bilkey, D.K. (1998c). Perirhinal cortex contributions to performance in the Morris water maze. *Behavioral Neuroscience*, **112**, 304–315.

McElree, B., Dolan, P.O., and Jacoby, L.R. (2000). Isolating the contributions of familiarity and source information to item recognition: a time course analysis. *Journal of Experimental Psychology: Learning, Memory, and Cognition*, **25**, 563–582.

Mandler, G. (1980). Recognizing: the judgment of previous occurrence. *Psychological Review*, **87**, 252–271.

Maunsell, J.H.R., Sclar, G., Nealey, T.A., and DePriest, D.D. (1991). Extraretinal representations in area V4 in the macaque monkey. *Visual Neuroscience*, **7**, 561–573.

Meunier, M., Bachevalier, J., Mishkin, M., and Murray, E.A. (1993). Effects on visual recognition of combined and separate ablations of the entorhinal and perirhinal cortex in rhesus monkeys. *Journal of Neuroscience*, **13**, 5418–5432.

Meunier, M., Hadfield, W., Bachevalier, J., and Murray, E.A. (1996). Effects of rhinal cortex lesions combined with hippocampectomy on visual recognition memory in rhesus monkeys. *Journal of Neurophysiology*, **75**, 1190–1205.

Meunier, M., Bachevalier, J., and Mishkin, M. (1997). Effects of orbital frontal and anterior cingulate lesions on object and spatial memory in rhesus monkeys. *Neuropsychologia*, **35**, 999–1015.

Mikami, A. and Kubota, B. (1980). Inferotemporal neuron activities and color discrimination with delay. *Brain Research*, **182**, 65–78.

Miller, E.K. (1999). The prefrontal cortex: complex neural properties for complex behavior. *Neuron*, **22**, 15–17.

Miller, E.K. and Desimone, R. (1994). Parallel neuronal mechanisms for short-term memory. *Science*, **263**, 520–522.

Miller, E.K., Gochin, P.M., and Gross, C.G. (1991). Habituation-like decrease in the responses of neurons in inferior temporal cortex of the macaque. *Visual Neuroscience*, **7**, 357–362.

Miller, E.K., Li, L., and Desimone, R. (1993). Activity of neurons in anterior inferior temporal cortex during a short-term memory task. *Journal of Neuroscience*, **13**, 1460–1478.

Miller, E.K., Erickson, C.A., and Desimone, R. (1996). Neural mechanisms of visual working memory in prefrontal cortex of the macaque. *Journal of Neuroscience*, **16**, 5154–5167.

Morris, R.G.M., Garrud, P., Rawlins, J.N.P., and O'Keefe, J. (1982). Place navigation impaired in rats with hippocampal lesions. *Nature*, **297**, 681–683.

Moser, E., Moser, M.B., and Andersen, P. (1993). Spatial-learning impairment parallels the magnitude of dorsal hippocampal-lesions, but is hardly present following ventral lesions. *Journal of Neuroscience*, **13**, 3916–3925.

Moser, M.B., Moser, E.I., Forrest, E., Andersen, P., and Morris, R.G.M. (1995). Spatial-learning with a minislab in the dorsal hippocampus. *Proceedings of the National Academy of Sciences of the United States of America*, **92**, 9697–9701.

Muller, R. (1996). A quarter of a century of place cells. *Neuron*, **17**, 813–822.

Mumby, D.G. (2001). Perspectives on object-recognition memory following hippocampal damage: lessons from studies in rats. *Behavioural Brain Research*, **127**, 159–181.

Mumby, D.G. and Pinel, J.P.J. (1994). Rhinal cortex lesions and object recognition in rats. *Behavioral Neuroscience*, **108**, 11–18.

Mumby, D.G., Wood, E.R., and Pinel, J.P.J. (1992). Object recognition memory in rats is only mildly impaired by lesions of the hippocampus and amygdala. *Psychobiology*, **20**, 18–27.

Mumby, D.G., Pinel, J.P.J., Kornecook, T.J., Shen, M.J., and Redila, V.A. (1995). Memory deficits following lesions of hippocampus or amygdala in rat: assessment by an object-memory test battery. *Psychobiology*, **23**, 26–36.

Murray, E.A. (1996). What have ablation studies told us about the neural substrates of stimulus memory? *Seminars in Neuroscience*, **8**, 13–22.

Murray, E.A. and Bussey, T.J. (1999). Perceptual-mnemonic functions of the perirhinal cortex. *Trends in Cognitive Neurosciences*, **3**, 142–151.

Murray, E.A. and Mishkin, M. (1998). Object recognition and location memory in monkeys with excitotoxic lesions of the amygdala and hippocampus. *Journal of Neuroscience*, **18**, 6568–6582.

Murray, E.A., Gaffan, D., and Mishkin, M. (1993). Neural substrates of visual stimulus-stimulus association in rhesus monkeys. *Journal of Neuroscience*, **13**, 4549–4561.

Murray, E.A., Baxter, M.G., and Gaffan, D. (1998). Monkeys with rhinal cortex damage or neurotoxic hippocampal lesions are impaired on spatial scene learning and object reversals. *Behavioral Neuroscience*, **112**, 1291–1303.

Nakamura, K. and Kubota, K. (1995). Mnemonic firing of neurons in the monkey temporal pole during a visual recognition memory task. *Journal of Neurophysiology*, **74**, 162–178.

Norman, K.A. and O'Reilly, R.C. (2001). *Modelling Hippocampal and Neocortical Contributions to Recognition Memory: A Complementary Learning Systems Approach.* Technical Report 01–02, University of Colorado, Boulder, CO.

O'Keefe, J. (1993). Hippocampus, theta rhythms and spatial memory. *Current Opinion in Neurobiology*, **3**, 917–924.

O'Keefe, J. and Nadel, L. (1978). *The Hippocampus as a Cognitive Map*. Oxford: Oxford University Press.

O'Keefe, J., Burgess, N., Donnett, J.G., Jeffery, K.J., and Maguire, E.A. (1998). Place cells, navigational accuracy, and the human hippocampus. *Philosophical Transactions of the Royal Society of London, Series B, Biological Sciences*, **353**, 1333–1340.

Otto, T. and Eichenbaum, H. (1992). Complementary roles of the orbital prefrontal cortex and the perirhinal–entorhinal cortices in an odor-guided delayed-nonmatching-to-sample task. *Behavioral Neuroscience*, **106**, 762–775.

Parker, A. and Gaffan, D. (1998). Interaction of frontal and perirhinal cortices in visual object recognition memory in monkeys. *European Journal of Neuroscience*, **10**, 3044–3057.

Riches, I.P., Wilson, F.A.W., and Brown, M.W. (1991). The effects of visual stimulation and memory on neurons of the hippocampal formation and the neighboring parahippocampal gyrus and inferior temporal cortex of the primate. *Journal of Neuroscience*, **11**, 1763–1779.

Ringo, J.L. (1996). Stimulus specific adaptation in inferior temporal and medial temporal cortex of the monkey. *Behavioural Brain Research*, **76**, 191–197.

Rolls, E.T., Perrett, D.I., Caan, A.W., and Wilson, F.A.W. (1982). Neuronal responses related to visual recognition. *Brain*, **105**, 611–646.

Rolls, E.T., Miyashita, Y., Cahusac, P.M.B., *et al.* (1989). Hippocampal neurons in the monkey with activity related to the place in which a stimulus is shown. *Journal of Neuroscience*, **9**, 1835–1845.

Rolls, E.T., Cahusac, P.M.B., Feigenbaum, J.D., and Miyashita, Y. (1993). Responses of single neurons in the hippocampus of the macaque related to recognition memory. *Experimental Brain Research*, **93**, 299–306.

Rolls, E.T., Treves, A., Robertson, R.G., Georges-François, P., and Panzeri, S. (1998). Information about spatial view in an ensemble of primate hippocampal cells. *Journal of Neurophysiology*, **79**, 1797–1813.

Scoville, W.B. and Milner, B. (1957). Loss of recent memory after bilateral hippocampal lesions. *Journal of Neurology, Neurosurgery and Psychiatry*, **20**, 11–21.

Seeck, M., Michel, C.M., Mainwaring, N., *et al.* (1997). Evidence for rapid face recognition from human scalp and intracranial electrodes. *Neuroreport*, **8**, 2749–2754.

Shi, C.J. and Cassell, M.D. (1997). Cortical, thalamic, and amygdaloid projections of rat temporal cortex. *Journal of Comparative Neurology*, **382**, 153–175.

Singer, W. and Gray, C.M. (1995). Visual feature integration and the temporal correlation hypothesis. *Annual Review of Neuroscience*, **18**, 555–586.

Sobotka, S. and Ringo, J.L. (1993). Investigations of long-term recognition and association memory in unit responses from inferotemporal cortex. *Experimental Brain Research*, **96**, 28–38.

Sohal, V.S. and Hasselmo, M.E. (2000). A model for experience-dependent changes in the responses of infero-temporal neurons. *Computations in Neural Systems*, **11**, 169–190.

Standing, L. (1973). Learning 10,000 pictures. *Quarterly Journal of Experimental Psychology*, **25**, 207–222.

Suzuki, W.A. (1996a). Neuroanatomy of the monkey entorhinal, perirhinal and parahippocampal cortices: organization of cortical inputs and interconnections with amygdala and striatum. *Seminars in Neuroscience*, **8**, 3–12.

Suzuki, W.A. (1996b). The anatomy, physiology and functions of the perirhinal cortex. *Current Opinion in Neurobiology*, **6**, 179–186.

Suzuki, W.A. and Eichenbaum, H. (2000). The neurophysiology of memory. *Annals of the New York Academy of Sciences*, **911**, 175–191.

Suzuki, W.A., Zola-Morgan, S., Squire, L.R., and Amaral, D.G. (1993). Lesions of the perirhinal and parahippocampal cortices in the monkey produce long-lasting memory impairment in the visual and tactual modalities. *Journal of Neuroscience*, **13**, 2430–2451.

Thompson, J., Brown, M.W., and Stewart, M.G. (2001). Measures of synaptic density in the perirhinal cortex of rats exposed to novel or familiar stimuli. *Abstracts—Society for Neuroscience*, **29**.

Vann, S.D., Brown, M.W., Erichsen, J.T., and Aggleton, J.P. (2000). Fos imaging reveals differential patterns of hippocampal and parahippocampal subfield activation in rats in response to different spatial memory tasks. *Journal of Neuroscience*, **20**, 2711–2718.

Vogels, R., Sary, G., and Orban, G.A. (1995). How task-related are the responses of inferior temporal neurons? *Visual Neuroscience*, **12**, 207–214.

Wan, H., Aggleton, J.P., and Brown, M.W. (1999). Different contributions of the hippocampus and perirhinal cortex to recognition memory. *Journal of Neuroscience*, **19**, 1142–1148.

Warburton, E.C., Koder, T., Cho, K., *et al.* (2003). Cholinergic neurotransmission is essential for perirhinal cortical plasticity and recognition memory. *Neuron*, **38**, 987–996.

Wiebe, S.P. and Staubli, U.V. (1999). Dynamic filtering of recognition memory codes in the hippocampus *Journal of Neuroscience*, **19**, 10562–10574

Wiener, S.I. (1996). Spatial, behavioral and sensory correlates of hippocampal CA1 complex spike cell activity: implications for information processing functions. *Progress in Neurobiology*, **49**, 335–361.

Wilson, F.A.W. and Rolls, E.T. (1990). Neuronal responses related to the novelty and familiarity of visual stimuli in the substantia innominata, diagonal band of Broca and the periventricular region of the primate basal forebrain. *Experimental Brain Research*, **80**, 104–120.

Witter, M.P., Groenewegen, H.J., Lopes da Silva, F.H., and Lohman, A.H.M. (1989). Functional organization of the extrinsic and intrinsic circuitry of the parahippocampal region. *Progress in Neurobiology*, **33**, 161–253.

Witter, M.P., Naber, P.A., Van Haeften, T., *et al.* (2000). Cortico-hippocampal communication by way of parallel parahippocampal-subicular pathways. *Hippocampus*, **10**, 398–410.

Wood, E.R., Didchenko, P.A., and Eichenbaum, H. (1999). The global record of memory in hippocampal neuronal activity. *Nature*, **397**, 613–616.

Xiang, J.-Z. and Brown, M.W. (1997). Processing visual familiarity and recency information: neuronal interactions in area TE and rhinal cortex. *Brain Research Abstracts*, **14**, 69.

Xiang, J.-Z. and Brown, M.W. (1998). Differential neuronal encoding of novelty, familiarity and recency in regions of the anterior temporal lobe. *Neuropharmacology*, **37**, 657–676.

Xiang, J.-Z. and Brown, M.W. (2004). Neuronal responses related to long-term recognition memory processes in prefrontal cortex. *Neuron* **42**, 817–829.

Young, B.J., Otto, T., Fox, G.D., and Eichenbaum, H. (1997). Memory representation within the parahippocampal region. *Journal of Neuroscience*, **17**, 5183–5195.

Zhu, X.O., Brown, M.W., and Aggleton, J.P. (1995a). Neuronal signalling of information important to visual recognition memory in rat rhinal and neighbouring cortices. *European Journal of Neuroscience*, **7**, 753–765.

Zhu, X.O., Brown, M.W., McCabe, B.J., and Aggleton, J.P. (1995b). Effects of novelty or familiarity of visual stimuli on the expression of the immediate early gene c-*fos* in rat brain. *Neuroscience*, **69**, 821–829.

Zhu, X.O., McCabe, B.J., Aggleton, J.P., and Brown, M.W. (1996). Mapping visual recognition memory through expression of the immediate early gene c-*fos*. *Neuroreport*, **7**, 1871–1875.

Zhu, X.O., McCabe, B.J., Aggleton, J.P., and Brown, M.W. (1997). Differential activation of the hippocampus and perirhinal cortex by novel visual stimuli and a novel environment. *Neuroscience*, **229**, 141–143.

Zola, S.M., Squire, L.R., Teng, E., Stefanacci, L., Buffalo, E.A., and Clark, R.E. (2000). Impaired recognition memory in monkeys after damage limited to the hippocampal region. *Journal of Neuroscience*, **20**, 451–463.

Zola-Morgan, S. and Squire, L.R. (1993). Neuroanatomy of memory. *Annual Review of Neuroscience*, **16**, 547–563.

Zola-Morgan, S., Squire, L.R., Amaral, D.G., and Suzuki, W.A. (1989). Lesions of perirhinal and parahippocampal cortex that spare the amygdala and hippocampal formation produce severe memory impairment. *Journal of Neuroscience*, **9**, 4355–4370.

Zola-Morgan, S., Squire, L.R., and Ramus, S.J. (1994). Severity of memory impairment in monkeys as a function of locus and extent of damage within the medial temporal lobe memory system. *Hippocampus*, **4**, 483–495.

Chapter 17

Unpacking explicit memory: the contribution of recollection and familiarity

Joel R. Quamme, Andrew P. Yonelinas, and
Neal E. A. Kroll

Introduction

Behavioural studies of recognition memory in humans have indicated that recognition reflects the operation of two processes: recollection of qualitative episodic information about prior events such as where or when an item was studied, and assessments of general memory strength or familiarity (reviewed by Yonelinas 2002; Rugg and Yonelinas 2003). Recollection supports the retrieval of details of an event that were previously bound in memory during a study episode, and it appears to contribute readily to most types of recognition because the qualitative information it provides is usually highly diagnostic that a particular item was studied. However, recollection is especially important for tasks where individuals must report details of a remembered episode, discriminate intact from recombined versions of studied associations, and discriminate items from different lists, sources, or other contexts. Familiarity, on the other hand, behaves in a fairly item-specific manner, providing graded feelings of familiarity or recency about individual studied items. Thus it is useful in discriminating between studied and new items, but is not well suited for recovering the details of a specific event or discriminating among associations, sources, and lists.

Studies of memory in rats and non-human primates have indicated that the hippocampus is critical for binding together episodic details of a learning event, whereas the parahippocampal gyrus is critical for strengthening single-item representations (reviewed in Chapter 16). In the current chapter, we focus on neuropsychological studies of memory in humans to ask whether these different medial temporal lobe regions also differentially support recollection and familiarity in human subjects. The neuropsychological results are found to be consistent with the animal studies and indicate that the hippocampus is necessary for recollection, but not familiarity, whereas the parahippocampal gyrus is necessary for familiarity.

It should be noted that there is good evidence that a number of other brain regions are involved in recollection and familiarity, most prominent among them being the prefrontal cortex (Milner and Petrides 1984; Shimamura 1996) and the thalamus (Zoppelt *et al.* 2003; Kishiyama *et al.* 2004), as well as the lateral occipital (Yonelinas *et al.* 2001) and parietal (Rugg and Allan 2000) regions. However, we will restrict our discussion primarily to the medial temporal lobe because this is the region that has been most carefully studied, and because it has been the focus of much current theorizing for several reasons. First and foremost, there is currently a fundamental disagreement among theorists over which areas of the temporal lobe are involved in recollection and familiarity (see Manns *et al.* (2003), Wixted and Squire (2004), and Yonelinas *et al.* (2002, 2004) for opposing positions). Secondly, with respect to the frontal lobe, although there is continued debate over the nature of the specific mechanisms supported by different areas of the prefrontal cortex, there is good agreement that the prefrontal cortex is somehow involved in both recollection and familiarity. Finally, the functional relationship of lateral occipital and parietal regions to explicit memory has not yet been as well specified, although existing evidence points to roles for these regions in familiarity (Yonelinas *et al.* 2001) and recollection (Rugg and Allan 2000), respectively.

In order to assess the brain regions involved in recollection and familiarity it is necessary first to develop methods of measuring these two processes. One approach, the task dissociation method, is to use memory tests that are expected to provide direct measures of a given memory process. For example, free recall is expected to rely primarily on recollection, and recognition is expected to rely more heavily on familiarity. Comparisons of these two tasks have been used extensively to assess the nature of recollection and familiarity (Mandler 1980; Aggleton and Shaw 1997). These methods have proved useful in showing that recollection and familiarity can be dissociated. However, task dissociation methods are limited in several important ways. First, a failure to find a dissociation between two such tests is difficult to interpret because the tests may not provide perfectly pure measures of the two processes. For example, recognition performance, which is often thought to rely most heavily on familiarity, can also be affected by recollection; and recall performance, thought to rely most on recollection, can also be influenced by a more familiarity-like retrieval process (Jacoby *et al.* 1993). Thus, if recall and recognition performance fail to dissociate in a given patient group, it could be because the two particular tests both happen to draw heavily on the same process. Secondly, the task dissociation approach often involves comparisons across tests that differ in various ways. For example, recall tests require subjects to generate items whereas recognition tests do not, and thus differences in performance between these tasks could reflect the operation of a generation process rather than the differential involvement of recollection or familiarity.

To overcome the limitations associated with task dissociation methods, several process estimation methods have been developed to provide quantitative estimates of recollection and familiarity. Several of these methods are described in detail below. Armed with these measurement tools, researchers have begun to uncover the brain regions involved in recollection and familiarity. Below, we focus on studies that have used these procedures to examine recollection and familiarity in amnesic patients with damage to different temporal lobe regions (for discussions of related studies using electrophysiological and neuroimaging methods see Yonelinas (2002), Rugg and Yonelinas (2003), and Chapters 18 and 19).

Studies of patients with damage to the hippocampus and parahippocampus

There have been numerous examinations of the effects of amnesia on recollection and familiarity using process estimation methods. In most of these studies, subjects have been selected because they had memory impairments, and thus they have included patients with fairly severe memory impairments and with damage to both the hippocampus and the parahippocampal gyrus of the medial temporal lobe. Studies of these patients have been important in examining whether the two processes are differentially dependent upon the medial temporal lobe region in general, but they are not particularly useful in separating the differential contribution of the hippocampus and the parahippocampal gyrus to recollection and familiarity. However, these studies have been useful in informing two theories of recollection and familiarity in amnesia. One theory is that both processes reflect different expressions of a single global medial temporal lobe memory system and that amnesia results in equivalent decreases in recollection and familiarity (Squire 1994). The other theory is that the medial temporal lobes are important for recollection whereas familiarity relies more on processes or memory systems outside the medial temporal lobes (Huppert and Piercy 1978; Tulving 1985; Mayes 1988). Thus, according to this theory, medial temporal lobe damage would be expected to produce a greater deficit in recollection than familiarity.

Results from a variety of process estimation studies indicate that both processes are reduced in amnesia, but that recollection is disrupted to a greater extent than familiarity. For example, several studies have made use of the remember–know procedure (Tulving 1985). In this procedure, subjects are presented with a recognition test list containing a mixture of new and previously studied items and, for each item, they are required to indicate whether the item was **remembered** (i.e. they could recollect some qualitative information about the study event such as when or where it was studied), was **known** (i.e. it was recognized on the basis of familiarity in the absence of recollection), or was **new** to the experiment. Importantly, the proportion of items given a 'remember' response is used as an index of recollection, and is taken to indicate the probability of subjectively experiencing the recovery of qualitative information about the study event that was bound to the representation of the study item. In contrast, because a 'know' response is made whenever an item is familiar but not recollected, familiarity is indexed as the proportion of non-remembered items that receive 'know' responses. To incorporate response bias, estimates for new items are subtracted from those for old items.

Figure 17.1(a) shows the estimates of recollection and familiarity for amnesics and age-matched controls averaged across several remember–know studies (Knowlton and Squire 1995; Schacter *et al.* 1996, 1997; Blaxton and Theodore 1997; Moscovitch and McAndrews 2002; Kishiyama *et al.* 2004). In all these studies the amnesic groups contained patients with extensive medial temporal lobe damage including the hippocampus and parahippocampal gyrus. As the figure indicates, both processes are disrupted, but recollection appears to be more disrupted than familiarity. Note that in four of the six studies the recollection deficits were much more pronounced than the familiarity deficits, and in two the deficit in familiarity was more comparable with that seen in recollection. In these latter studies (Blaxton and Theodore 1997; Moscovitch and McAndrews 2002), the data come from epileptic temporal lobectomy patients. These results suggest that there may be important differences between some patient subgroups. Unfortunately, the levels of false 'remember' responses to new items was exceptionally high relative to controls in these two studies, and this complicates the interpretation of these results. However, the results clearly indicate that amnesia disrupts both processes, and that recollection is often more disrupted than familiarity.

The remember–know results can be criticized because they rely exclusively on subjective reports of recollection and familiarity, i.e. it is possible that the differences between the amnesics and controls reflect differences in how the amnesics interpreted the remember–know instructions rather than true differences in the

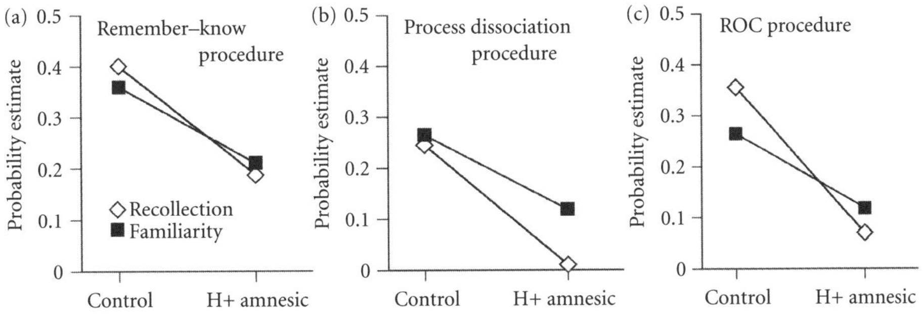

Figure 17.1 Estimates of recollection and familiarity in healthy controls and amnesic patients with damage to the hippocampus and parahippocampus. Plots show estimates from (a) the remember–know procedure, (b) the process dissociation procedure, and (c) the ROC modelling procedure.

underlying memory processes (Baddeley *et al.* 2001; Rajaram *et al.* 2002). Moreover, some amnesics may make 'remember' responses even when recollection fails because they have such low levels of recollection. For this reason it is important to verify these results using methods that do not depend on an individual's subjective reports of these two processes.

One such method is the process dissociation procedure (Jacoby 1991). In this procedure recollection is measured by the ability to determine from which of two different study lists a test item originated, and familiarity is measured as overall recognition performance conditionalized on recollection. In this case, the measure of recollection depends on successful binding of item and list context information in memory, whereas familiarity reflects successful retrieval of item information in the absence of list context information. This procedure was used to examine recognition memory in a group of amnesics with extensive medial temporal lobe damage (Verfaellie and Treadwell 1993). Estimates of recollection and familiarity from that study are presented in Figure 17.1(b), which shows that estimates from the process dissociation procedure leads to conclusions that are similar to those drawn from the remember–know experiments, i.e. medial temporal lobe amnesia led to a decrease in both recollection and familiarity, but recollection was reduced to a greater extent than familiarity.

Another method for estimating recollection and familiarity is the receiver operating characteristic (ROC) procedure (Yonelinas 1994). In this method, subjects make recognition confidence judgements that are used to plot ROCs (i.e. the relationship between hits and false alarms as a function of response confidence). ROCs for a group of amnesics and controls (Yonelinas *et al.* 1998) are presented in Figure 17.2(a). These amnesics were patients with damage to the

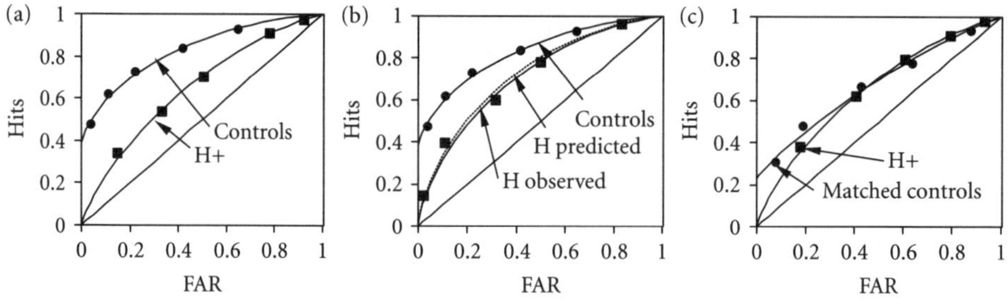

Figure 17.2 ROC curves for healthy controls and two types of amnesic patients: (a) fitted ROCs for controls and amnesics with damage to both the hippocampus and parahippocampus (H+ amnesics); (b) fitted ROCs for controls and hypoxic patients (H amnesics) with ROC curve predicted for H amnesics from best-fitting control curve; (c) fitted ROCs for controls and H+ amnesics when performance of the two groups was equated.

hippocampus and parahippocampal gyrus caused by posterior cerebral artery infarcts. A model-based equation was then fitted to the observed ROC points to estimate the contribution of recollection and familiarity. The model assumes that familiarity is a parameter in the equation that behaves as a signal detection process and gives the ROC a curvilinear aspect. Recollection is a parameter in the equation that gives the ROC an intercept, and determines the degree to which the ROC appears to be pushed up asymmetrically on the *y*-axis. The method is similar to a regression analysis except that, rather than estimating intercept and linear slope parameters, estimates are derived for an intercept (recollection) and a non-linear signal detection parameter (familiarity) (see Yonelinas *et al.* (1998) for more details of the equations and fitting procedure). The average parameter estimates from that study are presented in Figure 17.1(c). Amnesics again exhibited deficits in both recollection and familiarity, and again recollection was more severely disrupted than familiarity. Note that this method does not require that recollection depend on episodic binding *per se*, but that retrieval of episodic details would tend to increase highly confident hits, thus pushing the intercept up the *y*-axis.

In sum, the results from multiple studies using the remember–know, process dissociation, and ROC procedures converge in showing that both recollection and familiarity are disrupted in amnesic patients with extensive medial temporal lobe damage. Importantly, however, recollection is disrupted to a greater extent than familiarity in these individuals.

It might be argued that the disproportional recollection deficits seen in amnesia reflect scaling differences, i.e. it is possible that familiarity is less affected than recollection, because it is at a point on the scale that is less sensitive to change. However, this does not provide a full explanation of the results because the same pattern of results was observed across a large number of different studies in which the overall levels of recollection and familiarity varied quite widely. In fact, cross-over interactions were reported in several studies (e.g. Fig. 17.1(c)) which indicate that this type of scaling difference could not have produced the dissociations. Another potential explanation is that recollection might be more sensitive in general to manipulations than is familiarity. Support for this claim comes from studies showing that experimental manipulations, such as levels of processing and full versus divided attention, have larger effects on recollection than on familiarity (Gardiner and Parkin 1990; Toth 1996; Yonelinas 2001). However, other manipulations, such as masked priming, study–test lag, and response bias, have larger effects on familiarity than recollection (Rajaram 1993; Yonelinas 2001; Yonelinas and Levy 2002), showing familiarity is no less sensitive to change than is recollection.

The results are critical in showing that recollection is more disrupted by extensive medial temporal lobe damage than is familiarity. Thus it is not the case that both forms of memory rely equally on the medial temporal lobes (Squire 1994); rather, these regions are disproportionately important for recollection. Recollection was always severely reduced in these patients; in some cases the estimates were reduced effectively to zero. In contrast, although familiarity was generally reduced, patients exhibited some residual ability to use familiarity as a basis for recognition judgements. These results suggest that regions outside the medial temporal lobe may be capable of supporting a reasonable level of familiarity-based recognition memory (Huppert and Piercy 1978). However, these results do not allow us to address directly the question of whether the hippocampus and parahippocampal gyrus are equally important for recollection. In order to assess this question, it is necessary to examine patients with more selective damage.

Studies of patients with relatively restricted hippocampal damage

More recent research has focused on whether recollection and familiarity can be dissociated in patients with selective lesions of the medial temporal lobe. Relevant evidence comes primarily from patients with damage apparently restricted to the hippocampus. Almost invariably, these are patients who developed memory difficulties following a period of cerebral hypoxia (oxygen deprivation). The hippocampus is particularly vulnerable to hypoxic–ischaemic damage, and post-mortem studies as well as structural imaging studies have demonstrated that in mild cases neuronal loss is largely confined to this structure (Zola-Morgan *et al.* 1986; Hopkins *et al.* 1995; Gadian *et al.* 2000).

We recently examined a group of 56 cardiac arrest patients who suffered very mild hypoxic events, and examined recollection and familiarity using a variety of different methods (Yonelinas *et al.* 2002). Because these patients had defibrillators they could not be scanned in order to verify the hippocampal damage. However, the patient group was useful for the current purposes because it only included very mild cases of hypoxia and the patients had no lasting cognitive impairments other than explicit recall and recognition (Sauvé *et al.* 1996). Thus, based on aetiology and behavioural profile, the damage was expected to be restricted primarily to the hippocampus. Moreover, coma duration was recorded for each patient, which allowed us to examine the effect of hypoxic severity on memory performance.

As a preliminary analysis we first examined the recall and recognition deficits in the hypoxic patients by contrasting their memory scores with those from an aged-matched control group. If recollection is selectively disrupted in the hypoxic patients, and recall relies more heavily on recollection than does recognition, then the hypoxic patients should exhibit a more pronounced deficit in recall than recognition. This is, in fact, the pattern that we observed; both recall and recognition were lower in the hypoxic patients than in the controls, but their recall deficit was significantly greater than their recognition deficit. This pattern is suggestive but, as we pointed out previously, results from the task dissociation comparisons can be limited. For example, it is not clear from these results whether familiarity was completely, or just relatively, preserved in these patients.

We then examined partial correlations to determine how hypoxic severity was related to recall and recognition (Yonelinas *et al.* 2002). If hypoxia reduces recollection, but not familiarity, the severity of the hypoxic event should be related to recognition, but only through a variance component shared by recall (i.e. recollection). As expected, the correlation between recognition and coma duration was reduced from −0.30 to 0.03 when recall was partialled out, i.e. once recall-related variance was removed from recognition, recognition performance was no longer related to hypoxic severity. However, the correlation between recall and coma duration (−0.45) was still significant when recognition was partialled out (−0.26). This indicates that the relationship between recognition and coma duration is completely accounted for by a common correlation with recall, whereas the relationship between recall and coma duration is greater than a common correlation with recognition. This pattern of partial correlations is difficult to reconcile with the idea of a single explicit memory process. However, the pattern is exactly as would be predicted if recognition relies on two component processes, and only one is shared by recall and is affected by hypoxic severity.

We further tested these claims by examining the ability of a dual-process model to account for the covariance of recall, recognition, and coma duration. We did this by generating an explicit dual-process structural equation model that related recall and recognition directly to recollection and familiarity. In structural equation modelling, theoretical constructs are specified mathematically from theory as latent factors underlying the relationships among observed variables. The structural equation is a mathematical expression that predicts observed performance from sets of regression weights and correlations relating latent and observed variables to one another. The model is fitted directly to the covariance matrix of the observed variables to determine whether the model provides a statistically acceptable explanation of the observed relations among variables in the matrix. Additionally, estimates are obtained of the contribution of various theoretical processes to behaviour in the form of regression coefficients. Thus we could assess the adequacy of the dual-process model and directly examine how variables such as hypoxic severity influenced recollection and familiarity.

A simplified path diagram of a dual-process structural equation model is shown in Figure 17.3. The model assumes that recollection and familiarity contribute to recognition, whereas only recollection contributes to recall. The model also assumes that coma duration and age affect only recollection, and are not related to familiarity. Note that in testing this model and others discussed later, we included additional variables to constrain the model fits further, such as repeated measures of both recognition and recall and a test of verbal fluency, which are not shown in Figure 17.3 (Quamme *et al.* 2004). However, the model in Figure 17.3 contains all components relevant to the relations among coma duration, recall, and recognition. This model was found to fit the covariance matrix exceptionally well, and was not improved by adding parameters that would be inconsistent with dual-process theory. For example, no appreciable changes in fit or in the values of path coefficients were observed when recollection and familiarity were allowed to correlate or when age and coma duration were allowed to affect familiarity. These results are important because they indicate that the a priori restrictions inherent in the dual-process model were reasonable. In fact, when we conducted an extensive analysis of alterative structural equation models on this dataset, we failed to improve upon this simple model (Quamme *et al.* 2004). These alternatives and the details of their analyses will be discussed later.

Is recollection selectively impaired by mild hypoxia? This is the result one would expect if recollection, but not familiarity, relies on the integrity of the hippocampus, and if the hippocampus is selectively damaged by mild hypoxia.

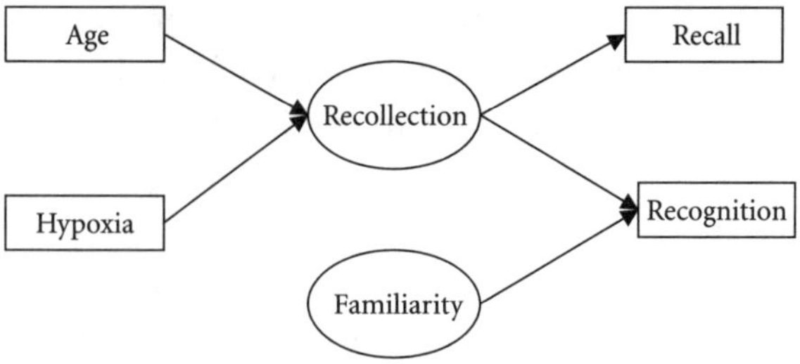

Figure 17.3 A dual-process structural equation model relating recall, recognition, age, and coma duration to recollection and familiarity in mild hypoxia.

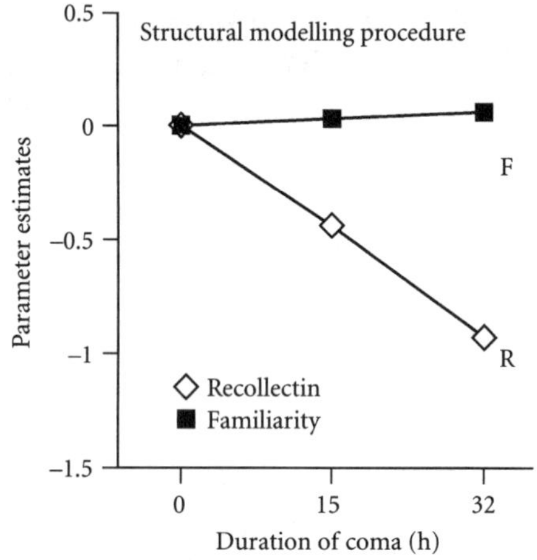

Figure 17.4 Best-fitting effects of coma duration on recollection and familiarity from the dual-process structural equation model of recall and recognition in mild hypoxia.

To examine this, we first allowed age and hypoxia to affect both familiarity and recollection in a modification of the structural model in Figure 17.3. Figure 17.4 shows estimates of recollection and familiarity from this model plotted for coma durations of 0 h, 16 h, and 32 h: a coma duration of 0 h represents the model's approximation to control subjects, and is just less than 1 standard deviation (SD) below the mean coma duration of the hypoxic sample; 32 h is 1 SD above the mean coma duration of the sample. Figure 17.4(a) shows that, according to the best-fitting estimates of the structural equation model, increases in hypoxic severity, as indexed by coma duration, are associated with decreases in recollection but not changes in familiarity.

To corroborate these model-generated estimates of recollection and familiarity we conducted a study of recollection and familiarity in a subgroup of hypoxic patients using the remember–know method, and another study using the ROC method (Yonelinas *et al.* 2002). Estimates of recollection and familiarity derived from remember–know reports indicated that the hypoxic patients exhibited a severe impairment in recollection relative to controls, but they did not exhibit deficits in familiarity. Estimates of recollection and familiarity from the ROC procedure also indicated that these patients suffered a severe deficit in recollection, but not familiarity. Note that both these studies tested memory for words, but similar effects have been reported in tests of recognition for pictures (Kishiyama *et al.* 2004).

The results from the recall–recognition contrasts, partial regression analysis, structural modelling, and the remember–know and ROC methods converge in showing that recollection is selectively affected by mild hypoxia. Although it is not possible to determine the precise lesion locations, there is good reason to believe that damage in these patients was specific to the hippocampus based on previous volumetric and histological studies of hypoxia (Zola-Morgan *et al.* 1986; Hopkins *et al.* 1995; Rempel-Clower *et al.* 1996). Thus the findings support the proposal that the hippocampus is critical for recollection but not familiarity.

It is important to note that these studies only examined the effects of mild hypoxia and the observed pattern of results might not be expected to generalize to more severe cases, i.e. it is well documented that as the hypoxic event becomes more severe, a variety of brain regions other than the hippocampus, such as the frontal lobes and thalamus, are also influenced (Smith *et al.* 1984; Caine and Watson 2000). Given that damage to the thalamus can disrupt both recollection and familiarity (Zoppelt *et al.* 2003; Kishiyama *et al.* 2004), and imaging results have implicated the frontal lobes in both recollection and familiarity (Henson *et al.* 1999; Eldridge *et al.* 2000), it follows that more severely hypoxic patients may suffer deficits in both recollection and familiarity. Evidence in support of this comes from a recent study by Manns *et al.* (2003) who found that a hypoxic amnesic group containing heroin overdose, CO_2 poisoning, and cardiac arrest patients, together with patients with unknown aetiologies, were equally impaired on both remember-based and know-based recognition responses. Unfortunately, the severity of the hypoxic events suffered by these patients was not reported. However, the patients were much more impaired on standardized memory tests (i.e. >3 SD below normal) compared with the mildly hypoxic patients examined by Yonelinas *et al.* (2002) and Quamme *et al.* (2004) (i.e. 0–3 SD below normal), suggesting more severe hypoxic damage in the former group. Moreover, although the hippocampus and parahippocampal gyrus were examined in these patients for evidence of atrophy, no other brain volume data was reported. Thus, it is difficult to determine what caused the memory impairments in that group.

In sum, the results from our studies of mildly hypoxic patients indicate that recollection can be disrupted in this group without reliable impairments in familiarity. This result is important in that it demonstrates the neuropsychological separability of these two recognition processes, and is consistent with models of medial temporal lobe function in which it is assumed that recollection, but not familiarity, relies on the hippocampus, whereas familiarity relies on the parahippocampal gyrus (Aggleton and Brown 1999).

Alternative models of memory and amnesia

Are there viable alternatives to the theory that recollection and familiarity rely differentially on the hippocampus and parahippocampus? The convergent results observed across a variety of measurement methods and patient groups provide strong evidence in support of the account we have provided. However, the value of any model is closely tied to how it performs relative to competing models, and thus it is critical to consider alternative accounts of the above results. In this section we consider two general classes of alternative theories that have been used to account for memory and amnesia: single-component strength theories and dual-process recall theories. We show that these theories do not provide an adequate account of the existing data. We will begin by considering the results from the remember–know, ROC, and process dissociation studies, and then use structural equation modelling to provide direct statistical tests of some competing models.

Alternative models of remember–know, ROC, and process dissociation results

There is a long history in experimental psychology of using single-component or single-process strength models to account for recognition memory performance (Murdock 1974). According to these models, recognition reflects the assessment of either a single underlying familiarity signal, or a single measure of how much information is retrieved about a studied item. This view of recognition has been applied to remember–know and confidence-based ROC data by assuming that 'remember' responses and high-confidence recognition responses simply reflect the most familiar items or those for which the subjects can retrieve the most episodic information (Donaldson 1996; Hirshman and Master 1997). Knowing responses or less confident recognition responses simply reflect weaker memories. A similar approach can be used to account for source memory and process dissociation results. Specifically, stronger items are those items for which the subjects can retrieve enough information about a study event to support source recognition, whereas more weakly remembered items fail to support such discriminations. In this case, recollection is simply a measure of how many items are strongly remembered, and familiarity is a measure of how many items are weakly remembered.

However, these single-component models fail to account for the existing amnesia results, because the recognition performance of amnesics differs not just quantitatively, but qualitatively, from that of healthy control subjects. Evidence for this difference was first obtained by Huppert and Piercy (1978) who showed that, unlike control subjects, amnesics tended to confuse more recently presented items with more frequently presented items, and vice versa. This holds true even when the controls are matched to amnesics for overall levels of recognition (Meudell *et al.* 1985). A single-process strength model would predict that controls and amnesics should have equivalent difficulty in discriminating these two types of items. However, these results are easily explained by the dual-process claim that amnesics base their recognition judgements on assessments of familiarity, whereas healthy subjects are able to use recollection to discriminate between recently presented and frequently presented items.

Additional evidence comes from our studies directly contrasting different groups of amnesics (Yonelinas *et al.* 2002). We found that, although overall recognition performance of hypoxic patients was comparable with that of patients with extensive left temporal lobe damage, their remember–know responses and recognition ROCs were quite different. The hypoxic patients had higher familiarity estimates but lower recollection estimates than the patients with extensive temporal lobe damage. This cross-over dissociation is difficult to explain from the perspective of a single-component model. However, the results are again quite consistent with the dual-process account. The high levels of familiarity in the hypoxic group reflect the fact that the parahippocampal gyrus was relatively preserved in this group. The greater recollection deficits in the hypoxic patients probably reflect the fact that the hippocampal damage in hypoxia is bilateral, whereas the temporal lobe group suffered only unilateral damage.

Converging evidence comes from an examination of recognition ROCs which indicate that recognition memory in healthy controls is qualitatively different from that seen in amnesics. Recall the previous discussion of Figure 17.2(a) which shows ROCs from controls and amnesics with damage to both hippocampus and parahippocampus (Yonelinas *et al.* 1998). Figure 17.2(b) shows ROCs of controls and hypoxic patients (Yonelinas *et al.* 2002). An examination of Figures 2(a) and 2(b) shows that the shapes of the ROCs of these amnesic groups differ from those of the controls in two important ways. First, the memory sensitivity is decreased (i.e. the amnesics' functions fall closer to the chance diagonal). Secondly, the controls' ROCs are asymmetrical along the diagonal (i.e. when the ROCs are plotted in *z*-space the slope is less than 1.0), whereas those of the amnesics' ROCs are symmetrical (i.e. the slope in *z*-space is not different from 1.0).

Can the differences between the control and amnesic ROC shapes be explained simply as a decrease in memory strength? If this were the case, we would expect the shapes of the control and amnesic ROCs to be identical when overall level of performance was equated, i.e. a single-process memory strength model would predict that ROCs of controls and amnesics would have the same shape when overall performance was matched. To address this question we examined ROCs for control subjects who were matched, using faster study rates, for overall recognition performance to amnesics with hippocampal and parahippocampal damage (Yonelinas *et al.* 1998). Figure 17.2(c) shows that even when the overall level of control performance was matched to that of the amnesics, the ROCs of these groups exhibited distinct shapes. As with the original analyses, the controls' ROCs were asymmetrical with a slope less than 1.0 in *z*-space, whereas the amnesics were symmetrical with a slope near 1 in *z*-space. No single-process memory strength model of which we are aware can explain the qualitative differences in recognition memory of controls and amnesics that we found. However, the observed differences in the ROCs in these two groups follows directly from the dual-process account of recognition, i.e. because amnesics should rely primarily on familiarity, their ROCs should be symmetrical (i.e. based on a signal detection process), but because controls can make use of both familiarity and recollection, the ROCs should be asymmetrical because the function is pushed up slightly on the *y*-axis by recollection.

Moreover, not only does the dual-process model account for the shapes of the amnesics' and controls' ROCs, it can also accurately predict the level of performance in the hypoxic amnesic group on the basis of analysing the shape of the controls' ROCs. That is, if the hypoxic patients exhibit a selective deficit in recollection, then we can simply remove the contribution of recollection from the control ROC by subtracting the intercept and arrive at the predicted level of performance for the hypoxic subjects. The dotted curve in Figure 17.2(b) represents this predicted level of performance for the hypoxic patients and the solid curve represents the observed function. The predicted and observed functions were virtually identical, indicating that the only difference between the controls and hypoxic patients is that the controls are able to use recollection to supplement their familiarity-based responses. Our ability to predict the shape of the hypoxic patients' ROCs and their absolute level of performance accurately leads us to have confidence in the accuracy of the ROC model and in the conclusion that mild hypoxia results in a selective disruption of recollection.

More complex strength-based recognition models may also account for the dissociations observed in amnesia, as long as they invoke at least two memory components. One example of such a model is the unequal-variance signal detection model. In this type of model old items are more familiar than new items, but there is an additional memory component that can vary independently of memory strength—the extent to which the variance of the old items' familiarity distribution is greater than that of the new item distribution. There is currently some debate regarding whether or not this model is falsified by the existing remember–know results in healthy subjects (MacMillan *et al.* 2003; Wixted and Stretch 2003), but it is now well documented that it cannot account for recognition ROC results in tests that rely heavily on recollection, such as source and associative recognition data (Yonelinas 1997, 1999; Rotello *et al.* 2000; Kelley and Wixted 2001; DeCarlo 2003). Thus, unequal-variance signal detection models do not provide an adequate account of human recognition memory. Note that more complex models have been proposed to account for these ROCs in healthy subjects (DeCarlo 2003; Kelley and Wixted 2001), but these models also assume that recognition involves at least one additional memory process. Thus the current viable alternatives to the dual-process model of recognition are in agreement that multiple processes are necessary to explain the range of observed recognition data.

Alternative structural equation models

As discussed earlier, structural equation modelling can be used to assess directly the fit of a model to data and to provide best-fitting estimates of the processes proposed by the model. Above, we reported the fit of the dual-process recognition model and the estimates of recollection and familiarity generated by the model that best explained the observed covariance of recall, recognition, age, and coma duration in our hypoxic group. One important caveat to keep in mind is that models cannot be confirmed by the data; they can only be disconfirmed. In fact, there may be any number of alternative models that fit the covariance matrix as well as or better than the dual-process model. Additionally, all models are false unless they correctly characterize *all* processes and their relationships that give rise to behaviour. This is, of course, an implausible criterion for models of any phenomenon as complex as human memory. Therefore, to reiterate, it is important to determine how well a given model accounts for the data, but it is equally, if not more, important to determine whether the model accounts for the data better than one or more plausible alternatives.

In this section we used data from the mildly hypoxic patients in the study by Yonelinas *et al.* (2002) to see if we could find a theoretically plausible alternative model that fared as well as or better than the dual-process model (for a complete description of these models and methods see Quamme *et al.* (2004)). The logic of the model comparison procedure is as follows. If an alternative model is a better characterization of the processes underlying memory, it should provide a fit that is better than the dual-process model, as well as parameter estimates that are consistent with the theory on which it is based. Further, for a model to be the preferred model, it should provide a statistical improvement over a simpler model and should not be improved further by adding parameters that are inconsistent with the theory. We assessed alternative models of performance by starting with a single-component memory model, and then added parameters to assess more complex multiprocess models.

A single-component model of memory is shown in Figure 17.5(a). The model assumes that there is only one form of explicit, or declarative, memory that underlies both recognition and recall (Squire 1994). Direct statistical tests of this model's ability to account for the covariation observed between these measured variables showed that the model provided a poor fit to the data and was statistically rejectable. Moreover, the fit of the model was improved significantly by simply adding an independent familiarity factor to recognition, as in the dual-process recognition model in Figure 17.3. The rejection of the single-component model may not be particularly surprising given the existing cognitive literature showing that two processes are involved in recognition memory (Yonelinas 2002). Nonetheless, it is useful to confirm that such a single-component model of explicit memory does not provide an adequate account of amnesia. Moreover, the model serves as a good baseline from which to compare more complex multicomponent models.

Next, we examined a dual-process model of recall (Fig. 17.5(b)). In this model there is a declarative memory component that contributes to recognition and recall, and additional controlled memory search component that also contributes

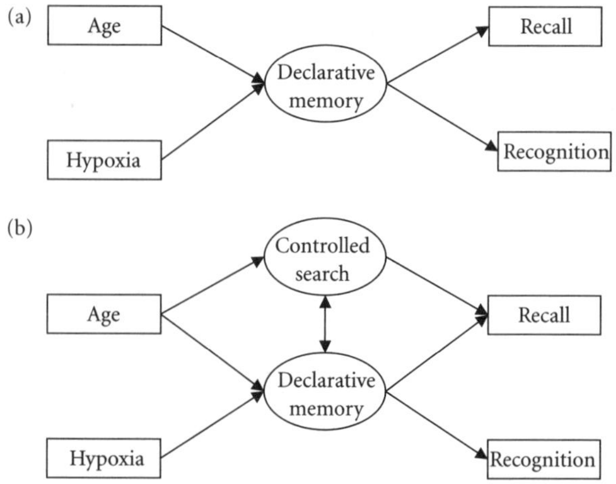

Figure. 17.5 Alternative structural equation models of the relationships among recall, recognition, coma duration, and age in mild hypoxia: (a) a single declarative memory process; (b) a dual-process model of recall.

to recall. The search component makes it possible for the model to account for dissociations between recall and recognition. Several versions of this model have been proposed in which the frontal lobes contribute executive processes to recall, but not recognition. These processes have been proposed to function in organizing a memory search (Squire and Zola 1998), inhibiting irrelevant responses (Shimamura 1995), and monitoring the products of memory retrieval (Moscovitch 1994). The model in Figure 17.5(b) makes the additional assumptions that mild hypoxia affects declarative memory, and that ageing affects declarative memory as well as controlled search processes. These additional assumptions were based on supportive neuropsychological findings, but are not critical for the current purposes because adopting various alternative assumptions about how these measures influence these two forms of memory did not change the outcome of the model evaluation.

When we fitted this model to the covariance matrix we found that it was statistically rejectable, indicating that, despite including two memory factors, the model did not account sufficiently for the relationships among these variables. However, as with the single-process model, when we added a familiarity factor, the fit improved significantly and the model was no longer rejectable. In fact, removing the effect of controlled search on recall did not significantly worsen the fit of the model. These comparisons indicate that a dual-process model of recall is not sufficient to explain the effects of hypoxia on recall and recognition. Thus it is not the case that the covariance matrix is explainable by just any two-factor model of memory; rather, two recognition processes are necessary.

These results should not be interpreted as showing that a frontally mediated search mechanism does not contribute to recall. There is compelling evidence that free recall relies on the integrity of frontal regions more than recognition does (Janowsky *et al.* 1989). The results simply show that the memory impairments seen in mild hypoxia are not due to a disruption of a frontally-mediated search mechanism that is unique to recall. Rather, the results reveal that recollection in both recall and recognition is disrupted, and that an unaffected familiarity process must be included in recognition in order to explain the observed relationships.

Conclusions

The studies of human amnesic patients we report here are consistent with studies of rats and non-human primates in indicating that the hippocampus is critical for recollection, whereas familiarity is dependent upon the parahippocampal gyrus. The results were based on convergent evidence from a variety of patient groups and measurement methods. The convergence of multiple measurement methods is striking given that each method assumes a very different operational definition of recollection and familiarity. A remarkably consistent story emerges when we examine estimates of recollection and familiarity derived from introspective reports of remembering and knowing (Tulving 1985), the process dissociation procedure (Jacoby 1991), confidence-rating ROCs (Yonelinas 1994), and covariance structures of recall and recognition (Yonelinas *et al.* 2002; Quamme *et al.* 2004).

Of course, all the methods we report make assumptions that can be questioned. One can always criticize the assumptions of a given method, and attribute the successful prediction of any particular data point or any single effect to artefacts to which the method is susceptible. However, when estimates derived from different methodological and analytical procedures begin to converge in favour of a particular theory, it becomes increasingly unlikely that success of the theory in accounting for a set of observations is the result of a set of artefacts. Indeed, at some point, it must be conceded that the particular collection of artefacts necessary to explain the range of data is so improbable that one has the choice of either acknowledging the theory's merit, or 'attributing replicable orderliness of observations to a damn strange coincidence' (Meehl 1990, p. 117). We believe that this point has been reached regarding the evidence that recollection and familiarity rely differentially on the hippocampus and parahippocampal gyrus in humans.

References

Aggleton, J.P. and Brown, M.W. (1999). Episodic memory, amnesia, and the hippocampal–anterior thalamic axis. *Behavioral and Brain Sciences*, **22**, 425–44.

Aggleton, J.P. and Shaw, C. (1996). Amnesia and recognition memory: a re-analysis of psychometric data. *Neuropsychologia*, **34**, 51–62.

Baddeley, A., Vargha-Khadem, F., and Mishkin, M. (2001). Preserved recognition in a case of developmental amnesia: implications for the acquisition of semantic memory? *Journal of Cognitive Neuroscience*, **13**, 357–369.

Blaxton, T.A. and Theodore, W.H. (1997). The role of the temporal lobes in recognizing visuospatial materials: remembering versus knowing. *Brain and Cognition*, **35**, 5–25.

Caine, D. and Watson, J.D.G. (2000). Neuropsychological and neuropathological sequelae of cerebral anoxia: a critical review. *Journal of the International Neuropsychological Society*, **6**, 86–99.

DeCarlo, L.T. (2003). An application of signal-detection theory with finite mixture distributions to source discrimination. *Journal of Experimental Psychology: Learning, Memory, and Cognition*, **29**, 767–778.

Donaldson, W. (1996). The role of decision processes in remembering and knowing. *Memory and Cognition*, **24**, 523–533.

Eldridge, L.L., Knowlton, B.J., Furmanski, C.S., Bookheimer, S.Y., and Engel, S.A. (2000). Remembering episodes: a selective role for the hippocampus during retrieval. *Nature Neuroscience*, **3**, 1149–1152.

Gadian, D.G., Aicardi, J., Watkins, K.E., Porter, D.A., Mishkin, M., and Vargha-Khadem, F. (2000). Developmental amnesia associated with early hypoxic-ischaemic injury. *Brain*, **123**, 499–507.

Gardiner, J.M. and Parkin, A.J. (1990). Attention and recollective experience in recognition memory. *Memory and Cognition*, **18**, 579–583.

Henson, R.N.A., Rugg, M.D., Shallice, T., Josephs, O., and Dolan, R.J. (1999). Recollection and familiarity in recognition memory: an event-related functional magnetic resonance imaging study. *Journal of Neuroscience*, **19**, 3962–3972.

Hirshman, E. and Master, S. (1997). Modeling the conscious correlates of recognition memory: reflections on the remember–know paradigm. *Memory and Cognition*, **25**, 345–351.

Hopkins, R.O., Kesner, R.P., and Goldstein, M. (1995). Item and order recognition memory in subjects with hypoxic brain injury. *Brain and Cognition*, **27**, 180–201.

Huppert, F.A. and Piercy, M. (1978). The role of trace strength in recency and frequency judgments by amnesic and control subjects. *Quarterly Journal of Experimental Psychology*, **30**, 347–354.

Jacoby, L.L. (1991). A process dissociation framework: separating automatic from intentional uses of memory. *Journal of Memory and Language*, **30**, 513–541.

Jacoby, L.L., Toth, J.P., and Yonelinas, A.P. (1993). Separating conscious and unconscious influences of memory: measuring recollection. *Journal of Experimental Psychology: General*, **122**, 139–154.

Janowsky, J.S., Shimamura, A.P., Kritchevsky, M., and Squire, L.R. (1989). Cognitive impairment following frontal lobe damage and its relevance to human amnesia. *Behavioral Neuroscience*, **103**, 548–560.

Kelley, R. and Wixted, J.T. (2001). On the nature of associative information in recognition memory. *Journal of Experimental Psychology: Learning, Memory, and Cognition*, **27**, 701–722.

Kishiyama, M.M., Yonelinas, A.P., and Lazzara, M.M. (2004). The von Restorff effect in amnesia: the contribution of the hippocampal system to novelty-related memory enhancements. *Journal of Cognitive Neuroscience*, **16**, 15–23.

Kishiyama MM, Yonelinas, A.P., Kroll, N.E.A., *et al.* (in press). Bilateral thalamic lesions affect recollection- and familiarity-based recognition judgments. *Cortex*.

Knowlton, B.J. and Squire, L.R. (1995). Remembering and knowing: two different expressions of declarative memory. *Journal of Experimental Psychology: Learning, Memory, and Cognition*, **21**, 699–710.

MacMillan, N.A., Rotello, C.M., and Verde, M.F. (2003). A', d', and the one-dimensional model of remember–know judgments. Paper presented at the 44th Annual Meeting of the Psychonomic Society, Vancouver, BC.

Mandler, G. (1980). Recognizing: the judgment of previous occurrence. *Psychological Review*, **87**, 252–271.

Manns, J.R. and Squire, L.R. (1999). Impaired recognition memory on the Doors and People Test after damage limited to the hippocampal region. *Hippocampus*, **9**, 495–499.

Manns, J.R., Hopkins, R.O., Reed, J.M., Kitchener, E.G., and Squire, L.R. (2003) Recognition memory and the human hippocampus. *Neuron*, **27**, 171–180.

Mayes, A.R. (1988). Amnesia and memory for contextual information. In *Memory in Context: Context in Memory* (ed G.M. Davies and D.M. Thomson). New York: John Wiley, pp. 193–213.

Meehl, P.E. (1990). Appraising and amending theories: the strategy of Lakatosian Defense and two principles that warrant it. *Psychological Inquiry*, **1**, 108–141.

Meudell, P.R., Mayes, A.R., Ostergaard, A., and Pickering, A. (1985). Recency and frequency judgments in alcoholic amnesics and normal people with poor memory. *Cortex*, **21**, 487–511.

Milner, B. and Petrides, M. (1984). Behavioural effects of frontal-lobe lesions in man. *Trends in Neuroscience*, **7**, 403–407.

Moscovitch, D.A. and McAndrews, M.P. (2002). Material-specific deficits in 'remembering' in patients with unilateral temporal lobe epilepsy and excisions. *Neuropsychologia*, **40,** 1335–1342.

Moscovitch, M. (1994). Memory and working with memory: evaluation of a component-process model and comparisons with other models. In *Memory Systems 1994* (ed D.L. Schacter and E. Tulving). Cambridge, MA: MIT Press, pp. 269–310.

Murdock, B.B. (1974). *Human Memory: Theory and Data*. Potomac, MD: Erlbaum.

Quamme, J.R., Yonelinas, A.P., Widaman K.F., *et al.* (2004). Recall and recognition in mild hypoxia: Using covariance structural modeling to test competing theories of explicit memory. *Neuropsychologia*, **42**, 672–691.

Rajaram, S. (1993). Remembering and knowing: two means of access to the personal past. *Memory and Cognition*, **21**, 89–102.

Rajaram, S., Hamilton, M., and Bolton, A. (2002). Distinguishing states of awareness from confidence during retrieval: evidence from amnesia. *Cognitive, Affective and Behavioral Neuroscience*, **2**, 227–235.

Rotello, C.M., Macmillan, N.A., and Van Tassel, G. (2000). Recall-to-reject in recognition: evidence from ROC curves. *Journal of Memory and Language*, **43**, 67–88.

Rotello C.M., Macmillan N.A., and Reeder J.A. (in press). A two-dimensional signal detection model of remember–know judgments. *Psychological Review*.

Rugg, M.D. and Allan, K. (2000). Event-related potential studies of memory. In *The Oxford Handbook of Memory* (ed F.I.M. Craik and E. Tulving). Oxford: Oxford University Press, pp.521–537.

Rugg, M.D. and Yonelinas, A.P. (2003). Human recognition memory: a cognitive neuroscience perspective. *Trends in Cognitive Sciences*, **7**, 313–319.

Sauvé, M.J., Doolittle, N., Walker, J.A., Paul, S.M., and Scheinmann, M.M. (1996). Factors associated with cognitive recovery after cardiopulmonary resuscitation. *American Journal of Critical Care*, **5**, 129–137.

Schacter, D.L., Verfaellie, M., and Pradere, D. (1996). The neuropsychology of memory Illusions: False recall and recognition in amnesic patients. *Journal of Memory and Language*, **35**, 319–334.

Schacter, D.L., Verfaellie, M., and Anes, M.D. (1997). Illusory memories in amnesic patients: conceptual and perceptual false recognition. *Neuropsychology*, **11**, 331–342.

Shimamura, A.P. (1995). Memory and frontal lobe function. In *The Cognitive Neurosciences* (ed M.S. Gazzaniga). Cambridge, MA: MIT Press, pp 803–813.

Shimamura, A.P. (1996). The role of prefrontal cortex in monitoring and controlling memory processes. In *Implicit Memory and Metacognition* (ed L. Reder). Mahwah, NJ: Erlbaum, pp. 259–274.

Smith, M.L., Auer, R.N., and Siesjo, B.K. (1984). The density and distribution of ischemic brain injury in the rat following 2–10 min of forebrain ischemia. *Acta Neuropathologica*, **64**, 319–332.

Squire, L.R. (1994). Declarative and nondeclarative memory: multiple brain systems supporting learning and memory. In *Memory Systems 1994* (ed D.L. Schacter and E. Tulving). Cambridge, MA: MIT Press, pp. 203–231.

Squire, L.R. and Zola, S. (1998). Episodic memory, semantic memory, and amnesia. *Hippocampus*, **8**, 205–211.

Toth, J.P. (1996). Conceptual automaticity in recognition memory: levels-of-processing effects on familiarity. *Canadian Journal of Experimental Psychology*, **50**, 123–138.

Tulving, E. (1985). Memory and consciousness. *Canadian Psychology*, **26**, 1–12.

Verfaellie, M. and Treadwell, J.R. (1993). The status of recognition memory in amnesia. *Neuropsychology*, **7**, 5–13.

Verfaellie M, Cermak LS, Letourneau L, and Zuffante P. (1991). Repetition effects in a lexical decision task: the role of episodic memory in the performance of alcoholic Korsakoff patients. *Neuropsychologia*, **29**, 641–657.

Wixted, J.T. and Squire, L. (2004). Recall and recognition are equally impaired in patients with selective hippocampal damage. *Cognitive, Affective and Behavioral Neuroscience*, **4**, 58–66.

Wixted, J.T. and Stretch, V. (2003). What signal-detection theory predicts about remember–know judgments. Paper presented at the 44th Annual Meeting of the Psychonomic Society, Vancouver, BC.

Yonelinas, A.P. (1994). Receiver-operating characteristics in recognition memory: evidence for a dual-process model. *Journal of Experimental Psychology: Learning, Memory, and Cognition*, **20**, 1341–1354.

Yonelinas, A.P. (1997). Recognition memory ROCs for item and associative information: the contribution of recollection and familiarity. *Memory and Cognition*, **25**, 747–763.

Yonelinas, A.P. (1999). The contribution of recollection and familiarity to recognition and source-memory judgments: a formal dual-process model and an analysis of receiver operating characteristics. *Journal of Experimental Psychology: Learning, Memory, and Cognition*, **25**, 1415–1434.

Yonelinas, A.P. (2001). Consciousness, control, and confidence: the 3 Cs of recognition memory. *Journal of Experimental Psychology: General*, **130**, 361–379.

Yonelinas, A.P. (2002). The nature of recollection and familiarity: a review of 30 years of research. *Journal of Memory and Language*, **46**, 441–517.

Yonelinas, A.P. and Levy, B.J. (2002). Dissociating familiarity from recollection in human recognition memory: different rates of forgetting over short retention intervals. *Psychonomic Bulletin and Review*, **9**, 575–582.

Yonelinas, A.P., Kroll, N.E.A., Dobbins, I., Lazzara, M., and Knight, R.T. (1998). Recollection and familiarity deficits in amnesia: convergence of remember–know, process dissociation, and receiver operating characteristic data. *Neuropsychology*, **12**, 323–339.

Yonelinas, A.P., Hopfinger, J.B., Buonocore, M.H., Kroll, N.E.A., and Baynes, K. (2001). Hippocampal, parahippocampal and occipital-temporal contributions to associative and item recognition memory: an fMRI study. *Neuroreport*, **12**, 359–363.

Yonelinas, A.P., Kroll, N.E.A., Quamme, J.R., *et al.* (2002). Effects of temporal lobe damage or mild hypoxia on recollection and familiarity. *Nature Neuroscience*, **5**, 1236–1241.

Yonelinas, A.P., Quamme, J.R., Widaman, K.F., Kroll, N.E.A., Sauvé M.-J., and Knight, R.T. (2004). Mild hypoxia disrupts recollection, not familiarity. *Cognitive, Affective and Behavioral Neuroscience*, **4**, 393–400.

Zola-Morgan, S., Squire, L.R., and Amaral, D.G. (1986). Human amnesia and the medial temporal lobe region: enduring memory impairment following a bilateral lesion limited to field CA1 of the hippocampus. *Journal of Neuroscience*, **6**, 2950–2967.

Zoppelt, D., Koch, B., Schwarz, M., and Daum, I. (2003). Involvement of the mediodorsal thalamic nucleus in mediating recollection and familiarity. *Neuropsychologia*, **41**, 1160–1170.

Chapter 18

Event-related potential explorations of dual processes in recognition memory

Tim Curran, Katharine L. Tepe, and Carley Piatt

Introduction

Most professors have plenty of first-hand experience of the distinction between recollection and familiarity. You might find yourself walking across campus and see a young woman who seems vaguely familiar as somebody you 'know' from somewhere, but often you are unable to recollect any detailed information about her. Is she a waitress at a favourite diner? Is she a student from a class? Which class? What was her grade? What is her name? Of course, at other times, you can recollect details about the person. This is Sophie who earned an A in my cognitive psychology class last semester, and so as she walks by you can confidently say, 'Hi Sophie, nice work on the final exam last semester'. The distinction between recollection and familiarity is the cornerstone of dual-process theories of recognition memory (reviewed by Yonelinas 2002). In general, recollection involves the retrieval of specific details associated with something recognized, whereas familiarity can underlie recognition without the retrieval of details.

In this chapter we will review recent event-related potential (ERP) work relevant to the dual-process perspective and examine the implications of this work for understanding binding in human memory. More comprehensive reviews of ERP memory research, each addressing the dual-process perspective to some extent, are available elsewhere (Johnson 1995; Rugg 1995; Allan *et al.* 1998; Friedman and Johnson 2000; Mecklinger 2000; Wilding and Sharpe 2003). In particular, we will review evidence relevant to the hypothesis that the 300–500 ms FN400 ERP old–new effect is related to familiarity, and the 400–800 ms parietal ERP old–new effect is related to recollection.[1]

ERPs recorded on the human scalp are obtained by averaging EEG activity across multiple trials designed to engage specific sensory, cognitive, or motor processes (for a methodological introduction, see Rugg and Coles (1995) and Fabiani *et al.* (2000)). By time locking the average to regularly occurring events (e.g. stimulus onset in most ERP recognition memory experiments), ERPs reflect the activity of brain processes that are regularly associated with stimulus processing. ERPs can be differentiated by their timing (with millisecond resolution) and scalp distribution, and so different neurocognitive processes can be identified with distinct spatiotemporal voltage patterns. ERP studies of the retrieval processes associated with recognition memory have typically compared ERPs elicited by studied (old) test items with those elicited by non-studied (new) test items. Because behavioural recognition memory performance involves discrimination between old and new items, ERP differences between old and new conditions potentially reflect the activity of brain processes contributing to recognition memory.

Previous ERP studies of recognition memory have been interpreted from dual-process perspectives. ERPs recorded over parietal sites from about 400 to 800 ms following stimulus onset are more positive for old than for new stimuli (reviewed by Johnson 1995; Rugg 1995; Allan *et al.* 1998; Friedman and Johnson 2000; Mecklinger 2000; Wilding and Sharpe 2003). Previous studies suggest that this parietal old–new effect is related to recollection (reviewed by Allan *et al.* 1998; Friedman and Johnson 2000; Mecklinger 2000; Wilding and Sharpe 2003).[2] When subjects are asked to introspectively differentiate words specifically 'remembered' from those that they merely 'know' to be old, larger parietal old–new effects are associated with 'remembering' than with 'knowing' (Smith 1993; Düzel *et al.* 1997; Rugg *et al.* 1998b; Trott *et al.* 1999; Curran 2004; Friedman, in press). The parietal old–new effect is sensitive to variables believed to affect recollection more than familiarity such as level of processing (Paller and Kutas 1992; Paller *et al.* 1995; Rugg *et al.* 1995) and word–pseudoword differences (Curran 1999). The parietal old–new effect is associated with the recollection of specific information such as study modality (Wilding *et al.* 1995; Wilding and Rugg 1997b), speaker's voice (Rugg *et al.* 1998b; Wilding and Rugg 1996, 1997a), and temporal source (Trott *et al.* 1997). More recent research, reviewed below, has upheld the hypothesized relationship between the parietal old–new effect and recollection, as well as suggesting that earlier mid-frontal ERP old–new effects may be related to familiarity.

Rugg *et al.* (1998a) were among the first to suggest that 300–500 ms mid-frontal old–new effects (here labelled 'FN400 old–new effects'[3]) are related to familiarity. A level-of-processing manipulation required subjects to study words with either a semantically 'deep' or a semantically 'shallow' encoding task. The 500–800 ms parietal old–new effect was greater for correctly recognized words following deep rather than shallow encoding, but a 300–500 ms frontal old–new effect did not differentiate between shallow and deep conditions. Rugg *et al.* suggested that the 300–500 ms frontal old–new effect may be related to familiarity because familiarity was presumed to be less sensitive than recollection to level of processing. Other evidence indicating a relationship between FN400 and familiarity was obtained in an experiment comparing recognition memory for words and pseudowords (Curran 1999). The 400–800 ms parietal old–new differences were larger for words than for pseudowords, but the 300–500 mid-frontal FN400 differences were similar for words and pseudowords. In addition to these old–new differences, FN400 showed a main effect of stimulus type such that it was more negative for pseudowords than for words. Thus FN400 appeared to be sensitive to both pre-experimental (pseudoword < word) and experimental (new < old) familiarity. Although the results of Rugg *et al.* (1998a) and Curran (1999) were consistent with the idea that 300–500 ms mid-frontal FN400 old–new effects are related to familiarity, these experiments did not provide particularly strong evidence because they were not originally designed to test this hypothesis.

Dissociating recollection and familiarity with study–test similarity

According to the global matching models of memory (Murdock 1982; Gillund and Shiffrin 1984; Hintzman 1988; Humphreys *et al.* 1989; Shiffrin and Steyvers 1997; Norman and O'Reilly 2003), familiarity is an assessment of the overall similarity between a test item and all study-list information in memory. Exploiting this putative property of familiarity by manipulating the similarity between studied and tested items has proved useful for dissociating familiarity from recollection. Hintzman and Curran developed a plurality recognition paradigm which provided behavioural evidence for separate recollection and familiarity processes (Hintzman *et al.* 1992; Hintzman and Curran 1994, 1995). The plurality recognition task required subjects to study plural and singular words (e.g. 'cats', 'jar') with the instruction to remember the plurality of each. The test list included studied words in their original plurality ('cats'), similar lures with reversed polarity ('jars'), and new words. The subjects were instructed to respond 'yes' for studied words, and 'no' for similar lures and new words. As expected, the false-alarm rate was much higher for similar than for new words, presumably because the similar lures were highly familiar. In several experiments items were studied a number of times (up to 20), and memory was tested with a frequency judgement test in which subjects judged how often each item was studied, but gave 'zero' estimates for similar and new words (Hintzman *et al.* 1992; Hintzman and Curran 1995). Frequency judgements increased with presentation frequency, but the false-alarm rate (frequency judgement greater than zero) to similar lures was minimally influenced by presentation frequency. These results suggested that the familiarity of studied and similar words increased with repetition (as indexed by increasing frequency judgements), whereas the ability to recollect specific information (i.e. plurality) was barely influenced (as indexed by false alarms to similar lures).

Hintzman and Curran (1994) examined the intuitively appealing notion that familiarity should act faster than recollection (Atkinson and Juola 1973; Mandler 1980). Plurality recognition was tested with a response-deadline procedure in which subjects were forced to make recognition judgements at various randomly determined times after stimulus onset (Reed 1973; Dosher 1984; Gronlund and Ratcliff 1989; Hintzman and Curran 1997). False alarms to similar lures showed an early increase (at fast response signals) followed by a later decrease (at slow response signals). Subjects discriminated studied from new words about 420 ms after stimulus onset, but studied–similar discrimination was delayed until about 520 ms. Hintzman and Curran (1994) interpreted these results from a dual-process perspective. Fast-acting familiarity processes were sufficient for discriminating studied from new words, but familiarity exacerbated false alarms to similar lures. Slower-acting recollection processes counteracted the familiarity of similar lures, and eventually allowed subjects to discriminate between studied and similar words.

Curran (2000) sought ERP evidence for separate familiarity and recollection processes by measuring ERPs during the plurality recognition task. Analyses focused on three conditions: studied words given a 'yes' response (Studied[yes]), similar words given a 'yes' response (Similar[yes]), and new words given a 'no' response (New[no]). The Studied[yes] condition was assumed to represent accurate plurality recollection and/or familiarity (hit rate, 66 per cent). The Similar[yes] condition was assumed to represent mostly familiarity with minimal recollection of word plurality (false-alarm rate, 41 per cent). The New[no] condition was assumed to represent minimal recollection and low familiarity (correct rejection rate, 79 per cent). As predicted, the parietal old–new effect behaved as would be expected of a recollection process (Fig. 18.1(a)). Parietal amplitudes (400–800 ms) were more positive in the condition associated with high recollection (Studied[yes]) than in the conditions with low recollection (Similar[yes], New[no]). Critically, the 300–500 ms FN400 old–new effect behaved more like a familiarity-related process (Fig. 18.1(b)). The FN400 amplitude was more negative for the least familiar condition (New[no]) than the more familiar conditions (Studied[yes], Similar[yes]). Topographic analyses confirmed that the differences related to familiarity (similar[yes]—new[no]) showed a qualitatively different pattern across the scalp than differences related

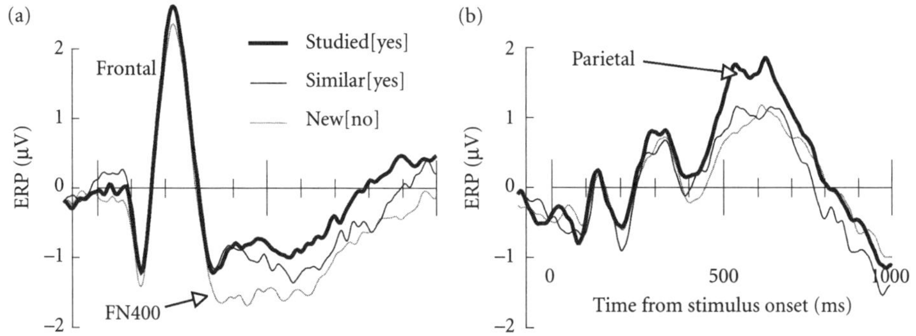

Figure 18.1 Primary results from Curran's (2000) plurality recognition experiment. (a) FN400 ERP effects hypothesized to be related to familiarity. Average ERPs from a cluster of left frontal sensors including the standard F3 location (Jasper 1958). Between 300 and 500 ms the FN400 was more negative for correctly rejected new items (New[no]) than for studied and similar items given 'yes' responses (Studied[yes], Similar[yes]). The Studied[yes] and Similar[yes] frontal ERPs did not differ between 300 and 500 ms. (b) Parietal ERP effects hypothesized to be related to recollection. Average ERPs from a cluster of left parietal sensors including the standard P3 location (Jasper 1958). Between 400 and 800 ms the parietal amplitude was more positive for the Studied[yes] than the Similar[yes] or New[no] conditions. The Similar[yes] and New[no] parietal ERPs did not differ between 400 and 800 ms.

to recollection (studied[yes]—similar[yes]) (Fig. 18.2(a)). Dissociating the two old–new effects according to the similarity manipulation, time, and topography provided strong evidence for separate familiarity and recollection processes.[4]

The impact of study–test similarity on familiarity and recollection was also found for pictures (Curran and Cleary 2003). Subjects studied grey-scale line drawings of various common objects, animals, people, and scenes, and were instructed to memorize the orientation of each. The recognition test included new pictures, identical studied pictures, and similar lures that were reversed in left–right orientation. The subjects were told to respond 'yes' only to pictures that were studied in their identical orientation, and to respond 'no' to similar (reversed orientation) lures and new pictures. Subjects were split into separate groups of 'good performers' and 'poor performers' based on their ability to discriminate between studied words and similar lures. Results from good performers replicated the plurality recognition results (Fig. 18.2(b)). The 300–500 ms FN400 effects were consistent with familiarity-related differences (New[no] < Similar[yes] = Studied[yes]) whereas the 400–800 ms parietal effects were consistent with recollection-related differences (New[no] = Similar [yes] < Studied[yes]). Poor performers showed similar FN400 familiarity effects, but 400–800 ms parietal differences showed no differentiation between studied and similar conditions (New[no] < Similar[yes] = Studied[no]).

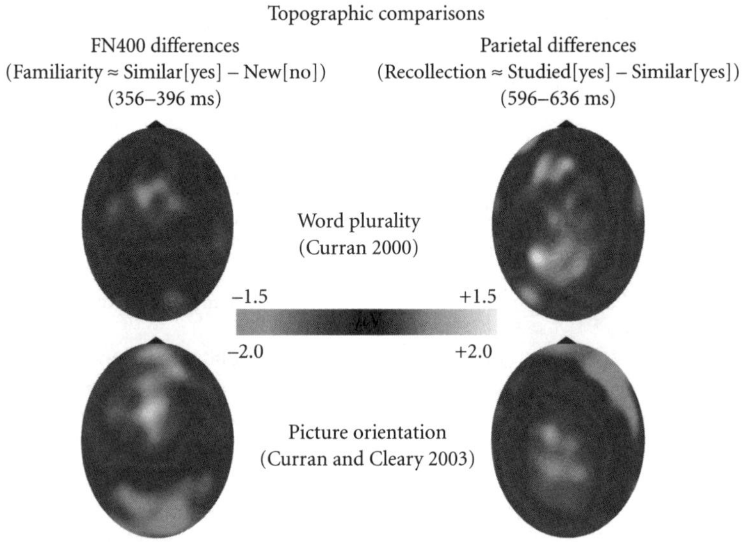

Figure 18.2 Topographical comparison of the FN400 familiarity effect with the parietal recollection effect. Each oval shows the head from above, so the nose is on top and the back of the head is on the bottom. Top figures from the plurality recognition experiment (Curran 2000). Bottom figures from the picture orientation recognition experiment (subjects with good studied–similar discrimination only) (Curran and Cleary 2003). The figures show ERP differences between conditions that should be particularly diagnostic of familiarity and recollection processes. In each case, data are plotted within a 40 ms window occurring at the peak of each difference. In the left panels, differences between the Similar[yes] and New[no] conditions are plotted that should be primarily attributable to familiarity because recollection should be minimal in each case. The familiarity-related differences are maximal over mid-frontal regions. In the right panels, differences between the Studied[yes] and Similar[yes] conditions are plotted that should be equally familiar, but differ in recollection. The recollection-related differences are maximal over left-parietal regions. See also colour plate section.

Thus parietal recollection effects were observed only for subjects with good ability to recollect the orientation of the pictures. FN400 familiarity effects were similar regardless of the recollection ability of the subjects.

Conceptual versus perceptual influences

The role of semantic–conceptual similarity was examined using the DRM false memory paradigm (Deese 1959; Roediger and McDermott 1995). In this paradigm, a series of semantically related words are studied (e.g. candy, sour, sugar, bitter, good, tooth, etc.) that are suggestive of a non-studied theme word ('similar lures', e.g. sweet). Subjects tend to falsely recognize similar lures nearly as often as they correctly recognize studied words. In an ERP extension of this paradigm, subjects studied a long list of words that were divided into semantically similar sets (Curran *et al.* 2001). After auditory presentation of the entire study list, the subjects completed a visual recognition test that included studied words, similar lures, and new words. The subjects responded 'yes' more often to studied words (63 per cent) than to similar lures (53 per cent), and responded 'yes' more often to similar lures than to new words (23 per cent).

As in previous experiments, ERP analyses focused on three conditions: hits to studied words (Studied[yes]), false alarms to similar lures (Similar[yes]), and correctly rejected new words (New[no]). It was expected that the 300–500 ms FN400, hypothesized to index familiarity, would show a basic old–new effect, but FN400 ERPs would not differ between Studied[yes] and Similar[yes] conditions. However, no FN400 effects were observed, not even the standard old–new effect. The parietal ERP was more positive for studied words than for lures. Additionally, late frontal ERP effects (1000–1500 ms, Studied[yes] = Lure[yes] > New[no]) were larger for good than for poor performers. Similar late frontal effects have been associated with strategic retrieval and evaluation processes (Johnson *et al.* 1996; Wilding and Rugg 1997a,b; Allan *et al.* 1998; Wilding 1999; Ranganath and Paller 2000; Curran and Friedman 2003).

Although the study of false recognition in the DRM paradigm by Curran *et al.* (2001) provided evidence that late frontal processes may be important for rejecting false memories, the results did not conform to expectations regarding the hypothesized relationship of the FN400 and parietal old–new effects to familiarity and recollection. However, Nessler *et al.* (2001) found a more consistent pattern of results in a similar experiment investigating false recognition of categorically related lures. A 300–500 ms mid-frontal FN400 showed the expected familiarity pattern (New[no] < Similar[yes] = Studied[yes]), whereas 500–700 ms parietal amplitudes showed a recollection pattern (New[no] < Similar[yes] < Studied[yes]). Notably, parietal differences between similar and new conditions suggest the possibility of 'false recollection' in this experiment, which was not observed in previous ERP experiments with similar lures (Curran 2000; Curran and Cleary 2003). Nessler *et al.* further split their subjects into groups with high versus low rates of false recognition. The group with high false recognition showed no FN400 or parietal differences between studied and similar words, but both conditions differed from new (similar to subjects with poor studied–similar discrimination in Curran and Cleary (2003)). The group with low false recognition showed typical FN400 and parietal studied–new differences, but no differences between similar and new.

In a second experiment, Nessler *et al.* (2001) tested the idea that different encoding strategies may have contributed to the group differences observed in their Experiment 1. When encoding focused on the conceptual similarity of the words, results were similar to those obtained for Experiment 1 subjects with high false-alarm rates. When encoding focused on the item-specific features, results were similar to those obtained for the Experiment 1 subjects with low false-alarm rates. Nessler and Mecklinger (2003) observed similar results in a subsequent experiment, except that FN400 similar–new differences were observed only after a short delay (40 s) and not after a long delay (80 s), as if the familiarity of lures declined across the delay. In summary, experiments by Nessler and colleagues (Nessler *et al.* 2001; Nessler and Mecklinger 2003) show that manipulating conceptual–semantic similarity leads to results very similar to manipulations of physical similarity (Curran 2000; Curran and Cleary 2003). In all cases, the 300–500 ms FN400 old–new effect is sensitive to familiarity (operationalized by differences between studied/similar, and new conditions), whereas the 400–800 ms parietal effect is sensitive to recollection (operationalized by differences between studied items and similar lures).

Evidence for 300–500 mid-frontal FN400 differences between new words and semantically similar lures suggests that the underlying processes are influenced by conceptual similarity (Nessler *et al.* 2001; Nessler and Mecklinger 2003). Indeed, it has been suggested that familiarity may primarily have a conceptual basis (Yonelinas 2002). However, research using novel visual objects called 'blobs' has suggested that FN400 old–new differences are also sensitive to perceptual similarity (Curran *et al.* 2002). Families (or categories) of blobs were created by a computer program that randomly generated a prototype and then procreated family members that were distortions of that prototype, similar to what has been done in studies of random dot classification (Posner and Keele 1968). In a training phase, subjects were shown the prototype and were asked to learn to identify a family of blobs whose members were physically similar to the prototype. Eight blobs which were in the family of the prototype were randomly intermixed with eight other blobs from outside the family, and each was presented 10 times in a task requiring subjects to categorize blobs as 'in' or 'out' of the family, with feedback. After each training set, EEG was recorded during two test lists with old and new blobs which could be either in the family or out of the family. Recognition test lists required subjects to make old–new judgements, whereas categorization test lists required subjects to make in–out judgements.

The experiment with blobs suggested that the 300–500 ms mid-frontal FN400 was sensitive to family membership as well as to recognition (Curran *et al.* 2002). FN400 was more negative to new than to old blobs, as well as being more negative to blobs outside the family than to blobs in the family. The 400–800 ms parietal effects differentiated between old and new blobs, but did not differentiate family members from non-members. Interestingly, an early (156–200 ms) N1 effect was more negative for family members than for non-members. Thus, taken as a whole, the experiment suggests a temporal transition such that earlier processes were sensitive to categorical discrimination (N1, 156–200 ms, in < out), intermediate processes were sensitive to both categorical and exemplar discrimination (FN400, 300–500 ms, in < out and new < old), and later processes were only sensitive to exemplar discrimination (parietal, 400–800 ms, old > new). The two earlier effects did not vary according to subject task (recognition versus categorization). In contrast, the parietal old–new difference was greater in the recognition than in the categorization task. The observation of task effects on parietal effects but not on FN400 effects is consistent with the perspective that recollection is particularly susceptible to intentional control, whereas familiarity is relatively automatic (Jacoby 1991; Yonelinas 2001). However, intentional retrieval may have less impact on the parietal recollection effect under less demanding conditions (Curran 1999).

Work described so far has suggested that FN400 familiarity effects are sensitive to dimensions of similarity ranging from purely perceptual (physically similar blobs (Curran *et al.* 2002)) to both perceptual and conceptual (similar words and pictures (Curran 2000; Curran and Cleary 2003)) to purely conceptual (categorically related words (Nessler *et al.* 2001; Nessler and Mecklinger 2003)). A more direct test of the relative importance of perceptual versus conceptual factors was undertaken in an experiment manipulating perceptual modality (Curran and Dien 2003). Subjects studied lists of words that were presented either visually or auditorily, and all recognition tests were visual. Both the 300–500 ms FN400 and the 400–800 ms parietal old–new effects were significant after both visual and auditory study. Thus neither effect appears to be influenced by changes in perceptual modality. Interestingly, an earlier (176–260 ms) frontal old–new difference was observed after visual but not after auditory study, and so it may be related to perceptual priming.

Challenges to the familiarity–recollection hypothesis of FN400 and parietal effects

Attention is an additional factor which may affect familiarity and recollection somewhat differently. Divided attention during study in behavioural experiments adversely affects familiarity and recollection, but affects recollection more strongly (Yonelinas 2001). Curran (2004) conducted two ERP experiments examining the effect of divided versus full attention at study on recognition of test items. Subjects studied two test lists of visually presented words. One list was studied with full attention, while the other was studied under divided attention.

To divide attention, numbers were presented auditorily and the subject pressed a button each time three consecutive odd numbers were heard. After the two study lists, the subject completed a recognition test with new words, divided attention words, and full attention words presented randomly.

Experiment 1 required subjects to discriminate between 'remembering' and 'knowing' at test (for a methodological review of the remember–know procedure see Gardiner and Richardson-Klavehn (2000)). Behavioural estimates of familiarity and recollection were both reduced by dividing attention, but divided attention had a stronger effect on recollection (replicating Yonelinas 2001). The 400–800 ms parietal ERP old–new effect was larger on trials associated with 'remembering' than with 'knowing' (replicating Smith 1993; Düzel *et al.* 1997; Rugg *et al.* 1998b; Trott *et al.* 1999), but the 300–500 ms FN400 old–new difference did not differ between 'knowing' and 'remembering'. On first consideration, one might expect the familiarity-related FN400 to be larger for 'knowing'. However, because 'knowing' is defined as the absence of 'remembering', familiarity levels for 'remember' and 'know' trials should be similar, i.e. items could be familiar regardless of whether or not they are recollected. Turning to the attention effects, the parietal old–new difference was larger after full attention during study than after divided attention, but the FN400 old–new difference was not influenced by dividing attention. This experiment appears to show an important difference between behavioural and electrophysiological indices of recollection and familiarity. Both behavioural estimates of recollection and the parietal ERP recollection effect were reduced by divided attention at study. However, the FN400 old–new difference was not influenced by divided attention, even though the behavioural estimate of familiarity was reduced.

Rather than collecting remember–know judgements at test, subjects in Experiment 2 (Curran 2004) rated their recognition responses on a four-point confidence scale (sure new, maybe new, maybe old, sure old). Words studied with full attention were recognized with greater confidence than those studied with divided attention (replicating Yonelinas 2001). Understanding how confidence influences the parietal old–new effect is important for reconciling single- and dual-process accounts of memory-related ERP effects. Some dual-process models conceptualize recollection as a high-threshold process that leads to high-confidence responses (Yonelinas 1994, 2001; Norman and O'Reilly 2003). From this perspective, conditions associated with higher recollection rates (e.g. full attention) would naturally foster higher confidence. However, from a single-process perspective that denies the existence of separate familiarity and recollection processes, confidence differences may be considered to reflect processes related more to decision-making than to memory retrieval *per se*. For example, Finnigan *et al.* (2002) have promoted the idea that different ERP old–new effects can be understood as a dissociation between a single memory process and relevant decision processes (a classic signal detection perspective) rather than separate memory processes of familiarity and recollection. Finnigan *et al.* found that a 300–500 ms N400 effect recorded over the parietal scalp varied with presentation frequency, so that the effect was considered to reflect familiarity (or 'strength' in their terminology). A later (500–800 ms) parietal effect varied with the accuracy of recognition judgements, and so it was interpreted as being related to decision processes. Thus Finnigan *et al.* essentially supported the FN400 familiarity hypothesis but challenged the parietal recollection hypothesis, favouring the idea that parietal old–new effects are merely related to decision processes. Measuring confidence can adjudicate between the recollection and decision process account of 400–800 ms parietal effects because confidence differences attributable to recollection should only be observed for old items, whereas confidence differences arising from genetic decision processes should be observed for both old and new items.

Curran's (2004) Experiment 2 supported the parietal recollection hypothesis, but support for the FN400 familiarity hypothesis was less clear. With regard to the recollection hypothesis, the 400–800 ms parietal ERP old–new difference was greater after full attention than after divided attention. Furthermore, confidence influenced 400–800 ms parietal amplitudes to old items but not to new items (replicating Rubin *et al.* 1999), and so the recollection hypothesis was supported over the decision-making hypothesis. With regard to 300–500 ms FN400 old–new effects, Experiment 2 (like Experiment 1) failed to find an effect of dividing attention, and so the FN400 did not respond in accord with expectations from behavioural estimates of familiarity. Curran speculated on the reasons for this null effect. First, power analyses indicated that the behavioural estimate of familiarity was more sensitive than FN400 to differences between full- and divided-attention conditions. Secondly, results from Experiment 2 suggest that confidence differences between the full- and divided-attention conditions may have obscured the influence of divided attention on FN400. Keeping in mind that confidence is higher after full attention than after divided attention, full-attention hits should be compared with high-confidence correct rejections and divided-attention hits should be compared with low-confidence correct rejections. These comparisons yielded significant FN400 old–new differences in the full-attention condition, but not in the divided-attention condition. Thus dividing attention appeared to have reduced FN400 old–new effects when confidence differences were taken into consideration.

A recent ERP study of the 'butcher on the bus' phenomenon raises important questions about the FN400 familiarity hypothesis (Yovel and Paller 2004).

Mandler (1980) noted that seeing familiar people in unfamiliar contexts, such as seeing your butcher on a bus, can lead to experiences of pure familiarity. Yovel and Paller (2004) studied a similar phenomenon experimentally by asking 12 subjects to study faces that were paired with verbally presented occupations. Subsequent recognition tests presented faces for old–new judgements. For faces judged old, subjects indicated whether they recollected the face's occupation, other specifics about studying the face, or no specifics. Recollection was inferred to be associated with correct recall of the occupation or other specifics. Pure familiarity was inferred from cases in which subjects correctly recognized the faces with no specifics. According to the FN400 familiarity hypothesis, 300–500 ms frontal old–new differences should be observed between old and new faces regardless of whether or not specifics were recollected. Contrary to this prediction, the results showed no evidence of 300–500 ms frontal old–new differences between any conditions. Yovel and Paller suggested that their results provide strong evidence against the familiarity hypothesis. Furthermore, it was suggested that 300–500 ms old–new differences that others have attributed to familiarity might be understood as being related to conceptual priming (see also Olichney *et al.* 2000) because FN400 old–new differences had been typically recorded in response to words or readily nameable pictures. However, other work has shown that the 300–500 ms FN400 old–new differences can be observed with novel visual objects (the 'blobs' described previously (Curran *et al.* 2002)) as well as faces (Norman *et al.* 2002; Nessler *et al.* 2005; Johansson *et al.*, in press). Given other demonstrations of FN400 old–new effects with faces, Yovel and Paller's results do not provide a very clear test of the familiarity hypothesis. A stronger test might be provided by an experiment showing typical FN400 old–new effects which did not behave in accord with familiarity, rather than demonstrating a null effect that could be attributed to innumerable experimental details. Understanding the conditions in which significant FN400 old–new effects are not observed (Curran *et al.* 2001; Yovel and Paller 2004) might further illuminate the nature of the underlying processes.

Olichney *et al.* (2000) similarly advanced the idea that 300–500 ms N400 old–new effects might be related to conceptual priming and/or short-term language comprehension processes. A mixed-aetiology group of amnesic patients completed a category verification task in which words were repeated with 0–13 intervening items. The amnesic patients showed normal 300–500 ms N400 old–new effects (comparing the first with repeated presentations), but impaired 500–800 ms parietal old–new effects. Only the parietal old–new effects were correlated with ability to recall and recognize the words later, and so the authors suggested that the N400 old–new effects might be related to conceptual priming and/or short-term language comprehension processes rather than to episodic memory. However, subsequent work challenges this hypothesis. First, experiments demonstrating significant 300–500 ms FN400 old–new effects with 'blobs' and faces suggests that a completely conceptual and linguistic basis is unlikely (Curran *et al.* 2002; Norman *et al.* 2002; Nessler *et al.* 2005; Johansson *et al.*, in press). Secondly, recent work has demonstrated that 300–500 ms old–new effects can be observed when memory for pictures is tested after a 1-day retention interval, so any short-term memory account of the FN400 is unlikely to be sufficient (Curran and Friedman 2004).

Brain mechanisms of familiarity and recollection

ERPs cannot precisely localize the brain mechanisms underlying familiarity and recollection processes, but other methods have yielded some relevant evidence (reviewed by Rugg and Yonelinas 2003). When groups of amnesic patients are tested without careful screening of the aetiology or anatomical origins of their functional deficits, impairment in both familiarity and recollection (more so) have been observed in experiments using behavioural estimation techniques such as the remember–know procedure, the process dissociation procedure, or receiver operating characteristic (ROC) procedures (Yonelinas *et al.* 1998). These results suggest that both familiarity and recollection are dependent upon some subset of the structures typically damaged in amnesia, such as the hippocampus and surrounding medial temporal cortex. In general, two different possibilities could be entertained. First, recollection and familiarity might depend on the same structures such that both processes would be impaired by damage to any component structure. Alternatively, recollection and familiarity might depend upon different structures such that damage limited to particular structures might selectively influence recollection and not familiarity, or vice versa. In general, Squire and colleagues have advanced the former view, arguing that both recollection and familiarity depend on the hippocampus and surrounding cortical regions (Manns *et al.* 2003; Stark and Squire 2003). Others have argued that recollection is specifically dependent on the hippocampus, whereas familiarity is dependent upon nearby temporal cortex (Aggleton and Brown 1999; Holdstock *et al.* 2002; Yonelinas 2002; Norman and O'Reilly 2003).

Several studies have shown that heterogenous forms of amnesia can diminish or abolish ERP old–new effects (Smith and Halgren 1989; Rugg *et al.* 1991; Mecklinger *et al.* 1998), but few studies have dissociated 300–500 ms FN400 and 400–800 ms parietal old–new effects in such patients. As mentioned previously, Olichney *et al.* (2000) found that a mixed group of amnesic patients showed normal short-term repetition effects on a 300–500 ms N400 component, but impaired 500–800 ms parietal repetition effects. To the extent to which these short-term repetition effects recorded during a category verification task are relevant to old–new effects observed in recognition memory experiments, this experiment suggests that the two ERP old–new effects are not dependent on equivalent brain mechanisms. Other evidence relating the 400–800 ms parietal ERP old–new effect to the hippocampus (Düzel *et al.* 2001) converges with the view that hippocampal activity is central to recollection (Rugg and Yonelinas 2003). An amnesic patient with seemingly isolated bilateral hippocampal damage sustained in childhood demonstrated a typical 300–500 ms FN400 old–new effect, but the 500–700 ms parietal old–new effect was absent (Düzel *et al.* 2001). These results are consistent with functional MRI (fMRI) studies indicating that hippocampal activity is specifically associated with 'remembering' rather than 'knowing' (Eldridge *et al.* 2000) and with source recollection (Dobbins *et al.* 2003).

Other fMRI evidence suggests that recollection-related activity originating from the parietal cortex itself may contribute to the parietal ERP old–new effect. Like the parietal ERP old–new effect (Smith 1993; Düzel *et al.* 1997; Rugg *et al.* 1998b; Trott *et al.* 1999; Curran 2004; Friedman, in press), fMRI studies have found that left parietal cortex activity is greater for 'remembering' than for 'knowing' (Henson *et al.* 1999; Eldridge *et al.* 2000; Wheeler and Buckner 2004). Furthermore, the parietal ERP old–new effect (Wilding *et al.* 1995; Wilding and Rugg 1996, 1997a,b; Trott *et al.* 1997; Rugg *et al.* 1998b) and parietal fMRI activation (Cansino *et al.* 2002; Dobbins *et al.* 2003) are both associated with accurate source memory. Evidence that both the hippocampus and the parietal cortex are related to the parietal ERP old–new effect is not necessarily incompatible because recollection is likely to involve the interaction between hippocampal and cortical networks (Norman and O'Reilly 2003).

Research using other recording and imaging techniques has suggested that familiarity and 300–500 ms FN400 old–new effects may arise from the anterior temporal (possibly perirhinal) cortex. Intracranial ERP old–new effects from epileptic patients show a 400 ms peak in anterior temporal regions (AMTL–N400) (Smith *et al.* 1986; Elger *et al.* 1997; Grunwald *et al.* 1998). Old–new effects recorded with magnetoencephalography (MEG) at latencies similar to FN400 (350–450 ms) have been estimated to arise within the left, anterior, and inferior temporal regions during recognition memory tests with words (Düzel *et al.* 2003). Recent fMRI research has documented perirhinal old–new differences thought to be related to familiarity because they were sensitive to neither intention–incidental task differences nor to the amount of contextual information retrieved (Henson *et al.* 2003).

Extensions to binding

Memory binding refers to the processes by which distinct aspects of a memory are linked together to form a coherent episode. In general, binding is similar to memory processes that others have called associative (Yonelinas *et al.* 2001), chunking (Wicklegren 1979), configural (Rudy and Sutherland 1994), conjunctive (O'Reilly and Rudy 2001), or relational (Eichenbaum and Cohen 2001). Although theoretical details differ among these authors, they all generally agree that the hippocampus and/or medial temporal cortex play an important role in memory binding. From a broader perspective, other memory phenomena requiring some type of binding include source recognition and context effects. For successful source recognition, information about the item must be bound to its source. Context effects are observed when item memory benefits from matching rather than mismatching study–test context (Godden and Baddeley 1980), and this requires some binding between item and context.

From a dual-process perspective, it has been claimed that familiarity is sufficient to support recognition of single items, yet recollection is necessary for associative recognition involving pairs of items (Yonelinas 1997, 1999; Hockley and Consoli 1999; Westerman 2001; Macken 2002). Indeed, much of the research supporting the recollection hypothesis of the 400–800 ms parietal ERP old–new effects can be conceptualized as requiring binding. When subjects are asked to recollect the modality (Wilding *et al.* 1995; Wilding and Rugg 1997b), speaker's voice (Rugg *et al.* 1998b; Wilding and Rugg 1996, 1997a), or temporal source (Trott *et al.* 1997) of studied words, the judgement requires binding between the words and these specific attributes. In all cases, the 400–800 ms parietal ERP old–new effect has been shown to depend upon recollection of these bound attributes. More direct evidence comes from studies of associative recognition in which subjects study pairs of words (e.g. table–shoe, pizza–cat, car–hammer) followed by associative recognition tests requiring discrimination between same pairs (table–shoe), rearranged pairs (pizza–hammer), and new pairs (pencil–lake). A 600–900 ms parietal ERP old–new effect is larger for correctly classified same pairs than for rearranged pairs (Donaldson and Rugg 1998, 1999).

A more contentious issue is whether or not familiarity can involve binding. Familiarity has sometimes been described as contextually insensitive (Atkinson and Juola 1974; Mandler 1980; Perfect *et al.* 1996; Tsivilis *et al.* 2001; Finnigan *et al.* 2002; Macken 2002), implying that item-context binding does not contribute to familiarity. Similarly, it has been suggested that associative recognition is influenced more by recollection than by familiarity (Yonelinas 1997; Rotello and Heit 2000). Although it may be true that familiarity is incapable of directly retrieving information about associated details such as source or context, nonetheless binding processes that link items together with associated information may contribute to the computation of familiarity. If we assume that the processes underlying familiarity operate similarly to the global matching models of memory, then it should be expected that familiarity is sensitive to contextual–associative variation. Although the associative–contextual mechanisms built into the global matching models have had difficulty accounting for detailed aspects of the empirical results and these difficulties have led some to favour dual-process accounts (reviewed by Clark and Gronlund 1996), it remains possible that familiarity is contextually–associatively sensitive. In general, according to the global matching perspective as well as the encoding specificity principle (Tulving and Thomson 1973), if items are encoded along with contextual–associative information, and contextual–associative information available at test is used to probe memory along with the test item, then familiarity should show contextual–associative effects. Indeed, the bind cue decided model of episodic memory (BCDMEM) suggests that the binding of items, contexts, and other information plays a central role in the computation of familiarity (Dennis and Humphreys 2001). A recent review found that the predictions made by global matching models are generally consistent with the pattern of effects found in environmental context-dependent memory (Smith and Vela 2001). The global matching models can also be extended to provide a more detailed account of context effects (Murnane *et al.* 1999). In summary, in principle there are reasons to believe that some form of binding may contribute to familiarity.

Tsivilis *et al.* (2001) have recently published an ERP experiment directly relevant to binding. Participants studied pictures of objects (e.g. radio, lantern, envelope) superimposed on unrelated scenes (e.g. lakes, mountains, valleys). A later recognition test specifically tested subjects' memory for the objects, but incidentally manipulated the background context. The object–context pairs were arranged into five conditions: same (studied object paired with studied scene), rearranged (studied object paired with a different studied scene), old–new (studied object paired with an unstudied scene), new–old (unstudied object paired with a studied scene), and new–new (both unstudied object and scene). When both parts (object and context) of the display were present at study and test (same and rearranged), the 300–500 ms FN400 differed from conditions in which the object and/or the context were new (old–new, new–old, new–new). The 700–900 ms parietal old–new effect differentiated between conditions associated with hits (same, rearranged, old–new) and those associated with correct rejection (new–old, new–new), regardless of the contextual manipulation. Regarding the notion of 'binding', comparing the same and rearranged conditions is critical because these conditions were equated for object familiarity and context familiarity. Differences between the same and rearranged conditions would indicate that the underlying memory processes are sensitive to the binding between objects and contexts. Tsivilis *et al.* did not observe any differences between the same and rearranged conditions, and so no evidence for binding was obtained.

One limitation of the study by Tsivilis *et al.* (2001) is that objects and contexts were not completely counterbalanced across the five conditions, and so the results may have been influenced by item effects. We recently replicated Tsivilis *et al.*'s experiment, but ensured complete counterbalancing of objects–contexts across subjects (Piatt, Curran, Collins, and Woroch, unpublished data). Only results from the same, rearranged, and new–new conditions are presented here because they are most pertinent to binding. Subjects were significantly more accurate in the same (83 per cent) than in the rearranged (78 per cent) conditions, and so their performance was sensitive to object–context binding. The new–new condition was more accurate (89 per cent) than either of the former conditions. The primary ERP results are shown in Figure 18.3. Condition (same, rearranged, new–new) × hemisphere analyses of variance (ANOVAs) were run on the 300–500 FN400 effects recorded over frontal regions (electrode clusters around F3 and F4) (Jasper 1958) and on the 400–800 ms parietal effects over parietal regions (electrode clusters around P3 and P4) (Jasper 1958). Condition effects were significant for both components: FN400, $F(2, 29) = 10.07$, MSE $= 2.23$, $P < 0.001$; parietal, $F(2, 29) = 6.04$, MSE $= 2.57$, $P < .01$. Critically, the difference between same and the rearranged conditions was significant for FN400 ($F(2, 29) = 6.97$, MSE $= 2.23$, $P = 0.01$) and marginally significant for

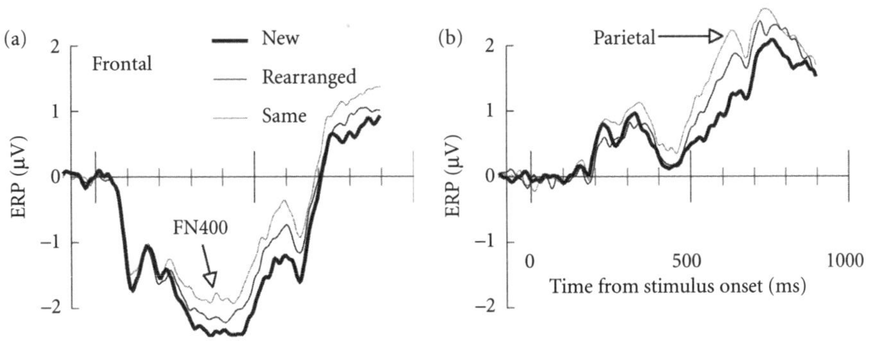

Figure 18.3 Primary results from Piatt, Curran, Collins, and Woroch (unpublished data). ERPs were computed from correct trials only. (a) Average ERPs from a cluster of left frontal sensors including the standard F3 location (Jasper 1958). (b) Average ERPs from a cluster of left parietal sensors including the standard P3 location (Jasper 1958).

the parietal effects ($F(2, 29) = 3.94$, MSE $= 2.57$, $P = 0.06$. These results suggest that, given the assumption that FN400 is related to familiarity, familiarity was sensitive to the binding of objects with contexts.

More work is needed to explore further the extent to which binding may influence the ERP correlates of recognition memory. For example, Donaldson and Rugg (1998, 1999) have observed 600–900 ms parietal ERP differences between same and rearranged conditions in experiments with word pairs, but did not report early differences that might be related to FN400. Another recent study with same, rearranged, and new word pairs reported widespread 300–600 ms same–rearranged differences (Van Petten *et al.* 2002). Although Van Petten *et al.* interpret their 300–600 ms results as replicating Donaldson and Rugg's (1998, 1999) 600–900 ms results, the temporal offset of these effects raises the question of whether their effects are more related to the 300–500 ms FN400 effects or the 400–800 ms parietal effects. Some have argued that associative effects on familiarity will occur to the extent to which the information to be associated can be encoded as a single unitized representation (Murnane *et al.* 1999; Yonelinas *et al.* 1999). It seems likely that the procedure of combining objects and contexts used by Tsivilis *et al.* (2001) is likely to foster more unitization than unrelated words, so this could explain why we were able to observe significant 300–500 ms FN400 same–rearranged differences with this method. Furthermore, subjects were specifically instructed to reject rearranged pairs in the associative recognition studies with words, whereas rearranged object–context pairs should be given 'yes' responses in the method of Tsivilis *et al.* because judgements were based on objects alone, regardless of context. Further research will be needed to test the relevance of these various factors, but the results of Piatt *et al.* (unpublished) clearly establish an influence of binding under the particular conditions of that experiment.

Binding may play a more important role in recollection than familiarity, but it may be overly simplistic to suggest that it influences only the former process. Norman and O'Reilly (2003) have developed a biologically plausible dual-process model suggesting that the hippocampus primarily contributes to recollection whereas adjacent cortical regions contribute to familiarity. Both the hippocampal recollection network and the cortical familiarity network support binding, but they do so in different ways. Familiarity may involve low-order cortical binding by conjoining only a small number of features, whereas recollection may benefit from higher-order binding within the hippocampus (O'Reilly *et al.* 2003). If, as we have argued, distinct ERP components are associated with recollection and familiarity, future ERP research may be useful for testing such theoretical perspectives on binding.

Acknowledgements

This research was supported by NIMH grant MH64812, the McDonnell–Pew Program in Cognitive Neuroscience, and the James S. McDonnell Foundation.

Notes

1. In addition to the 300–800 ms ERP old–new effects that are the focus of this review, late (roughly 800–1500 ms) right frontal ERP old–new effects are often observed. Their precise functional significance is unclear, but they are often associated with some sort of post-retrieval evaluation processes (reviewed by Allan *et al.* 1998; Friedman and Johnson 2000; Rugg and Allan 2000; Wilding and Sharpe 2003).
2. The 400–800 ms parietal ERP old–new effect co-occurs with the P300 component (Bentin and McCarthy 1994; Spencer *et al.* 2000), and has been variously labelled the P300 old–new difference (Johnson 1995), the late ERP old–new effect (Rugg 1995), the P600 old–new effect (Rugg and Doyle 1992; Curran 1999), and the late positive complex (LPC) (Olichney *et al.* 2000) old–new effect.
3. The 300–500 ms FN400 old–new effect has elsewhere been called the mid-frontal (Tsivilis *et al.* 2001), medial frontal (Friedman and Johnson 2000), or early frontal (Mecklinger 2000) old–new effect.
4. We have measured EEG with a 128-channel geodesic sensor net (Tucker 1993) and used an average-reference transformation to analyse ERPs (Curran *et al.* 1993; Dien 1998). With respect to the mastoid reference that is often used in ERP studies of memory, old–new effects are usually characterized by more positive amplitudes for old than for new items over superior regions of the scalp. With respect to the average reference, we typically find that the superior old > new differences are accompanied by inferior differences of opposite polarity (new < old), as can be see in Figure 18.2. Thus, when both superior and inferior regions are analysed, old–new effects are characterized by old–new × superior–inferior interactions. These interactions have been the focus of our earlier work, but we have generally found the superior aspects more reliable. Thus, for simplicity and comparability with mastoid reference results from other laboratories, we primarily focus on the superior effects in this review.

References

Aggleton, J.P. and Brown, M.W. (1999). Episodic memory, amnesia, and the hippocampal-anterior thalamic axis. *Behavioral and Brain Sciences*, **22**, 425–489.

Allan, K., Wilding, E.L., and Rugg, M.D. (1998). Electrophysiological evidence for dissociable processes contributing to recollection. *Acta Psychologica*, **98**, 231–252.

Atkinson, R.C. and Juola, J.F. (1973). Factors influencing speed and accuracy of word recognition. In *Attention and Performance IV* (ed S. Kornblum). New York: Academic Press, pp. 583–612.

Atkinson, R.C. and Juola, J.F. (1974). Search and decision processes in recognition memory. In *Contemporary Developments in Mathematical Psychology. I: Learning, Memory, and Thinking* (ed D.H. Krantz, R.C. Atkinson, R.D. Luce, and P. Suppes). San Francisco, CA: Freeman, pp. 243–293.

Bentin, S. and McCarthy, G. (1994). The effects of immediate stimulus repetition on reaction time and event-related potentials in tasks of different complexity. *Journal of Experimental Psychology: Learning, Memory, and Cognition*, **20**, 130–149.

Cansino, S., Maquet, P., Dolan, R.J., and Rugg, M.D. (2002). Brain activity underlying encoding and retrieval of source memory. *Cerebral Cortex*, **12**, 1048–1056.

Clark, S.E. and Gronlund, S.D. (1996). Global matching models of recognition memory: how the models match the data. *Psychonomic Bulletin and Review*, **3**, 37–60.

Curran, T. (1999). The electrophysiology of incidental and intentional retrieval: ERP old/new effects in lexical decision and recognition memory. *Neuropsychologia*, **37**, 771–785.

Curran, T. (2000). Brain potentials of recollection and familiarity. *Memory and Cognition*, **28**, 923–938.

Curran, T. (2004). Effects of attention and confidence on the hypothesized ERP correlates of recollection and familiarity. *Neuropsychologia*, **42**, 1088–1106.

Curran, T. and Cleary, A.M. (2003). Using ERPs to dissociate recollection from familiarity in picture recognition. *Cognitive Brain Research*, **15**, 191–205.

Curran, T. and Dien, J. (2003). Differentiating amodal familiarity from modality-specific memory processes: an ERP study. *Psychophysiology*, **40**, 979–988.

Curran, T. and Friedman, W.J. (2003). Differentiating location- and distance-based processes in memory for time: an ERP study. *Psychonomic Bulletin and Review*, **10**, 711–717.

Curran, T. and Friedman, W.J. (2004). ERP old/new effects at different retention intervals in recency discrimination tasks. *Cognitive Brain Research*, **8**, 107–120.

Curran, T., Tucker, D.M., Kutas, M., and Posner, M.I. (1993). Topography of the N400: brain electrical activity reflecting semantic expectation. *Electroencephalography and Clinical Neurophysiology*, **88**, 188–209.

Curran, T., Schacter, D.L., Johnson, M.K., and Spinks, R. (2001). Brain potentials reflect behavioral differences in true and false recognition. *Journal of Cognitive Neuroscience*, **13**, 201–216.

Curran, T., Tanaka, J.W., and Weiskopf, D.M. (2002). An electrophysiological comparison of visual categorization and recognition memory. *Cognitive, Affective, and Behavioral Neuroscience*, **2**, 1–18.

Deese, J. (1959). On the prediction of occurrence of particular verbal intrusions in immediate recall. *Journal of Experimental Psychology*, **58**, 17–22.

Dennis, S. and Humphreys, M.S. (2001). A context noise model of episodic word recognition. *Psychological Review*, **108**, 452–478.

Dien, J. (1998). Issues in the application of the average reference: review, critiques, and recommendations. *Behavior Research Methods, Instruments and Computers*, **30**, 34–43.

Dobbins, I.G., Rice, H.J., Wagner, A.D., and Schacter, D.L. (2003). Memory orientation and success: separable neurocognitive components underlying episodic recognition. *Neuropsychologia*, **41**, 318–333.

Donaldson, D.I. and Rugg, M.D. (1998). Recognition memory for new associations: electrophysiological evidence for the role of recollection. *Neuropsychologia*, **36**, 377–395.

Donaldson, D.I. and Rugg, M.D. (1999). Event-related potential studies of associative recognition and recall: electrophysiological evidence for context dependent retrieval processes. *Cognitive Brain Research*, **8**, 1–16.

Dosher, B.A. (1984). Degree of learning and retrieval speed: study time and multiple exposures. *Journal of Experimental Psychology: Learning, Memory, and Cognition*, **10**, 541–574.

Düzel, E., Yonelinas, A.P., Mangun, G.R., Heinze, H.-J., and Tulving, E. (1997). Event-related potential correlates of two states of conscious awareness in memory. *Proceedings of the National Academy of Sciences of the United States of America*, **94**, 5973–5978.

Düzel, E., Vargha-Khadem, F., Heinze, H.-J., and Mishkin, M. (2001). Brain activity evidence for recognition without recollection after early hippocampal damage. *Proceedings of the National Academy of Sciences of the United States of America*, **98**, 8101–8106.

Düzel, E., Habib, R., Schott, B., *et al.* (2003). A multivariate, spatiotemporal analysis of electromagnetic time-frequency data of recognition memory. *NeuroImage*, **18**, 185–197.

Eichenbaum, H. and Cohen, N.J. (2001). *From Conditioning to Conscious Recollection: Memory Systems of the Brain*. New York: Oxford University Press.

Eldridge, L.L., Knowlton, B.J., Furmanski, C.S., Bookheimer, S.Y., and Engel, S.A. (2000). Remembering episodes: a selective role for the hippocampus during retrieval. *Nature Neuroscience*, **3**, 1149–1152.

Elger, C.E., Grunwald, T., Lehnertz, K., *et al.* (1997). Human temporal lobe potentials in verbal learning and memory processes. *Neuropsychologia*, **35**, 657–667.

Fabiani, M., Gratton, G., and Coles, M.G.H. (2000). Event-related brain potentials. In *Handbook of Psychophysiology* (2nd edn) (ed J.T. Cacioppo). New York: Cambridge University Press, , pp. 53–84.

Finnigan, S., Humphreys, M.S., Dennis, S., and Geffen, G. (2002). ERP 'old/new' effects: memory strength and decisional factor(s). *Neuropsychologia*, **40**, 2288–2304.

Friedman, D. ERP studies of recognition memory: differential effects of familiarity, recollection, and episodic priming. *Cognitive Sciences*, , in press.

Friedman, D. and Johnson, R., Jr (2000). Event-related potential (ERP) studies of memory encoding and retrieval: a selective review. *Microscopy Research and Technique*, **51**, 6–28.

Gardiner, J.M. and Richardson-Klavehn, A. (2000). Remembering and knowing. In *Oxford Handbook of Memory* (ed E. Tulving and F.I.M. Craik). New York: Oxford University Press, pp. 229–244.

Gillund, G. and Shiffrin, R.M. (1984). A retrieval model for both recognition and recall. *Psychological Review*, **91**, 1–67.

Godden, D.R. and Baddeley, A.D. (1980). When does context influence recognition memory? *British Journal of Psychology*, **71**, 99–104.

Gronlund, S.D. and Ratcliff, R. (1989). Time course of item and associative information: Implications for global memory models. *Journal of Experimental Psychology: Learning, Memory, and Cognition*, **15**, 846–858.

Grunwald, T., Lehnertz, K., Heinze, H.J., Helmstaedter, C., and Elger, C.E. (1998). Verbal novelty detection within the human hippocampus proper. *Proceedings of the National Academy of Sciences of the United States of America*, **95**, 3193–3197.

Henson, R.N.A., Rugg, M.D., Shallice, T., Josephs, O., and Dolan, R.J. (1999). Recollection and familiarity in recognition memory: an event-related functional magnetic resonance imaging study. *Journal of Neuroscience*, **19**, 3962–3972.

Henson, R.N., Cansino, S., Herron, J.E., Robb, W.G., and Rugg, M.D. (2003). A familiarity signal in human anterior medial temporal cortex? *Hippocampus*, **13**, 301–304.

Hintzman, D.L. (1988). Judgments of frequency and recognition memory in a multiple-trace memory model. *Psychological Review*, **95**, 528–551.

Hintzman, D.L. and Curran, T. (1994). Retrieval dynamics of recognition and frequency judgments: evidence for separate processes of familiarity and recall. *Journal of Memory and Language*, **33**, 1–18.

Hintzman, D.L. and Curran, T. (1995). When encoding fails: instructions, feedback, and registration without learning. *Memory and Cognition*, **23**, 213–226.

Hintzman, D.L. and Curran, T. (1997). Comparing retrieval dynamics in recognition memory and lexical decision. *Journal of Experimental Psychology: General*, **126**, 228–247.

Hintzman, D.L., Curran, T., and Oppy, B. (1992). Effects of similarity and repetition on memory: Registration without learning? *Journal of Experimental Psychology: Learning, Memory, and Cognition*, **18**, 667–680.

Hockley, W.E. and Consoli, A. (1999). Familiarity and recollection in item and associative recognition. *Memory and Cognition*, **27**, 657–664.

Holdstock, J.S., Mayes, A.R., Roberts, N., ***et al.*** (2002). Under what conditions is recognition spared relative to recall after selective hippocampal damage in humans? *Hippocampus*, **12**, 341–351.

Humphreys, M.S., Bain, J.D., and Pike, R. (1989). Different ways to cue a coherent memory system: a theory for episodic, semantic, and procedural tasks. *Psychological Review*, **96**, 208–233.

Jacoby, L.L. (1991). A process dissociation framework: separating automatic from intentional uses of memory. *Journal of Memory and Language*, **30**, 513–541.

Jasper, H.A. (1958). The ten–twenty system of the International Federation. *Electroencephalography and Clinical Neurophysiology*, **10**, 371–375.

Johansson, M., Mecklinger, A., and Treese, A. Recognition memory for emotional and neutral faces: an event-related potential study. *Journal of Cognitive Neuroscience*, in press.

Johnson, M.K., Kounios, J., and Nolde, S.F. (1996). Electrophysiological brain activity and memory source monitoring. *Neuroreport*, **7**, 2929–2932.

Johnson, R.J. (1995). Event-related potential insights into the neurobiology of memory systems. In *Handbook of Neuropsychology*, Vol. 10 (ed F. Boller and J. Grafman). Amsterdam: Elsevier, pp. 135–163.

Macken, W.J. (2002). Environmental context and recognition: the role of recollection and familiarity. *Journal of Experimental Psychology: Learning, Memory, and Cognition*, **28**, 153–161.

Mandler, G. (1980). Recognizing: the judgment of previous occurrence. *Psychological Review*, **87**, 252–271.

Manns, J.R., Hopkins, R.O., Reed, J.M., Kitchener, E.G., and Squire, L.R. (2003). Recognition memory and the human hippocampus. *Neuron*, **37**, 171–180.

Mecklinger, A. (2000). Interfacing mind and brain: a neurocognitive model of recognition memory. *Psychophysiology*, **37**, 565–582.

Mecklinger, A., von Cramon, D.Y., and Matthes-von Cramon, G. (1998). Event-related potential evidence for a specific recognition memory deficit in adult survivors of cerebral hypoxia. *Brain*, **121**, 1919–1935.

Murdock, B.B. (1982). A theory of the storage and retrieval of item and associative information. *Psychological Review*, **89**, 609–626.

Murnane, K., Phelps, M.P., and Malmberg, K. (1999). Context-dependent recognition memory: the ICE theory. *Journal of Experimental Psychology: General*, **128**, 403–415.

Nessler, D. and Mecklinger, A. (2003). ERP correlates of true and false recognition after different retention delays: stimulus- and response-related processes. *Psychophysiology*, **40**, 146–159.

Nessler, D., Mecklinger, A., and Penney, T.B. (2001). Event related brain potentials and illusory memories: the effects of differential encoding. *Cognitive Brain Research*, **10**, 283–301.

Nessler, D., Mecklinger, A., and Penney, T.B. (2005). Perceptual fluency, semantic familiarity, and recognition-related familiarity: an electrophysiological exploration. *Cognitive Brain Research*, **22**, 265–288.

Norman, K.A. and O'Reilly, R.C. (2003). Modeling hippocampal and neocortical contributions to recognition memory: a complementary learning systems approach. *Psychological Review*, **110**, 611–646.

Norman, K.A., Curran, T., and Tepe, K. (2002). Event-related potential correlates of interference effects on recognition memory. Paper presented at the 43rd Annual Meeting of the Psychonomic Society, Kansas City, MO.

Olichney, J.M., Van Petten, C., Paller, K.A., Salmon, D.P., Iragui, V.J., and Kutas, M. (2000). Word repetition in amnesia: electrophysiological measures of impaired and spared memory. *Brain*, **123**, 1948–1963.

O'Reilly, R.C. and Rudy, J.W. (2001). Conjunctive representations in learning and memory: principles of cortical and hippocampal function. *Psychological Review*, **108**, 311–345.

O'Reilly, R.C. Busby, R.S., and Soto, R. (2003). Three forms of binding and their neural substrates: alternatives to temporal synchrony. In *The Unity of Consciousness: Binding, Integration, and Dissociation* (ed A. Cleeremans). Oxford: Oxford University Press, pp. 168–192.

Paller, K.A. and Kutas, M. (1992). Brain potentials during memory retrieval provide neurophysiological support of the distinction between conscious recollection and priming. *Journal of Cognitive Neuroscience*, **4**, 375–391.

Paller, K.A., Kutas, M., and McIsaac, H.K. (1995). Monitoring conscious recollection via the electrical activity of the brain. *Psychological Science*, **6**, 107–111.

Perfect, T.J., Mayes, A.R., Downes, J.J., and Van Eijk, R. (1996). Does context discriminate recollection from familiarity in recognition memory? *Quarterly Journal of Experimental Psychology*, **49**, 797–813.

Posner, M.I. and Keele, S.W. (1968). On the genesis of abstract ideas. *Journal of Experimental Psychology*, **77**, 353–363.

Ranganath, C. and Paller, K.A. (2000). Neural correlates of memory retrieval and evaluation. *Brain Research: Cognitive Brain Research*, **9**, 209–222.

Reed, A.V. (1973). Speed–accuracy tradeoff in recognition memory. *Science*, **181**, 574–576.

Roediger, H.L.I. and McDermott, K.B. (1995). Creating false memories: remembering words not presented in lists. *Journal of Experimental Psychology: Learning, Memory, and Cognition*, **21**, 803–814.

Rotello, C.M. and Heit, E. (2000). Associative recognition: a case of recall-to-reject processing. *Memory and Cognition*, **28**, 907–922.

Rubin, S.R., Van Petten, C., Glisky, E.L., and Newberg, W.M. (1999). Memory conjunction errors in younger and older adults: event-related potential and neuropsychological data. *Cognitive Neuropsychology*, **16**, 459–488.

Rudy, J.W. and Sutherland, R.J. (1994). The memory-coherence problem, configural associations, and the hippocampal system. In *Memory Systems 1994* (ed D.L. Schacter and E. Tulving). Cambridge, MA: MIT Press, pp. 119–146.

Rugg, M.D. (1995). ERP studies of memory. In *Electrophysiology of Mind* (ed M.D. Rugg and M.G.H. Coles). New York: Oxford University Press, pp. 132–170.

Rugg, M.D. and Allan, K. (2000). Event-related potential studies of memory. In *Oxford Handbook of Memory* (ed E. Tulving and F.I.M. Craik). New York: Oxford University Press, pp. 521–537.

Rugg, M.D. and Coles, M.G.H. (ed) (1995). *Electrophysiology of Mind*. New York: Oxford University Press.

Rugg, M.D. and Doyle, M.C. (1992). Event-related potentials and recognition memory for low- and high-frequency words. *Journal of Cognitive Neuroscience*, **5**, 69–79.

Rugg, M.D., and Yonelinas, A.P. (2003). Human recognition memory: a cognitive neuroscience perspective. *Trends in Cognitive Sciences*, **7**, 313–319.

Rugg, M.D., Roberts, R.C., Potter, D.D., Pickles, C.D., and Nagy, M.E. (1991). Event-related potentials related to recognition memory. effects of unilateral temporal lobectomy and temporal lobe epilepsy. *Brain*, **114**, 2313–2332.

Rugg, M.D., Cox, C.J.C., Doyle, M.C., and Wells, T. (1995). Event-related potentials and the recollection of low and high frequency words. *Neuropsychologia*, **33**, 471–484.

Rugg, M.D., Mark, R.E., Walla, P., Schloerscheidt, A.M., Birch, C.S., and Allan, K. (1998a). Dissociation of the neural correlates of implicit and explicit memory. *Nature*, **392**, 595–598.

Rugg, M.D., Schloerscheidt, A.M., and Mark, R.E. (1998b). An electrophysiological comparison of two indices of recollection. *Journal of Memory and Language*, **39**, 47–69.

Shiffrin, R.M. and Steyvers, M. (1997). A model of recognition memory: REM—retrieving effectively from memory. *Psychological Bulletin and Review*, **4**, 145–166.

Smith, M.E. (1993). Neurophysiological manifestations of recollective experience during recognition memory judgments. *Journal of Cognitive Neuroscience*, **5**, 1–13.

Smith, M.E. and Halgren, E. (1989). Dissociation of recognition memory components following temporal lobe lesions. *Journal of Experimental Psychology: Learning, Memory, and Cognition*, **15**, 50–60.

Smith, M.E., Stapleton, J.M., and Halgren, E. (1986). Human medial temporal lobe potentials evoked in memory and language tasks. *Electroencephalography and Clinical Neurophysiology*, **63**, 145–159.

Smith, S.M. and Vela, E. (2001). Environmental context-dependent memory: a review and meta-analysis. *Psychonomic Bulletin and Review*, **8**, 203–220.

Spencer, K.M., Vila Abad, E., and Donchin, E. (2000). On the search for the neurophysiological manifestation of recollective experience. *Psychophysiology*, **37**, 494–506.

Stark, C.E. and Squire, L.R. (2003). Hippocampal damage equally impairs memory for single items and memory for conjunctions. *Hippocampus*, **13**, 281–292.

Trott, C.T., Friedman, D., Ritter, W., and Fabiani, M. (1997). Item and source memory: differential age effects revealed by event-related potentials. *NeuroReport*, **8**, 3373–3378.

Trott, C.T., Friedman, D., Ritter, W., Fabiani, M., and Snodgrass, J.G. (1999). Episodic priming and memory for temporal source: event-related potentials reveal age-related differences in prefrontal functioning. *Psychology and Aging*, **14**, 390–413.

Tsivilis, D., Otten, L.J., and Rugg, M.D. (2001). Context effects on the neural correlates of recognition memory: an electrophysiological study. *Neuron*, **31**, 497–505.

Tucker, D.M. (1993). Spatial sampling of head electrical fields: the geodesic sensor net. *Electroencephalography and Clinical Neurophysiology*, **87**, 154–163.

Tulving, E. and Thomson, D.M. (1973). Encoding specificity and retrieval processes in episodic memory. *Psychological Review*, **80**, 352–373.

Van Petten, C., Luka, B.J., Rubin, S.R., and Ryan, J.P. (2002). Frontal brain activity predicts individual performance in an associative memory exclusion test. *Cerebral Cortex*, **12**, 1180–1192.

Westerman, D.L. (2001). The role of familiarity in item recognition, associative recognition, and plurality recognition on self-paced and speeded tests. *Journal of Experimental Psychology: Learning, Memory, and Cognition*, **27**, 723–732.

Wheeler, M.E. and Buckner, R. L. (2004). Functional-anatomic correlates of remembering and knowing. *NeuroImage*, **21**, 1337–1349.

Wicklegren, W.A. (1979). Chunking and consolidation: a theoretical synthesis of semantic networks, configuring in conditioning, S-R versus cognitive learning, normal forgetting, the amnesic syndrome, and the hippocampal arousal system. *Psychological Review*, **86**, 44–60.

Wilding, E.L. (1999). Separating retrieval strategies from retrieval success: an event-related potential study of source memory. *Neuropsychologia*, **37**, 441–454.

Wilding, E.L. and Rugg, M.D. (1996). An event-related potential study of recognition memory with and without retrieval of source. *Brain*, **119**, 889–905.

Wilding, E.L. and Rugg, M.D. (1997a). Event-related potential and the recognition memory exclusion task. *Neuropsychologia*, **35**, 119–128.

Wilding, E.L. and Rugg, M.D. (1997b). An event-related potential study of recognition memory for words spoken aloud or heard. *Neuropsychologia*, **35**, 1185–1195.

Wilding, E.L. and Sharpe, H. (2003). Episodic memory encoding and retreival: Recent insights from event-related potentials. In *The Cognitive Electrophysiology of Mind And Brain* (ed A. Zani and A.M. Proverbio). San Diego, CA: Academic Press, pp. 169–196.

Wilding, E.L., Doyle, M.C., and Rugg, M.D. (1995). Recognition memory with and without retrieval of context: an event-related potential study. *Neuropsychologia*, **33**, 743–767.

Yonelinas, A.P. (1994). Receiver-operating characteristics in recognition memory: evidence for a dual-process model. *Journal of Experimental Psychology: Learning, Memory, and Cognition*, **20**, 1341–1354.

Yonelinas, A.P. (1997). Recognition memory ROCs for item and associative information: The contribution of recollection and familiarity. *Memory and Cognition*, **25**, 747–763.

Yonelinas, A.P. (1999). The contribution of recollection and familiarity to recognition and source-memory judgments: a formal dual-process model and an analysis of receiver operating characteristics. *Journal of Experimental Psychology: Learning, Memory, and Cognition*, **25**, 1415–1434.

Yonelinas, A.P. (2001). Consciousness, control, and confidence: the 3 Cs of recognition memory. *Journal of Experimental Psychology: General*, **130**, 361–379.

Yonelinas, A.P. (2002). The nature of recollection and familiarity: a review of 30 years of research. *Journal of Memory and Language*, **46**, 441–517.

Yonelinas, A.P., Kroll, N.E., Dobbins, I., Lazzara, M., and Knight, R.T. (1998). Recollection and familiarity deficits in amnesia: convergence of remember–know, process dissociation, and receiver operating characteristic data. *Neuropsychology*, **12**, 323–339.

Yonelinas, A.P., Kroll, N.E., Dobbins, I.G., and Soltani, M. (1999). Recognition memory for faces: when familiarity supports associative recognition judgments. *Psychonomic Bulletin and Review*, **6**, 654–661.

Yonelinas, A.P., Hopfinger, J.B., Buonocore, M.H., Kroll, N.E., and Baynes, K. (2001). Hippocampal, parahippocampal and occipital-temporal contributions to associative and item recognition memory: an fMRI study. *Neuroreport*, **12**, 359–363.

Yovel, G. and Paller, K.A. (2004). The neural basis of the butcher-on-the-bus phenomenon: when a face seems familiar but is not remembered. *NeuroImage*, **21**, 789–800.

Chapter 19

Mnemonic binding in the medial temporal lobe

Barbara J. Knowlton and Laura L. Eldridge

Introduction

It has long been known that the medial temporal lobe (MTL) is critical for conscious, or declarative, memory. However, debate continues to surround the precise role of the neural components of this region. The MTL is comprised of several interconnected structures known to be involved in memory, including the hippocampus and the entorhinal, perirhinal, and parahippocampal cortices. Recent evidence suggests that these different structures may make functionally dissociable contributions to memory processes. In this chapter we will consider the distinction between different forms of declarative memory while reviewing the current evidence regarding the specific role of the hippocampus in these processes.

In order to understand the role of the MTL in declarative memory, it is important to consider the anatomical connections of the component structures (Figure 19.1). The hippocampus, one structure of the MTL, has featured prominently in theories of declarative memory (Rempel-Clower *et al.* 1996). However, it is clear that adjacent cortical regions (the entorhinal, perirhinal, and parahippocampal cortices) also play a prominent role. In general, the surrounding cortical structures send input to the hippocampus and also receive the output of the hippocampal system (Amaral 1993). The entorhinal cortex serves as the primary gateway to the hippocampus proper, projecting to the dentate gyrus. Neurons then project in a loop through the hippocampus, beginning with field CA3, then progressing to field CA1, the subiculum, and finally back to entorhinal cortex. The MTL circuit is completed as the entorhinal cortex sends output to the parahippocampal and perirhinal cortices, which in turn send projections to a number of temporal, frontal, and parietal lobe regions (Rosene and Van Hoesen 1977).

In addition to this simple circuit, there are other important projections within the MTL. Some entorhinal cells bypass the dentate gyrus to synapse on cells

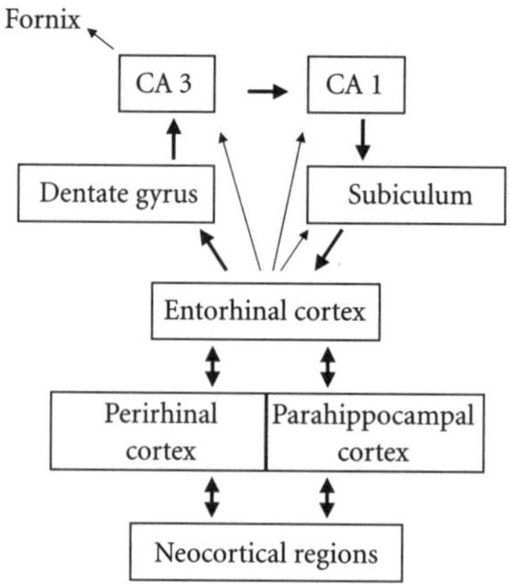

Figure 19.1 Diagram of components and connections within the medial temporal lobe system.

within CA3, CA1, and the subiculum (Amaral 1993). Projections from the hippocampus reach subcortical structures via the fornix to innervate diencephalic structures, including the mammillary and septal nuclei of the hypothalamus (Amaral 1993). Damage to these diencephalic structures, as seen in patients with Korsakoff's syndrome, can produce amnesia that is very similar to that seen after MTL damage (Kopelman 1989). In addition, cells in the CA1 and subicular regions send direct projections to the frontal, temporal, and parietal cortices (Insausti and Munoz 2001).

The fact that the hippocampus is the ultimate recipient of a convergence of information from several association cortices suggests that it is well suited to bind together disparate elements of an experience during memory formation. The reciprocal output pattern of the hippocampus is also consistent with the idea that it reactivates cortical sites of memory storage during the retrieval of memories. Based on anatomical connections, MTL cortical structures not only appear to provide the hippocampus with input, but the extensive connections that these structures have with other cortical regions suggest that they may also make independent contributions to memory function. The examination of patients with MTL damage has been critical for deducing the function of these structures.

Neuropsychological data

Anterograde amnesia

Ever since Milner (1958) reported the case of HM, a young man who underwent brain surgery to treat intractable epilepsy, it has been clear that the MTL plays a critical role in the formation and storage of newly acquired memories. Large portions of the MTL were excised bilaterally to remove the neural focus of HM's seizures, and this resulted in a profound anterograde amnesia. The lesions caused by HM's surgery were extensive and affected several structures within the MTL, including the hippocampus, surrounding cortical structures, and the amygdala. As a result of the diffuse lesions, it was not clear what roles individual structures might play in memory processes. However, this striking case served to focus investigators on the critical role that the MTL region plays in the formation and storage of new memories.

Neuropsychological tests of patients with focal MTL lesions reveal selective impairments to memory, while other cognitive functions remain intact (Zola-Morgan *et al.* 1986). The memory deficits associated with amnesia typically extend to both verbal and non-verbal domains (Zola-Morgan *et al.* 1986; Squire 1992; Rempel-Clower *et al.* 1996). Although amnesic patients may be able to recall information after very brief delays, they are severely impaired when the delays are increased to only a few minutes. Patients with lesions limited to the hippocampal region exhibit amnesia; however, it is generally much milder than the degree of deficit in patients with more extensive medial temporal lobe damage. For example, focal hippocampal patient RB was able to recall several details of a prose passage immediately after it had been read, but could not recall the passage after a delay of 12 min (Zola-Morgan *et al.* 1986). Nevertheless, this patient was able to score above chance levels on easier memory tasks.

A key question in the neuropsychology of memory is whether patients with selective hippocampal damage have relative preservation of some declarative memory abilities or a qualitatively similar amnesia to patients with more extensive damage. Consistent with the former, some evidence indicates that patients with damage limited to the hippocampus exhibit a selective impairment of memory for episodes, with relatively preserved memory for recognizing items and recalling facts (Vargha-Khadem *et al.* 1997). According to this view, memory for episodes relies on a distinct neural system. Because episodic memories are linked to a specific time and place, allowing one to re-experience the original event, these memories reflect the retrieval of a bound representation of the spatiotemporal context in which encoding occurred. In contrast, some retrieved memories may be accompanied only by a feeling of familiarity. These 'non-episodic', or familiarity-based, memories lack the rich recollective component that is the hallmark of episodic memory (Tulving 1985). For example, knowledge of facts about the world or the retrieval of one's semantic memories may not be accompanied by the recollection of the episode in which the facts were learned.

Although episodic and semantic memory may represent different forms of memory, there is conflicting evidence from neuropsychological patients as to whether they are functionally dissociable in the MTL. Some evidence indicates that damage restricted to the hippocampus is sufficient to impair both episodic and semantic memory performance (Ostergaard and Squire 1990; Rempel-Clower *et al.* 1996; Squire and Zola 1998; Manns *et al.* 2003). For example, a subset of patients identified as having damage restricted primarily to the hippocampal region (although in some cases damage to the entorhinal cortex was also noted) exhibited impairments on episodic and non-episodic memory tasks (Rempel-Clower *et al.* 1996). While these data suggest that the hippocampus is necessary for both episodic and semantic memory, it is virtually impossible to rule out the possibility that these global declarative memory deficits were the result of damage beyond the hippocampus.

There has also been some neuropsychological evidence suggesting that the hippocampus selectively supports episodic memories (Moscovitch 1995; Vargha-Khadem *et al.* 1997; Tulving and Markowitsch 1998; Aggleton and Brown 1999). For example, a study of amnesic patients who had sustained damage restricted to the hippocampal formation early in life (neonatally or early in childhood) revealed that, despite profound episodic memory deficits, they were able to acquire new semantic knowledge (Vargha-Khadem *et al.* 1997). These individuals were able to progress through standard schools, although they were unable to remember virtually any episodic information, such as the events of the day or where they had placed their house keys. Strikingly, these children not only acquired language, but also learned to read and write, learned social norms, and were even able to perform in the low average range of standardized tests in school (Vargha-Khadem *et al.* 1997). These findings suggest that focal hippocampal damage may result in a profound inability to acquire episodic memories, while the acquisition of non-episodic information is relatively spared.

One difficulty in interpreting these data is that tests of episodic and semantic memory generally differ in terms of difficulty. Episodic memories are comprised of multiple elements and occur only once, while semantic memories may be fairly simple and can be supported by multiple learning trials. Squire and Zola (1998) have argued that the patients with selective hippocampal damage during childhood may have demonstrated some sparing of episodic memory, which may have made it possible for them to slowly acquire semantic knowledge. In addition, plasticity following damage early in life could potentially explain the ability to acquire semantic knowledge following hippocampal damage that would otherwise not occur (Squire and Zola 1998). In these patients, MTL structures outside the MTL may have been able to assume memory functions subserved by the hippocampus in neurologically intact individuals. However, fairly selective episodic memory deficits have also been noted in hippocampal patients who sustained damage later in life (Verfaellie *et al* 2000; Mayes *et al.* 2002). Thus the role of the hippocampus in episodic and semantic memory remains under debate.

It should be noted that studies of neuropsychological patients cannot fully dissociate impairments in the encoding, storage, and retrieval of information. It is clear that patients with circumscribed hippocampal damage have impairments in their ability to learn new information, and they may also have difficulty in retrieving information normally. The issue of the nature of memory encoding is of particular importance when considering whether hippocampal damage results in a differential impairment to episodic memory. The re-experience of time and place during retrieval is a critical feature which differentiates episodic memories from other forms of declarative memory, but it is unclear whether memories are all initially encoded as episodes. Some memories may become non-episodic with time, as memory for the incidental details supporting the memory and the links between them decay (Squire and Zola 1998). For example, meeting a new person may initially result in a strong episodic memory for the encounter, although eventually the person may merely evoke a sense of familiarity. In addition, repeated similar experiences may result in the loss of distinctiveness for the elements of an episodic memory, eventually leading to a transition to semantic knowledge. For example, the first time a new fact is recalled it may be retrieved in the context of its learning episode, while the retrieval of repeatedly encountered familiar facts may not elicit the same contextual detail. In contrast, in another view, some memories may be encoded independently of their spatiotemporal context and thus will never available to be retrieved as part of an episode (Tulving and Markowitsch 1998; Aggleton and Brown 1999).

These different theories of the relative independence of episodic and non-episodic memories make different predictions regarding the effect of hippocampal damage. If all declarative memories are encoded as episodes, then hippocampal damage may lead to a general memory impairment, potentially accompanied by a disproportionate difficulty in reinstantiating the learning episode. In contrast, if memories can be encoded separately from the learning episode in which they occur, non-episodic memory ought to be relatively spared in patients with selective hippocampal damage. Unfortunately, previous studies have been unable to determine conclusively the extent of hippocampal involvement in these mnemonic processes.

Retrograde amnesia

Although the inability to form new memories is a hallmark of amnesia, the additional loss of memories preceding damage also provides important insight into the functions of the MTL. Many amnesic patients suffer from a retrograde amnesia that accompanies their anterograde amnesia (Reed and Squire 1998). The characteristics of retrograde amnesia vary between reports; in some cases retrograde amnesia is described as extensive, affecting both remote and recent memories (Kopelman *et al.* 1999), while most cases are described as temporally graded, in which more remote memories are spared (Alvarez *et al.* 1995; Reed and Squire 1998). It appears that lesions restricted primarily to the hippocampus generally result in the loss of declarative memories for a limited time period prior to the lesion, and as the extent of the MTL lesion increases so does the extent of the retrograde amnesia (Reed and Squire 1998). It is difficult to assess which regions of the MTL may be most important for declarative retrieval using neuropsychological patients, in part because it is difficult to determine whether newly formed memories could be retrieved normally if the memories were never adequately encoded. In addition, the rather diffuse lesions make it difficult to determine the differential contributions of individual structures.

Reed and Squire (1998) reported that hippocampal patients with limited retrograde amnesia can have intact autobiographical memories for periods that occurred before their memory was affected, suggesting that episodic memories can become independent of the hippocampus. However, these autobiographical memories may not be entirely normal. The patients tended to have a longer latency between cue presentation and the recollection of an episodic memory and also required more prompts to retrieve the episodic memory than controls. This suggests that, at the very least, these patients were having some difficulty in accessing their episodic memories. It is also possible that the retrieved memories differ qualitatively from those of individuals with intact MTL systems, but the way to compare the qualitative nature of these memories is not readily apparent.

There is some question regarding whether retrograde amnesia resulting from MTL damage selectively affects episodic memories (Nadel and Moscovitch 1997) or impairs both episodic and semantic memory retrieval similarly (Rempel-Clower *et al.* 1996). It may be that the nature of the retrograde amnesia, and not only the degree, is affected by the specific structures damaged within the MTL. Damage to the hippocampus alone may affect retrograde episodic memories disproportionately, while more extensive MTL damage results in retrograde amnesia for episodic and semantic information. However, the extent to which episodic and semantic memories are differentially affected is often difficult to assess because of the lack of standardized tests of episodic memories, which are unique to each individual. In addition, the quality and accuracy of episodic memories cannot be reliably determined because it is difficult to know whether a memory has been fabricated or was in fact experienced. It is also difficult to assess whether subjects are truly experiencing older memories as episodes or, rather, are recalling semantic information about events that had happened to them. While it is difficult to assess the nature of episodic and non-episodic memory, the use of neuroimaging provides some additional insight into the contribution of MTL structures to the different forms of declarative memory.

Functional MRI studies

Encoding

Neuroimaging techniques provide a means of measuring patterns of neural activity associated with encoding and retrieval processes in normal healthy participants. Several recent studies have used functional neuroimaging in order to identify MTL regions that are important for establishing memories. The encoding tasks typically require that the participants intentionally memorize the stimulus items, although in some cases the memorization is incidental. These studies have revealed robust activations within the MTL region, as reflected by the large number of studies which have reported encoding related MTL activations using positron-emission tomography (PET) (Haxby *et al.* 1996; Vandenberghe *et al.* 1996; Dolan and Fletcher 1997) and functional MRI (fMRI) (Stern *et al.* 1996; Gabrieli *et al.* 1997; Brewer *et al.* 1998; Kelley *et al.* 1998; Wagner *et al.* 1998b; Dolan and Fletcher 1999; Fernández *et al.* 1999; Davachi *et al.* 2003; Kensinger *et al.* 2003; Zeineh *et al.* 2003; reviewed by Lepage *et al.* 1998; Schacter and Wagner 1999). Owing to the complexity of structures within the MTL, precise anatomical localization of activity is critical. Because PET studies lack the spatial resolution necessary to make strong claims regarding MTL contributions to memory, this review will focus primarily on fMRI data which can more reliably discern the contribution of individual MTL structures.

Because of technical limitations initial investigations into the neural correlates of encoding were restricted to blocked trial designs. In these studies, subjects viewed alternating blocks of novel and familiar items and the levels of MR activity during these two types of blocks were compared. For example, Stern *et al.* (1996) found greater posterior hippocampal and parahippocampal activity during the intentional encoding of novel visual scenes compared with the encoding of familiar visual scenes that had been presented prior to scanning. In addition, Gabrieli *et al.* (1997) reported greater activity bilaterally in the parahippocampal cortex during the incidental encoding of novel pictures compared with familiar pictures, leading to the suggestion that MTL activations may reflect novelty detection.

Consistent with neuropsychological studies, subsequent evidence has indicated that the role of the MTL during encoding is greater than simply the detection of novelty (Brewer *et al.* 1998; Fernández *et al.* 1998; Wagner *et al.* 1998b; Davachi *et al.* 2003; Zeineh *et al.* 2003). MTL activity appears to reflect encoding processes that are critical for later retrieval. For example, a blocked trial fMRI study revealed MTL activity in the hippocampal region during encoding that was correlated with the ability to retrieve the studied information later (Fernández *et al.* 1998). A recent high-resolution fMRI study increased the specificity of previous findings, indicating that the CA2, CA3, and the dentate gyrus may play a distinct role in the storage of new associations (Zeineh *et al.* 2003). The level of activity in the CA fields and dentate gyrus changed during learning, decreasing in step with the decreasing number of new face–name associations to be learned across blocks in the study, thus supporting the idea that the hippocampus plays an integral role in binding together information to form new associations.

The use of event-related designs further extends the utility of neuroimaging studies by making it possible to compare the magnitude of MTL activity during encoding associated with items that are later remembered versus those that are later forgotten. This retrieval comparison has been made using familiar words (Wagner *et al.* 1998b) and pictures (Brewer *et al.* 1998). Wagner *et al.* (1998b) found greater activity in the left parahippocampal gyrus for words that were subsequently recognized with high confidence than for words that were forgotten. Brewer *et al.* (1998) additionally probed participants during retrieval to assess their ability to recall episodic detail using the remember–know recognition task. In this task, subjects evaluate the content of their recognition memories as to whether they are able to remember the specific time and place in which the item was encountered or whether the subject simply 'knows' that the item occurred in the absence of specific recollections about the moment of learning (Tulving 1985). Greater activity in the parahippocampal cortex, bilaterally, was evident for items later labelled as 'remembered' (episodic) rather than 'known' (familiarity based), and also for items labelled as 'known' rather than forgotten. The results from both studies suggest that the extent to which the parahippocampal region is engaged may be one critical factor that influences the later memorability of information.

More recent evidence suggests that the hippocampus proper is engaged during learning only when detailed information is encoded that is able to support later recollection. Kensinger *et al.* (2003) used a divided-attention paradigm to vary the amount of detail that participants would encode by manipulating the difficulty of an auditory discrimination task. While the left anterior hippocampus was engaged during the easy encoding condition, in which more detail could be encoded, the left inferior parahippocampus was active during both the easy and the hard encoding conditions. Davachi *et al.* (2003) compared MTL encoding activity for items that would later be recognized with and without the recollection of contextual source information. Similar to the results reported by Kensinger *et al.* (2003), activity in the hippocampus during encoding was correlated with the ability to recall the source of the memory later. In addition, the posterior parahippocampal cortex exhibited a similar pattern of responses to the hippocampus. These data suggest a clear role for the hippocampus in establishing episodic memory traces, but leave open the extent to which the parahippocampus is involved in more general encoding processes. Thus, while these studies together suggest a clear role for the hippocampus in establishing episodic memory traces, the role of other MTL structures remains elusive. It is possible that there are dual mechanisms for encoding, with the parahippocampal cortex supporting non-episodic encoding. Further experiments are needed to determine whether these dual-encoding routes are independent, or whether the parahippocampal cortex contributes to both episodic and non-episodic encoding.

The perirhinal cortex may also be involved in memory encoding (Davachi *et al.* 2003; Strange *et al.* 2002). Results from subdural event-related potential (ERP) recording in humans have revealed responses within the rhinal cortex (as well as within the hippocampus) that differentiated whether an item was later remembered or forgotten (Fernández *et al.* 1999). A more recent neuroimaging study, in which subjects encoded items using rote rehearsal, revealed a subsequent memory effect localized to the perirhinal cortex (Strange *et al.* 2002). It appears that the role of the perirhinal cortex in encoding is not tied to the ability to recall episodic detail of the source of the memory later (Davachi *et al.* 2003). Davachi *et al.* found that, while the hippocampus and parahippocampus may be involved in binding features of an event to establish an episodic memory, the perirhinal cortex may be more generally involved in establishing a memory trace for the item. It is not clear whether the perirhinal cortex and the parahippocampal cortex play fundamentally different roles in memory encoding, or whether they are differentially affected by the materials or encoding task used.

In summary, fMRI studies of MTL have revealed different neural signatures within the hippocampus, parahippocampus, and perirhinal cortex during encoding. Although early investigators described the role of the MTL in terms of novelty detection, more recent neuroimaging results, consistent with neuropsychological evidence, point to a more complex involvement in encoding processes. Indeed, novel items should engender greater encoding processes than items previously seen because there is no pre-existing memory representation for these items. Thus it appears likely that novelty responses in the MTL reflect encoding processes. A related interpretation is that the detection of novelty provides a cue that triggers encoding processes (Tulving *et al.* 1996). Support for this idea comes from the fact that later recognition of items that are novel in a particular situation is better than later recognition of items that are familiar in that context (Habib *et al.* 2003).

Retrieval

The ability to assess the neural substrate of declarative retrieval processes when information has been properly encoded is a unique advantage of neuroimaging studies. Although neuropsychological studies have revealed both anterograde and retrograde amnesia following MTL damage, many early neuroimaging studies (primarily using PET) failed to detect MTL activity and instead revealed robust responses in the frontal regions (Kapur *et al.* 1995; Tulving *et al.* 1996; Fletcher *et al.* 1998a,b, 1999). However, subsequent studies have reported MTL activity during the retrieval of test stimuli (Aguirre and D'Esposito 1997; Henson *et al.* 1999; Eldridge *et al.* 2000; Stark and Squire 2000), supporting the notion that MTL structures are involved in retrieval.

Investigators have attempted to distinguish whether MTL structures are involved in the retrieval of both episodic and non-episodic memories. This question is particularly relevant at retrieval because it is at this point that episodic memory is differentiated from other forms of declarative memory, as the complex conjunction of features that comprised the encoding context are reinstated as a bound representation. To date, studies have not fully resolved whether the hippocampus is critical for all forms of declarative memory or is really only necessary for processing episodic memories. Several studies have relied upon recognition tasks in which the subject makes old–new judgements for each item (e.g. Wagner *et al.* 1998a). Because a simple recognition task collapses across items that are recognized based on familiarity and those that are accompanied by episodic recollection, it is difficult to reveal the precise role of the MTL. In an attempt to probe the nature of recognition, some studies have employed the remember–know task. Henson *et al.* (1999) found MTL activity memory retrieval, but did not find evidence of a distinction between 'remembered' (episodic) and 'known' (non-episodic) memories. In contrast, Eldridge *et al.* (2000) found that the hippocampus was selectively active during retrieval for the recollection of episodic memories. Importantly, hippocampal activity did not differ either from baseline or from one another for 'known', correctly rejected, or forgotten items. The difference in results between the two studies may be due to key differences in task instructions. The remember–know task as administered by Henson *et al.* (1999) may not have adequately differentiated episodic and familiarity-based recognition because the instructions used by the experimenters tend to induce subjects to operationalize 'remember' and 'know' in terms of confidence, rather than as different forms of declarative memory. It appears that it is easier for subjects to evaluate the nature of their recognition response if they first decide whether they confidently recognize the item, and then decide whether their recognition decision is based on episodic recollection or familiarity, rather than making a three-alternatives decision between 'remember', 'know', and 'new' (Eldridge *et al.* 2002).

Manipulations of encoding to influence the likelihood of later episodic retrieval further suggest that the hippocampus may be selectively involved at retrieval in supporting episodic memories. In the same study that found differential hippocampal responses during the encoding of episodic memories, the left hippocampus was also found to be active during the retrieval of items that were encoded in a manner that facilitated the formation of episodic memories (Kensinger *et al.* 2003). The left anterior hippocampus was selectively engaged during the retrieval of words that had been encoded under 'easy' conditions that would increase the chance that the memory would be episodic rather than familiarity based. In contrast, the left parahippocampal cortex was active during retrieval, regardless of encoding conditions and the level of detail subsequently available at retrieval (Kensinger *et al.* 2003). Thus there is some evidence that the hippocampus may play a differential role in retrieving episodic memories, while other surrounding MTL structures are involved more generally in declarative memory retrieval.

Evidence from neuroimaging studies indicates a specific role for the perirhinal cortex in signalling stimulus familiarity (Henson *et al.* 2003). Over the course of several fMRI studies conducted by a single laboratory, a striking pattern of decreased perirhinal activity for familiar items relative to novel items became evident. In these studies stimulus familiarity was signalled as a decrease relative to baseline, similar to human electrophysiology results (Fried *et al.* 2002). The perirhinal cortex and adjacent parahippocampal cortex are well positioned to signal stimulus familiarity, based on both their relative anatomical relationship with the hippocampus and the response properties of neurons that comprise the structures (Brown and Aggleton 2001). Neurons within the perirhinal cortex have been found to change their firing rate following a single stimulus presentation (Brown *et al.* 1987), consistent with a system that tracks the relative familiarity of particular items.

One difficulty in interpreting activation in the MTL during memory retrieval is that it is likely that the retrieval cues and the information that has been retrieved by the subject are in fact automatically encoded into memory. Thus spontaneously occurring encoding-related activity may be interpreted as reflecting underlying retrieval processes. Consistent with this idea, overlapping hippocampal, parahippocampal, and perirhinal regions were found to be active during both encoding and retrieval (Stark and Okado 2003), potentially reflecting automatic encoding responses during retrieval. Although the same structures seem to be involved in encoding and retrieval, it is possible that subregions within these MTL structures may participate in distinct functions. Within the hippocampus, differences in connectivity of the separate subregions suggest that they make different contributions to memory performance. In the study by Stark and Okada (2003), it was impossible to differentiate the contribution of discrete components of the hippocampus. A more recent study using high-resolution fMRI techniques indicates that while subregions of the hippocampal circuit (CA2, CA3 and the dentate gyrus) were engaged during encoding, a subregion later in the circuit (subiculum) was engaged during episodic retrieval (Eldridge *et al.* 2005). Similarly, as discussed previously, Zeineh *et al.* (2003) found that while activity in the CA2, CA3, and the dentate gyrus appeared to reflect the acquisition of new associations, the subiculum was recruited during the retrieval of those associations. Thus earlier neuroimaging findings regarding the overlapping role of the hippocampus in encoding and retrieval may reflect the relative contributions of individual subcomponents to episodic memory.

Retrieval of remote memories

Based on the phenomenon of temporally graded retrograde amnesia that has been demonstrated following MTL damage, one would predict that there may be differences in the level of activation in the MTL during retrieval depending on the age of the memory. The retrieval of old memories may be accompanied by a lower fMRI signal than during the retrieval of recently acquired memories. Because retrograde memory gradients are particularly steep following damage limited to the hippocampus, one might predict that hippocampal signal increases during retrieval may be restricted to fairly recently acquired memories. In fact, findings from fMRI studies have not been reliably consistent with results from lesion studies, for the most part because of the difficulties inherent in retrospectively assessing memories and interpreting fMRI signals. Although the MTL has been found to be active during the retrieval of retrograde memories, clear evidence of a temporal gradient has sometimes been elusive. Using a test of recall of the names of famous faces, Haist *et al.* (2001) found a clear temporal gradient of activation in the entorhinal cortex, with activation greater for faces that had become famous in the previous decade compared with faces that had become famous 20 years earlier. In the hippocampus, activation accompanied the retrieval of faces from the previous decade, but this was not significantly higher than the activation during retrieval of the more remote time periods, which was not significantly above baseline levels. These results suggest that the hippocampus itself may not be involved in the consolidation of memories over decades, but that the entorhinal cortex may have such a role. These results are consistent with neuropsychological data showing that damage limited to the hippocampus results in mild retrograde amnesia for only a few years before the damage, while lesions that include adjacent cortical regions result in retrograde amnesia which can include decades before the insult. The results obtained by Haist *et al.* (2001) demonstrate a temporal gradient in the involvement of MTL structures in retrieving memories. However, only semantic memory for the names of famous faces was assessed in this study. It may be that a different pattern would emerge for episodic memories, which require the recollection of the specific time and place that memories were formed.

Some evidence indicates a lack of a temporal gradient in hippocampal activation for memories of personal experiences (Ryan *et al.* 2001). Although robust activations were found in the hippocampus during retrieval of personal events, there was no difference between remote and recent events. The authors interpret this finding as consistent with the idea that the hippocampus plays an enduring role in binding together the different contextual elements that comprise an episodic memory. By this view, the role of the hippocampus in episodic memory retrieval is not time limited. However, in this study the experimenters elicited specific detailed episodic memories from subjects immediately before they entered the scanner and these memories were then cued during the scanning session. Given the proximity of the screening and scanning sessions, it appears quite possible that subjects were retrieving memories of the recent event in which they recounted their memories, in addition to the actual remote event. Thus the hippocampal activation detected may reflect the retrieval of the proximal event.

In contrast, some evidence suggests a temporal gradient for spatial episodic memories. In a more recent fMRI study (Niki and Luo 2002), subjects were asked at least a day before the scanning session to list places they had visited either recently (within the last year) or remotely (about 10 years ago). During the scanning session, they were asked to recall the events that occurred during these visits. In contrast with the findings of Ryan *et al* (2001), there was a significantly greater activation when subjects were recalling the newer events than when they recalled the old events. This activation was centred in the parahippocampal cortex, but included parts of the hippocampus as well. Importantly, this difference persisted even when recent and remote memories were controlled for the number of details retrieved. Because of the longer delay between the screening and scanning sessions, it is more likely that subjects were retrieving the original events during scanning. These results are consistent with the idea that memories consolidate with time, in that they become independent of the MTL. Because the study by Niki and Luo focused on memories of visits, the spatial setting was an extremely important part of the memory, with place names and landmarks used to cue memories of these visits. The emphasis on locations in this experiment may explain the localization of activity to the parahippocampal gyrus, a region that has been implicated in memory for scenes. Although the activation extended into the hippocampus, it was unclear whether retrieval of these memories resulted in robust activation in the hippocampus itself.

Maguire and Frith (2003) solicited detailed memories of specific events from subjects with a procedure similar to that used by Ryan *et al.* (2001). However, this interview took place several weeks before the scanning session, and subjects reported that they did not recollect the interview when asked about their memories during the scanning session. There was significant activation in the hippocampus during memory retrieval, but there was an interesting effect of laterality in terms of the effect of the age of the memories. The right hippocampus showed a clear temporal gradient, with recall of more remote memories associated with less activation than retrieval of recent memories. However, the left hippocampus did not show evidence of such a gradient (Maguire and Frith 2003). These results suggest that right hippocampal involvement in recalling old episodic memories decreases with time, while also suggesting that the left hippocampus contributes to the retrieval of episodic memories throughout the lifespan.

Although studies of neuropsychological patients suggest that remote autobiographical memories can still be retrieved after damage to the left MTL, this region may play a role in the quality of these memories and the ability to retrieve them as part of one's personal past. However, a viable alternative is that the left hippocampal activity reflected the encoding of the event of retrieving these memories during scanning. It will be difficult to eliminate this alternative explanation until it is possible to differentiate encoding and retrieval-related activity in the hippocampus.

Electrophysiological studies

Although fMRI studies have been one of the primary sources of information about the role of different MTL structures in memory processing, it is not completely clear how the blood oxygenation-dependent (BOLD) signal relates to neuronal functions. For example, decreases in BOLD signal may indicate neuronal inhibition, but in some cases increases in inhibitory synaptic activity could lead to an increased BOLD signal. Because of these ambiguities in interpreting fMRI results, it is also important to study directly patterns of neuronal firing in the MTL during learning and memory performance. Although most single-unit recording studies of the MTL have been performed in rats, there are a growing number of electrophysiological studies using non-human primates. In addition, there are several recent studies of patients with pharmacologically intractable epilepsy who have been implanted with electrodes in the MTL in an attempt to localize the seizure focus. Studies of these patients have provided a fascinating glimpse into the properties of individual neurons in the human MTL and have indicated that there is striking convergence between species.

Electrophysiological data have been particularly informative in developing the idea that the perirhinal cortex plays a role in processing stimulus familiarity. Electrophysiological recordings in animals have revealed that a significant proportion of perirhinal neurons decrease their firing rate when a stimulus is repeatedly presented (Xiang and Brown 1998), suggesting that a neural correlate of familiarity may be a decrement in activity to previously presented items. It appears that this property may be fairly specific to the perirhinal cortex, as such response reductions are relatively uncommon in the hippocampus. Hippocampal neurons exhibit response modulations for recognition tasks that require the use of information with a spatial or associational component (Rolls *et al.* 1989; Eichenbaum 2000). For example, an extremely robust finding from electrophysiological studies of freely moving rats is that hippocampal neurons commonly respond to spatial information in the environment, and as a result they have been labelled 'place cells' (O'Keefe 1976). These neurons are likely to play a role in allowing the rat to navigate by supporting representations of different locations in the environment. Recently, hippocampal recordings in patients with epilepsy have revealed similar place-sensitive cells that fire when the patients visit certain locations in a virtual reality computer game (Ekstrom *et al.* 2003).

However, neurons in the hippocampus may be sensitive to more than just spatial information. For example, hippocampal neurons in non-human primates have been found to respond to the combination of stimulus familiarity and spatial location (Miyashita *et al.* 1989). In rats, neurons in the CA1 field have been shown to respond differently based on what had occurred in the previous trial, even when the rat was in the same location (Wood *et al.* 2000). Hippocampal neurons also appear to change their firing to stimuli as they become associated with a particular response to obtain a goal (Wirth *et al* 2003). In this study, hippocampal neurons showed changes in their firing to specific pictures as monkeys learned to associate the picture with a particular eye movement to obtain a juice reward. Similarly, single-unit recordings in humans have revealed that a subset of hippocampal neurons may code the conjunction of stimulus features, even though these stimuli lacked strong spatial information (Kreiman *et al.* 2000). Firing in human hippocampal neurons has also been shown to be responsive to locations in conjunction with the goal that is currently being sought, such as finding a particular shop in a virtual reality town (Ekstrom *et al.* 2003).

The majority of existing electrophysiological data suggest that hippocampal neurons may be particularly sensitive to location. This finding is consistent with the idea that it plays an important role in supporting episodic memory, for which the spatial context of the event is a key feature. However, episodic memories are defined not simply by the spatial context of learning, but also by the conjunction of external environment features and internally generated thoughts that co-occur during the learning event. Thus it is not surprising that hippocampal neurons also respond to non-spatial conjunctions. In Interestingly, the sensitivity of hippocampal neurons to the current goal being sought may reflect the role memory plays in directing actions.

In parallel with fMRI studies, electrophysiological studies support the idea that different components of the MTL make different contributions to memory processes. While the perirhinal cortex may have a specific role in supporting feelings of familiarity, the hippocampus plays a role in supporting the binding together of the elements of an episode, particularly the spatial context in which the memory occurred. Neuronal responses in the hippocampus also appear different from those recorded from the parahippocampal cortex. It appears that cells in the parahippocampal cortex fire when viewing specific landmarks regardless of one's spatial position in a virtual reality game (Ekstrom *et al.* 2003). Such information about features of the environment may converge in the hippocampus to form a representation of space.

Conclusions

Across the different experimental approaches discussed in this chapter, some consistencies have emerged regarding the roles of different MTL structures in declarative memory. While the hippocampus appears to play a selective role in episodic memory, including recall and recollection, surrounding MTL cortical regions appear able to support recognition based on feelings of familiarity. However, this issue is not completely settled, in part because of the introspective nature of the distinction between recollection and familiarity. Indeed, it is a matter of debate whether recollection and familiarity represent distinct types of recognition or are merely weak and strong forms of recognition memory arising from a single neural process. Nevertheless, the idea that the hippocampus plays a selective role in episodic memory has found particularly strong support from neuroimaging studies (Eldridge *et al.* 2000; Davachi *et al.* 2003).

A potentially selective role of the hippocampus in episodic memory is consistent with the idea that this structure plays a critical role in binding together the incidental disparate elements of the spatiotemporal context that comprise memory for an event. This binding process occurs both at the time of learning, and when the event is re-experienced at retrieval. Although surrounding MTL cortical structures also play a critical role in declarative memory, they may not necessarily facilitate the cohesion of mnemonic traces that is critical to support the rapid acquisition and retrieval of distinct episodes. While these cortical structures may support familiarity-based recognition, it is still unclear to what extent hippocampal-based episodic memory depends on familiarity processes subserved by MTL cortical regions. The hippocampus receives almost all of its input from MTL cortical regions via the entorhinal cortex. Thus it is possible that familiarity signals for particular items that are computed in the MTL cortex are a necessary input to the hippocampus during the retrieval of the episodic memory surrounding those items. If so, one might predict a redundant relationship between familiarity and episodic memory such that all retrieved elements of an episodic memory also feel familiar. On the other hand, it seems quite possible that the neural substrate of familiarity is independent of the cortical input to the hippocampus.

Computational models of memory may help to clarify the constraints under which the MTL memory system must operate. The complementary learning systems (CLS) model represents one attempt to computationally account for the familiarity and recollective processes that characterize recognition memory (O'Reilly and Rudy 2001; O'Reilly and Norman 2002; Norman and O'Reilly 2003). The core of the CLS model builds upon the broad division of labour between the hippocampus and surrounding cortices suggested by Aggleton and Brown (1999) and further characterizes the differential contributions of individual MTL structures. The fundamental idea of the CLS framework is that there must be two declarative memory systems, one which is responsible for keeping track of specific events and one which extracts generalities about the environment. Consistent with the ideas outlined by Aggleton and Brown (1999), Norman and O'Reilly (2003) suggest that the hippocampus is specialized for quickly memorizing specific events, and the cortical MTL structures are specialized for learning similarities across events. As is the case with a number of models of hippocampal function (e.g. Marr 1971), a key feature of the CLS model is that information in the dentate gyrus and CA3 is sparsely represented. This follows from the fact that there are many more cells in the dentate gyrus and CA3 than in the superficial layers of the entorhinal cortex that give rise to hippocampal input. This divergence of input allows the dentate and CA3 region to support distinctive, non-overlapping memory representations (O'Reilly and Rudy 2001). The elements of these representations are bound together as a distinct episodic memory representation through the strengthening of recurrent collaterals in area CA3 that interconnect the representations of the different elements of the representation. This process is termed 'pattern separation' in that the resulting episodic memory representations are cohesive, yet are distinct from each other. During retrieval a process referred to as 'pattern completion' occurs when an input (such as a word presented during a recognition test) serves to reactivate the representation of the entire learning episode because these elements had been bound together during encoding. When an episodic memory is successfully retrieved through the pattern completion process in CA3, representations in CA1 and the MTL cortex should also be activated.

Based on the properties of the hippocampal circuit in the CLS model, one would predict that the CA3 and dentate regions would be particularly active during the successful encoding of episodic memories. Recent fMRI results using high-resolution scanning methods have been consistent with this prediction (Zeineh *et al.* 2003; Eldridge *et al.* 2005). According to the CLS model, familiarity-based memories would not be encoded in the hippocampus, but would be encoded in the MTL cortex. These cortical representations are formed through a sharpening process such that representations of repeated stimuli involve fewer neurons than representations for novel stimuli, but these neurons respond more intensely. This aspect of the model is conceptually similar to views of perceptual priming that suggest that the repetition of stimuli results in a sharpening of the representation of that stimulus in sensory cortex (Wiggs and Martin 1998). However, unlike perceptual priming, familiarity-based recognition memory is declarative in the sense that subjects are aware of their memory. Although perceptual priming and feelings of familiarity may be supported by distinct brain regions, it is an intriguing possibility that they are based on similar neural mechanisms.

Support for the CLS model has been found in single-unit recording studies showing that some perirhinal neurons decrease their firing rates to repeated presentation of stimuli (Brown and Xiang 1998). Evidence that a small subset of perirhinal neurons increase their firing to familiar stimuli has not yet been found, although according to the model the cells contributing to the sharpened representation may be relatively few compared with those that are inhibited. Although the CLS model holds that the formation of these representations is hippocampal independent, the fact that these MTL cortical regions are the major recipients of hippocampal output via the entorhinal cortex suggests that feedback from the hippocampal system may influence these representations.

A full understanding of how the MTL system is able to encode and retrieve declarative memories will be based on knowledge of the anatomical interrelations between the subcomponents of this system. Computational models that take into account the anatomical and physiological properties of the MTL will be useful to the extent that they generate testable predictions. Advances in high-resolution neuroimaging techniques coupled with creative behavioural paradigms will make it possible to test such predictions.

References

Aggleton, J.P., and Brown, M.W. (1999). Episodic memory, amnesia, and the hippocampal-anterior thalamic axis. *Behavioral and Brain Sciences*, **22**, 425–489.

Aguirre, G.K. and D'Esposito, M. (1997). Environmental knowledge is subserved by separable dorsal/ventral neural areas. *Journal of Neuroscience*, **17**, 2512–2518.

Alvarez, P., Zola-Morgan, S., and Squire, L. R. (1995). Damage limited to the hippocampal region produces long-lasting memory impairment in monkeys. *Journal of Neuroscience*, **15**, 3796–3807.

Amaral, D.G. (1993). Emerging principles of intrinsic hippocampal organization. *Current Opinion in Neurobiology*, **3**, 225–229.

Brewer, J.B., Zhao, Z., Desmond, J.E., Glover, G.H., and Gabrieli, J.D. (1998). Making memories: brain activity that predicts how well visual experience will be remembered [see comments]. *Science*, **281**, 1185–1187.

Brown, M.W. and Aggleton, J.P. (2001). Recognition memory: what are the roles of the perirhinal cortex and hippocampus? *Nature Reviews Neuroscience*, **2**, 51–61.

Brown, M.W. and Xiang, J.Z. (1998). Recognition memory: neuronal substrates of the judgment of prior occurrence. *Progress in Neurobiology*, **55**, 149–189.

Brown, M.W., Wilson, F.A., and Riches, I.P. (1987). Neuronal evidence that inferomedial temporal cortex is more important than hippocampus in certain processes underlying recognition memory. *Brain Research*, **409**, 158–162.

Davachi, L., Mitchell, J.P., and Wagner, A.D. (2003). Multiple routes to memory: distinct medial temporal lobe processes build item and source memories. *Proceedings of the National Academy of Sciences of the United States of America*, **100**, 2157–2162.

Dolan, R.J. and Fletcher, P.C. (1997). Dissociating prefrontal and hippocampal function in episodic memory encoding. *Nature*, **388**, 582–585.

Dolan, R.J. and Fletcher, P.F. (1999). Encoding and retrieval in human medial temporal lobes: an empirical investigation using functional magnetic resonance imaging (fMRI). *Hippocampus*, **9**, 25–34.

Eichenbaum, H. (2000). Hippocampus: mapping or memory? *Current Biology*, **10**, R785–787.

Ekstrom, A.D., Kahana, M.J., Caplan, J.B., *et al.* (2003). Cellular networks underlying human spatial navigation. *Nature*, **425**, 184–188.

Eldridge, L.L., Knowlton, B.J., Furmanski, C.S., Bookheimer, S.Y., and Engel, S.A. (2000). Remembering episodes: a selective role for the hippocampus during retrieval. *Nature Neuroscience*, **3**, 1149–1152.

Eldridge, L.L., Sarfatti, S., and Knowlton, B.J. (2002). The effect of testing procedure on remember–know judgments. *Psychonomic Bulletin and Review*, **9**, 139–145.

Eldridge, L.L., Engel, S., Zeineh, M.M., Bookheimer, S.Y., and Knowlton, B.J. (2005). A dissocation of encoding and retrieval processes in the human hippocampus. *Journal of Neuroscience*, **25**, 3280–3286.

Fernández, G., Weyerts, H., Schrader-Bölsche, M., *et al.* (1998). Successful verbal encoding into episodic memory engages the posterior hippocampus: a parametrically analyzed functional magnetic resonance imaging study. *Journal of Neuroscience*, **18**, 1841–1847.

Fernández, G., Brewer, J.B., Zhao, Z., Glover, G.H., and Gabrieli, J.D. (1999). Level of sustained entorhinal activity at study correlates with subsequent cued-recall performance: a functional magnetic resonance imaging study with high acquisition rate. *Hippocampus*, **9**, 35–44.

Fletcher, P.C., Shallice, T., and Dolan, R.J. (1998a). The functional roles of prefrontal cortex in episodic memory. I. Encoding. *Brain*, **121**, 1239–1248.

Fletcher, P.C., Shallice, T., Frith, C.D., Frackowiak, R.S., and Dolan, R.J. (1998b). The functional roles of prefrontal cortex in episodic memory. II. Retrieval. *Brain*, **121**, 1249–1256.

Fletcher, P., Buchel, C., Josephs, O., Friston, K., and Dolan, R. (1999). Learning-related neuronal responses in prefrontal cortex studied with functional neuroimaging. *Cerebral Cortex*, **9**, 168–178.

Fried, I., Cameron, K.A., Yashar, S., and Morrow, J.W. (2002). Inhibitory and excitatory responses of single neurons in the human medial temporal lobe during recognition of faces and objects. *Cerebral Cortex*, **12**, 575–584.

Gabrieli, J.D., Brewer, J.B., Desmond, J.E., and Glover, G.H. (1997). Separate neural bases of two fundamental memory processes in the human medial temporal lobe. *Science*, **276**, 264–266.

Habib, R., MacIntosh, A.R., Wheeler, M.A., and Tulving, E. (2003). Memory encoding and hippocampally-based novelty/familiarity discrimination networks. *Neuropsychologia*, **41**, 271–279.

Haist, F., Bowden Gore, J, and Mao, H. (2001). Consolidation of human memory over decades revelaed by functional magnetic resonance imaging. *Nature Neuroscience*, **4**, 1139–1145.

Haxby, J.V., Ungerleider, L.G., Horwitz, B., Maisog, J.M., Rapoport, S.I., and Grady, C.L. (1996). Face encoding and recognition in the human brain. *Proceedings of the National Academy of Sciences of the United States of America*, **93**, 922–927.

Henson, R.N., Rugg, M.D., Shallice, T., Josephs, O., and Dolan, R.J. (1999). Recollection and familiarity in recognition memory: an event-related functional magnetic resonance imaging study. *Journal of Neuroscience*, **19**, 3962–3972.

Henson, R.N.A., Cansino, S., Herron, J.E., Robb, W.G.K., and Rugg, M.D. (2003). A familiarity signal in human anterial medial temporal cortex? *Hippocampus*, **13**, 301–304.

Insausti, R. and Munoz, M. (2001). Cortical projections of the non-entorhinal hippocampal formation in the cynomolgus monkey (*Macaca fascicularis*). *European Journal of Neuroscience*, **14**, 435–451.

Kapur, S., Craik, F.I., Jones, C., Brown, G.M., Houle, S., and Tulving, E. (1995). Functional role of the prefrontal cortex in retrieval of memories: a PET study. *Neuroreport*, **6**, 1880–1884.

Kelley, W.M., Miezin, F.M., McDermott, K.B., *et al.* (1998). Hemispheric specialization in human dorsal frontal cortex and medial temporal lobe for verbal and nonverbal memory encoding. *Neuron*, **20**, 927–936.

Kensinger, E.A., Clarke, R.J., and Corkin, S. (2003). What neural correlates underlie successful encoding and retrieval? A functional magnetic resonance imaging study using a divided attention paradigm. *Journal of Neuroscience*, **23**, 2407–2415.

Kopelman, M.D. (1989). Remote and autobiographical memory, temporal context memory and frontal atrophy in Korsakoff and Alzheimer patients. *Neuropsychologia*, **27**, 437–460.

Kopelman, M.D., Stanhope, N., and Kingsley, D. (1999). Retrograde amnesia in patients with diencephalic, temporal lobe or frontal lesions. *Neuropsychologia*, **37**, 939–958.

Kreiman, G., Koch, C., and Fried, I. (2000). Category-specific visual responses of single neurons in the human medial temporal lobe. *Nature Neuroscience*, **3**, 946–953.

Lepage, M., Habib, R., and Tulving, E. (1998). Hippocampal PET activations of memory encoding and retrieval: the HIPER model. *Hippocampus*, **8**, 313–322.

Maguire, E.A. and Frith, C.D. (2003). Lateral asymmetry in the hippocampal response to the remoteness of autobiographical memories. *Journal of Neuroscience*, **23**, 5302–5307.

Manns, J.R., Hopkins, R.O., Reed, J.M., Kitchener, E.G., and Squire, L.R. (2003). Recognition memory and the human hippocampus. *Neuron*, **37**, 171–180.

Marr (1971). Simple memory: a theory for archicortex. *Philosophical Transactions of the Royal Society, London*, **262**, 23–81

Mayes, A.R., Holdstock, J.S., Isaac, C.L., Hunkin, N.M., and Roberts, N. (2002). Relative sparing of item recognition memory in a patient with adult-onset damage limited to the hippocampus. *Hippocampus*, **12**, 325–340.

Milner, B. (1958). Psychological defects produced by temporal lobe excision. *Research Publications of the Association for Research in Nervous and Mental Disease*, **36**, 244–257.

Miyashita, Y., Rolls, E.T., Cahusac, P.M., Niki, H., and Feigenbaum, J.D. (1989). Activity of hippocampal formation neurons in the monkey related to a conditional spatial response task. *Journal of Neurophysiology*, **61**, 669–678.

Moscovitch, M. (1995). Recovered consciousness: a hypothesis concerning modularity and episodic memory. *Journal of Clinical and Experimental Neuropsychology*, **17**, 276–290.

Nadel, L. and Moscovitch, M. (1997). Memory consolidation, retrograde amnesia and the hippocampal complex. *Current Opinion in Neurobiology*, **7**, 217–227.

Niki, K. and Luo, J. (2002). An fMRI study on the time limited role of the medial temporal lobe in long-term topographic autobiographical memory. *Journal of Cognitive Neuroscience*, **14**, 500–507.

Norman, K.A. and O'Reilly, R.C. (2003). Modeling hippocampal and neocortical contributions to recognition memory: a complementary-learning-systems approach, *Psychological Review*, **110**, 611–646.

O'Keefe, J. (1976). Place units in the hippocampus of the freely moving rat. *Experimental Neurology*, **51**, 78–109.

O'Reilly, R.C. and Norman, K.A. (2002). Hippocampal and neocortical contributions to memory: advances in the complementary learning systems framework. *Trends in Cognitive Sciences*, **6**, 505–510.

O'Reilly, R.C. and Rudy, J.W. (2001). Conjunctive representations in learning and memory: principles of cortical and hippocampal function. *Psychological Review*, **108**, 311–345.

Ostergaard, A.L. and Squire, L.R. (1990). Childhood amnesia and distinctions between forms of memory: a comment on Wood, Brown, and Felton. *Brain and Cognition*, **14**, 127–133.

Reed, J.M. and Squire, L.R. (1998). Retrograde amnesia for facts and events: findings from four new cases. *Journal of Neuroscience*, **18**, 3943–3954.

Rempel-Clower, N.L., Zola, S.M., Squire, L.R., and Amaral, D.G. (1996). Three cases of enduring memory impairment after bilateral damage limited to the hippocampal formation. *Journal of Neuroscience*, **16**, 5233–5255.

Rolls, E.T., Miyashita, Y., Cahusac, P.M., *et al.* (1989). Hippocampal neurons in the monkey with activity related to the place in which a stimulus is shown. *Journal of Neuroscience*, **9**, 1835–1845.

Rosene, D.L., and Van Hoesen, G.W. (1977). Hippocampal efferents reach widespread areas of cerebral cortex and amygdala in the rhesus monkey. *Science*, **198**, 315–317.

Ryan, L., Nadel, L., Keil, K., *et al.* (2001). Hippocampal complex and retrieval of recent and very remote autobiographical memories: evidence from functional magnetic resonance imaging in neurologically intact people. *Hippocampus*, **11**, 707–714.

Schacter, D.L. and Wagner, A.D. (1999). Medial temporal lobe activations in fMRI and PET studies of episodic encoding and retrieval. *Hippocampus*, **9**, 7–24.

Squire, L.R. (1992). Memory and the hippocampus: a synthesis from findings with rats, monkeys, and humans. *Psychological Review*, **99**, 195–231.

Squire, L.R. and Zola, S.M. (1998). Episodic memory, semantic memory, and amnesia. *Hippocampus*, **8**, 205–211.

Stark, C.E.L. and Okado, Y. (2003). Making memories without trying: medial temporal lobe activity associated with incidental memory formation during recognition. *Journal of Neuroscience*, **23**, 6748–6753.

Stark, C.E. and Squire, L.R. (2000). fMRI activity in the medial temporal lobe during recognition memory as a function of study–test interval. *Hippocampus*, **10**, 329–337.

Stern, C.E., Corkin, S., Gonzalez, R.G., *et al.* (1996). The hippocampal formation participates in novel picture encoding: evidence from functional magnetic resonance imaging. *Proceedings of the National Academy of Sciences of the United States of America*, **93**, 8660–8665.

Strange, B.A., Otten, L.J., Josephs, O., Rugg, M.D., and Dolan, R.J. (2002). Dissociable human perirhinal, hippocampal, and parahippocampal roles during verbal encoding. *Journal of Neuroscience*, **22**, 523–528.

Tulving, E. (1985). Memory and consciousness. *Canadian Psychology*, **26**, 1–12.

Tulving, E. and Markowitsch, H.J. (1998). Episodic and declarative memory: role of the hippocampus. *Hippocampus*, **8**, 198–204.

Tulving, E., Markowitsch, H.J., Craik, F.E., Habib, R., and Houle, S. (1996). Novelty and familiarity activations in PET studies of memory encoding and retrieval. *Cerebral Cortex*, **6**, 71–79.

Vandenberghe, R., Price, C., Wise, R., Josephs, O., and Frackowiak, R.S. (1996). Functional anatomy of a common semantic system for words and pictures [see comments]. *Nature*, **383**, 254–256.

Vargha-Khadem, F., Gadian, D.G., Watkins, K.E., Connelly, A., Van Paesschen, W., and Mishkin, M. (1997). Differential effects of early hippocampal pathology on episodic and semantic memory [see comments]. *Science*, **277**, 376–380. Erratum, *Science*, **277**, 1117, 1997.

Verfaellie, M., Koseff, P., and Alexander, M.P. (2000). Acquisition of novel semantic information in amnesia: effects of lesion location. *Neuropsychologia*, **38**, 484–492.

Wagner, A.D., Desmond, J.E., Glover, G.H., and Gabrieli, J.D. (1998a). Prefrontal cortex and recognition memory. Functional-MRI evidence for context-dependent retrieval processes. *Brain*, **121**, 1985–2002.

Wagner, A.D., Schacter, D.L., Rotte, M., *et al.* (1998b). Building memories: remembering and forgetting of verbal experiences as predicted by brain activity [see comments]. *Science*, **281**, 1188–1191.

Wiggs, C.L. and Martin, A. (1998). Properties and mechanisms of perceptual priming. *Current Opinion in Neurobiology*, **8**, 227–233.

Wirth, S., Yanike, M., Frank, L.M., Smith, A.C., Brown, E.N., and Suzuki, W.A. (2003). Single neurons in the monkey hippocampus and learning of new associations. *Science*, **300**, 1578–1581.

Wood, E.R., Dudchenko, P.A., Robitsek, R.J., and Eichenbaum, H. (2000). Hippocampal neurons encode information about different types of memory episodes occurring in the same location. *Neuron*, **27**, 623–633.

Xiang, J.Z. and Brown, M.W. (1998). Differential neuronal encoding of novelty, familiarity and recency in regions of the anterior temporal lobe. *Neuropharmacology*, **37**, 657–676.

Zeineh, M.M., Engel, S.A., Thompson, P.M., and Bookheimer, S.Y. (2003). Dynamics of the hippocampus during encoding and retrieval of face–name pairs. *Science*, **299**, 577–580.

Zola-Morgan, S., Squire, L.R., and Amaral, D.G. (1986). Human amnesia and the medial temporal region: enduring memory impairment following a bilateral lesion limited to field CA1 of the hippocampus. *Journal of Neuroscience*, **6**, 2950–2967.

Chapter 20

Functional imaging studies of intentional and incidental reactivation: implications for the binding problem

Lars Nyberg

Introduction

A remarkable feature of memory is its ability to group related experiences and differentiate them from the wealth of other, often similar, experiences that are also stored. In effect, when we see the face of a person we know we may recall his or her profession, we may recollect events that occurred when we last met the person, and certain feelings and bodily states which relate to how we feel about the person may be induced. If, in the past, we shared a delicious dinner with the person, it is even possible that gustatory and olfactory sensations from that experience will be induced when we see the face. Thus, at least under certain circumstances, various features or elements of an episode seem to be integrated in memory such that the subsequent remembering of one element can trigger several other related elements.

The issue of how information that belongs to the same experience is bound in memory has attracted substantial interest, and it has been addressed in numerous publications including this book. In the present chapter we will approach this 'binding problem' from the aspect of functional brain imaging studies of **reactivation.** The common feature of such studies is that they explore whether the way the brain is activated during initial encoding/perception is subsequently reflected, wholly or in part, in the way that the brain is activated at the time of retrieval (i.e. whether parts of the activation pattern at encoding/perception are reactivated during retrieval).

The discussion of empirical studies is organized on the basis of a distinction between **intentional** and **incidental** reactivation (Nyberg *et al.* 2000). In studies of intentional reactivation, the test instructions to the participants explicitly mention retrieval of the stimulus dimension of interest (e.g. recollection of sounds on the basis of visual cue words). In contrast, in studies of incidental reactivation, there is no explicit mention of retrieval of the dimension of interest (e.g. simple name recognition, where some names have been associated with face information in a previous encoding phase and the focus of the analysis is on activation of the face area).

Before turning to the empirical studies, some methodological issues that are critical in studies of reactivation will be commented on (for a more detailed discussion see Nyberg 2002). Finally, some speculations are offered on how the results from reactivation studies may shed some light on the binding problem.

Methodological considerations

The brain activation data that are discussed in this chapter were obtained using positron-emission tomography (PET) or functional MRI (fMRI). A common feature of PET and fMRI studies is that brain activity is monitored during intentional or incidental encoding of information, as well as during subsequent episodic memory retrieval of information from the previous encoding event. By registering brain activity during both encoding and retrieval it is possible to quantify the degree of overlap in activation patterns at each stage of the memory process.

When the degree of overlap is evaluated it may be difficult to determine whether brain regions that are activated at each stage are a result of memory-related or sensory-related processes. That is, if the encoding phase consists of intentional encoding of visual words and the retrieval phase of a visual word recognition test, it is difficult to determine whether common activations at each stage reflect reactivation processes at retrieval or simply sensory–perceptual activity associated with visual word processing at each stage. One approach that has been used to overcome this problem involves varying the way of presenting items at encoding and retrieval (e.g. visual word presentation during encoding and auditory presentation during test). This approach will be exemplified below.

A possibly more difficult problem relates to the potential confounding effects of selective attention. It is well documented that selective attention towards a specific modality or stimulus dimension is associated with increased activity in brain regions that would be engaged if information of that kind or in that modality was actually presented (reviewed by Cabeza and Nyberg 2000). Therefore, if a person is presented with a family name and asked whether he or she can visualize the face of the person who was paired with that specific name during a previous encoding episode, it would not be possible to take a finding of increased activity in the face area of the fusiform gyrus as unequivocal evidence for reactivation; it could simply be the process of covertly attending to face information that resulted in such activity. For example, participants might imagine faces as a way of solving the task, but none of these faces may actually represent the target face. A possible approach to resolving confounding effects of selective attention is to use an event-related design in an fMRI study. Such a design would permit analyses of correct responses (hits) relative to incorrect responses (misses or false alarms), and could thus show whether overlap of retrieval-related brain activity with encoding-related brain activity is specific for the correct response.

Another approach that is relevant in this context relates to how the retrieval instructions are construed. If, as in the above example on name–face memory, the retrieval instruction orients participants towards the dimension of interest (in this case, faces), the risk for attentional influences are obvious. If, instead, the retrieval instructions probe another dimension, the risk may be reduced. For example, the retrieval instructions could ask participants to decide whether the family names presented were also presented during the encoding phase (i.e. there is no explicit mention of face information). A possible outcome of such a study could be that correct recognition of names is associated with relative increased activity in the face area. It might be argued that such activity could be a reflection of an intentional strategy to use remembered face information as a means of determining whether names had previously been encountered (i.e. the effect might still reflect selective attention rather than memory). However, if the effect were simply a reflection of strategy use, it is reasonable to assume that such a strategy should also be used for names that had not been paired with faces during the encoding phase (i.e. new names). If the response is selective or stronger for names that actually were paired with faces during encoding, then the argument that the effect simply reflects attention is considerably weakened. The latter approach towards resolving the effects of selective attention relates to the distinction between intentional and incidental reactivation (Nyberg *et al.* 2000).

Brain imaging studies of encoding–retrieval overlap

Intentional reactivation

An early PET study examined neural correlates of encoding and retrieval of three different kinds of event information; item, temporal, and spatial information (Nyberg *et al.* 1996). Multivariate analyses indicated that general encoding and retrieval networks, i.e. networks that were engaged during episodic encoding and retrieval for all three kinds of information, were operating. In addition, information-specific activation patterns were observed at both encoding and retrieval. Detailed analyses of common features in information-specific activity between the encoding and retrieval phases provided evidence for encoding–retrieval overlap (Persson and Nyberg 2000). In keeping with much prior evidence (Cabeza and Nyberg 2000), the encoding condition that specifically asked the participants to memorize the spatial position of study words and the subsequent retrieval condition that involved memory of spatial information were jointly associated with increased activity in the bilateral parietal cortex, i.e. in the 'where?' pathway (for related observations, see Moscovitch *et al.* 1995; Köhler *et al.* 1998).

Evidence for intentional reactivation in the auditory domain was provided in a PET study of encoding and retrieval of visual and auditory information (Nyberg *et al.* 2000). In brief, the design that was used in two independent experiments was as follows. The participants were given two encoding conditions. In one condition, they were presented with pairs of visual words and unrelated sounds (e.g. the word 'table' paired with the sound of a plane during take-off). They were asked to try to memorize the pairs so that later on, when they were cued with one member of the pair, they would be able to retrieve the other member. In the other encoding condition, subjects were presented with visual words only and asked to memorize them for a later test. The encoding conditions were followed by two retrieval conditions (in a counterbalanced order). In both conditions, visual words were presented and subjects were asked to press one mouse button for words they recognized and thought had been presented alone at study, to press another mouse button when they recognized a word and remembered that it had been paired with a sound at study, and to press no button if they did not recognize a word. Thus, in both retrieval conditions, subjects intentionally had to remember whether visual words had been paired with sounds during encoding. Therefore the conditions should not have differed with regard to selective attention to the auditory modality. The only difference between the retrieval conditions related to the type of words that were presented during the scan interval: In one retrieval condition, the words were paired with sounds during study (paired condition); in the other condition, they were presented alone during study (unpaired condition).

To examine whether brain regions activated during perception–encoding of auditory information were reactivated during retrieval of auditory information, the encoding condition involving words and sounds was contrasted with the encoding condition involving words only. As expected, in both experiments the former condition was associated with increased activity in bilateral auditory regions in the temporal lobe compared with the latter condition. The activation map from the encoding contrast was then used as a mask for a subsequent contrast between the paired and unpaired retrieval conditions. In both experiments, retrieval of sound information was associated with increased activity in auditory association areas in the temporal cortex. This finding provided support for the idea that some of the brain regions that are active during encoding of information are reactivated during subsequent retrieval of that information from memory.

A study by Wheeler *et al.* (2000) provided further evidence for intentional reactivation in the auditory domain by showing that retrieval of auditory information based on visual labels engaged auditory brain regions. In addition, these authors examined intentional reactivation for visual information by asking subjects to retrieve pictorial information on the basis of verbal labels. They observed retrieval-related activity in several visual areas that were also activated during initial perception–encoding, including the medial occipito-parietal cortex (for a related finding based on encoding and retrieval of visual geometrical patterns, see Roland and Gulyás (1995)).

Incidental reactivation

As was noted at the beginning of the chapter, the definition of incidental reactivation is that it is observed under conditions where the test instruction does not direct the participants towards retrieval of the stimulus dimension that is of primary interest. The design of Nyberg *et al.*'s (2000) second experiment is in keeping with this definition. Following encoding of single visual words or word–sound pairs, as described above, the participants were tested for visual word recognition. The instructions stated that they had to indicate by pressing one of two response buttons whether they thought that the words had been part of the previous encoding lists. The main difference between the test conditions was that for one of them no word–sound associations had been established during the encoding phase, whereas word–sound associations of varying strength had been created for the other two conditions (i.e. these words had been paired with sounds during the encoding phase and the number of pairings was varied to manipulate the strength of associations). Importantly, however, the participants were simply instructed to indicate whether they recognized the visual words—there was no mention of auditory information.

The main interest of the experiment was whether visual word recognition would be associated with activation of auditory brain regions for the conditions where the words had been associated with sounds. Such a pattern of results would qualify as evidence for incidental reactivation. A contrast between the conditions for which a sound association existed with the no-sound conditions indeed revealed increased activity in auditory responsive regions of bilateral temporal cortex. Thus the results provided support for incidental reactivation.

Support for incidental reactivation is also provided by studies of whether motor areas of the brain are activated when one episodically remembers previous motor actions (i.e. declarative memory of information that has procedural components). Nyberg *et al.* (2001) used PET to monitor brain activity during encoding and retrieval of simple commands (for related studies, see Nilsson *et al.* 2000; Russ *et al.* 2003). The commands were constructed in such a way that they were possible to perform with the right hand while lying in the PET scanner. In one experimental condition, the participants were instructed that the actions described by each command were to be executed/enacted (using imaginary objects whenever a command mentioned external objects). Thus this condition involved right arm/hand motor activity at the time of encoding. In another experimental condition, the subjects were instructed to encode the commands by means of maintenance rehearsal. This latter condition qualified as a non-motor encoding condition.

Both encoding conditions were followed by tests of cued recall where the verbs from the commands were presented and the subjects were asked to try to remember the noun that had been paired with each verb. Importantly, in keeping with the definition of incidental reactivation, the test instructions did not focus the subjects' attention on the fact that the encoding of some commands had involved motor activity. The main interest in the data analysis was whether retrieval of information that had been encoded by means of enactment would be associated with increased activity in motor areas relative to the verbal condition. It was found that some of the brain regions that showed increased activity during enacted encoding, including the left premotor and parietal cortex, were reactivated during retrieval. Thus these results can be taken as additional evidence for incidental reactivation.

Table 19.1 summarizes the results from various studies of intentional and incidental reactivation as a function of type of event information and select

Table 20.1 Functional brain imaging studies of reactivation

Type of event information	Select overlap sites
Auditory information	
Nyberg *et al.* (2000)	Bilateral auditory responsive cortex (BA 21/22)
Wheeler *et al.* (2000)	Left superior temporal cortex (BA 22)
Visual information	
Roland and Gulyás (1995)	Precuneus and angular gyrus
Wheeler *et al.* (2000)	Precuneus (BA 7) and left fusiform cortex (BA 19)
Spatial information	
Köhler *et al.* (1998)	Right inferior parietal cortex (BA 39/40)
Moscovitch *et al.* (1995)	Right inferior parietal cortex (BA 39/40)
Persson and Nyberg (2000)	Bilateral inferior parietal cortex (BA 39/40)
Motor information	
Nyberg *et al.* (2001)	Left ventral motor cortex (BA 4/6)

BA, Brodmann area

overlap sites (for a more complete review of PET and fMRI reactivation studies, see Nyberg (2002)).

Concluding comments

The PET and fMRI studies reviewed above provide support for the view that the way the brain is activated during the initial perception–encoding of an event is in part reproduced when episodic information is subsequently retrieved. In other words, the activity pattern at encoding is reactivated at test. These observations of reactivation, in particular incidental reactivation, have potential implications for our understanding of the binding problem.

The test of incidental reactivation in the study by Nyberg *et al.* (2000) was based on the hypothesis that when different components of a complex event (e.g. visual, haptic, and auditory components) have been consolidated in memory, functional connections are established between the neuronal ensembles in the neocortex where the different components are represented (Alvarez and Squire 1994; McClelland *et al.* 1995). As a result of these connections, triggering of one component during retrieval (by internal or external cues) will lead to activation of the other components, similar to the idea of 'spread of activation' in semantic networks and the idea of 'redintegration' (Tulving and Madigan 1970). Hence incidental reactivation of motor or auditory brain regions during retrieval of verbal information may be based on neural connections between regions involved in representing the verbal information and regions representing motor or auditory information.

Results from studies of the neural basis of conditioning are consistent with the general idea that functional interactions between distributed brain regions constitute the basis for triggering associated information in memory when a subset of an integrated stimulus complex is activated (Cahill *et al.* 1996; McIntosh *et al.* 1998). In addition, recent neuronal recordings from four different neocortical areas of macaque monkeys provide strong evidence that neuronal interactions are changed by experience (Hoffman and McNaughton 2002). The monkeys were trained to perform tasks that coactivated the four areas, and neuronal activity was recorded when they performed the trained tasks and also when they rested. Strikingly, the same set of neurons, distributed across the four neocortical sites, was activated during both task performance and rest but not during a pre-task control condition. The finding of task-specific neuronal activation during rest can be interpreted as reflecting consolidation of declarative memory (i.e. establishing the relevant connections between involved regions).

It is likely that the consolidation phase is critical for what will be bound in memory over the long term, and it is possible that the nature of the encoding process has consequences for the consolidation process and hence ultimately for what is bound in memory (Moscovitch 1995). Slow gradual learning, as in the above examples of conditioning and training, might facilitate the consolidation process in comparison with single-trial episodic encoding. Indeed, consideration of the encoding process may shed light on the critical issue of the circumstances under which remembering some aspects of a complex event will trigger associated information that was acquired during the same event (i.e. the boundary conditions for redintegration).

In the section on incidental reactivation, activation of auditory brain regions during visual word recognition was discussed. In this case, the encoding instructions emphasized that word–sound associations had to be established during encoding. It seems likely that such encoding conditions, when one is actively trying to relate distinct pieces of information, will promote strong visual–auditory binding that is subsequently manifested as incidental reactivation of auditory regions. In the studies of activation of motor regions following enacted encoding, the participants were not asked to remember motor information. However, there is much data suggesting that motor information will automatically be represented after enacted encoding (e.g. Engelkamp 1998). Hence, this example may also have included an encoding condition that supported the formation of a strong link between the information of interest (i.e. motor information) and the verbal information in the commands.

In contrast with these examples, episodic retrieval can be more piecemeal in that only some specific details of a complex event are retrieved. One example of this is when one is remembering information from a conversation with a group of people, without remembering who contributed that information. Or one may recall going to the cinema with someone a few weeks previously without being able to remember the actual film. In short, sometimes we are able to remember some pieces of information from an event without being able to remember related information which one might expect to be strongly associated with the remembered information. One hypothesis is that the remembered and forgotten information were not sufficiently strongly linked at the time of encoding, and therefore different pieces of information from the same event were not strongly related at the time of retrieval. Moscovitch (1995) has suggested **cohesion** as a process by which various elements and corresponding brain structures are bound into a memory trace at the time of encoding. On this view, the pattern of brain activity during encoding may in principle predict which elements will be bound in memory. This hypothesis, as well as similar hypotheses related to the binding problem, could be addressed in future functional neuroimaging studies of intentional and incidental reactivation.

References

Alvarez, P. and Squire, L.R. (1994). Memory consolidation and the medial temporal lobe: a simple network model. *Proceedings of the National Academy of Sciences of the United States of America*, **91**, 7041–7045.

Cabeza, R. and Nyberg, L. (2000). Imaging cognition. II: An empirical review of 275 PET and fMRI studies. *Journal of Cognitive Neuroscience*, 12, 1–47.

Cahill, L., Ohl, F., and Scheich, H. (1996). Alteration of auditory cortex activity with a visual stimulus through conditioning: a 2-deoxyglucose analysis. *Neurobiology of Learning and Memory*, **65**, 213–222.

Engelkamp, L. (1998). *Memory for Actions.* Hove, UK: Psychology Press.

Hoffman, K.L. and McNaughton, B.L. (2002). Coordinated reactivation of distributed memory traces in primate neocortex. *Science*, **297**, 2070–2073.

Köhler, S., Moscovitch, M., Winocur, G., Houle, S., and McIntosh, A. R. (1998). Networks of domain-specific and general regions involved in episodic memory for spatial location and object identity. *Neuropsychologia*, **36**, 129–142.

McClelland, J.L., McNaughton, B.L., and O'Reilly, R.C. (1995). Why there are complementary learning systems in the hippocampus and neocortex: insights from the successes and failures of connectionist models of learning and memory. *Psychological Review*, **102**, 419–457.

McIntosh, A.R., Cabeza, R., and Lobaugh, N.J. (1998). Analysis of neural interactions explains the activation of occipital cortex by an auditory stimulus. *Journal of Neurophysiology*, **80**, 2790–2796.

Moscovitch, M. (1995). Recovered consciousness: a hypothesis concerning modularity and episodic memory. *Journal of Clinical and Experimental Neuropsychology*, **17**, 276–290.

Moscovitch, M., Kapur, S., Köhler, S., and Houle, S. (1995). Distinct neural correlates of visual long-term memory for spatial location and object identity: A positron emission tomography study in humans. *Proceedings of the National Academy of Sciences of the United States of America*, **92**, 3721–3725.

Nilsson, L.-G., Nyberg, L., Klingberg, T., Åberg, C., Persson, J., and Roland, P.E. (2000). Activity in motor areas while remembering action events. *Neuroreport*, **11**, 2199–2201.

Nyberg, L. (2002). Where encoding and retrieval meet in the brain. In *Neuropsychology of Memory* (ed L.R. Squire and D.L. Schacter). New York: Guilford Press, pp. 193–203.

Nyberg, L., McIntosh, A.R., Cabeza, R., Habib, R., Houle, S., & Tulving, E. (1996). General and specific brain regions involved in encoding and retrieval of events: What, where, and when. *Proceedings of the National Academy of Sciences, USA*, **93**, 11280–11285.

Nyberg, L., Habib, R., McIntosh, A.R., and Tulving, E. (2000). Reactivation of encoding-related brain activity during memory retrieval. *Proceedings of the National Academy of Sciences of the United States of America*, **97**, 11120–11124.

Nyberg, L., Petersson, K.-M., Nilsson, L.-G., Sandblom, J., Åberg, C., and Ingvar, M. (2001). Reactivation of motor brain areas during explicit memory for actions. *NeuroImage*, **14**, 521–528.

Persson, J. and Nyberg, L. (2000). Conjunction analysis of cortical activations common to encoding and retrieval. *Microscopy Research and Technique*, **51**, 39–44.

Roland, P.E. and Gulyás, B. (1995). Visual memory, visual imagery, and visual recognition of large field patterns by the human brain: functional anatomy by positron emission tomography. *Cerebral Cortex*, **5**, 79–93.

Russ, M.O., Mack, W., Grama, C.-R., Lanfermann, H., and Knopf, M. (2003).Enactment effect in memory: evidence concerning the supramarginal gyri. *Experimental Brain Research*, **149**, 497–504.

Tulving, E. and Madigan, S.A. (1970). Memory and verbal learning. *Annual Review of Psychology*, **21**, 437–484.

Wheeler, M.E., Petersen, S.E., and Buckner, R.L. (2000). Memory's echo: vivid remembering reactivates sensory-specific cortex. *Proceedings of the National Academy of Sciences of the United States of America*, **97**, 11125–11129.

Chapter 21

Binding memory fragments together to form declarative memories depends on cross-cortical storage

Ken A. Paller

Introduction

What happens in your brain to allow you to remember a recent acquaintance, your favourite film, your last summer vacation, or your first kiss? Investigations of such phenomena are founded on contemporary classification systems for memory abilities. The category of **declarative memory** refers to the ability to remember prior autobiographical episodes and complex facts, as assessed by tests of recall or recognition (Squire 1987). Declarative memory provides each of us with a vast but imperfect storehouse of information, and a basis for our own life story.

What would constitute a comprehensive scientific understanding of declarative memory? Relevant evidence concerning declarative memory includes physiological recordings in animals, cognitive modelling with computers, neuroimaging in patients with memory disorders, reversible magnetic neurodisruption in willing human volunteers, and more. A long-standing and venerable approach to exploring both neural and psychological underpinnings of memory is to investigate memory deficits in neurological patients.

Neuropsychological investigations of amnesia have provided many insights into memory functions of the human brain (Schacter and Tulving 1994; Schacter 1996; Squire and Kandel 1999; Eichenbaum and Cohen 2001; Squire and Schacter 2002). Contemporary theoretical explanations of declarative memory based on this evidence generally describe how memory storage depends on representations distributed across networks in the cerebral cortex. Although it is beyond the scope of the present chapter to summarize each of these theories, I will attempt to present some views on declarative memory that fit well within the current zeitgeist.

A core goal of research into declarative memory is to answer the question: 'How is declarative memory different from all other types of memory?' By analogy with the 'Four Questions' traditionally recited by the youngest child at Passover celebrations, consider the following answers to this overarching question (Paller 2002), which will be elaborated on in subsequent sections.

1. Declarative memory is behaviourally distinct in that it is assessed using recall and recognition tests for facts and episodes.
2. Declarative memory has distinct subjective characteristics in that it is often accompanied by the experience of conscious recollection.
3. Declarative memory has a distinct cognitive structure that entails retrieving a conjunction of discrete informational fragments.
4. Declarative memory has a distinct neural basis that depends on storage across a set of neocortical modules, with enduring storage dependent upon a cross-cortical consolidation process mediated by cortico-hippocampal and cortico-thalamic networks.

Although each of these four points is important, I take the position that our understanding of declarative memory can be significantly improved by striving to elucidate the connections between them. Thus binding is at the core of this understanding. Cross-cortical storage is a way to bind together the distinct neocortical ensembles that comprise a declarative memory. At the same time, these ensembles represent a set of discrete informational fragments that must be bound together. This **neurocognitive binding** of declarative memories is essential for the recall and recognition of facts and episodes, and it may also be a critical ingredient for the experience of conscious recollection.

Neurocognitive foundations of declarative memory

Investigations of **amnesia** have focused on patients who experience memory difficulties, but whose intellectual functioning is otherwise preserved. An amnesic patient may carry on an intelligent and detailed conversation but, shortly afterwards, be unable to remember that the conversation ever occurred. On the other hand, such patients often produce completely normal performance when it comes to a set of other memory phenomena collectively referred to as **non-declarative memory** (Table 21.1). The selective deficits in amnesia imply that certain neural computations are essential for recalling and recognizing episodes and facts, but not for perceiving and manipulating the same types of information in other ways. Indeed, it appears that cortical networks play a major role in perceiving and manipulating the information inherent in an episode, whereas alterations in connections among neurons in these same networks are responsible for declarative memory storage.

Table 21.1 Comparing declarative memory with other types of memory

Type of memory	Definition	Findings in circumscribed amnesia
Declarative memory	Recall and recognition of episodes and facts (i.e. episodic memory and semantic memory)	Impairment in storage, producing deficits in new learning (anterograde amnesia) and in remembering information acquired prior to illness or injury (retrograde amnesia)
Immediate memory	Information kept in mind by continuous rehearsal (e.g. verbal working memory)	Preserved
Non-declarative memory[a]		Generally preserved, but with some notable exceptions
Perceptual priming	Speeded or more accurate responses to a stimulus when repeated, based on altered perceptual representations	Preserved if performance is not contaminated by declarative memory (i.e. implicit memory testing with no explicit retrieval)
Conceptual priming	Speeded or more accurate responses to a stimulus when repeated, based on altered conceptual representations	Preserved in some cases, but further investigation is required, particularly across stimulus domains
Skills	Behaviours that improve gradually with practice, including cognitive skills (e.g. reading mirror-reversed text) and motor skills	Preserved when skill acquisition is accomplished without reliance on declarative memory (which is not the case for many skills learned outside the laboratory)
Classical conditioning	Learned associations between two stimuli, one of which elicits an automatic response	Preserved under conditions with temporal overlap between conditioned and unconditioned stimuli

[a] Also includes non-associative learning, habits, category learning, and artificial grammar learning.

Here I will articulate a theoretical explanation for such memory disorders that postulates a core defect in a process called **cross-cortical storage.** This process is assumed to be essential for connecting the fragments of an episode or the various features of a complex fact together into a coherent and sturdy representation in the brain (Paller 1997, 2002). For example, fragments linked together in the cerebral cortex to form an enduring memory of an episode might include representations of various sights, sounds, smells, a spatial layout of objects, people, actions, emotional colouring, a set of precipitating events, consequences of the episode, and so on. Cortical regions are clearly specialized for processing these different types of information.

The cross-cortical storage process is believed to depend on a group of representations instantiated not in a single brain region but rather in many neocortical networks, each specialized for a different set of computations. The fundamental characteristic of declarative memory is taken to be its dependence on a linking together of discrete representations in multiple neocortical zones. I propose that this fundamental neural characteristic strongly influences the form of the other characteristics of declarative memory: its cognitive characteristics, its behavioural characteristics, and its association with conscious recollection.

Binding is a key aspect of declarative memory, but the term 'binding' can take on substantively different meanings in different contexts. For example, binding of a different sort, feature integration, occurs during visual object perception when distinct features present at the same spatial location are processed such that representations of feature conjunctions are formed (see Chapter 12). Binding also occurs in immediate memory as multimodal and multidimensional representations of sensory input are formed and manipulated. With respect to declarative memory, binding concerns representational elements in memory that can be brought back together in a unitized way when a specific episode or fact is retrieved. Declarative memory binding (cross-cortical storage) is accomplished through network interactions that are not well understood but that probably involve changes in neuronal connectivity among various neocortical regions and the medial temporal region, as well as between the neocortex and the medial diencephalon. This hypothesis is based on the fact that amnesia generally results from damage to either the medial temporal or the medial diencephalic regions of the brain.

Furthermore, cross-cortical storage is not finalized immediately after a learning episode; rather, it can evolve over an extended time course as the information becomes integrated with knowledge already accrued as well as with information acquired subsequently. This process of **cross-cortical consolidation** may continue for many years for a fact or event that is re-evaluated, re-interpreted, and repeatedly integrated with other information. Cross-cortical consolidation may proceed not only during waking, but also during sleep (Maquet *et al.* 2003; Paller and Voss 2004). It may also continue beyond a point in time when the memory has become **cortically self-sufficient**, which is when the memory would not be disrupted by hippocampal damage because cortical storage sites would be sufficient to support retrieval. This brain damage leads to difficulties in remembering declarative memories that are not cortically self-sufficient, including memories formed prior to the onset of amnesia (retrograde amnesia) and memories formed after the onset of amnesia (anterograde amnesia). Because memories are less likely to be cortically self-sufficient if acquired recently, retrograde amnesia is typically worse for recently acquired information. Many amnesic patients can remember episodes from their childhood and early adulthood as well as anyone.

Normal declarative memory is a by-product of three stages of information processing. **Encoding** refers to the initial stage, when information arrives in the brain following sensory analysis or via imagination. The term encoding has been used to refer to the input and comprehension of this information (which is not problematic for amnesic patients), as well as to the transformation of the experience into a memory (which is impaired in amnesia).

As described above, declarative memory formation is often not finalized at encoding but rather can continue over a prolonged storage period when memory is subject to change, consolidation, interference, distortion, and forgetting. **Storage** denotes this second stage of information processing, which may actually begin as soon as new information is acquired.

The final stage, **retrieval**, takes place when memory is accessed and used. Amnesic patients are generally able to retrieve some memories, particularly those already consolidated to the point of cortical self-sufficiency. However, memory retrieval can be quite demanding and require effortful search strategies, such as when one searches for a relatively insignificant childhood memory. In such cases, contributions from the prefrontal cortex are especially important with respect to conducting a systematic search, evaluating products of retrieval, escaping from the present moment to bring a prior experience to mind, maintaining information in working memory, inhibiting the intrusion of irrelevant information, constructing a remembered experience based on retrieved information, evaluating the suitability of each bit of retrieved information, and so on. Accordingly, prefrontal damage alone can lead to memory retrieval difficulties as well as memory encoding difficulties, and when combined with medial temporal damage can lead to exacerbated memory deficits.

The evidence that amnesic patients can show intact performance when it comes to various types of non-declarative memory (Table 21.1) supports the idea that declarative memory depends on special storage mechanisms. Non-declarative memory does not require the linking of distinct representations across multiple neocortical zones. Often, tests of non-declarative memory do not make explicit reference to prior learning episodes; such tests are called implicit memory tests. For instance, behavioural responses to a specific stimulus may be faster or more accurate as a result of prior experience, even when a person is unable to remember that prior experience. This behavioural effect constitutes **priming** (also known as item-specific implicit memory). With respect to the concept of binding, declarative memory retrieval can be conceptualized as requiring the reinstatement of cross-cortically bound information; in contrast, priming may depend on locally bound information within discrete cortical networks. Evidence relevant to this idea can be obtained in functional neuroimaging experiments that succeed in dissociating these two types of memory and, ideally (as described below), contrasting them within the same experiment while other stimulus and task factors are held constant. EEG measures of neural synchrony (e.g. von Stein *et al.* 1999; Weiss and Rappelsberger 2000, chapter 5, 6) may also prove relevant for contrasting binding across multiple cortical regions in declarative memory retrieval as opposed to the more localized processing in priming. Ultimately, explorations of the fundamental differences between declarative and non-declarative memory should shed much light on the neuro-cognitive mechanisms unique to declarative memory.

Furthermore, understanding special cases when non-declarative memory is not preserved in amnesia can provide pivotal insights into the core defect. Future research may be able to test one particular prediction that follows from the foregoing discussion, namely that priming should be preserved in amnesia only when performance can be mediated through neural plasticity within one or more isolated neocortical zones. Special tests in which priming is mediated through neural plasticity connecting separate neocortical zones (see discussion of cross-domain conceptual priming below) should show that priming is impaired in amnesia.

Electrophysiology of declarative memory

To gain further insight into the distinct cognitive functions that combine to support declarative memory, it will be crucial to be able to measure these functions independently. Recordings of the electrical activity of the brain have shown that such measures can indeed be obtained so as to track relevant memory functions on a millisecond-by-millisecond basis. I will outline this evidence below, emphasizing findings from my laboratory.

The EEG is a summation of electrical fields produced by the activity of vast numbers of neurons and recorded using electrodes placed harmlessly on an individual's head. Time-locked average responses known as event-related potentials (ERPs) can be calculated based on EEG responses to different categories of stimuli presented to the individual in a suitable experimental setting (for reviews of ERP studies of memory see Friedman and Johnson 2000; Mecklinger 2000; Paller 2000; Rugg and Wilding 2000; for a general review of ERP methods see Münte *et al.* 2000). ERPs can be characterized in terms of their latency (when they occur relative to the onset of a stimulus), their polarity (positive or negative at the recording location relative to a distant reference location), their amplitude (size of a potential deflection), and their topography (distribution of potential amplitudes across the head).

The extant findings suggest that future prospects are strong for using electrophysiological measures of brain activity in healthy individuals to test and advance theoretical frameworks developed from neuropsychological studies of memory disorders. Despite the emphasis on ERP research, the general approach advocated here also holds for other methods of directly or indirectly measuring brain activity, including neuromagnetic, haemodynamic, and optical neuroimaging.

Transforming experience into memory

One way of investigating the formation of declarative memories is to contrast neural activity at encoding that predicts successful versus unsuccessful memory performance. Brain potentials that predict successful subsequent recall and recognition have been observed in many experiments. These potentials generally have a positive polarity over parietal or frontal brain regions relative to a distant reference location, reach maximal amplitudes 400–800 ms or so after stimulus onset, and have larger amplitudes for remembered stimuli (reviewed by Wagner *et al.* 1999; Paller and Wagner 2002). Similar ERPs have been observed in a few experiments in which electrodes were implanted in the medial temporal region of the brain in patients who were candidates for surgery to relieve medically intractable epilepsy (Fernandez *et al.* 1999, 2002). ERPs have also been identified that predict whether a person will remember seeing a common object, as well as whether a person will claim to have seen an object than was not actually seen but rather was imagined (Gonsalves and Paller 2000). Stimuli to be remembered in the majority of these ERP studies have been visual words, but other stimuli that have been used include pictures of objects, faces, abstract patterns, spoken names, and environmental sounds.

In one experiment, words were presented visually in an encoding phase followed by either an implicit or an explicit memory test (Paller 1990). In the implicit memory test, participants were instructed to complete three-letter stems with the first word to come to mind. The extent to which their completions matched words from encoding, compared with a baseline completion rate, provided a measure of priming. In the explicit memory test, participants attempted to recall words from the encoding phase to complete the stems. ERPs from the encoding phase were more positive for words recalled later than for words not recalled later. This systematic difference in brain potentials can be referred to as **Dm-recall** (an ERP **D**ifference based on later **m**emory performance on a **recall** test). On the other hand, ERPs did not reliably predict later priming. These findings, together with others, are consistent with the idea that Dm-recall indexed encoding activity specific to declarative memory formation, most likely

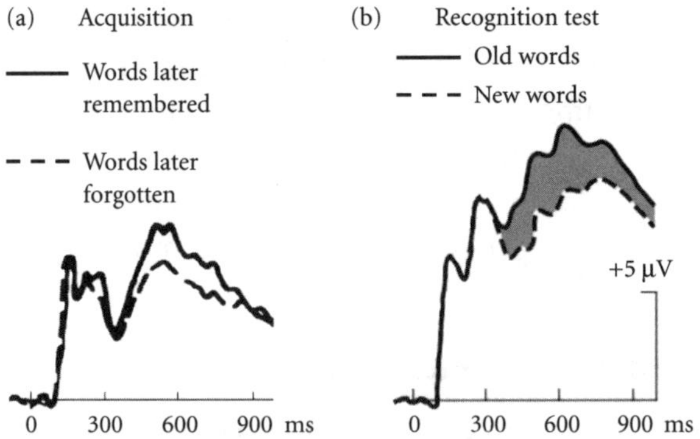

Figure 21.1 Examples of ERPs investigated in memory paradigms demonstrating (a) a subsequent memory effect and (b) an old–new effect. ERPs were elicited by words presented visually in the study and test phases of the same experiment (Paller *et al.* 1987). The recordings shown were obtained from electrodes located at the midline parietal scalp location in a group of 16 young adults. During the study phase (acquisition), participants responded to each word according to task requirements in four different tasks. During the test phase (recognition test), participants made yes–no recognition judgements followed by a three-choice confidence rating. The subsequent memory effect was observed by averaging ERPs recorded during acquisition as a function of later recognition performance. The ERP difference between responses to subsequently remembered and subsequently forgotten words (Dm) was apparent from about 400–800 ms after word onset. The old–new effect was recorded during the recognition test and is shaded in (b). ERPs elicited by old words were more positive than ERPs elicited by new words. Results also showed that this old–new effect was greater for words recognized with high confidence. However, old–new effects of this sort cannot be unequivocally linked to declarative memory, given that priming also occurs (see Fig. 21.2). (Adapted from Paller ***et al.*** 1987.)

pertaining to the meaning of each word rather than merely to its visual appearance. Similar Dm phenomena have also been observed using recognition tests, as shown in Figure 21.1(a).

In an experiment with faces, ERPs at initial encoding predicted not only whether later recognition was successful, but also the experiential quality of the recognition experience (Yovel and Paller 2003). Positive ERPs from parietal regions over both hemispheres predicted recognition accompanied by retrieval of episodic detail, whereas only right-parietal ERPs predicted successful recognition without episodic detail, a phenomenon referred to as **pure familiarity**, because it occurs when a face seems familiar but is not remembered.

Other studies of ERPs, frequency-domain EEG measures, functional magnetic resonance images of brain activity, and spiking from single neurons have suggested that many cortical regions can be involved in memory encoding, and that hippocampal activity may be particularly relevant for the storage of declarative memories (Cameron *et al.* 2001; Fell *et al.* 2002; Paller and McCarthy 2002; Reber *et al.* 2002; Sederberg *et al.* 2003).

Many different types of processing at encoding can promote successful memory storage. Accordingly, many avenues of investigation will be required to understand the formation and preservation of declarative memories. Measures of neural activity predictive of subsequent memory, such as Dm-recall, provide a valuable perspective on this problem, and will ultimately be most useful to the extent that connections can be built between these measures and specific neurocognitive processes. This goal will require analysing neural activity as a function of successful versus unsuccessful encoding in conjunction with experimental manipulations that systematically affect memory encoding and storage.

Memory retrieval

The effectiveness of encoding and storage becomes evident only when stored information is subsequently accessed. In studies of retrieval, differences between ERP responses to new and old items in recognition tests have been researched in considerable detail. These so-called **old–new ERP** effects are generally positive shifts in ERPs to old items relative to ERPs to new items, as shown in Figure 21.1(b). Early experiments on old–new ERP effects prompted a range of conclusions without leading to consensus. In retrospect, firm interpretations were difficult because remembering in these circumstances generally involves a variety of different cognitive processes such that multiple brain potentials are produced in overlapping time intervals. As a result, functionally distinct brain signals within old–new ERP effects were difficult to isolate from one another.

For example, consider two memory phenomena that can co-occur when a person views a face: retrieval of prior episodes involving the same face, and faster or more accurate processing due to prior perceptual analysis of that same face, as indexed by the behavioural phenomenon of perceptual priming. Thus, special tactics are needed to isolate ERPs associated with these different sorts of memory (Fig. 21.2). Indeed, it is notoriously difficult to prevent people from systematically recalling prior episodes when stimuli are repeated, and this incidental retrieval can contaminate neural analyses of priming.

One approach to this problem made use of a condition in which faces were encoded only to a minimal extent (Paller *et al.* 2003a). Each face was presented at a central location for 100 ms while participants were required to make a difficult visual discrimination at another location. When the face disappeared, a noise stimulus appeared centrally to limit further face encoding. On a subsequent recognition test, participants' performance was no better than would be expected if they were purely guessing. However, priming was still observed for these faces in an implicit memory test. Thus, ERPs elicited by these faces were associated with priming uncontaminated by conscious remembering. Within the same

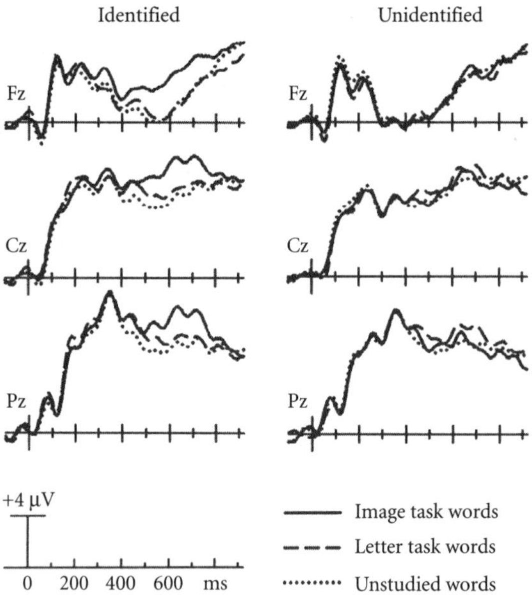

Figure 21.2 Specific electrophysiological correlates of recollection were first isolated by examining ERP old–new effects based on a study phase manipulation that dissociated priming and recollection (Paller and Kutas 1992). In general, ERP differences between old and new items cannot unequivocally be associated with declarative memory, but in the experiment conducted by Paller and Kutas (1992) two types of old items were compared to achieve this goal. Memory results were critical in showing that recall and recognition were superior for words studied in the image task compared with words studied in the letter task, whereas equivalent levels of word-identification priming were observed in these two conditions. ERP elicited during the test phase, when this priming test was given, differed very little for words that could not be identified correctly (right). However, words that participants identified (left) elicited ERPs that differed systematically between conditions. The usual old–new effect was observed, in that ERPs were more positive for old words than for new words. Importantly, the ERP difference between image task words and letter task words (two conditions with matched priming results) showed for the first time that this portion of the old–new effect beginning at a latency of 500 ms was associated specifically with declarative memory retrieval. Moreover, given that the manipulation influenced free recall performance, recollection was implicated. This ERP correlate of recollection was shown to be functionally distinct from an earlier portion of the old–new effect that was present for both types of old words and visible from 400–500 ms. Recordings shown were from midline frontal (Fz), central (Cz), and parietal (Pz) locations. (Adapted from Paller and Kutas 1992.)

experimental runs of this experiment, other faces were presented for a longer duration with no competing stimulus discrimination requirement to limit encoding; these faces were remembered well by the participants. The two conditions provide for a direct comparison between ERPs associated with conscious memory for faces and ERPs associated with priming. As illustrated in Figure 21.3, recognizing a repeated face was associated with positive ERPs at the rear of the head 400 to 800 ms after face onset (Fig. 21.3(a)), whereas priming was

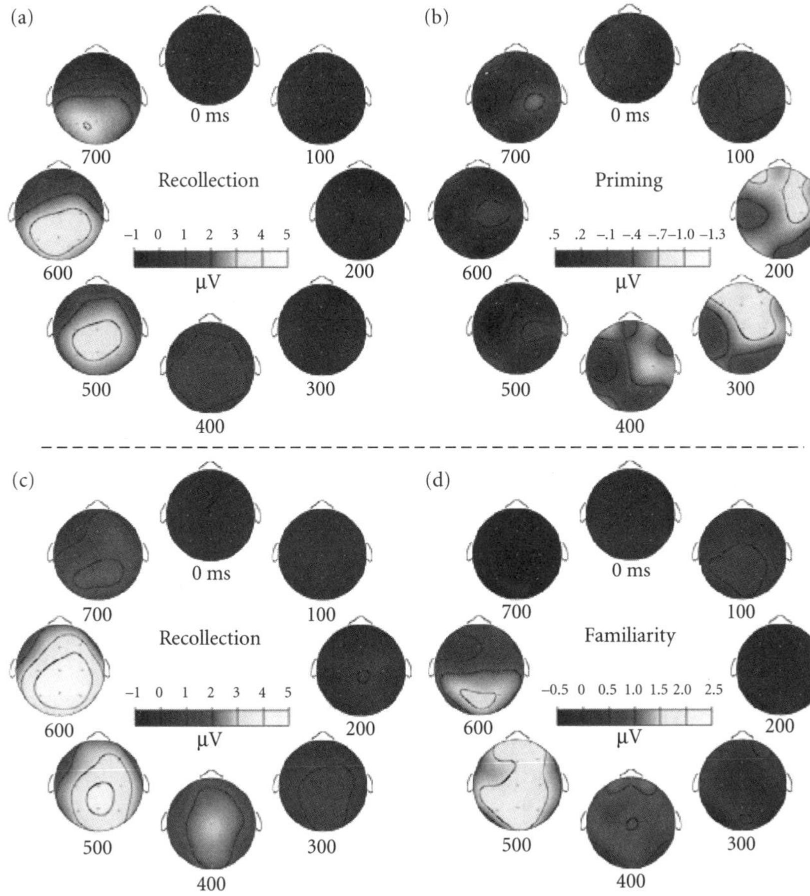

Figure 21.3 Topographic maps of brain potentials associated with different memory phenomena: (a) recollection and (b) perceptual priming in one experiment (Paller 2003a); (c) recollection and (d) pure familiarity in another experiment (Yovel and Paller *et al*. 2004). Differences in potentials between pairs of conditions are shown on schematic heads as if viewed from above (nose at the top), interpolated from 21 scalp locations. Measurements were made over eight 100-ms intervals beginning at the time shown below each map, where time 0 is the time of stimulus onset. Thus each panel shows potential differences for eight time intervals, arranged like a stopwatch that runs for 800 ms. Potentials are displayed according to a different microvolt scale in each panel, together with isopotential lines. In all panels, the largest differences are signified by the lightest colours (yellow and white). Polarity is negative only in (b), and values beyond the negative range of the scale in the 700–800 ms map in (d) are shown as black. In one experiment (Paller *et al*. 2003a), subtractions were computed to isolate potentials associated with (a) recollection prompted by faces and (b) perceptual priming with faces. The two contrasts were between remembered faces and new faces, and between primed but forgotten faces and new faces, respectively. Quite different electrical signals were observed; priming was associated with negativity at 200–400 ms towards the front of the head, whereas recollection was associated with positivity at 400–800 ms towards the rear of the head. In the other experiment (Yovel and Paller 2004), subtractions were computed to isolate potentials associated with (c) recollection and (d) pure familiarity for faces. These two contrasts were between faces remembered with associative information and new faces, and between faces recognized without episodic retrieval and new faces, respectively. Electrical signals of pure familiarity did not resemble electrical signals of face priming, but rather seemed like reduced-amplitude versions of signals of face recollection. (Adapted from Paller *et al*. 2003a; Paller 2004; Yovel and Paller 2004.) See also colour plate section.

associated with negative ERPs at the front of the head, particularly on the right side, 200 to 400 ms after face onset (Fig. 21.3(b)).

In another experiment we used a different strategy to isolate signals associated with face recollection (Paller *et al.* 1999). At encoding, participants attempted to memorize 20 faces accompanied by a spoken vignette (to simulate actually meeting the individual pictured) and were told to forget 20 other faces. One vignette, for example, was: 'I'm Alison; I won the Boston Marathon twice.' Later recognition was superior for the former compared with the latter faces, but the magnitude of priming observed during implicit memory testing was the same for the two groups of faces. In the implicit memory test face identification was made difficult by obscuring portions of each face with superimposed black pixels. In order to perform the famous–non-famous face discriminations required in this test, face identification was required, and prior exposure to a face presumably facilitated the processing of these partially obscured faces. Priming effects were observed as both faster response times and high response accuracy for faces repeated from the encoding phase compared with new faces. Therefore comparing ERPs for the two kinds of repeated faces revealed a neural signal of face recollection uncontaminated by face priming. This neural signal of recollection bore a strong resemblance to the spatiotemporal electrical patterns associated with face recollection in other studies (e.g. Fig. 21.3(a)). Analogous results have been obtained using verbal stimuli to obtain ERP correlates of recollection cued by words, as shown in Figure 21.2.

In one follow-up study using ERP and functional MRI methods in different groups of subjects, a contrast between remembered faces learned with a spoken vignette and new faces revealed left hippocampal, cortical (left insula and left temporal), and cerebellar activity (Paller *et al.* 2003b). Another experiment juxtaposed electrical signals of remembering a face *per se* and remembering a face together with corresponding biographical facts learned at encoding (Paller *et al.* 2000), such as the name Alison and the winning of the Boston Marathon. Brain activity was observed over posterior brain regions in both situations, whereas additional activity that was slightly more anterior was observed only when biographical retrieval occurred. Recalling person-specific information, as in the latter case, is dependent on a very high degree of binding, as diverse types of information must be linked together, and thus is perhaps a prototypical example of the sort of declarative memory retrieval that would naturally give rise to conscious recollection.

Awareness of remembering

Despite the strong connection between declarative memory and the experience of remembering, these phenomena need not always occur together. Declarative memory provides some of the necessary precursors at memory retrieval, but it is not sufficient to produce the awareness of remembering. Rather, conscious memory depends on a further inference—the explicit idea that the current contents of consciousness are derived from memory retrieval.

Thus dysfunctional cross-cortical storage in amnesia has an indirect impact on awareness of remembering. A strong and rather selective disruption of declarative memory will also disrupt awareness of remembering because memory for the spatiotemporal context of an episode is a critical factor that can help one to infer that a memory for a prior event has been retrieved (Johnson and Chalfonte 1994). This function falls within the aforementioned category of prefrontal functions that contribute to memory retrieval, together with strategic search, evaluation, and working memory (or 'working-with-memory' (Moscovitch 1992)). Indeed, frontal brain potentials associated with retrieval functions have been identified in many studies (Ranganath and Paller 1999; Rugg and Wilding 2000).

Accordingly, neural signals of memory must be evaluated with respect to the possibility that declarative memory retrieval need not necessarily give rise to awareness of remembering. Sometimes a stimulus can seem familiar even in the absence of conscious remembering. This experience is called **pure familiarity**. The epitome of a pure familiarity experience is the so-called butcher-on-the-bus phenomenon (Mandler 1980), which is when one believes that a person is familiar (often upon seeing their face in an atypical context) while failing to recall any information whatsoever about that person. Indeed, when the butcher is encountered in the context of a bus, very few clues are available concerning the identity of the butcher compared with those typically present when the butcher is encountered in the butcher's shop.

Particularly informative results were obtained by comparing circumstances when a face provoked a full-blown recollective experience driven by remembering contextual features associated with that face with circumstances when a face provoked the unsubstantiated impression of memory known as pure familiarity (Yovel and Paller 2004). In comparison with electrical signals associated with face-induced recollection (Fig. 21.3(c)), electrical signals associated with pure familiarity with faces (Fig. 21.3(d)) were similar but exhibited reduced amplitudes. Notably, electrophysiological correlates of pure familiarity with faces and of priming with faces (Fig. 21.3(d) and Fig. 21.3(b), respectively) were highly divergent, consistent with the notion that familiarity is not a straightforward outcome of priming, despite superficial similarities between familiarity and priming. Pure familiarity can instead be conceived of as a result of limited stimulus recognition without contextual retrieval adequate for triggering episodic recollection.

Border areas of declarative memory

Current theories of memory address a variety of memory phenomena and their neural implementation, but many questions remain open. Some subtle but critical questions concern memory phenomena at the border between declarative and non-declarative memory, such as some subtypes of priming. If amnesia fundamentally entails a disruption of memory functions dependent upon cross-cortical storage, as proposed, priming should remain preserved only if mediated within single neocortical zones.

Conceptual priming is one subtype of priming that deserves further study; it is believed to arise from altered representations of the meaning of a stimulus rather than merely the physical features of a stimulus. Conceptual priming can cross stimulus domains, such as when hearing a word primes its meaning so as to facilitate processing of that meaning when subsequently reading that word, or when reading the name of a famous person primes knowledge of their identity so as to facilitate processing of person identity when subsequently viewing that person's face. Indeed, a putative electrical signal of conceptual priming with words has been identified and shown to be preserved in patients with deficient declarative memory (Olichney *et al.* 2000; see also Yovel and Paller 2004). This signal may reflect a component of exactly the type of memory that allows amnesic patients to engage fully in complex conversations, all the while maintaining their comprehension abilities and focus on the topic at hand.

The neural processing responsible for conceptual priming is not well understood. Moreover, it may be useful to assume that there are multiple types of conceptual priming. For example, conceptual priming may in some circumstances reflect activation of the representation of the meaning of a word, in which case it is plausible that such a representation may be instantiated entirely within the neurons of a discrete neocortical zone. Likewise, in some cases new associations may be learned to the point where relevant information takes the form of a unitized representation dependent on a single neocortical zone. On the other hand, there may be many cases when conceptual priming depends on links among multiple neocortical zones, such as when very different types of perceptual objects are associated with one another. According to the present account, priming in such circumstances would be expected to depend on hippocampal processing and to be impaired in amnesic patients. Testing these predictions empirically will not be easy, but doing so will have important theoretical implications and thus may help to advance our understanding of the neural substrates of memory.

Conclusions

We now have the ability to record neural signals associated with several of the many processes that contribute to declarative and non-declarative memory. These neural signals provide a vital window on the physiology of memory that will become increasingly important for further explorations of the neurocognitive substrates of remembering.

Therefore, future efforts should be aimed at elucidating exactly how declarative memory differs from priming and other types of non-declarative memory. What is unique about declarative encoding, storage, and retrieval? What memory processes support priming when is it preserved in amnesia, and how do they differ from those that support declarative memory? Does remembering in the absence of contextual retrieval, as exemplified by pure familiarity experiences, rely on any memory processing in common with priming, or is it more closely allied with declarative memory? What processing underlies priming phenomena that are impaired in amnesia, and what might this processing have in common with declarative memory?

A promising strategy to promote progress on these and related issues is to isolate and characterize neurophysiological events specifically responsible for memory functions. A variety of techniques for measuring brain activity can be used together to study human memory and memory disorders, and to provide data needed to advance and refine neurobiological hypotheses concerning memory, such as those outlined above. This approach may also lead to an eventual understanding of how neurocognitive processing gives rise to the conscious experience of remembering. We might thereby obtain a modicum of insight into the neurocognitive substrates of human awareness in general—a supreme challenge that has historically remained out of the reach of humankind but which now appears to be gradually yielding to determined scientific pursuit.

Acknowledgements

Portions of this chapter were extracted or adapted with permission from a paper published in *Current Directions in Psychological Science* (Paller 2004). Research support from the US National Institutes of Health is gratefully acknowledged.

References

Cameron, K.A., Yashar, S., Wilson, C.L., and Fried, I. (2001). Human hippocampal neurons predict how well word pairs will be remembered. *Neuron*, **30**, 289–298.

Eichenbaum, H. and Cohen, N.J. (2001). *From Conditioning to Conscious Recollection: Memory Systems of the Brain*. New York: Oxford University Press.

Fell, J, Klaver, P., Elger, C.E. and Fernandez, G. (2002). The interaction of rhinal cortex and hippocampus in human declarative memory formation. *Reviews in the Neurosciences*, **13**, 299–312.

Fernandez, G., Effern, A., Grunwald, T., *et al.* (1999). Real-time tracking of memory formation in the human rhinal cortex and hippocampus. *Science*, **285**, 1582–1585.

Fernandez, G., Klaver, P., Fell, J., Grunwald, T., and Elger, C.E. (2002). Human declarative memory formation: segregating rhinal and hippocampal contributions. *Hippocampus*, **12**, 514–519.

Friedman, D. and Johnson, R., Jr (2000). Event-related potential (ERP) studies of memory encoding and retrieval: a selective review. *Microscopy Research and Technique*, **51**, 6–28.

Gonsalves, B. and Paller, K.A. (2000). Neural events that underlie remembering something that never happened. *Nature Neuroscience*, **3**, 1316–1321.

Johnson, M.K. and Chalfonte, B.L. (1994). Binding complex memories: the role of reactivation and the hippocampus. In *Memory Systems 1994* (ed D.L. Schacter and E. Tulving). Cambridge, MA: MIT Press, pp. 311–350).

Mandler, G. (1980). Recognizing: the judgment of previous occurrence. *Psychological Review*, **87**, 252–271.

Maquet, P., Smith, S., and Stickgold, R. (ed) (2003). *Sleep and Brain Plasticity*. New York: Oxford University Press.

Mecklinger, A. (2000). Interfacing mind and brain: a neurocognitive model of recognition memory. *Psychophysiology*, **37**, 565–582.

Moscovitch, M. (1992). Memory and working-with-memory: a component process model based on modules and central systems. *Journal of Cognitive Neuroscience*, **4**, 257–267.

Münte, T.F., Urbach, T.P., Düzel, E., and Kutas, M. (2000). Event-related brain potentials in the study of human cognition and neuropsychology. In *Handbook of Neuropsychology*, Vol. 1 (ed F. Boller, J. Grafman, and G. Rizzolatti). Amsterdam: Elsevier, pp. 139–234.

Olichney, J.M., Van Petten, C., Paller, K.A., Salmon, D.P., Iragui, V.J., and Kutas, M. (2000). Word repetition in amnesia: electrophysiological measures of impaired and spared memory. *Brain*, **123**, 1948–1963.

Paller, K.A. (1990). Recall and stem-completion priming have different electrophysiological correlates and are modified differentially by directed forgetting. *Journal of Experimental Psychology: Learning, Memory, and Cognition*, **16**, 1021–1032.

Paller, K.A. (1997). Consolidating dispersed neocortical memories: the missing link in amnesia. *Memory*, **5**, 73–88.

Paller, K.A. (2000). Neural measures of conscious and unconscious memory. *Behavioural Neurology*, **12**, 127–141.

Paller, K.A. (2002). Cross-cortical consolidation as the core defect in amnesia: prospects for hypothesis-testing with neuropsychology and neuroimaging. In *Neuropsychology of Memory* (3rd edn) (ed L.R. Squire and D.L. Schacter). New York: Guilford Press, pp. 73–87).

Paller, K.A. (2004). Electrical signals of memory and of the awareness of remembering. *Current Directions in Psychological Science*, **13**, 49–55.

Paller, K.A. and Kutas, M. (1992). Brain potentials during memory retrieval: neurophysiological indications of the distinction between conscious recollection and priming. *Journal of Cognitive Neuroscience*, **4**, 375–391.

Paller, K.A. and McCarthy, G. (2002). Field potentials in the human hippocampus during the encoding and recognition of visual stimuli. *Hippocampus*, **12**, 415–420.

Paller, K.A. and Voss, J.L. (2004). Memory reactivation and consolidation during sleep. *Learning and Memory*, **11**, 655–660.

Paller, K.A. and Wagner, A.D. (2002). Observing the transformation of experience into memory. *Trends in Cognitive Sciences*, **6**, 93–102.

Paller, K.A., Kutas, M., and Mayes, A.R. (1987). Neural correlates of encoding in an incidental learning paradigm. *Electroencephalography and Clinical Neurophysiology*, **67**, 360–371.

Paller, K.A., Bozic, V.S., Ranganath, C., Grabowecky, M., and Yamada, S. (1999). Brain waves following remembered faces index conscious recollection. *Cognitive Brain Research*, **7**, 519–531.

Paller, K.A., Gonsalves, B., Grabowecky M., Bozic, V.S., and Yamada, S. (2000). Electrophysiological correlates of recollecting faces of known and unknown individuals. *NeuroImage*, **11**, 98–110.

Paller, K.A., Hutson, C.A., Miller, B.B., and Boehm, S.G. (2003a). Neural manifestations of memory with and without awareness. *Neuron*, **38**, 507–516.

Paller, K.A., Ranganath, C., Gonsalves, B., *et al.* (2003b). Neural correlates of person recognition. *Learning and Memory*, **10**, 253–260.

Ranganath, C. and Paller, K.A. (1999). Frontal brain potentials during recognition are modulated by requirements to retrieve perceptual detail. *Neuron*, **22**, 605–613.

Reber, P.J., Siwiec, R.M., Gitelman, D.R., Parrish. T.B., Mesulam, M.-M., and Paller, K.A. (2002). Neural correlates of successful encoding identified using functional magnetic resonance imaging. *Journal of Neuroscience*, **22**, 9541–9548.

Rugg, M.D. and Wilding, E.L. (2000). Retrieval processing and episodic memory. *Trends in Cognitive Science*, **4**, 108–115.

Schacter, D.L. (1996). *Searching for Memory: The Brain, the Mind, and the Past.* New York: BasicBooks.

Schacter, D.L. and Tulving E. (ed) (1994). *Memory Systems 1994.* Cambridge, MA: MIT Press.

Sederberg, P.B., Kahana, M.J., Howard, M.W., Donner, E., and Madsen, J.R. (2003). Theta and gamma oscillations during encoding predict subsequent recall. *Journal of Neuroscience*, **23**, 10809–10814.

Squire, L.R. (1987). *Memory and Brain.* New York: Oxford University Press.

Squire, L.R. and Kandel, E.R. (1999). *Memory: From Mind to Molecules.* New York: Scientific American Library.

Squire, L.R. and Schacter, D.L. (ed) (2002). *Neuropsychology of Memory* (3rd edn). New York: Guilford Press.

von Stein, A., Rappelsberger, P., Sarnthein, J., and Petsche, H. (1999). Synchronization between temporal and parietal cortex during multimodal object processing in man. *Cerebral Cortex*, **9**, 137–150.

Wagner, A.D., Koutstaal, W., and Schacter, D.L. (1999). When encoding yields remembering: insights from event-related neuroimaging, *Philosophical Transactions of the Royal Society of London, Series B, Biological Sciences*, **354**, 1307–1324.

Weiss, S. and Rappelsberger, P. (2000). Long-range EEG synchronization during word encoding correlates with successful memory performance. *Cognitive Brain Research*, **9**, 299–312.

Yovel, G. and Paller, K.A. (2004). The neural basis of the butcher-on-the-bus phenomenon: when a face seems familiar but is not remembered. *NeuroImage*, **21**, 789–800.

Chapter 22

Retrieval inhibition in episodic recall: effects on feature binding

Karl-Heinz Bäuml

Introduction

Benefits and costs of episodic processing

Many types of episodic processing show a mixture of induced benefits and costs, increasing later recall of the processed material and reducing recall of the unprocessed material. One such prominent class of cases is the strengthening of episodic material, whereby the binding between items and their cue(s) and/or the binding of intra-item features is enhanced. Results from a large body of research have shown that recall of learned material can be greatly improved if the number of study trials, or study time, of the material to be learned is increased (Roberts 1972). However, such benefits of enhancing the binding level of episodic material may be accompanied by costs if only part of the material is strengthened. In fact, if study time or study trials are increased for only a subset of the learned material, then such strengthening will increase recall for the strengthened material but decrease it for the non-strengthened material (Tulving and Hastie 1972; Ratcliff *et al.* 1990).

A similar picture is obtained if an increase in binding level occurs through repeated retrieval. Prior work has demonstrated that the retrieval of learned material improves later recall of the retrieved material (Hogan and Kintsch 1971). Again, however, such benefits may be accompanied by costs if only part of the material is practised. If subjects repeatedly retrieve a subset of previously learned material, later recall of the non-retrieved material is worse than in a control condition in which no retrieval practice takes place (Anderson *et al.* 1994; Anderson and Spellman 1995). Obviously, enhancing the cue-item or intra-item binding, be it through relearning or retrieval, is not only beneficial for episodic recall but can also be detrimental.

It might appear that cueing represents a special form of episodic processing in so far as it can only be beneficial, and not detrimental, for recall, in contrast with the mixture of benefits and costs obtained by the strengthening of episodes.

Indeed, cueing has been found to facilitate recall in many situations. For instance, if a categorized list with several items from each category is presented to participants and, at test, the category names are provided as retrieval cues, such cueing typically improves recall performance compared with unaided free recall (Tulving and Pearlstone 1966) (see Tulving (1974) for further examples).

However, cueing is not always facilitatory. If participants learn a categorized list and, at test, receive the category names of half the learned categories as retrieval cues, such part-list cueing improves recall of items from the cued categories but impairs recall of items from the uncued categories (Roediger 1978). Detrimental effects of cueing also occur within subjective units. If subjects learn a categorized list and, at test, receive the category name plus a subset of the category items as retrieval cues, recall of the remaining category exemplars is poorer than recall of the same items if only the category name is provided as a retrieval cue (Slamecka 1968; Roediger 1973). Obviously, just like the strengthening of episodes, cueing is beneficial in some cases, but detrimental in others (reviewed by Roediger and Neely 1982; Nickerson 1984).

Mechanisms underlying the detrimental effects of strengthening and cueing

A simple account of the detrimental effects of strengthening and cueing is provided by the concept of strength-dependent competition. According to this concept, memories bound to a common cue (e. g. FRUIT–apple, FRUIT–orange) compete for renewed binding when that cue is presented. Corresponding evidence has

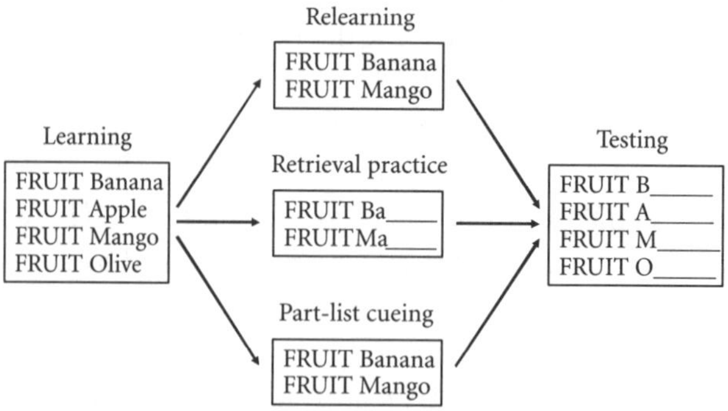

Figure 22.1 Three forms of reprocessing episodic material. Relearning: a subset of the previously studied material is re-exposed for additional learning. Retrieval practice: the word stems of a subset of the previously studied material are presented and subjects are asked to retrieve the items that correspond to the cues. Part-list cueing: a subset of the previously studied material is re-exposed for use as a retrieval cue at test. Note that the presentation of the cue items may also occur as part of the testing procedure; in this case only the non-cue items are to be recalled. For details see Bäuml and Aslan (2004).

been provided by a number of studies in which it was shown that the cued recall of an item decreases as the number of items bound to the same cue increases (reviewed by Watkins 1975). Moreover, the competition is often assumed to be strength dependent, i.e. the cued recall of an item is assumed to decrease (increase) as a function of the increase (decrease) in the level of the binding of its competitors to the common cue. Correspondingly, recall chances for FRUIT–apple should decrease if, during learning, FRUIT–orange is studied twice rather than once (Rundus 1973; Raaijmakers and Shiffrin 1981; Anderson 1983; Mensink and Raaijmakers 1988).

The concept of strength-dependent competition is theoretically attractive because it offers a unified account of the detrimental effects of both strengthening and cueing. Indeed, according to this concept, the strengthening of material, be it through relearning or retrieval, increases the binding level of the reprocessed items and thus makes these items stronger competitors for the material which has not been reprocessed. Because of this change in competition conditions for renewed binding, recall of the strengthened material improves and recall of the non-strengthened material becomes worse compared with a condition in which no strengthening takes place at all (Raaijmakers and Shiffrin 1981; Mensink and Raaijmakers 1988). In a similar way, strength-dependent competition also provides an explanation for why part-list cueing can cause forgetting. If the presentation of part-list cues increases the binding level of the cue items in a very similar way to that produced by relearning or retrieval (Rundus 1973; Roediger 1973), this enhancement should induce a competition bias and thus reduce recall of non-cue items. If this is true, the same mechanism would mediate the detrimental effects of relearning, retrieval, and cueing.

At least two properties of the strength-dependence account are challenging. One property is the assumption that forgetting leaves the memory representation of the forgotten material unchanged. In fact, the material is neither inhibited nor degraded in any way, so that it is assumed that no change in binding level or binding structure occurs. Rather, episodic forgetting arises only because new competing material is bound to the same cue, or competing material already bound to the common cue is strengthened in its binding level. The second property is that the account does not distinguish between changes in binding level as they occur through relearning and changes in binding level as they occur through retrieval. Indeed, this proposed equivalence between learning and retrieval is part of many computational models (Rundus 1973; Raaijmakers and Shiffrin 1981; Mensink and Raaijmakers 1988). In addition, the account does not distinguish between changes in binding level as they occur through relearning and changes as they occur through part-list cueing. Such an equivalence between learning and cueing is part of Rundus's (1973) computational framework.

A third property of strength dependence appears noteworthy. Forgetting episodic material is assumed to occur only if other material bound to the same cue is strengthened. For instance, if RED–blood, RED–cherry, FOOD–radish, FOOD–bread, etc. are learned, strengthening RED–blood should lead to impaired recall of RED–cherry but not to impaired recall of FOOD–radish or FOOD–bread. Indeed, increasing the level of binding between the practised item and its cue should reduce chances for the other item which is bound to the same cue, but should not impair recall of items which are bound to a different cue (e.g. FOOD–radish). This property of cue-dependent forgetting is part of many computational models of the past years (Rundus 1973; Raaijmakers and Shiffrin 1981; Mensink and Raaijmakers 1988). Of course, the adequacy of strength dependence and the computational models which rely on it depend on the empirical soundness of all these properties. However, until recently these properties have not been tested directly.

Aim of the present chapter

In the past 10 years, evidence has accumulated that strength-dependent competition is not the mechanism underlying the detrimental effects of strengthening and cueing. Rather, a more complex picture of episodic forgetting has arisen. This new picture challenges all three properties of the strength-dependence account outlined above, indicating that (a) episodic forgetting does not arise from enhancing the binding level of competing material and is often, although not always, caused by retrieval inhibition of the non-processed material, (b) the proposed equivalence between learning, retrieval, and cueing is wrong and at least learning on the one hand and retrieval and cueing on the other differ, and (c) forgetting may cross cue boundaries and be cue independent. Because of these results, a substantial modification of our picture of episodic forgetting has emerged.

The aim of this chapter is to outline some of the landmarks of this recent development by showing how our understanding of episodic forgetting has changed in the light of new experimental evidence. This outline is provided separately for the three forms of episodic forgetting discussed in the present chapter, i.e. relearning, retrieval, and cueing. Then episodic forgetting is discussed on the basis of two-stage models of recall (Raaijmakers and Shiffrin 1981; Mensink and Raaijmakers 1988; Rohrer 1996), before some conclusions are offered about how forgetting affects feature binding.

Detrimental effects of relearning

Interference studies

The relationship between an increase in binding level as it occurs through relearning part of a studied list and episodic forgetting has been studied using a variety of experimental paradigms. Many of these studies were interference studies, examining how the recall of target material varies as a function of either some prior learning (proactive interference) or of some subsequent learning (retroactive interference). In retroactive interference, for instance, the typical finding has been that a higher degree of interpolated learning induces greater interference than a lower degree (Briggs 1957; Barnes and Underwood 1959). This finding agrees with strength-dependent competition, as higher degrees of interpolated learning should increase the binding level of the interpolated material, make these items stronger competitors, and thus the previously learned target material to be forgotten. In fact, almost no exceptions from this pattern have been reported.

All the studies showing an effect of the degree of interpolated learning used the anticipation procedure during acquisition of the interpolated task (Crowder 1976). In this procedure, subjects must learn to give the response member of a paired associate when presented with the stimulus member of the pair. In each trial the stimulus member is presented as a cue to which subjects attempt to recall or 'anticipate' the associated response. Following the response, feedback regarding the correct pairing is given. By cueing recall in this manner, subjects are engaged in retrieval practice with every trial of the learning task.

Using this procedure, the degree of interpolated learning is manipulated by varying the number of study trials for the interpolated task. However, as more study opportunities are given, more prescribed retrieval efforts are also being made, thus increasing the retrieval practice on the interpolated task. Because retrieval of material can cause forgetting of non-retrieved material (Anderson *et al.* 1994; see also below), the retrieval practice on the interpolated task may have caused the forgetting of the original task, with a higher amount of retrieval practice leading to stronger forgetting.

Bäuml (1996) examined the issue in two free-recall experiments. He let subjects study one original and then four interpolated lists. The degree of interpolated learning was manipulated by varying exposure time. In Experiment 1, where the typical confounding of retrieval practice and degree of interpolated learning was present, greater interpolated learning induced greater retroactive interference, which is consistent with prior research. However, in Experiment 2, where the degree of interpolated learning was manipulated without concomitant variation in retrieval practice, retroactive interference was the same, whether the interpolated lists had been learned well or poorly. Therefore greater interpolated learning did not increase the amount of retroactive interference, a finding which challenges the strength dependence account (see DaPolito (1966) for a related result in proactive interference.)

The list-strength effect

A more recent illustration of the apparent relationship between an enhancement in binding level as it occurs through relearning and episodic forgetting comes from a series of studies of what has been termed the list-strength effect (Ratcliff *et al.* 1990). Using a mixed-pure paradigm, Ratcliff *et al.* presented subjects with three kinds of item lists: pure-strong lists containing strong items only, pure-weak lists containing weak items only, and mixed lists containing half weak and half strong items. Strengthening was accomplished by increasing either the exposure time or the number of repetitions of the items to be strengthened. In free-recall tests Ratcliff *et al.* found that relatively more strong items were recalled from the mixed lists than from the pure-strong lists, and relatively more weak items were recalled from the pure-weak lists than from the mixed lists, a pattern consistent with strength-dependent competition.

However, the results obtained by Ratcliff *et al.* might also have been induced by uncontrolled retrieval practice. Indeed, if the strong items from a mixed list are retrieved earlier than the weak items (Anderson *et al.* 1994; Wixted *et al.* 1997), recall performance of strong items from mixed lists should be higher than from pure-strong lists. In fact, in the pure-strong lists the retrieval of items in the first testing positions should lead to recall impairment of the items still to be remembered, yielding lower performance, on average, than in the mixed lists. Similarly, recall performance of weak items from mixed lists should be lower than from pure-weak lists, because, on average, there is less retrieval-induced recall impairment for the weak items in the pure-weak lists than in the mixed lists. Thus the list-strength effect found by Ratcliff *et al.* need not necessarily have been the result of strength-dependent competition but might have been caused by output-order biases and a process of retrieval-induced forgetting.

Bäuml (1997) reported an experiment in which categorizable lists were employed and some categories in each list contained strong items only, some weak items only, and some both strong and weak items. Strengthening was accomplished by varying the exposure time of the items. The testing sequence of the items from each category was controlled by the use of category-plus-first-letter cues. When the typical confounding of strengthening and output order was mimicked, list-strength effects were found, which is consistent with prior

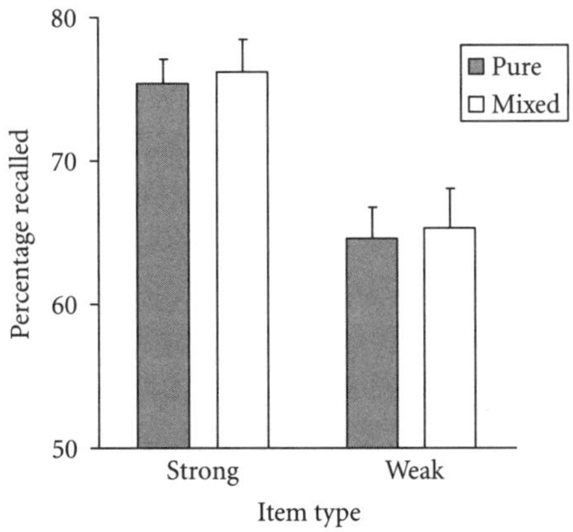

Figure 22.2 Recall percentages and standard errors on a category-plus-first-letter cued recall test as a function of item type and category composition. In pure categories all items are strong or all items are weak; in mixed categories half the items are strong and half are weak. (Reproduced from K.-H. Bäuml, *Psychonomic Bulletin and Review*, **4**, 260–264, 1997.)

research. However, when this confounding was eliminated, the list-strength effects disappeared: Neither the recall of strong nor the recall of weak items varied with the strength of the other category exemplars (Fig. 22.2). These results indicate that enhancing the binding level of a subset of previously learned material *per se* does not impair recall of the unprocessed material, an indication which is in line with results from other work (Ciranni and Shimamura 1999; Anderson *et al.* 2000a).

Summary

The results from a number of recent studies have demonstrated that enhancing the binding level of a subset of previously learned material through additional learning may or may not cause the unreprocessed material to be forgotten. Whether it causes forgetting or not depends on the recall task and on whether output order at test is controlled. If output order is not controlled and subjects recall the reprocessed material first and the unreprocessed material last, which is the preferred output order in free recall (Wixted *et al.* 1997), the typical relationship between additional learning and impairment arises. However, if output order is controlled and subjects recall the unreprocessed material first, reprocessing does not cause impairment. These results challenge strength-dependent competition as a general explanation of the detrimental effects accompanied by increases in item binding levels. Rather, they suggest that such effects arise from a non-control of retrieval factors at test. The importance of retrieval for episodic forgetting is stressed in the next section.

Detrimental effects of retrieval

Recall-specific forgetting

The relationship between an increase in binding level as it occurs through the retrieval of part of a studied list and episodic forgetting has generally been studied using the retrieval-practice paradigm (Anderson *et al.* 1994; Anderson and Spellman 1995; reviewed by Levy and Anderson 2002). In this paradigm, subjects are presented with a categorized list containing several items in each category (e.g. FRUIT–apple, FRUIT–orange), and subsequently retrieve half of the items from each category given partial word stems of these items as retrieval cues (e.g. FRUIT–ap).

Strengthening the retrieved items in this way typically impairs later recall of the non-retrieved items (e.g. FRUIT–orange) relative to a control condition in which there is no such retrieval practice. This pattern is consistent with strength-dependent competition, because the retrieval practice increased the binding level of the practised items (e.g. FRUIT–apple) and thus made these items stronger competitors for the unpractised material (e.g. FRUIT–orange) (Raaijmakers and Shiffrin 1981; Mensink and Raaijmakers 1988).

However, there is evidence that retrieval-induced forgetting is not caused by an increase in binding level of the practised material. This evidence comes partly from the studies cited above. In these studies, it was demonstrated that an increase in binding level *per se* does not cause forgetting and that possible detrimental effects of relearning arise only as a result of output order biases at test. However, detrimental effects of retrieval have been reported both when output order at test was not controlled and when it was controlled (Anderson *et al.* 1994; Anderson and Spellman 1995). Therefore, retrieval-induced forgetting should not be due to changes in binding level of the retrieved material.

A study by Anderson *et al.* (2000a) addressed the issue more directly. They let subjects learn a categorized list (e.g. FRUIT–apple, FRUIT–orange). Then subjects either retrieved a subset of a category's items given the word stem of the items as a retrieval cue (e.g. FRUIT–ap—) (competitive condition) or were provided the same items intact and were asked to recall the appropriate category name by using the exemplar and a stem as cues (e.g. FR— -apple) (non-competitive condition). Although the two conditions led to comparable strengthening of the practised items (apple), only the competitive condition induced forgetting of the non-strengthened material (orange) in a final recall test. This finding indicates that retrieval-induced forgetting is not caused by the strengthening of competitors *per se* but rather is due to a recall-specific process (for a related result see Ciranni and Shimamura 1999).

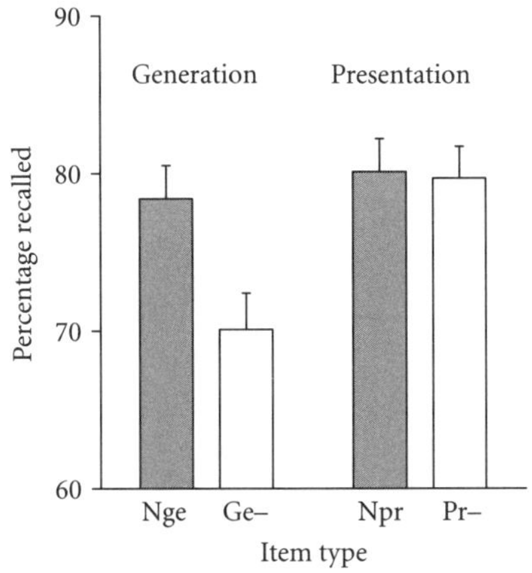

Figure 22.3 Recall percentages and standard errors on a category-plus-first-letter cued-recall test as a function of item type and experimental condition: Ge, items for which related material was generated from semantic memory; Nge, items for which no related material was generated from semantic memory. Pr, items for which related material was presented for study; Npr, items for which no related material was presented for study. (Reproduced from K.-H. Bäuml, *Psychological Science*, **13**, 357–361, 2002.)

Bäuml (2002) provided further evidence for recall-specific processes in retrieval-induced forgetting by investigating a situation in which the retrieved and non-retrieved items are not part of the same experiential episode and task. Subjects learned a categorized list (e.g. FRUIT–apple, FRUIT–orange) which they had to recall later in the experiment. In a separate intermediate phase they repeatedly generated related items from semantic memory (e.g. FRUIT–pin—, FRUIT–ki—), or were presented with the same items intact for study (e.g. FRUIT–pineapple, FRUIT–kiwi). Only the semantic generation of items but not their presentation for study induced forgetting of the initially learned items (Fig. 22.3). This result indicates that semantic generation can cause recall-specific episodic forgetting, thus generalizing the findings of Ciranni and Shimamura (1999) and Anderson *et al.* (2000a) from episodic to semantic practice.

Retrieval-induced forgetting as retrieval inhibition

There is a surprising role of item strength in retrieval-induced forgetting. Results obtained by Anderson *et al.* (1994) indicate that items which are strongly bound to a common cue are subject to retrieval-induced forgetting, whereas items which are weakly bound to the common cue do not show forgetting. Indeed, if subjects are presented categorized material with the categories consisting either of high-frequency (FRUIT–apple) or low-frequency (FRUIT–olive) category members, then retrieval practice on a subset of the items has been found to impair later recall of a category's strong items (e.g. FRUIT–apple) but not the weak items (e.g. FRUIT–olive) (for related results see Bäuml 1998). This pattern appears to be independent of whether the practised items are strongly or weakly bound to the common cue.

This difference between strongly and weakly bound items was interpreted as evidence for the action of a retrieval-inhibition mechanism. This view rests on the assumption that, during retrieval of the items to be practised, items which are not to be practised and are bound to the same cue interfere and need to be inhibited to guarantee successful recovery of the items to be practised. Because items strongly bound to the common cue are assumeded to induce more interference than items weakly bound to that cue, they should be subject to more inhibition than the weakly bound items. This role of item strength is interesting as it poses an additional challenge to strength dependence as a possible explanation of retrieval-induced forgetting. According to strength dependence, weakly bound items should suffer proportionally more forgetting than strongly bound items (Anderson *et al.* 1994, Appendix A), which is not the case.

In another challenge to strength dependence, Anderson and Spellman (1995) provided evidence that retrieval-induced forgetting is cue independent. They let subjects study lists consisting of items like GREEN–emerald, GREEN–lettuce, SOUP–mushroom, and SOUP–minestrone. The participants then repeatedly retrieved GREEN–emerald and thus caused GREEN–lettuce to be forgotten on a later recall test. More importantly, the repeated retrieval of GREEN–emerald also caused SOUP–mushroom to be forgotten, although not SOUP–minestrone. According to Anderson and Spellman, this finding suggests that, because lettuce and mushroom are vegetables and thus share a number of semantic features, the inhibition of lettuce spread to the representation of mushroom and thus impaired recall of SOUP–mushroom. The fact that mushroom was forgotten although the cue at test (SOUP) was different from the cue used in the retrieval-practice phase (GREEN) indicates that retrieval-induced forgetting suppresses an item's memory representation itself and therefore is cue independent (for a related result see Ciranni and Shimamura 1999).

Retrieval-induced forgetting and integration

Retrieval-induced forgetting can be greatly reduced or even eliminated if participants enhance the binding between competing memories, a process called integration. For instance, Anderson and McCulloch (1999) found that encouraging participants to interrelate the exemplars of studied categories during the study phase greatly reduced retrieval-induced forgetting. In studies of the fan effect, Radvansky (1999) found a similar pattern of less forgetting when participants integrated propositional knowledge into what he called location schemata.

Analogously, retrieval-induced forgetting was found to be reduced or eliminated if there was a high degree of semantic similarity between practised and unpractised items (Anderson *et al.* 2000b; Bäuml and Hartinger 2002). By enhancing the binding between items by integrating facts into more cohesive representations, participants appear to experience less interference between related facts, require less inhibition, and thus are protected from impairment (Smith *et al.* 1978; Anderson and Bell 2001). Anderson and Spellman's (1995) feature inhibition theory provides a rationale for these results (for details see Anderson *et al.* 2000b).

All these findings are consistent with recent work employing Deese–Roediger–McDermott (DRM) lists (Deese 1959; Roediger and McDermott 1995). DRM lists consist of items which are all strongly bound to a critical item. When presented to participants, such lists can create high levels of false recall of the unstudied critical item. For instance, if participants study words like pillow, bed, silence, etc., all of which are the strongest semantic associates to the unpresented critical item, sleep, they are highly likely to recall the critical item falsely. DRM lists differ substantially in the degree to which they cause false memories (Stadler *et al.* 1999). Because this variation in false-recall level is largely due to differences in the binding between the critical item of the list and the non-critical items (Roediger *et al.* 2001), high false-recall lists should show more integration than low false-recall lists and thus show less retrieval-induced forgetting.

Bäuml and Kuhbandner (2003) confirmed this prediction. They performed two experiments in which they examined the effect of retrieval practice on a subset of the items from DRM lists on recall of the critical items. In Experiment 1, the critical items were part of the studied lists; thus the veridical recall of these items was addressed. In Experiment 2, the critical items were not studied; thus the false recall of these items was addressed. As predicted, retrieval practice induced an integration effect in veridical recall, with substantial forgetting of critical items in lists with low false-recall levels and no forgetting in lists with high false-recall levels. However, retrieval practice reduced not only the veridical recall of critical items but also their false recall. This latter result is consistent with the hypothesis that false recall reflects activation during study (Kimball and Bjork 2002; Reysen and Nairne 2002) and that retrieval of related items can lead to inhibition of the activated, unstudied critical items very similar to how retrieval inhibits studied material.

Summary

Results from recent research show that increasing the binding level of a subset of previously learned material through retrieval practice can lead to forgetting the unreprocessed material. However, this forgetting is not caused by the reprocessing *per se* but rather by recall-specific inhibition, whereby interfering material, which is not to be retrieved, is inhibited to guarantee successful recovery of material which is to be retrieved. Retrieval inhibition is particularly strong if the interference potential of the material not to be practised is high, and if the similarity between practised and unpractised items is only moderate. It applies to both veridical and false memories. Retrieval inhibition affects the unpractised items by reducing the binding between the items and their cue(s) and/or reducing the intra-item binding, as suggested by the finding of cue independence.

Detrimental effects of cueing

Retrieval competition

The detrimental effects of cueing have been shown in a number of different paradigms. Subjects are often presented with a categorized list and, at test, receive the category name and a subset of a category's items as a retrieval cue for recall of the remaining items. Typically, such cueing impairs recall of the remaining items compared with a control condition in which only the category name is provided as a retrieval cue (Slamecka 1968; Roediger 1973). The detrimental effect of part-list cueing has been found to be fairly robust, occurring with both categorized and uncategorized lists, and with either intra- or extra-list items as cues (reviewed by Roediger and Neely 1982; Nickerson 1984).

A still very popular account of part-list cueing is retrieval competition (Rundus 1973; Kimball and Bjork 2002). This account, which is consistent with strength-dependent competition, assumes that part-list cueing strengthens the binding level of the cue items and thus leads participants to covertly retrieve (the more strongly bound) cue items before (the more weakly bound) non-cue items at test. In this way, a competition bias for renewed binding is introduced, favouring covert retrieval of cue items at the expense of retrieval of non-cue items. Because each retrieval of a cue item reflects a failure to retrieve a new non-cue item and the retrieval process is assumed to stop after a critical number of failures, this bias can reduce recall chances for the non-cue items, and thus cause the detrimental effect of part-list cueing.

If part-list cueing is really mediated through strengthening-induced output order biases at test, forgetting should disappear if the bias is eliminated. Exactly such a pattern has been found in the list-strength effect, which is caused by increasing the binding level of part of a list through relearning (Bäuml 1997; see above). In a recent study, Bäuml and Aslan (2004) directly compared the effects of cueing and relearning when controlling for output order biases. Subjects learned category exemplars consisting of target and non-target items. In a subsequent phase, the non-target items were re-exposed, either for relearning or for

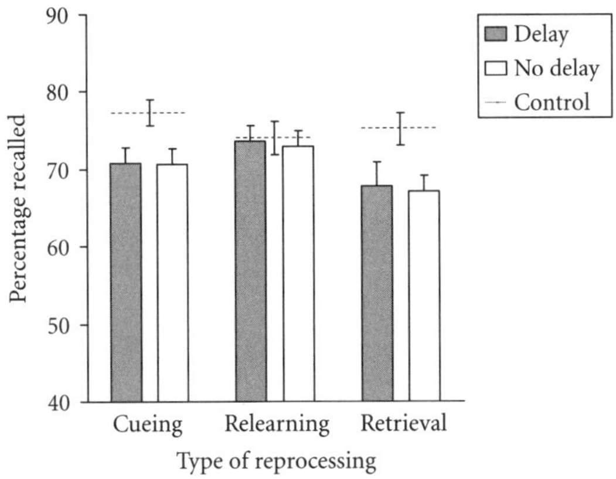

Figure 22.4 Mean target item recall and standard errors on a category-plus-first-letter cued-recall test as a function of type of reprocessing and delay between reprocessing and test. The broken lines indicate performance in the control condition in which no reprocessing took place. (Reproduced from K.-H. Bäuml and A. Aslan, *Memory and Cognition*, **32**, 610–617, 2004.)

use as a retrieval cue at test. This re-exposure occurred immediately before testing, mimicking typical part-list cueing, or separated from testing by a distractor task, mimicking typical part-list relearning. In the test, the category-plus-first-letter cues of the target items were presented and subjects were instructed to recall the target items, thus controlling for output order.

The results replicated prior work by showing that part-list relearning has no detrimental effect on target material if output order is controlled. In contrast, a detrimental effect of part-list cueing was found. This held true both when re-exposure occurred immediately before testing and when it was separated from testing by a distractor task (Fig. 22.4). This finding disagrees with the proposal that part-list cueing is due to competition bias caused by increases in the binding level of the cue items.

Strategy disruption and retrieval inhibition

Two other prominent accounts of part-list cueing have been suggested in recent years. The first of these is strategy disruption. According to this hypothesis (Basden *et al.* 1977; Basden and Basden 1995), the presentation of cue items disrupts retrieval by forcing a serial recall order that is inconsistent with subjects' inter-item bindings in a list. Following this line of reasoning, part-list cueing induces a change in the retrieval process from a more effective one when cues are absent to a less effective one when they are present (for related suggestions see Raaijmakers and Shiffrin 1981; Sloman *et al.* 1991). Therefore part-list cueing should be mediated by quite a different mechanism than retrieval-induced forgetting.

The other account of part-list cueing is retrieval inhibition (Anderson *et al.* 1994). Like retrieval competition, this account assumes that the presentation of cue items leads to an increase in the binding level of these items and that this increase induces early covert retrieval of the cue items at test. In contrast with Rundus's (1973) account, however, this covert retrieval is assumed to cause forgetting not because of biased retrieval competition but, rather, because of retrieval inhibition. Other work has shown that overt retrieval of a subset of previously learned material can cause retrieval inhibition of the non-retrieved material (see above). If covert retrieval of items has a similar effect on non-retrieved items to that of the overt retrieval of items, then the covert retrieval of cue items should cause retrieval inhibition of non-cue items as well. As a result, part-list cueing and retrieval-induced forgetting should show a number of parallels.

Indeed, the results from several recent studies suggest that the detrimental effects of retrieval practice and part-list cueing have many things in common. For instance, Bäuml *et al.* (2002) showed that the effect of item strength which is present in retrieval-induced forgetting also holds in part-list cueing. They found detrimental effects of part-list cueing for items strongly bound to the common cue but not for items weakly bound to the cue. Hicks and Starns (2004) demonstrated that retrieval-induced forgetting occurs not only in recall but also in recognition, a result which mimics a similar finding in part-list cueing (Todres and Watkins 1981). Furthermore, it was shown that not only the presentation of semantically related extra-list items as retrieval cues (Watkins 1975; Roediger *et al.* 1977) but also the generation of such extra-list items (Bäuml 2002) can cause forgetting of previously learned material.

Bäuml and Kuhbandner (2003) provided a direct comparison of the effects of retrieval practice and part-list cueing in DRM lists. They compared the effects of retrieval practice on a subset of the items and of the presentation of those items as retrieval cues at test on veridical and false recall of the critical items of the lists. Just as in retrieval practice (see above), cueing induced an integration effect in veridical recall, with substantial forgetting in DRM lists with low false-recall levels and no forgetting in DRM lists with high false-recall levels. Just as in retrieval practice, cueing reduced not only the veridical recall of critical items but also their false recall (Fig. 22.5). These parallels held in both pattern and size. They are consistent with the view that the mechanism that mediates retrieval-induced forgetting also underlies part-list cueing. Thus the results challenge the strategy-disruption account and favour a retrieval-inhibition account of part-list cueing.

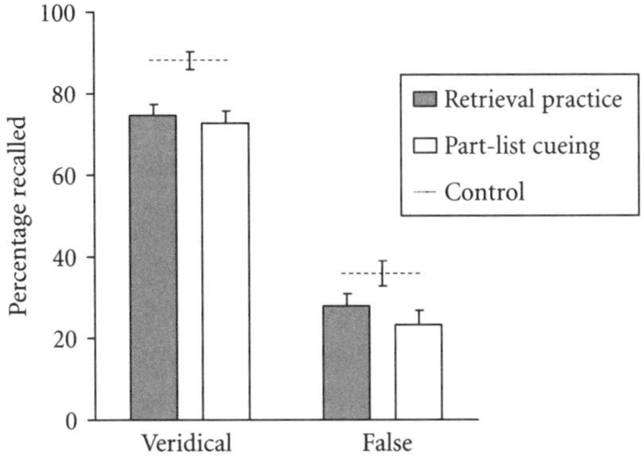

Figure 22.5 Recall percentages and standard errors for veridical and false recall of critical items as a function of recall condition (retrieval practice, part-list cueing, control condition). Veridical recall refers to the case in which both the non-critical and the critical items were part of the studied DRM lists; false recall refers to the case in which only the non-critical but not the critical items were part of the studied lists. The results shown are based on 16 DRM lists, including lists with relatively high false-recall levels and lists with relatively low false-recall levels. (Reproduced from K.-H. Bäuml and C. Kuhbandner, *Memory and Cognition*, **31**, 1188–1197, 2003.)

Instructed retrieval inhibition

The original retrieval-inhibition account of part-list cueing (Anderson *et al.* 1994) assumes that, just like retrieval competition, the presentation of cue items leads to an increase in the binding level of these items, this increase induces early covert retrieval of the cue items at test, and this covert retrieval of the cue items causes retrieval inhibition of the non-cue items. In this sense, the retrieval-inhibition account depends on the validity of the proposal that part-list cueing is due to the increase in binding level of the cue items, a proposal which is challenged by the finding of Bäuml and Aslan (2004).

Although the Bäuml–Aslan finding rules out all types of strengthening accounts of part-list cueing, it is consistent with the view that covert retrieval of cue items is at the heart of the part-list cueing effect (Roediger 1973; Rundus 1973; Anderson *et al.* 1994). However, unlike previous accounts, the finding suggests that this covert retrieval is not caused by enhancing the binding level of cue items but rather reflects an instructional effect. In fact, by directly comparing the effects of part-list relearning (i.e. the re-exposure of items for additional learning) and part-list cueing (i.e. the re-exposure of the same items for use as a retrieval cue at test) Bäuml and Aslan were able to demonstrate that the detrimental effect of part-list cueing is caused by instruction. The instruction to use items as cues apparently induces covert retrieval of the cue items and thus leads to retrieval inhibition of non-cue items.

Patient data

The detrimental effect of part-list cueing in amnesic and schizophrenic patients has been examined in two recent studies. Using categorized lists, Bäuml *et al.* (2002) demonstrated that, while in healthy people the detrimental effect of part-list cueing is restricted to items strongly bound to the category cue, in amnesia patients the forgetting extends to items which are weakly bound to the cue. This finding was independent of the presence of executive dysfunction in some of the patients. On the basis of the retrieval-inhibition account of part-list cueing, these results indicate that amnesic patients show more retrieval inhibition than healthy controls. They also suggest that the detrimental effect of part-list cueing is primarily mediated by medial temporal lobe structures.

In a more recent study, Kissler and Bäuml (2005) used the same experimental set-up to examine part-list cueing in schizophrenic patients. Like the amnesic patients, the schizophrenic patients showed substantial recall deficits. However, unlike the amnesic patients, they did not exhibit increased susceptibility to part-list cueing effects, indicating that schizophrenic patients do not show enhanced retrieval inhibition. Moreover, because schizophrenic patients have repeatedly been shown to exhibit deficits in executive control and response suppression related to prefrontal cortex functioning (Braver *et al.* 1999; Perlstein *et al.* 2003), this result suggests that it is not the frontal lobe structures which mediate the detrimental effect of part-list cueing. This suggestion agrees with the finding that amnesic patients with executive dysfunctions show the same detrimental effect as amnesic patients without executive dysfunctions (Bäuml *et al.* 2002).

Together, the results for the amnesic and schizophrenic patients indicate that a certain type of feature-binding process in temporal lobe structures, and not strategic control mechanisms mediated by the frontal lobes, is responsible for the detrimental effect of part-list cueing. This pattern of results provides another parallel between the detrimental effects of part-list cueing and retrieval practice. Indeed, examining inhibitory control mechanisms in patients with lesions to the frontal and temporal lobes, Conway and Fthenaki (2003) recently found that retrieval-induced forgetting was affected in patients with temporal lobe lesions whereas patients with frontal lobe lesions showed normal retrieval-induced forgetting. These findings are consistent with the proposal that part-list cueing and retrieval-induced forgetting are mediated by similar mechanisms.

Summary

The results from recent research indicate that the detrimental effect of part-list cueing is not caused by biases in items' competition for renewed binding or strategy disruption. Instead, the results support the view that part-list cueing is caused by retrieval inhibition. It is suggested that the cueing instruction leads to covert retrieval of the cue items at test, and this covert retrieval then causes retrieval inhibition of the non-cue items. The inhibition supposedly reduces the binding level of the items and thus reduces their recall chances. As a corollary, this proposal claims that retrieval-induced forgetting and part-list cueing are mediated by similar mechanisms. Consistent with this view, a number of quantitative and qualitative parallels between the two forms of forgetting have emerged in recent work.

Forgetting mechanisms

Inhibitory mechanisms

Models of recall are often two-stage models, where in the first stage an item's relative strength and in the second stage an item's absolute strength are of importance for recall (Raaijmakers and Shiffrin 1981; Gronlund and Shiffrin 1986; Rohrer 1996; Wixted *et al.* 1997). In the first stage, an item is sampled from a set of items according to a relative-strength rule, which determines the item's response latency: A high relative strength leads to a fast response and a low one to a slow response. In the second stage, a sampled item is recovered into consciousness if its absolute strength exceeds some threshold. Thus, whereas an item will eventually be sampled, it may not be recovered because its memory representation may be too weak to exceed threshold.

On the basis of such two-stage models of recall, the question arises of whether retrieval inhibition prevents an item from being sampled at all, or whether it permits sampling but prevents recovery. This would occur if inhibition reduced the absolute strength of the inhibited item so that it no longer exceeded the recovery threshold. If a reduction in binding level was equivalent to a reduction in the item's absolute strength, then retrieval inhibition should reflect a recovery problem and not prevent the item from being sampled.

As Rohrer and colleagues (Wixted and Rohrer 1994; Rohrer *et al.* 1995; Rohrer 1996) demonstrated, response latency analysis can be used to examine whether a change in recall performance is due to a change in sampling or a change in recovery. Indeed, if the absolute strength of items is reduced while their relative strength is maintained, which may occur if retrieval inhibition reduces the binding level of the unpractised items, recall frequency of the unpracticed items should decrease and their response latency should not be influenced.

Bäuml *et al.* (2005) reported an experiment in which they measured recall frequencies and response latencies of retrieval-practised and non-retrieval-practised items. They let participants study categorized lists in which each category (e.g. ANIMALS) consisted of exemplars from two different semantic subcategories (e.g. PREDATORS, HOOFED ANIMALS). In the retrieval-practice phase, subjects repeatedly retrieved the items from one of the two subcategories of a category (e.g. PREDATORS) before, in the final test, they separately recalled the items from both subcategories (e.g. HOOFED ANIMALS, PREDATORS). As expected, retrieval practice improved later recall of the practised items (e.g. PREDATORS) but impaired recall of the unpractised items (e.g. HOOFED ANIMALS). Most interestingly, neither type of item showed any change in response latency compared with a control condition in which no items were practised at all. This result, which was replicated in a second experiment, is consistent with the view that retrieval inhibition reduces the binding level of items and thus reduces their absolute strength. As a result, the inhibited items may eventually be sampled but they no longer exceed the recovery threshold (for related results see Zellner and Bäuml 2004a).

Retrieval competition

The results from the retrieval-induced forgetting experiments contrast sharply with those from interference studies. As in retrieval-induced forgetting, interference leads to reduced recall frequencies. However, unlike retrieval-induced forgetting, interference leads to a strong increase in response latencies. Wixted and Rohrer (1994) demonstrated such a pattern in a proactive-interference paradigm, and Rohrer (1996) showed the same point when varying the amount of material to be learned within lists. This increase in response latency suggests that interference is already acting at the sampling stage: The binding of new material reduces the relative strength of the target material and thus reduces the material's chances of being sampled. These findings are consistent with the view that interference and retrieval-induced forgetting are caused by quite different mechanisms. Interference reflects enhanced competition for renewed binding, which reduces the relative strength of items and thus reduces their chances of being sampled. Retrieval-induced forgetting is due to retrieval inhibition, which reduces the binding level of items and thus reduces their absolute strength and chances for being recovered.

Summary

The results from recent work suggest that retrieval inhibition does not prevent inhibited items from being sampled. Rather, by reducing the binding level of the items, inhibition reduces the absolute strength of inhibited items so that they can no longer be recovered. Thus retrieval inhibition is quite different from retrieval competition, where the binding of additional material induces forgetting by increasing the competition between items for renewed binding. This increased competition leads to a reduction in the relative strength of the items and reduces sampling chances. Thus retrieval competition reflects a failure at the sampling stage of recall, whereas retrieval inhibition reflects a failure at the recovery stage.

Conclusions

Experimental results from the past decade clearly demonstrate that the detrimental effects of (re)learning, retrieval, and cueing are not due to strength-dependent competition. According to strength dependence, forgetting of an episode arises because new material is bound to the common cue or material already bound to the common cue is strengthened in its binding level. Because (re)learning, retrieval, and cueing lead to an increase in the binding level of items, it has been argued that it is this increase which is at the heart of the detrimental effects of the three forms of episodic reprocessing (Rundus 1973; Raaijmakers and Shiffrin 1981; Mensink and Raaijmakers 1988). However, this prediction could not be confirmed for any of the three forms of forgetting.

Recent results from interference studies suggest a modification of strength-dependent competition to non-strength-dependent competition. Indeed, strong competitors have been found to induce the same amount of forgetting of target material as weak competitors. This has been demonstrated when using both classical interference paradigms (DaPolito 1966; Bäuml 1996) and within-list strength manipulations (Bäuml 1997; Ciranni and Shimamura 1999; Anderson *et al.* 2000a). These results suggest that interference effects are caused by the binding of new material to a common cue but not by increasing the binding level of competitors that are already bound. The change in the binding structure enhances competition and thus reduces the relative strength of single items (Wixted and Rohrer 1994). This change affects item sampling and thus causes forgetting.

Results from retrieval-induced forgetting studies point to retrieval inhibition rather than any variants of (strength-dependent) competition as the major source of the recall impairment. According to inhibition, retrieval suppresses interfering material not to be retrieved in order to guarantee the recovery of material to be retrieved (Anderson *et al.* 1994; Anderson and Spellman 1995). As opposed to interference effects, retrieval-induced forgetting reflects a change in the binding level of forgotten items. This change does not exclude inhibited items from the sampling process but rather leads to failure in the item recovery process (Bäuml *et al.* 2005).

Recent work on part-list cueing indicates that the detrimental effects of both retrieval and cueing are caused by retrieval inhibition. However, unlike retrieval-induced forgetting, which is caused by overt retrieval, part-list cueing appears to be caused by covert retrieval. Indeed, experimental results indicate that the instruction to use items as cues induces covert retrieval of the cue items at test and thus leads to retrieval inhibition of non-cue items (Bäuml and Aslan 2004). Consistent with this view, a number of quantitative and qualitative parallels between the detrimental effects of retrieval and cueing have been reported in recent research (Bäuml and Kuhbandner 2003; Hicks and Starns 2004; Zellner and Bäuml 2004b).

In this chapter we focused on unintentional episodic forgetting. In fact, it is not typically the aim of subjects to impair later recall of the unprocessed material in interference or retrieval-induced forgetting or part-list cueing. In this sense, these forms of forgetting differ from other forms in which subjects intentionally wish to forget material. Such intentional forgetting, as occurs for instance in the directed-forgetting paradigm (Bjork 1970, 1989), has also been explained in terms of retrieval inhibition (reviewed by MacLeod 1998). However, there is recent evidence that retrieval inhibition in intentional forgetting is not the same as retrieval inhibition in unintentional forgetting (Kimball and Bjork 2002; Perfect *et al.* 2002). Discovering exactly how the two types of inhibition are related and how they differ in their effects on feature binding is an important task for future research.

Acknowledgements

The research reported here was supported by grants from the Deutsche Forschungsgemeinschaft to K.-H.B. (Ba-1382/4 and FOR 448).

References

Anderson, J.R. (1983). *The Architecture of Cognition*. Hillsdale, NJ: Erlbaum.

Anderson, M.C. and Bell, T. (2001). Forgetting our facts: the role of inhibitory processes in the loss of propositional knowledge. *Journal of Experimental Psychology: General*, **130**, 544–570.

Anderson, M.C. and McCulloch, K.C. (1999). Integration as a general boundary condition on retrieval-induced forgetting. *Journal of Experimental Psychology: Learning, Memory, and Cognition*, **25**, 608–629.

Anderson, M.C. and Spellman, B.A. (1995). On the status of inhibitory mechanisms in cognition: memory retrieval as a model case. *Psychological Review*, **102**, 68–100.

Anderson, M.C., Bjork, R.A., and Bjork, E.L. (1994). Remembering can cause forgetting: retrieval dynamics in long-term memory. *Journal of Experimental Psychology: Learning, Memory, and Cognition*, **20**, 1063–1087.

Anderson, M.C., Bjork, E.L., and Bjork, R.A. (2000a). Retrieval-induced forgetting: evidence for a recall-specific mechanism. *Psychonomic Bulletin and Review*, **7**, 522–530.

Anderson, M.C., Green, C., and McCulloch, K.C. (2000b). Similarity and inhibition in long-term memory: evidence for a two-factor theory. *Journal of Experimental Psychology: Learning, Memory, and Cognition*, **26**, 1141–1159.

Barnes, J.M. and Underwood, B. J. (1959). 'Fate' of first-list associations in transfer theory. *Journal of Experimental Psychology*, **58**, 95–105.

Basden, D.R. and Basden, B.H. (1995). Some tests of the strategy disruption hypothesis of part-list cuing inhibition. *Journal of Experimental Psychology: Learning, Memory, and Cognition*, **21**, 1656–1669.

Basden D.R., Basden, B.H., and Galloway, B. C. (1977). Inhibition with part-list cuing. *Journal of Experimental Psychology: Human Learning and Memory*, **3**, 100–108.

Bäuml, K.-H. (1996). Revisiting an old issue: retroactive interference as a function of the degree of original and interpolated learning. *Psychonomic Bulletin and Review*, **3**, 380–384.

Bäuml, K.-H. (1997). The list-strength effect: strength-dependent competition or suppression? *Psychonomic Bulletin and Review*, **4**, 260–264.

Bäuml, K.-H. (1998). Strong items get suppressed, weak items do not: the role of item strength in output interference. *Psychonomic Bulletin and Review*, **5**, 459–463.

Bäuml, K.-H. (2002). Semantic generation can cause episodic forgetting. *Psychological Science*, **13**, 357–361.

Bäuml, K.-H. and Aslan, A. (2004). Part-list cuing as instructed retrieval inhibition. *Memory and Cognition*, **32**, 610–617.

Bäuml, K.-H. and Hartinger, A. (2002). On the role of item similarity in retrieval-induced forgetting. *Memory*, **10**, 215–224.

Bäuml, K.-H. and Kuhbandner, C. (2003). Retrieval-induced forgetting and part-list cuing in associatively structured lists. *Memory and Cognition*, **31**, 1188–1197.

Bäuml, K.-H., Kissler, J., and Rak, A. (2002). Part-list cuing in amnesic patients: evidence for a retrieval deficit. *Memory and Cognition*, **30**, 862–870.

Bäuml, K.-H., Zellner, M., and Vilimek, R. (2005). When remembering causes forgetting: retrieval-induced forgetting as recovery failure. *Journal of Experimental Psychology: Learning, Memory, and Cognition*, **31**, 1221–1234.

Bjork, R.A. (1970). Positive forgetting: the noninterference of items intentionally forgotten. *Journal of Verbal Learning and Verbal Behavior*, **9**, 255–268.

Bjork, R.A. (1989). Retrieval inhibition as an adaptive mechanism in human memory. In *Varieties of Memory and Consciousness* (ed H.L. Roediger and F.I.M. Craik). Hillsdale, NJ: Erlbaum, pp. 309–330.

Braver, T.S., Barch, D.M., and Cohen, J.D. (1999). Cognition and control in schizophrenia: a computational model of dopamine and prefrontal function. *Biological Psychiatry*, **46**, 312–328.

Briggs, G.E. (1957). Retroactive inhibition as a function of the degree of original and interpolated learning. *Journal of Experimental Psychology*, **53**, 60–67.

Ciranni, M.A. and Shimamura, A.P. (1999). Retrieval-induced forgetting in episodic memory. *Journal of Experimental Psychology: Learning, Memory, and Cognition*, **25**, 1403–1414.

Conway, M.A. and Fthenaki, A. (2003). Disruption of inhibitory control of memory following lesions to the frontal and temporal lobes. *Cortex*, **39**, 667–686.

Crowder, R.G. (1976). *Principles of Learning and Memory*. New York: John Wiley.

DaPolito, F.J. (1966). Proactive effects with independent retrieval of competing responses. Unpublished doctoral dissertation, Indiana University.

Deese, J. (1959). On the prediction of occurence of particular verbal intrusions in immediate recall. *Journal of Experimental Psychology*, **58**, 17–22.

Gronlund, S.D. and Shiffrin, R.M. (1986). Retrieval strategies in recall of natural categories and categorized lists. *Journal of Experimental Psychology: Learning, Memory, and Cognition*, **12**, 550–561.

Hicks, J.L. and Starns, J.J. (2004). Retrieval-induced forgetting occurs in tests of item recognition. *Psychonomic Bulletin and Review*, **11**, 125–130.

Hogan, R.M. and Kintsch, W. (1971). Differential effects of study and test trials on long-term recognition and recall. *Journal of Verbal Learning and Verbal Behavior*, **10**, 562–567.

Kimball, D.R. and Bjork, R.A. (2002). Influences of intentional and unintentional forgetting on false memories. *Journal of Experimental Psychology: General*, **131**, 116–130.

Kissler, J. and Bäuml, K.-H. (2005). Memory retrieval in schizophrenia–evidence from part-list cuing. *Journal of the International Neuropsychological Society*, **11**, 273–280.

Levy, B.J. and Anderson, M.A. (2002). Inhibitory processes and the control of memory retrieval. *Trends in Cognitive Sciences*, **6**, 299–305.

MacLeod, C.M. (1998). Directed forgetting. In *Intentional Forgetting: Interdisciplinary Approaches* (ed J.M. Golding and C.M. MacLeod). Mahwah, NJ: Erlbaum, pp. 1–57.

Mensink, J.-G. and Raaijmakers, J.G.W. (1988). A model of interference and forgetting. *Psychological Review*, **95**, 434–455.

Nickerson, R.S. (1984). Retrieval inhibition from part-set cuing: a persisting enigma in memory research. *Memory and Cognition*, **12**, 531–552.

Perfect, T.J., Moulin, C.J.A., Conway, M.A., and Perry, E. (2002). Accessing the inhibitory account of retrieval-induced forgetting with implicit-memory tests. *Journal of Experimental Psychology: Learning, Memory, and Cognition*, **28**, 1111–1119.

Perlstein, W.M., Dixit, W.K., Carter, C.S., Noll, D.C., and Cohen, J.D. (2003). Prefrontal cortex dysfunction mediates deficits in working memory and prepotent responding in schizophrenia. *Biological Psychiatry*, 53, 25–38.

Raaijmakers, J.G.W. and Shiffrin, R.M. (1981). Search of associative memory. *Psychological Review*, **88**, 93–134.

Radvansky, G.A. (1999). Memory retrieval and suppression: the inhibition of situation models. *Journal of Experimental Psychology: General*, **128**, 563–579.

Ratcliff, R., Clark, S.E., and Shiffrin, R.M. (1990). The list-strength effect. I: Data and discussion. *Journal of Experimental Psychology: Learning, Memory, and Cognition*, **16**, 163–178.

Reysen, M.B. and Nairne, J.S. (2002). Part-set cuing of false memories. *Psychonomic Bulletin and Review*, **9**, 389–393.

Roberts, W.A. (1972). Free recall of word lists varying in length and rate of presentation: a test of total-time hypotheses. *Journal of Experimental Psychology*, **92**, 365–372.

Roediger, H.L., III (1973). Inhibition in recall from cueing with recall targets. *Journal of Verbal Learning and Verbal Behavior*, **12**, 644–657.

Roediger, H.L., III (1978). Recall as a self-limiting process. *Memory and Cognition*, **6**, 54–63.

Roediger, H.L., III and McDermott, K.B. (1995). Creating false memories: remembering words not presented in lists. *Journal of Experimental Psychology: Learning, Memory, and Cognition*, **21**, 803–814.

Roediger, H.L., III and Neely, J.H. (1982). Retrieval blocks in episodic and semantic memory. *Canadian Journal of Psychology*, **36**, 213–242.

Roediger, H.L., III, Stellon, C.C., and Tulving, E. (1977). Inhibition from part-list cues and rate of recall. *Journal of Experimental Psychology: Human Learning and Memory*, **3**, 174–188.

Roediger, H.L., III, Watson, J.M., McDermott, K.B., and Gallo, D.A. (2001). Factors that determine false recall: a multiple regression analysis. *Psychonomic Bulletin and Review*, **8**, 385–407.

Rohrer, D. (1996). On the relative and absolute strength of a memory trace. *Memory and Cognition*, **24**, 188–201.

Rohrer, D., Wixted, J.T., Salmon, D.P. and Butters, N. (1995). Retrieval from semantic memory and its implications for Alzheimer's disease. *Journal of Experimental Psychology: Human Learning and Memory*, **21**, 1127–1139.

Rundus, D. (1973). Negative effects of using list items as recall cues. *Journal of Verbal Learning and Verbal Behavior*, **12**, 43–50.

Slamecka, N.J. (1968). An examination of trace storage in free recall. *Journal of Experimental Psychology*, **76**, 504–513.

Sloman, S.A., Bower, G.H., and Rohrer, D. (1991). Congruency effects in part-list cuing. *Journal of Experimental Psychology: Learning, Memory, and Cognition*, **17**, 974–982.

Smith, E.E., Adams, N., and Schorr, D. (1978). Fact retrieval and the paradox of interference. *Cognitive Psychology*, **10**, 438–464.

Stadler, M. A., Roediger, H.L., III, and McDermott, K.B. (1999). Norms for word lists that create false memories. *Memory and Cognition*, **27**, 494–500.

Todres, A.K. and Watkins, M.J. (1981). A part-set cuing effect in recognition memory. *Journal of Experimental Psychology: Human Learning and Memory*, **2**, 91–99.

Tulving, E. (1974). Cue-dependent forgetting. *American Scientist*, **62**, 74–82.

Tulving, E. and Hastie, R. (1972). Inhibition effects of intralist repetition in free recall. *Journal of Experimental Psychology*, **92**, 297–304.

Tulving, E. and Pearlstone, Z. (1966). Availability versus accessibility of information in memory for words. *Journal of Verbal Learning and Verbal Behavior*, **5**, 381–391.

Watkins, M.J. (1975). Inhibition in recall with extra-list 'cues'. *Journal of Verbal Learning and Verbal Behavior*, **14**, 294–303.

Wixted, J.T. and Rohrer, D. (1994). Analyzing the dynamics of free recall: an integrative review of the empirical literature. *Psychonomic Bulletin and Review*, **1**, 89–106.

Wixted, J.T., Ghadisha, H., and Vera, R. (1997). Recall latency following pure- and mixedstrength lists: a direct test of the relative strength model of free recall. *Journal of Experimental Psychology: Learning, Memory, and Cognition*, **23**, 523–538.

Zellner, M. and Bäuml, K.-H. (2004a). Retrieval inhibition in episodic recall. In *Bound in Memory: Insights from Behavioral and Neuropsychological Studies* (ed A. Mecklinger, H. Zimmer, and U. Lindenberger), pp. 1–26. Aachen: Shaker Verlag.

Zellner, M. and Bäuml, K.-H. (2004b). Intact retrieval inhibition in children's episodic recall. *Memory and Cognition*, **33**, 396–404.

Section 5

Binding in the ageing brain

Chapter 23

Remembering items and their contexts: effects of ageing and divided attention

Fergus I. M. Craik

Introduction

Human memory is a complex business! Cognitive psychologists have proposed various schemes to organize the many observations and experimental findings that have accrued over the past 100 years or so; some of the more salient proposals are shown in Table 23.1. The notion of different memory *stores* dominated the field from the emergence of the cognitive perspective in the 1950s until the late 1970s (e.g. Murdock 1967), and is still a popular shorthand way of referring to a variety of memory phenomena. The 'systems' view was given its major impetus by the formulation of the distinction between episodic and semantic memory (Tulving 1972, 1983), and it was fleshed out by the later addition of procedural memory (Tulving 1983), working memory (Baddeley 1986), and the perceptual representational systems (Tulving and Schacter 1990). Whereas the earlier viewpoint focused on the structural characteristics of the various postulated memory stores, the systems view involves both structures and processes. The move towards processing accounts of memory, attention, and related cognitive phenomena was given a boost by the publication of the 'levels of processing' article by Craik and Lockhart (1972). We took the position that rather than thinking of memory as a 'thing' in the head, researchers should view remembering as an *activity of mind*, thereby endorsing the earlier suggestions of Bartlett (1932) and others.

These different approaches to understanding memory have implications for views of memory disorders. For example, patterns of memory loss can be thought of as reflecting the specific impairment of a particular memory store or system. From the processing point of view, mild memory impairments can be regarded as reflecting inefficiencies of a specific set of processes. Craik (1983, 1986) further suggested that remembering necessarily involves the external environment as well as processes that are initiated from within the brain. In this sense, remembering is similar to perceiving; the final set of neural and mental

Table 23.1 Understanding human memory

1. Memory stores		Structures
	Sensory memory stores	
	Short-term memory store	
	Long-term memory store	
2. Memory systems		Structures/processes
	Episodic memory	
	Semantic memory	
	Procedural memory	
3. Memory processes		Mental/neural activities
	Levels of processing	
	Self-initiated activities	
	Environmental support	

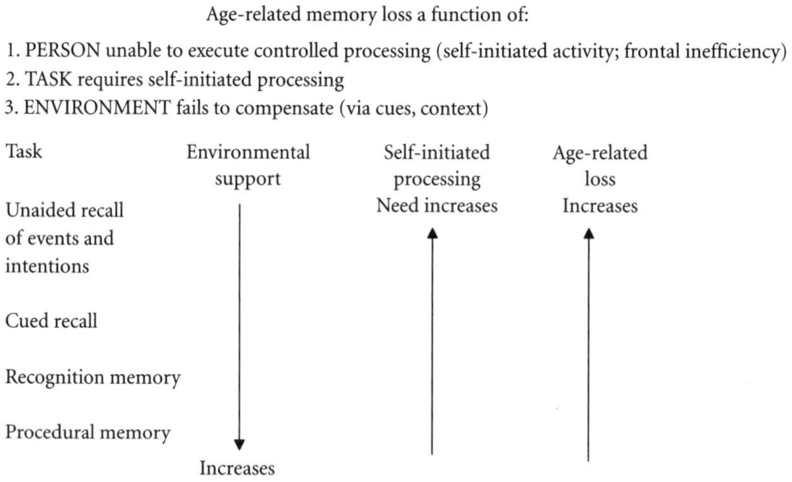
Age-related memory loss a function of:
1. PERSON unable to execute controlled processing (self-initiated activity; frontal inefficiency)
2. TASK requires self-initiated processing
3. ENVIRONMENT fails to compensate (via cues, context)
Task
Environmental support
Self-initiated processing
Age-related loss
Unaided recall of events and intentions
Need increases
Increases
Cued recall
Recognition memory
Procedural memory
Increases

Figure 23.1 Hypothetical scheme linking age-related memory loss to tasks and environmental support.

products reflect interactions between patterns of sensory input (perceptual stimulation, retrieval cues, or reinstatement of context) and activated schemas. Craik's (1983, 1986) suggestion was that successful remembering involves some mixture of externally driven 'environmental support' and internally generated 'self-initiated activities'. Craik further suggested that ageing is associated with a gradual decline in the ability to organize and execute self-initiated processing, and therefore older people must rely more on environmental support. Different memory tasks arguably require greater or lesser amounts of self-initiated processing as the environmental contribution varies. Figure 23.1 lists a number of common memory paradigms arranged in order of increasing environmental support and the concomitant decreasing need for self-initiated processing. If older adults are less able to carry out self-initiated processing, perhaps as a consequence of declining frontal lobe function (Prull *et al.* 2000; Raz 2000), they should show greatest age-related performance losses on such tasks as free recall and time-based prospective memory that involve the least support from external stimulation. In general, this is the pattern of performance that is typically observed (Craik and Jennings 1992; Zacks *et al.* 2000).

In a more recent article (Craik 2002) I raised a further question with regard to ageing and memory. Many researchers have noted that two major problems encountered by older people are difficulty in recollecting the source of learned information (told by a friend? read it in a newspaper? saw it on television?) or the context in which an event occurred (Schacter *et al.* 1984) and difficulty with retrieval, often of words and even more often of specific names. I speculated that these two age-related problems might reflect one common underlying problem, namely a difficulty in both encoding and retrieving specific detail, as opposed to encoding and retrieving general information—the gist of an experienced event or transmitted message. One way of representing this state of affairs is shown in Figure 23.2(a). The basic idea is that knowledge representations in the brain/mind are organized hierarchically. Single events (episodes) are perceived and experienced together with many specific details of their contexts of occurrence, and the commonalities among sets of similar events are then represented as higher-order nodes. This process continues as children and adults learn about

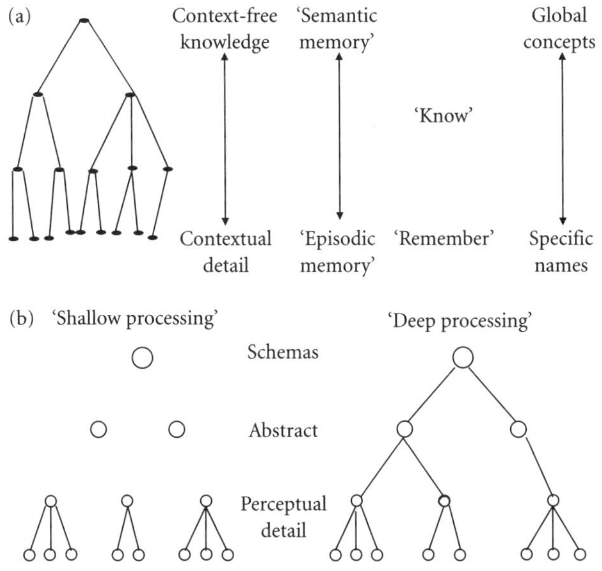

Figure 23.2 Hierarchical model showing representations at various levels of specificity (see text for details): (a) hierarchical model; (b) processing hierarchy.

the world until many such levels of representation exist, running from representations of specific instances involving autobiographical details of time and place, through representations of features common to a number of specific instances, to higher nodes representing abstract decontextualized facts about the world.

Figure 23.2(a) also makes the point that the lowest, most specific, levels of representation correspond to the notion of episodic memory in Tulving's (1972) terms, and higher levels correspond to semantic memory. However, in this scheme there is no categorical break between the two systems; instead there are degrees of specificity that gradually shade off into abstract representations. A case in point involves the study of recognition memory in the laboratory. Participants study a list of words and are later presented with original target words mixed with distractor items; their task is to select the original words. In one popular variant, participants are also asked to judge whether they 'remember' the recognized word, i.e. can recollect studying it because of some mental or contextual association, or simply 'know' it was on the list (Tulving 1985; Gardiner and Richardson-Klavehn 2000). It has been argued that the two types of awareness associated with remember and know judgements are products of the episodic and semantic memory systems, respectively (Tulving 1983, 1985). However, when a participant says he 'knows' that a word was on the list, such a judgement is far from abstract; on the contrary, the participant recollects that he encountered the word in a specific list in the laboratory during the current experiment. There is a great deal of contextual information involved in the know–recognition judgement. My point is that there are degrees of abstraction and degrees of contextual specificity, and that people access whichever level of representation is appropriate to their present purpose. I can ask a friend such questions as 'In your experience is John Smith a trustworthy person?' or 'Is John Smith in your discussion group at the university?' or 'Tell me about the last time you talked to John Smith'. These various enquiries necessitate access to various levels of contextual specificity. Other questions ('Do you enjoy living in Toronto?' 'Which city is the capital of Iran?') tap even more abstract and decontextualized representations. Further evidence that forgetting involves movement of encoded information from being 'remembered' to simply 'known' is discussed by Gardiner and Richardson-Klavehn (2002). It is worth stressing that these ideas do not negate the usefulness of the episodic–semantic *distinction*, but suggest that there is a *continuum* of representational abstractness rather than a categorical difference between the two types of memory. The terms (in my view) refer to areas of the continuum rather than to separate systems.

With regard to ageing, the present suggestion is that older people have cognitive systems that are less efficient both at encoding new episodic representations and at retrieving representations at the specific terminals of the knowledge hierarchy. Thus new experiences are encoded less richly and elaborately by older adults (Craik and Byrd 1982; Craik 1983), presumably because incoming patterns of sensory data are 'interpreted' less fully by existing knowledge structures, and perhaps less well integrated with them (Fig. 23.2(b)). At the time of retrieval, older adults have difficulty in retrieving (or reactivating) records of specific episodes, although higher abstract levels present fewer problems, perhaps because higher-level representations have a richer network of associative links to other parts of the knowledge system. As an extension of this argument, conceptual knowledge may be organized similarly to autobiographical knowledge; if so, general common features of known people, places, and objects may be represented at higher levels, and specific features (e.g. names) may be represented at the terminal nodes. Speculatively then, one way of understanding the difficulty that older adults have in recollecting both episodic contextual detail and names of people and objects is that they have difficulty in 'resolving' their retrieval processes to the level of specificity required.

Figure 23.2(b) shows how this hierarchical scheme might accommodate the notion of depth of processing (Craik and Lockhart 1972; Craik and Tulving 1975). Shallow processing can be seen as a case in which an incoming stimulus pattern is 'perceived', in the sense that the person is aware of its basic perceptual features, but not fully 'comprehended', in the sense that the pattern is not well integrated with existing schematic knowledge. Deep processing, in contrast, is a case in which the new stimulus or event is well integrated with existing knowledge. This process of integration is one case of *binding* in the cognitive system. The overall suggestion is that older adults typically process incoming information in a 'shallower' fashion (Craik and Simon 1980; Craik and Byrd 1982) as a result of the smaller amounts of processing resource at their disposal. Figure 23.2(b) makes the point that such shallower processing can also be regarded as an age-related inefficiency in binding new events to existing schemas (Chalfonte and Johnson 1996), resulting in an age-related associative deficit (Naveh-Benjamin 2000). If new events are not fully bound to existing schemas, one implication is that events will not be fully interpreted and therefore will not be well differentiated from each other. In turn, such inefficient encoding will result in products that lack distinctiveness and are therefore more difficult to retrieve at a later time (Craik and Simon 1980; Hunt and Einstein 1981; Craik 1983; Li *et al.* 2001). In addition to their encoding deficiencies, older adults also exhibit retrieval difficulties, given that they have problems retrieving information (such as names of friends and public figures) that was encoded many years ago. The present suggestion is that the retrieval difficulty can be characterized as an age-related inability to access the 'terminal twigs' of knowledge representations.

Given that the overall theme of this book is binding, one further speculation will be offered. This is the idea that just as attentional–conceptual processing varies from shallow to deep, depending on the participant's abilities and purposes, so binding can also be regarded as performing various functions at various levels of processing. For example, perceptual binding is necessary to integrate sensory and perceptual features into holistic objects; incoming information (words, gestures, actions, sequences of events) must bind to existing knowledge in order that meaning may be achieved. In the case of memory, new information must be perceived and comprehended deeply and elaborately to yield a distinctive memory record; it also seems likely that further neural processes of consolidation must occur to ensure longevity of the record. In other words, just as it is possible to refer to 'levels of processing', we can also refer to 'levels of binding', and it will be helpful to keep this distinction in mind when formulating comprehensive theories of binding processes.

Empirical illustrations

In this part of the chapter, I discuss some experiments that were conducted within the general theoretical framework outlined in the previous section. I will first describe some work from my laboratory that provides empirical backing for the claim that the effects of ageing on memory can be mimicked (in part at least) by dividing attention in young adults between a memory task and a secondary task. I then describe an experiment whose results suggest that as attention is progressively diverted away from a memory task at the time of learning, the qualitative nature of the encoding processes changes from relatively deep to relatively shallow. This result can be melded with the previous result to conclude speculatively that ageing is associated with a progressive loss of processing resources, and that memory encoding will become progressively 'shallower' (less well bound?) in nature. If the processes of binding items to their contexts and items to each other become less efficient in the course of ageing, it could be argued that older adults will show a greater loss in associative information than in item information (Murdock 1974), and this result was reported by Naveh-Benjamin (2000). However, Naveh-Benjamin also claimed that this asymmetry between item loss and associative loss was not obtained when full and divided attention in young adults was compared, thereby throwing doubt on the similarity between ageing and divided attention. I will describe an experiment from my laboratory (Castel and Craik 2003) that examines this issue. Finally, is it the case that processing resources simply determine the qualitative types of processing that can be carried out at encoding (shallow–deep, amount of elaboration, degree of binding etc.), and that the resulting encoded trace determines the memorability of the item or event? Alternatively, are there further factors that must be considered in order to understand the different outcomes of various encoding and retrieval combinations? These questions are addressed briefly before attempting to bind the various experimental results into a coherent theoretical whole.

Comparing the effects of ageing and divided attention

How similar are the effects of ageing and divided attention (DA) on memory performance? Anderson *et al.* (1998) reported a study that demonstrates a striking equivalence between the performance of older adults and young adults working under conditions of DA at the time of encoding. In one condition, participants heard lists of 15 unrelated common nouns and then attempted to recall as many words as possible in any order (free recall) after performing an arithmetic filler task for 30 s. Younger and older adults attempted to learn the lists either under full attention (FA) conditions or while also performing a continuous four-choice visual reaction time (RT) task. Retrieval was done orally and was performed under FA. In different lists, the RT task was performed under one of three emphasis conditions; participants were instructed to do *both* tasks to the best of their ability, but to pay most attention to memory encoding, pay equal attention to the memory task and the RT task, or to pay most attention to the RT task. In a second condition to be reported, participants listened to lists of 12 pairs of unrelated words and attempted to learn them. This encoding phase was again carried out by groups of younger and older adults either under FA or while performing the visual four-choice RT task in each of the three conditions of emphasis. In this case, the retrieval task was cued recall (the 12 first words in each pair were re-presented randomly as cues for the second words) and retrieval was again performed under FA conditions.

The results from groups of 24 younger and 24 older adults are shown in Table 23.2. The values of memory are the proportions of words recalled by the two age groups after studying the lists under either FA or DA when the emphasis was placed on the RT task, i.e. when attention was most fully diverted from the memory encoding task. The values for the RT task are the average RTs in milliseconds for each choice. The RT task was 'continuous' in the sense that each correct key press immediately brought up the next stimulus; therefore the values shown in Table 23.2 are mean values over the length of the encoding phase (75 s for free recall and 84 s for cued recall). Also, the RT values shown for DA are those from the condition in which emphasis was placed primarily on the memory task, i.e. when attention was most fully diverted from the RT task. The

Table 23.2 Proportions correct and reaction time scores for free recall and cued recall tests as a function of age and full or divided attention

Experimental condition	**Memory**		**Reaction time**	
	Young	**Old**	**Young**	**Old**
Free recall				
Full attention	0.82	**0.53**	408	**570**
Divided attention	**0.51**	0.28	**530**	815
Cued recall				
Full attention	0.85	**0.49**	404	**510**
Divided attention	**0.50**	0.25	**502**	745

Reproduced from Anderson *et al.* 1998.

values shown in bold type compare memory and RT performance between older adults working under FA and younger adults working under the DA condition in which attention was maximally diverted to the other task. The table shows a close correspondence between the two groups for both memory recall and (surprisingly) RT performance.

One interesting implication of the finding that RT performance in young adults working under DA conditions slows to the speed shown by older adults is that an age-related attentional resource deficit may be the primary cause of the general slowing of performance shown by the elderly. That is, rather than slowing itself being the fundamental problem underlying age-related cognitive decline (Salthouse 1996), perhaps slowing is an effect of a more fundamental loss in available processing resources. In any event, the general conclusion is that a good correspondence exists between the effects of ageing and the effects of DA on younger adults. The hypothetical reason for the correspondence is that both conditions involve a reduction in available processing (or attentional) resources.

What is the nature of these 'resources'? This question is still under debate, but it seems clear that one or more neurobiological mechanisms underlie the very replicable results that are obtained. Plausible candidates for such mechanisms include declining efficiency of cortical tissue, reduced blood flow to relevant cortical areas, inefficient glucose utilization by ageing cells, or age-related changes in psychopharmacological systems (e.g. those concerned with acetylcholine or dopamine).

Divided attention and memory encoding

It is well established that performance of a secondary task during the encoding phase of a memory task results in a reduction in later memory performance (Murdock 1965; Anderson and Craik 1974; Craik *et al.* 1996), but the exact reasons for the finding are less clear. Given the many studies that have shown memory performance to be a function of depth and elaboration of processing during encoding (e.g. Craik and Tulving 1975), it is a reasonable speculation that DA acts to reduce depth of processing and so leads to a reduction in later memory. A study was performed in my laboratory that gathered some evidence on this possibility (Naveh-Benjamin *et al.* 2000). In one set of conditions, participants were presented auditorily with lists of 10 unrelated word pairs at rates of 2, 3, 4, or 6 s per pair to learn for a later memory test. The word pairs were presented under FA and the later memory test was cued recall—the first words were given as cues for their associated second words. During the encoding phase, participants processed the word pairs in either a shallow, medium, or deep fashion as suggested to them in encoding instructions: for the shallow level of processing, the participants were asked to judge which of the two words in the presented pair was first alphabetically; for the medium level, they were asked to judge whether the two words had no, some, or many phonemes in common; for the deep task, they were asked to judge the degree of semantic association between the words in each pair. The combination of three levels of processing and four presentation rates thus yielded 12 conditions combining depth and rate. The corresponding recall levels are shown in Figure 23.3. The 6 s rate gave

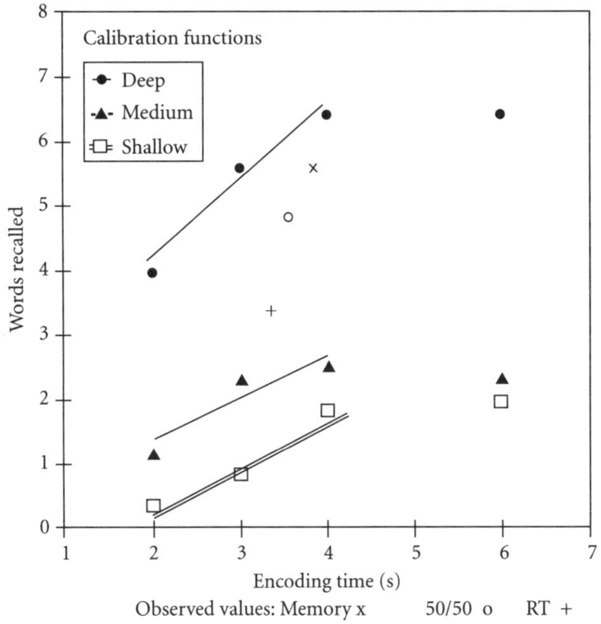

Figure 23.3 Mean numbers of words recalled as a function of encoding time under FA (calibration functions). The graph also shows observed values for divided attention when emphasis was on memory, both tasks equally (50/50), or RT (Reproduced from M. Naveh-Benjamin *et al.*, *Memory and Cognition*, **28**, 965–976, 2000).

no further recall advantage over the 4 s rate, but the 2, 3, and 4 s conditions yielded linear increases in recall that varied in slope and in level of performance as a function of depth of initial processing. These three 'calibration functions' are obviously arbitrary, and our more general point is that there is presumably a family of such functions relating encoding time to encoding depth.

The dual-task part of the experiment was carried out in a separate session. In this part, participants performed a visual four-choice RT task while also attempting to learn further lists of word pairs under free learning instructions. As in the experiment by Anderson *et al.* (1998), participants again performed the dual task under three different emphasis conditions (attend primarily to the RT task, attend primarily to the memory encoding task, or divide attention equally). The word pairs were presented auditorily at a rate of 6 s. Finally, the visual RT task was also performed under single task conditions; it was a continuous RT task, in the sense that a correct response caused the next stimulus to appear immediately, and so the measure was the average inter-response time over the encoding phase for each list.

Following the shared time model discussed by Craik *et al.* (1996), we assumed that the functional time available for memory encoding in the DA conditions can be calculated from the difference in time between the RT task performed alone and in the dual-task conditions. That is, the RT task was performed more slowly in dual-task than in single-task conditions, and it is this 'extra' time that is used to encode the word pairs (for more details see Craik *et al.* 1996; Naveh-Benjamin *et al.* 2000). Thus although the nominal time allowed to encode each word pair was 6 s, the functional times for encoding in the three different emphasis conditions were as follows: memory emphasis, 3.96 s; 50/50 emphasis, 3.87 s; RT emphasis, 3.61 s. When recall levels for the three emphasis conditions are plotted as a function of those functional encoding times, the points fall systematically between the deep and medium calibration functions shown in Figure 23.3. Thus it appears that when functional encoding time is withdrawn during memory encoding, the consequent recall levels do not fall off by following one of the depth-related calibration functions, but rather fall between the functions. The implication is that as resources are withdrawn during encoding, the depth of processing achieved is necessarily reduced, and that in the present experiment as attention was withdrawn from the memory encoding task, the encoding achieved dropped from being similar to the deep level–4 s combination to being similar to the medium level–3 s combination.

The point of this somewhat laborious exercise is that the results lend some weight to the argument that one reason for poorer memory performance when attention is divided at encoding is that the qualitative type of processing achieved becomes shallower and less elaborate as attentional resources are withdrawn. The further point is that by combining this conclusion with the previous conclusion that the ageing process can be mimicked by dividing attention in dual-task situations in young adults (as in the present experiment), it can be argued that one reason for age-related memory loss is that a reduction in available processing resources results in less deep and elaborate encoding processes and therefore in lower levels of subsequent memory.

An age-related binding deficit?

There is good evidence that the binding mechanisms of older adults are less effective, resulting in poorer integration of events with their contexts of occurrence, and also in the creation of weaker associative links between items themselves (Chalfonte and Johnson 1996; Naveh-Benjamin 2000). In particular, Naveh-Benjamin (2000) has argued that older adults show a greater loss in associative information than in item information relative to younger adults; thus older people remember facts and events, but have greater difficulty than younger adults in remembering their contexts of occurrence. Older adults also show a deficit in the ability to form associative links between items; names and faces might be an example. On the other hand, Naveh-Benjamin *et al.* (2003) have shown that DA during encoding in young adults has the effect of reducing memory for item and associative information equally, i.e. DA at encoding, unlike normal ageing, does not result in a differential loss of associative information.

These findings obviously cast doubt on, or at least set limits to, the equivalence of DA and ageing, and so we set out to check these facts and results in our own laboratory. Castel conducted an experiment to explore these issues (Castel and Craik 2003). Participants learned lists of unrelated pairs of nouns and were then given a recognition test, either for the second words of the pairs ('item test') or for word pairs ('associative test'). If original presented word pairs are designated A–B and C–D, the pairs that were presented in the recognition test were Y–Z pairs ('new', both new words), A–X pairs ('item', first word old but second word new), A–D pairs ('conjunction', both words old but in a rearranged pairing), or A–B pairs ('old', both words old in the original pairing). In the part of the experiment testing item information, the participant's task was to decide whether the second word in the pair presented at test was an old word (regardless of the first word). Thus for the item test both A–B pairs and A–D pairs should be 'yes' responses; the only difference was that B words appeared in their initial context (A–B) whereas D words were in a new context. However, only A–B pairs were correct for the word pair test; a 'yes' response to other pairs constituted a false

Table 23.3 Proportions of 'old' responses corrected for baseline false alarms

	Single-word test			Word-pair test		
	Item (A–X)	**Conj. (A–D)**	**Old (A–B)**	**Item (A–X)**	**Conj. (A–D)**	**Old (A–B)**
Young–FA	–0.3	0.37	0.52	0.03	0.12	0.58
Young–DA_1	0.04	0.35	0.44	0.07	0.16	0.52
Old–FA	0.08	0.38	0.41	0.11	0.28	0.49
Young–DA_2	0.02	0.16	0.21	0.06	0.13	0.24

Conj., conjunction pairs.

In the single-word test, 'old' responses to conjunction and old items are hits; 'old' responses to item pairs are false alarms. In the word-pair test, 'old' responses to old items are hits; 'old' responses to item and conjunction pairs are false alarms.

Reproduced from Castel and Craik 2003.

alarm. We expected more false alarms to A–D pairs since both words were old and therefore 'familiar'.

In this study the word pairs were presented visually at both the encoding and retrieval phases. The secondary task was auditory; it consisted of a very long string of digits between zero and nine spoken by a female voice at a 1.5-s rate. In condition DA_2 (Table 23.3) the participant's task was to monitor the digit sequence for targets defined as 'three successive odd digits' (e.g. 519, 171, 935) and to repeat such sequences aloud. As shown by the hit rates in Table 23.3, this secondary task was very difficult, and so a second group of young adults also performed the experiment but with the difference that they monitored the digit string for any occurrences of the single digit nine. This group is labelled Young–DA_1 in Table 23.3. The results from four groups of 32 participants are shown in Table 23.3. The groups were younger (mean age, 21 years) and older (mean age, 70 years) participants who performed the memory task under FA conditions (no secondary task), and two further groups of comparable young adults who encoded the word lists while performing either the easy secondary task (DA_1) or the difficult secondary task (DA_2).

The results shown in Table 23.3 are the proportions of responding 'old' to test items minus the proportion of responding 'old' to 'new' test pairs (Y–Z). Thus the scores are corrected for baseline false alarms (see also Jones and Jacoby 2001). In the single-word test, both A–B and A–D should be answered 'old,' whereas only A–B pairs are hits in the word-pair test. One similarity between older adults and younger (DA_2) adults in the single-word test is that B items were answered correctly only slightly more than D items. However, A–B pairs conferred a substantial benefit for younger adults under FA, presumably because they were able to take advantage of the reinstatement of the B word's original encoding 'context' A–B. Thus both ageing and DA are associated with a reduced ability to take advantage of re-presented context, arguably because participants in these groups 'bound' the original A–B items together into a cohesive unit less well than did the FA younger group.

In the word-pair test, the best measure of associative information is the difference between conjunction pairs (A–D) and old pairs (A–B). The difference was 0.46 for the young FA group, 0.36 for the easy DA group, 0.21 for the older adults, and 0.11 for the difficult DA group. Thus the ability to discriminate A–B from A–D pairs declined as attention was diverted from the word pairs during encoding. The older adults performed at a level intermediate between the levels shown by the easy and difficult Young–DA groups, suggesting that older adults also have fewer processing resources at their disposal. Again, it is possible to argue that both ageing and DA are associated with less efficient binding of the word pairs at the time of encoding.

The other noteworthy feature of the word-pair test results is the very high false-alarm rate to conjunction pairs shown by the older adult group; the raw scores for conjunction errors (i.e. before subtracting baseline false alarms) were 0.17 for FA young participants but 0.40 for the older group. This result suggests strongly that older adults based their recognition decision largely on familiarity rather than on more analytical processes of recollection (Jacoby *et al.* 1996; Jones and Jacoby 2001). However, this tendency to commit many false-positive responses to A–D pairs was not shared by the Young–DA groups. Therefore one possible account of the data shown in Table 23.3 is that both ageing and DA are associated with less efficient memory encoding processes. Speculatively, such reduced efficiency involves less effective binding of items and events to local contexts and to each other; it may also result in shallower encoding, as suggested in Figure 23.2(b), implying less integration with and modification by relevant schematic knowledge structures. I have previously suggested that such inefficient encoding processes result in encoded records that are less distinctive and therefore less well retrieved by specific retrieval cues; ageing and DA are associated with encoded traces that are general and stereotyped, rather than being richly differentiated by the specific context or by specific semantic interpretations (Craik and Simon 1980; Craik and Byrd 1982; see also Moscovitch and Craik 1976; Simon 1979). However, the results shown in Table 23.3 make it clear that older adults also differ from Young–DA participants by making many more false-positive responses to items that are similar to target items and thus feel familiar. Older adults process events in a more general, less analytical, fashion at *both* encoding and retrieval.

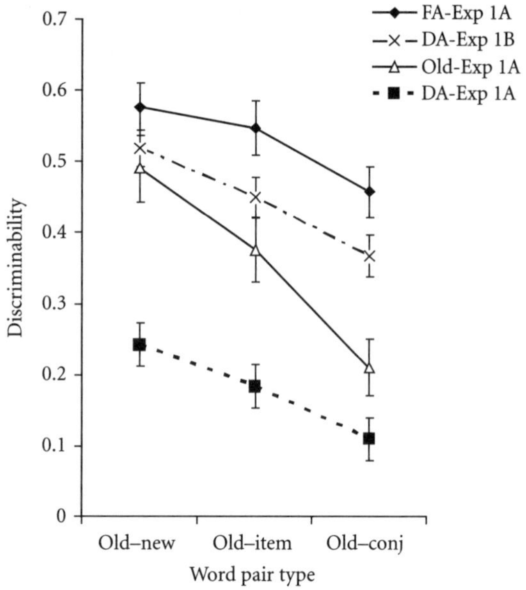

Figure 23.4 Discriminability between old word pairs and other distractor types as a function of age and attentional condition (Reproduced from A.D. Castel and F.I.M. Craik, *Psychology and Aging*, **18**, 873–885, 2003).

The difference between the effects of ageing and DA is seen clearly when the data from the word-pair test are plotted in terms of the ability to discriminate between old target items (A–B pairs) and the other three types of test item (Y–Z, A–X, and A–D pairs). Figure 23.4 shows these discriminability functions (simply the differences between the probability of saying 'old' to A–B pairs and each of the three types of distractor pairs) as a function of the four groups of participants. Discriminability drops from Y–Z pairs to A–D pairs, and the figure shows that the drop in discriminability for the two DA groups is parallel to the drop for the FA young group; overall level is determined simply by the difficulty of the DA task. However, the figure also shows that the discriminability function for older adults is not parallel to the other groups; discriminability drops off more quickly, again showing that older adults have a greater difficulty in discriminating A–B pairs from A–D pairs.

A final question concerns the loss of item and associative information by older and Young–DA groups relative to the levels shown by young adults under FA. Naveh-Benjamin's work (Naveh-Benjamin 2000; Naveh-Benjamin *et al.* 2003) has suggested that, whereas older adults have a particular problem with associative information, DA in young adults results in an equivalent loss of item and associative information. Castel and Craik (2003) proposed that item information in their experiments could be measured as the difference between the probabilities of saying 'yes' to new word pairs (Y–Z) and conjunction word pairs (A–D) in the single-word test; this procedure yields a 'hits minus false alarms' measure of item information. They also proposed that associative information could be measured as the difference between the probabilities of saying 'yes' to conjunction pairs (A–D) and old pairs (A–B). Once these measures were obtained, estimates of item loss and associative loss were calculated as the differences between these measures in older adults and Young–DA_2 adults on the one hand, and the corresponding measures in young FA adults on the other hand.

The estimates of item and associative loss for the older adults were −0.01 and 0.24, respectively, and the corresponding estimates of loss for the Young–DA_2 group were 0.21 and 0.34, respectively. Statistical treatment of these results yielded a main effect of type of information (greater associative loss than item loss), a significant effect of group (greater losses for the DA_2 group), and an interaction between group and type showing that the difference between item and associative loss was greater for the older adults than for the Young–DA group. Thus these results confirm Naveh-Benjamin's claim that ageing is associated with greater losses of associative information than of item information, but differ from the results of Naveh-Benjamin *et al.* (2003) in showing that DA was also associated with a significantly greater loss of associative information than of item information (0.34 versus 0.21, $t(31) = 4.66$, $P < .001$). Statistics were not run on losses for the easier DA_1 group, but their losses were 0.02 and 0.10 for item and associative information, respectively, and so again there was a comparatively greater loss of associative information. Thus these findings differ from those of Naveh-Benjamin and colleagues in that both ageing and DA were associated with greater deficits in associative than in item information, but the two sets of findings agree that ageing is associated with a differentially greater loss of associative information.

Are depth and elaboration sufficient?

This final empirical illustration concerns some further thoughts about the mechanism by which ageing and DA act to reduce memory performance. So far, I have suggested that both ageing and DA are associated with reduced processing resources, and that this reduction acts to reduce the depth and elaboration of processing that occur during the encoding phase (Naveh-Benjamin *et al.* 2002) and may also act to impair binding processes. Therefore a plausible formulation is one that states that a reduction of processing resources leads to impaired encoding processes, and that subsequent memory performance will reflect whatever degrees of depth, elaboration, distinctiveness, and binding were in fact achieved. However, we have some evidence that questions this reasonable formulation. This further evidence suggests that when depth and elaboration are equated between FA and DA, subsequent memory performance is still inferior in the DA condition.

This somewhat tentative (and to me surprising) conclusion is based on the results of some unpublished experiments conducted in my laboratory over the last few years. The general method was to present word pairs or single words to encode under either FA or DA conditions in a manner that enabled us to estimate the depth or elaboration of processing achieved. We then gave participants a test of recall or recognition (under FA conditions) and examined the data to see whether memory performance was reduced by the DA manipulation even after any reduction in elaboration was partialled out.

In the first experiment, participants were presented with 70 pairs of common nouns on a computer screen and instructed to attempt to form some meaningful association between members of each pair. They were also asked to rate the meaningfulness of the association on a scale from 0 to 5, where 0 indicated no meaningful connection and 5 indicated that a strong meaningful connection had been achieved. Two groups of 18 young adults performed this incidental encoding task, one under FA conditions and the other while carrying out a DA task (the 'three successive odd digits' task described previously). Two surprise memory tests (both under FA conditions) followed the encoding phase. In a cued recall test the first words from each pair were presented as cues for the second words, and in a subsequent test the 70 second words from the original pairs were presented along with 70 new words in a yes–no recognition task. The results of both tests are shown in Table 23.4(a). The data were pooled over meaningfulness ratings 0 and 1, and also over ratings 4 and 5, as there were relatively few responses in the 0 and 5 rating categories. The table shows that both cued recall and recognition performance increased as a function of meaningfulness, and that this increase occurred for both FA and DA groups. Interestingly, both recall and recognition scores were lower for the DA group despite the apparent equivalence of the semantic processing carried out at encoding. Statistically, there were strong effects of the meaningfulness ratings and the FA–DA manipulation for both cued recall and recognition, but no trace of an interaction in either case. Thus it seems that diversion of attention reduced memory performance despite the equivalence of initial processing.

An obvious objection to this conclusion is that the ratings of meaningfulness may not be equivalent under FA and DA conditions; it is possible that DA reduces depth and elaboration but that participants allocate the full 0–5 range of subjective ratings to span their own experienced range. It seemed necessary to obtain a more objective measure of semantic processing. Accordingly, we carried out a second experiment in which 16 undergraduates were presented with pairs

Table 23.4 Mean proportions correct for cued recall and recognition tests as a function of meaningfulness

	(a) Meaningfulness rating			
	0 + 1	**2**	**3**	**4 + 5**
Cued recall				
Full attention	0.36	0.47	0.50	0.61
Divided attention	0.10	0.17	0.23	0.31
Recognition memory				
Full attention	0.71	0.77	0.78	0.85
Divided attention	0.56	0.56	0.63	0.66
	(b) Degree of elaboration			
	0 + 1	**2**	**3 + 4**	
Cued recall				
Full attention	0.50	0.67	0.70	
Divided attention	0.36	0.53	0.57	

Reproduced from Craik and Kester 2000.

of unrelated concrete nouns auditorily, and were asked to generate a rich meaningful sentence linking the two words in each pair. They were told that the experiment was on creativity and the effects of attention on creativity; they were given 12 s to generate and then speak their generated sentences aloud into a tape recorder. The participants were given 36 word pairs under FA conditions and 36 under DA conditions; in this experiment the DA task was again the 'three odd digits' task, but presented visually to avoid interfering with the auditory presentation of word pairs and spoken responses. Finally, participants were given the 72 first words from both the FA and DA conditions mixed randomly, and asked to recall the paired second words.

In this experiment, the sentences generated in the first phase were transcribed, mixed randomly between FA and DA conditions, and given to three judges who scored each sentence for elaboration, meaningfulness, and cohesiveness on a scale from 0 to 4. Cued recall scores were then calculated as a function of attentional condition and judged degree of semantic elaboration. Table 23.4(b) shows the results; ratings 0 and 1, and also 3 and 4, were pooled because of the small frequencies in the extreme categories. The findings were very similar to those of the first experiment in the series, i.e. cued recall levels increased as sentence elaboration increased, the DA condition was associated with lower scores than the FA condition, and there was no interaction between the variables. Again, it appears as if DA does more than reduce the depth and elaboration of initial processing; final memory scores are lower for DA even when the degree of encoding elaboration is equated between FA and DA.

One other objection that might be made to the conclusion that DA at encoding reduces memory over and above its effects on semantic processing is that DA might reduce the effectiveness of higher levels of organization on other types of between-pair processing. Such reduced effectiveness would lead to impaired memory, but would not be picked up by our measures of within-pair elaboration. To address this possibility, Kester devised and ran a study in my laboratory in which 24 young adults were presented with two lists of 42 words, one under FA and one under DA conditions. The word lists were presented visually, and the DA task was again the auditorily presented three odd digit task. Each word list consisted of six exemplars from each of seven semantic categories (e.g. vegetables), with the exemplars randomly mixed throughout the list. The participants' task was to generate a mental image of each word and then rate the elaborateness of each generated image on a scale of 0–6; the categorical structure of the list was not mentioned. Each list was followed by a 60-s arithmetic task, and participants were then given a free recall test. In this case 'elaboration' was measured in terms of participants' ratings, and 'organization' was measured by the Adjusted Ratio of Clustering (ARC) score (Roenker *et al.* 1971). This clustering score estimates organization by examining the order in which the participant recalls list words; if participants organize words in terms of categories, they are likely to recall words clustered according to the categories.

DA had the effect of reducing both rated elaborateness of generated images (2.9 versus 3.5) and the ARC measure of organization (0.50 versus 0.65), but when recall scores are plotted as a function of elaboration rating (Fig. 23.5) it is again obvious that DA acted to reduce subsequent recall. To assess the effects of organization on recall, participants in each condition were split at the median into high-organization and low-organization subgroups (also shown in Fig. 23.5). High organization was associated with a recall benefit in the DA group but not in the FA group (with the exception of the lowest level of elaboration). However, the high-organization subgroup in the DA condition had a mean ARC score of 0.72, substantially higher than the low-organization subgroup in the FA condition (0.47), and so it appears that DA was associated with low recall despite equivalent elaboration and a higher level of organization in the FA group.

Taken together, these three experiments strongly suggest that, whereas part of the deleterious effect of DA on subsequent memory is attributable to a reduction in the depth and elaboration of encoding achieved (Naveh-Benjamin *et al.* 2000), a further part is attributable to other factors. One possibility is that these other factors are physiological mechanisms that do not have cognitive correlates

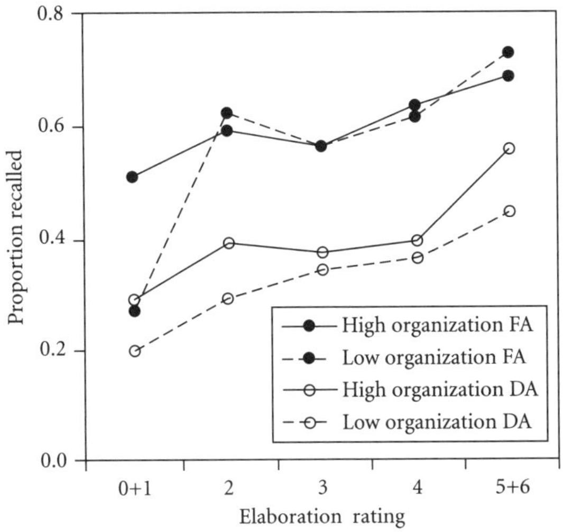

Figure 23.5 Proportions of words recalled as a function of elaboration rating, organization, and either FA or DA. (Data from Craik and Kester 2000.)

(e.g. consolidation processes), i.e. DA may act to reduce the effectiveness of both cognitive correlates and neurological correlates of successful memory encoding.

This possibility is given added credibility when some more obviously biologically based conditions are considered. For example, both alcoholic intoxication (Birnbaum *et al.* 1978) and depressive drugs (Curran 1991) are associated with impaired subsequent memory, although immediate cognitive processes may show relatively slight amounts of impairment. Amnesia patients provide further evidence that memory can be grossly impaired despite relatively intact abilities to process and elaborate meaning in the course of conversation, thinking, or problem solving. Therefore the present speculation is that the negative effects of DA, and perhaps also ageing, on memory are partly a function of reduced ability to process information deeply, elaborately, and in an organized fashion, but partly also a function of the reduced efficiency of the biological mechanisms subsumed under the label of 'consolidation'.

Concluding comments

In this chapter I have set out my current ideas on some of the factors underlying age-related decrements in memory. It seems likely, in fact, that many age-related changes converge to influence final performance, although some factors may conveniently be grouped together until we develop the analytic tools to tease apart their effects. Thus, while various researchers have argued that age-related declines in cognitive performance are primarily attributable to general slowing, or to a decline in processing resources, or to declines in associative efficiency or the efficiency of inhibitory mechanisms, the more likely scenario is that all of these factors play some part in the overall picture of abilities that decline and those that hold up well with increasing age. It also seems likely that such broad concepts as inhibition, associative deficit, and processing resources are themselves determined by a number of concurrent changes in the underlying neurobiology. Given our limited knowledge at present, it is probably useful to continue to use such shorthand concepts as 'processing resources', but we should also be alert for opportunities to refine our concepts and postulated mechanisms of change.

In this spirit, I have suggested a number of factors that appear to underlie age-related decrements in memory. Some of these factors come into play at encoding and others have their effects at retrieval, although it may be that a smaller number of common causes affect both encoding and retrieval. In this chapter I have suggested that knowledge is represented hierarchically, as a continuous series of levels of representation running from highly context-specific representations of episodic events to increasingly abstract and generalized representations of concepts, facts, and ideas. Good episodic memory depends first on the encoding of experienced events as distinctive representations that are both well differentiated from other similar events and well integrated into existing schematic knowledge structures (see Ausubel (1962) for a similar suggestion). The present argument is that older people have fewer processing resources at their disposal (owing to age-related neurobiological changes that are not yet well understood) and that this drop in resources results in encoded representations that are relatively shallow (Fig. 23.2(b)) and not well differentiated from other similar representations. Just as older adults rely more on feelings of general familiarity than on specific recollections at the time of retrieval (Jacoby and Hay 1998); so older adults may analyze incoming stimuli and events in more general ways at the time of encoding, with the result that the encoded records are less modulated and specified by the current context. This age-related change may be considered a partial failure of binding processes, but note that it is not simply a case of well-bound versus poorly-bound, but rather that the new event is 'comprehended' in a more general way.

The claim that processing resources decline with increasing age in adulthood is supported by the qualitative similarity of age-related effects to those resulting from division of attention in young adults (Anderson *et al.* 1998), although the two cases may not be identical (Naveh-Benjamin *et al.* 2003). The suggestion that a drop in the availability of processing resources results in shallower encodings is supported by the results shown in Figure 23.3 (Naveh-Benjamin *et al.* 2000). Finally, the point that events are less well bound to their contexts as a function of both ageing and DA is supported by the finding of Castel and Craik (2003) that, whereas young adults benefit substantially from a reinstatement of encoding context in the case of item recognition, older adults and Young–DA adults benefit to a lesser extent. The final experiments reported in the chapter showed that DA results in lower memory performance even when drops in elaboration and organization are taken into account. These results led to the speculation that division of attention (and thus perhaps ageing also) results in a failure of consolidation—a set of neurophysiological processes that may have no experiential correlates. In this sense, age-related memory problems may resemble a mild form of the amnesic syndrome, i.e. the memory deficit may be greater than that predicted from a decline in the quality of the cognitive operations performed during the activities of perceiving, attending, comprehending, and learning.

I have concentrated on encoding processes rather than on retrieval processes, but it is clear that age-related inefficiencies of retrieval also play a part in the poorer memory abilities of older adults. First, of course, if the encoded trace is less well bound to schematic knowledge, and less well differentiated from other similar representations, the older retrieval system is already at a disadvantage. However, older people also experience problems in retrieving well-encoded information, so that other factors must be operating. In Figure 23.1, the idea is set out that older adults are less able to generate self-initiated retrieval processes, and so must rely more on environmental support. This difficulty may be a function of an age-related decline in the efficiency of the frontal lobes (Grady and Craik 2000). In addition, such frontal inefficiency may result in poorer 'resolving power' in the processes needed to access the highly specific information represented in the lowest branches of knowledge hierarchies (Fig. 23.2(a)). That is, older adults (like depressed patients; Williams 1996) appear to have particular difficulties in accessing and retrieving specific types of knowledge, whether 'episodic' or 'semantic' in nature.

Jacoby and colleagues (Jacoby *et al.* 1996; Jacoby and Hay 1998) have made a persuasive case for the point that older adults rely more on general familiarity than on specific recollection as a basis for recognition memory, and this case fits well with my overall argument. Jacoby's view also predicts that older adults will commit more false-positive errors when presented with information that is correct in its general aspects although wrong in specific aspects. This prediction is upheld by the very high false-positive rates observed with conjunction (A–D) items in the pair recognition part of the study by Castel and Craik (2003). Other observations of inflated false-alarm rates in the elderly are also in line with Jacoby's viewpoint (Balota *et al.* 1999; Jacoby 1999; Benjamin 2001).

In summary, it seems likely that age-related changes in a number of cognitive processes underlie the inefficiencies of memory that accompany normal ageing.

Some of these processes involve binding mechanisms; including for example the formation of associations between items, the integration of events with their contexts of occurrence, and the integration of events with existing knowledge bases. However, as suggested earlier, binding mechanisms exist at different 'levels of binding' running from perceptual feature binding to the formation of new concepts, ideas, and even theories, and it seems likely that 'binding' is a general term for a set of somewhat different processes. Other age-related memory problems are attributable to quite different processing impairments; two examples are the difficulty in accessing specific information at retrieval and (speculatively) an impairment in consolidation. Any complete theory of age-related changes in memory must bind these and other factors into a coherent final model.

References

Anderson, C.M.B. and Craik, F.I.M. (1974). The effect of a concurrent task on recall from primary memory. *Journal of Verbal Learning and Verbal Behavior*, **13**, 107–113.

Anderson, N.D., Craik, F.I.M., and Naveh-Benjamin, M. (1998). The attentional demands of encoding and retrieval in younger and older adults. I: Evidence from divided attention costs. *Psychology and Aging*, **13**, 405–423.

Ausubel, D.P. (1962). A subsumption theory of meaningful verbal learning and retention. *Journal of General Psychology*, **66**, 213–224.

Baddeley, A. (1986). *Working Memory*. Oxford: Oxford University Press.

Balota, D.W., Cortese, M.J., Duchek, J.M., *et al.* (1999). Veridical and false memories in healthy older adults and dementia of the Alzheimer's type. *Cognitive Neuropsychology*, **16**, 361–384.

Bartlett, F.C. (1932). *Remembering*. Cambridge: Cambridge University Press.

Benjamin, A.S. (2001). On the dual effects of repetition on false recognition. *Journal of Experimental Psychology: Learning, Memory, and Cognition*, **29**, 691–697.

Birnbaum, I.M., Parker, E.S., Hartley, J.T., and Noble, E.P. (1978). Alcohol and memory: Retrieval processes. *Journal of Verbal Learning and Verbal Behavior*, **17**, 325–335.

Castel, A.D. and Craik, F.I.M. (2003). The effects of aging and divided attention on memory for item and associative memory. *Psychology and Aging*, **18**, 873–885.

Chalfonte, B.L. and Johnson, M.K. (1996). Feature memory and binding in young and older adults. *Memory and Cognition*, **214**, 403–416.

Craik, F.I.M. (1983). On the transfer of information from temporary to permanent memory. *Philosophical Transactions of the Royal Society, Series B, Biological Sciences*, **302**, 341–359.

Craik, F.I.M. (1986). A functional account of age differences in memory. In *Human Memory and Cognitive Capabilities, Mechanisms and Performances* (ed F.Klix and H. Hagendorf). Amsterdam: Elsevier, pp. 409–422.

Craik, F.I.M. (2002). Human memory and aging. In *Psychology at the turn of the Millenium* (ed L. Bäckman and C. von Hofsten). Hove, UK: Psychology Press, pp. 261–280.

Craik, F.I.M. and Byrd, M. (1982). Aging and cognitive deficits: the role of attentional resources. In *Aging and Cognitive Processes* (ed F.I.M. Craik and S. Trehub). New York: Plenum, pp. 191–211.

Craik, F.I.M. and Jennings, J.J. (1992). Human memory. In *The Handbook of Aging and Cognition* (ed F.I.M. Craik and T.A. Salthouse). Hillsdale, NJ: Erlbaum, pp. 51–110.

Craik, F.I.M. and Kester, J.D. (2000). Divided attention and memory: impairment of processing or consolidation? In *Memory, Consciousness, and the Brain* (ed E.Tulving). Philadelphia, PA: Psychology Press, pp. 38–51.

Craik, F.I.M. and Lockhart, R.S. (1972). Levels of processing: a framework for memory research. *Journal of Verbal Learning and Verbal Behavior*, **11**, 671–684.

Craik, F.I.M. and Simon, E. (1980). Age differences in memory: the roles of attention and depth of processing. In *New Directions in Memory and Aging* (ed L. Poon., J.L. Fozard, L.S. Cermak, D. Arenberg, and L.W. Thompson). Hillsdale, NJ: Erlbaum, pp. 95–112.

Craik, F.I.M. and Tulving, E. (1975). Depth of processing and the retention of words in episodic memory. *Journal of Experimental Psychology: General*, **104**, 268–294.

Craik, F.I.M., Naveh-Benjamin, M., Govoni, R., and Anderson, N.D. (1996). The effects of divided attention on encoding and retrieval processes in human memory. *Journal of Experimental Psychology: General*, **125**, 159–180.

Curran, H.V. (1991). Benzodiazepines, memory and mood: a review. *Psychopharmacology*, **105**, 1–8.

Gardiner, J.M. and Richardson-Klavehn, A. (2000). Remembering and knowing. In *The Oxford Handbook of Memory* (ed E. Tulving and F.I.M. Craik). New York: Oxford University Press, pp. 229–244.

Grady, C. L. and Craik, F.I.M. (2000). Changes in memory processing with age. *Current Opinion in Neurobiology*, **10**, 224–231.

Hunt, R.R. and Einstein, G.O. (1981). Relational and item-specific information in memory. *Journal of Verbal Learning and Verbal Behavior*, **20**, 497–514.

Jacoby, L.L. (1999). Ironic effects of repetition: measuring age-related differences in memory. *Journal of Experimental Psychology: Learning, Memory, and Cognition*, **25**, 3–22.

Jacoby, L.L. and Hay, J.F. (1998). Age-related deficits in memory: theory and application. In *Theories of memory* (ed M.A. Conway, S.E. Gathercole, and C. Cornoldi). Hove, UK: Psychology Press, pp. 111–134.

Jacoby, L.L., Jennings, J.M., and Hay, J.F. (1996). Dissociating automatic and consciously-controlled processes: implications for diagnosis and rehabilitation of memory deficits. In *Basic and Applied Memory Research: Theory in Context* (ed D.J. Herrmann, M.K. Johnson, C.L. McEvoy, C. Hertzog, and P.Hertel). Hillsdale, NJ: Erlbaum, pp. 161–193.

Jones, T.C. and Jacoby, L.L. (2001). Feature and conjunction errors in recognition memory: evidence for dual-process theory. *Journal of Memory and Language*, **45**, 82–102.

Li, S.-C., Lindenberger, U., and Sikstroem, S. (2001). Aging cognition: from neuromodulation to representation. *Trends in Cognitive Sciences*, **5**, 479–486.

Moscovitch, M. and Craik, F.I.M. (1976). Depth of processing, retrieval cues, and uniqueness of encoding as factors in recall. *Journal of Verbal Learning and Verbal Behavior*, **15**, 447–458.

Murdock, B.B.J. (1965). Effects of a subsidiary task on short-term memory. *British Journal of Psychology*, **56**, 413–419.

Murdock, B.B.J. (1967). Recent developments in short-term memory. *British Journal of Psychology*, **58**, 421–433.

Murdock, B.B.J. (1974). *Human Memory: Theory and Data*. Potomac, MD: Erlbaum.

Naveh-Benjamin, M. (2000). Adult age differences in memory performance: tests of an associative deficit hypothesis. *Journal of Experimental Psychology: Learning, Memory, and Cognition*, **26**, 1170–1187.

Naveh-Benjamin, M., Craik, F.I.M., Gavrilescu, D., and Anderson, N.D. (2000). Asymmetry between encoding and retrieval processes: evidence from divided attention and a calibration analysis. *Memory and Cognition*, **28**, 965–976.

Naveh-Benjamin, M., Craik, F.I.M., and Ben-Shaul, L. (2002). Age-related differences in cued recall: Effects of support at encoding and retrieval. *Aging, Neuropsychology and Cognition*, **9**, 276–287.

Naveh-Benjamin, M., Guez, J., and Marom, M. (2003). The effects of divided attention at encoding on item and associative memory. *Memory and Cognition*, **31**, 1021–1035.

Prull, M.W., Gabrieli, J.D.E., and Bunge, S.A. (2000). Age-related changes in memory: a cognitive neuroscience perspective. In *The Handbook of Aging and Cognition* (2nd edn) (ed F.I.M. Craik and T.A. Salthouse). Mahwah, NJ: Erlbaum, pp. 91–153.

Raz, N. (2000). Aging of the brain and its impact on cognitive performance: integration of structural and functional findings. In *The Handbook of Aging and Cognition* (2nd edn) (ed F.I.M. Craik and T.A. Salthouse). Mahwah, NJ: Erlbaum, pp. 1–90.

Roenker, D.L., Thompson, C.P., and Brown, S.C. (1971). A comparison of measures for the estimation of clustering in free recall. *Psychological Bulletin*, **76**, 45–48.

Salthouse, T.A. (1996). The processing-speed theory of adult age differences in cognition. *Psychological Review*, **103**, 403–428.

Schacter, D.L., Harbluk, J.L., and McLachlan, D. (1984). Retrieval without recollection: an experimental analysis of source amnesia. *Journal of Verbal Learning and Verbal Behavior*, **23**, 593–611.

Simon, E. (1979). Depth and elaboration of processing in relation to age. *Journal of Experimental Psychology: Learning, Memory, and Cognition*, **5**, 115–124.

Tulving, E. (1972). Episodic and semantic memory. In *Organization of Memory* (ed E. Tulving and W. Donaldson). New York: Academic Press, pp. 382–404.

Tulving, E. (1983). *Elements of Episodic Memory*. New York: Oxford University Press.

Tulving, E. (1985). Memory and consciousness. *Canadian Psychology*, **26**, 1–12.

Tulving, E. and Schacter, D.L. (1990). Priming and human memory systems. *Science*, **247**, 301–306.

Williams, J.M.G. (1996). Depression and the specificity of autobiographical memory. In *Remembering our past: Studies in autobiographical memory* (ed D. Rubin). Cambridge, UK: Cambridge University Press.

Zacks, R.T., Hasher, L., and Li, K.Z.H. (2000). Human memory. In *The Handbook of Aging and Cognition* (2nd edn) (ed F.I.M. Craik and T.A. Salthouse). Mahwah, NJ: Erlbaum, pp. 293–357.

Chapter 24

Prefrontal and medial temporal lobe contributions to relational memory in young and older adults

Roberto Cabeza

Introduction

When we remember a past event, we typically remember not only the various components of the event, or **item memory** (IM), but also the associations among these components, or **relational memory** (RM). RM is more sensitive than IM to several memory disorders, including those associated with healthy ageing. In fact, age effects on RM are about twice as large as those on IM (Spencer and Raz 1995). Studies with animals, human patients, and neuroimaging techniques have shown that RM depends prominently on the prefrontal cortex (PFC) and the medial temporal lobes (MTLs). Although age-related RM deficits are most likely due to PFC and/or MTL dysfunction, direct evidence for this causal link is very scarce. In this chapter we review ideas and findings concerning the neural correlates of RM and how they change as a function of ageing. In the first section we introduce some basic concepts, in the second section we describe theories and evidence linking RM to PFC and MTL function, and in the third section we consider the effects of ageing on the PFC and MTL substrates of RM. Finally, in the fourth section we discuss several open issues.

Basic concepts

There are different forms of RM. For example, our memory for a statement that we heard at a party may involve associations between the statement and other aspects of the event, including the topic of the conversation (semantic RM), the voice of the speaker (featural RM), our location in the room (spatial RM), and the sequence of the events in the party (temporal RM). These various forms of RM are likely to depend on different neural correlates and to be differentially affected by ageing.

In the laboratory, semantic RM has been typically investigated using word pairs. In a typical paradigm, participants study pairs of unrelated words (tree–horse, tuxedo–lamp, cake–stapler, . . .), and their memory is tested with item recognition and associative recognition tests (e.g. Hockley 1992). In the item recognition test, participants decide whether single words (e.g. cake) are old or new. In the associative recognition test, they decide whether word pairs are identical with studied pairs (e.g. tree–horse) or are made up of words previously studied in different pairs (e.g. tuxedo–stapler). Dissociations between item and associative recognition tests can be used to distinguish the cognitive and/or neural mechanisms of IM and RM. Spatial, temporal, featural, and source RM have typically been investigated under the rubric 'context memory' or 'source memory' (reviewed by Johnson *et al.* 1993). In the standard paradigm, participants study single items (e.g. words) in two or more locations (e.g. left versus right side of the screen), times (e.g. first versus second study list), formats (e.g. red versus blue letters), or sources (e.g. male versus female speaker), and then perform an item and a context (or source) memory task. In the item memory task, they indicate what items were presented (e.g. old–new recognition), whereas in the context memory task, they indicate where (spatial RM), when (temporal RM), or how (featural RM; source RM) they were presented.

Given that tasks are never pure, item memory tasks always involve a certain amount of relational memory. Actually, recognition memory tasks are assumed to involve two processes: recollection and familiarity (reviewed by Yonelinas 2002). Recollection refers to the retrieval of a past event that is accompanied by the recovery of specific associations or contextual details (i.e. IM plus RM), whereas familiarity refers to the feeling that an event occurred in the past in the absence of specific associations or contextual details (i.e. IM without RM). Among other methods, recollection and familiarity can be distinguished using the remember–know procedure (Tulving 1985; reviewed by Gardiner 2001), in which participants use introspection to decide whether their recognition decision was based on recollection ('remember' responses) or familiarity ('know' responses).

Although the recollection–familiarity distinction approximately maps onto the RM–IM distinction, we tend to prefer the latter terminology for three reasons. First, the recollection–familiarity distinction applies mainly to retrieval, whereas the RM–IM distinction can be applied to both encoding and retrieval. Secondly, the recollective experience is complex and may be based on different types of information. For example, in a study in which participants were asked to describe the basis of their 'remember' responses (Perfect *et al.* 1996), they reported the retrieval of external associations (25.5 per cent of 'remember' responses), inter-item associations (22.1 per cent), spatial associations (13.5 per cent), temporal associations (15 per cent), featural associations (22 per cent), etc. Since there is evidence that memory for these different kinds of associations involves distinct MTL and PFC regions, we prefer to describe them as different forms of RM rather than treating them as different aspects of the same recollection process. Finally, whereas recollection refers to an explicit form of memory, the term relational memory can be applied to implicit forms of memory dependent on hippocampal function (Ryan *et al.* 2000).

Prefrontal cortex and medial temporal lobe contributions to relational memory

In a strict sense, all forms of memory are relational, and hence the distinction between RM and IM is only a matter of degree. Thus the standard research strategy for investigating RM has been to compare conditions which involve both RM and IM but emphasize one over the other. This has been an effective method, as attested by numerous studies showing functional, developmental, lesion, and functional neuroimaging dissociations between RM and IM conditions. Only a subset of these studies is reviewed in this chapter. First, the review focuses on the MTL and PFC regions, and does not cover the important contributions of other brain regions, such as the role of the ventral temporal regions in featural RM, the role of the parietal regions in spatial RM, or the role of lateral temporal regions in semantic RM. Secondly, the review focuses on functional neuroimaging and lesion data, and does not cover other types of data, such as single-cell recordings. Finally, only some of the many ideas and theories proposed about RM are mentioned and discussed.

Prefrontal cortex

It is generally accepted that the PFC plays a supervisory role over the function of other brain regions including the MTL (Norman and Shallice 1986; Miller and Cohen 2001). During encoding, the PFC is assumed to implement the strategies that organize the input to the MTL, and during retrieval, it is assumed to control search and monitoring operations (Moscovitch 1992). Consistent with the idea that these working-with-memory functions (Moscovitch 1992) are more critical for RM than for IM, PFC lesions tend to yield larger deficits on RM than on IM (reviewed by Stuss *et al.* 1994; Wheeler *et al.* 1995; Shimamura 2002; Yonelinas 2002). For example, PFC damage has been associated with pronounced temporal RM deficits in both recency discrimination tasks (Milner 1971; McAndrews and Milner 1991; Milner *et al.* 1991; Butters *et al.* 1994; Kesner *et al.* 1994) and order recall tasks (Shimamura *et al.* 1990; Mangels 1997a) (reviewed by Milner *et al.*

1985; Schacter 1987; Petrides 1994). Also, PFC lesions tend to impair recollection more than familiarity (reviewed by Yonelinas 2002; Wheeler and Stuss 2003). In monkeys, PFC damage has been associated with greater deficits on spatial and temporal RM than on IM (reviewed by Petrides 1994). The PFC lesions that lead to RM deficits are often in the dorsolateral cortex (Milner *et al.* 1991; Petrides 1994), whereas lesions in the ventromedial cortex may be more important for IM (Bachevalier and Mishkin 1986).

The results of functional neuroimaging studies suggest that semantic RM is associated with activity in the left PFC during both encoding (Mottaghy *et al.* 1999; Fletcher *et al.* 2000; Lepage *et al.* 2000; Henson *et al.* 2002) and retrieval (Badgaiyan *et al.* 2002). The lateralization of PFC activity during context memory is less clear. Compared with IM conditions, the left PFC was more activated when participants remembered whether a studied item was seen or imagined (Nolde *et al.* 1998b), was seen on the left or the right of the screen (Rugg *et al.* 1999), or was larger or smaller than a probe item (Ranganath *et al.* 2000). Moreover, the left PFC was more activated for recollection than for familiarity (Henson *et al.* 1999b; Dobbins *et al.* 2003). However, other studies have associated context memory with the right PFC. For example, right PFC activity was linked to the recovery of spatial-order information (Henson *et al.* 1999a; Kostopoulos and Petrides 2003) and temporal-order information (Cabeza *et al.* 1997b, 2003). The reasons for these inconsistencies in the lateralization of RM-related PFC activity are still unclear, but they may be related to the type of information retrieved and/or the nature of retrieval processes recruited by the task.

Regarding the type of information retrieved, a recent study by Dobbins and Wagner (2005) found that that a semantic RM decision (what type of semantic encoding task was associated with each item) yielded activations in left PFC activity whereas a featural RM decision (how large was each item on the screen during encoding) yielded activations in right PFC activity. Of course, this finding fits very well with the well-known hemispheric asymmetry between semantic–linguistic processing versus pictorial–spatial processing. Regarding the nature of retrieval processes, we recently found a hemispheric asymmetry in PFC activity between two RM tasks—word-pair cued recall and context recognition. As illustrated in Figure 24.1, whereas the left PFC was more activated for recall than for context recognition, the right PFC showed the converse pattern. Given that the stimuli were verbal in both cases, this hemispheric asymmetry seems to reflect a difference in retrieval processes rather than a difference in information type. In particular, we proposed that recall tasks are more dependent on information production processes mediated by the left PFC, whereas recognition tasks are more

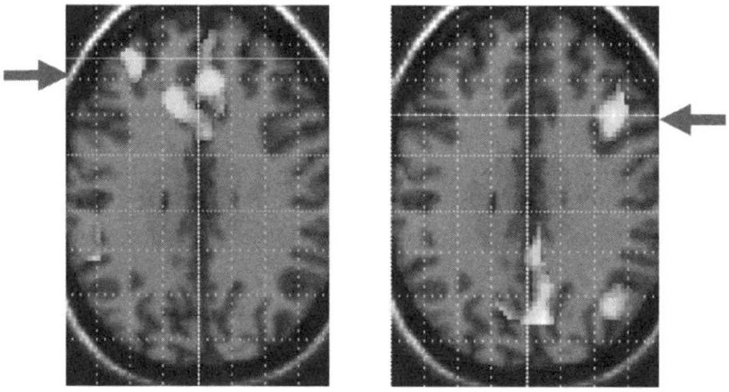

Figure 24.1 Hemispheric asymmetry in PFC activity between two RM tasks: word-pair cued recall and context recognition. Left PFC activity was greater for cued recall than for context recognition, possibly reflecting greater production demands, whereas right PFC activity was greater for context recognition than for cued recall, possibly reflecting greater monitoring demands. See colour plate section. (Reproduced from R. Cabeza *et al.*, *Journal of Cognitive Neuroscience*, **15**, 249–259, 2003.)

dependent on monitoring and verification processes mediated by right PFC activity (Cabeza *et al.* 2003).

Thus there is evidence that the lateralization of PFC activity during RM may reflect the nature of the information retrieved as well as the nature of the retrieval processes. It is still uncertain whether the conceptual–perceptual and production–monitoring dimensions are orthogonal or whether they could be integrated. For example, it is possible that production processes depend more on conceptual than on perceptual information, whereas the converse occurs for monitoring processes.

Medial temporal lobe

The MTL memory system has a hierarchical organization; inputs from various sensory association cortices are channelled through the parahippocampal region (the perirhinal cortex and the parahippocampal cortex) to the entorhinal cortex, and from there to the hippocampus, which sits at the top of the hierarchy (Squire and Zola-Morgan 1991).There is an ongoing debate about whether various MTL regions contribute differently to RM and IM. According to the **hippocampal–RM view**, the hippocampus is more critical for RM than for IM (Eichenbaum *et al.* 1994; Kroll *et al.* 1996; Mishkin *et al.* 1998; Aggleton and Brown 1999; Eldridge *et al.* 2000; Brown and Aggleton 2001). In its strongest version, this view assumes that the hippocampus is not necessary for simple IM tasks, such as old–new recognition. Instead, IM is assumed to depend on the parahippocampal region, particularly the perirhinal cortex (Aggleton and Brown 1999; Brown and

Aggleton 2001). The hippocampal–RM view fits very well with the hierarchical organization of the MTL memory system. At the same time, the fact that most connections among MTL regions are reciprocal suggests that these regions operate in a highly integrated fashion. Thus an alternative view of the MTL memory system does not assume marked differences between the roles of various MTL subregions in declarative memory (Squire and Knowlton 1995). According to this **unified MTL view**, the hippocampus is critical not only for RM but also for IM, including simple recognition tasks (Reed and Squire 1994; Stark and Squire 2001, 2003; Broadbent *et al.* 2002; Stark *et al.* 2002). Although there is evidence supporting both the hippocampal–RM and the unified MTL view, at present the field seems to be leaning towards the former.

Aggleton and Brown (Aggleton and Brown 1999; Brown and Aggleton 2001) reviewed a large amount of evidence demonstrating that hippocampal lesions produce greater deficits in RM whereas perirhinal/parahippocampal lesions yield greater deficits in IM. For example, Kroll *et al.* (1996) found that hippocampal patients were not impaired in recognizing standard items but made more false alarms to items composed of parts previously seen in other items (conjunction errors), suggesting that these parts were not properly bound during encoding. Likewise, a recent study found that amnesic patients were impaired in associative recognition when stimuli had to be integrated (word pairs) but not when they were already integrated (compound words) (Giovanello *et al.* 2003). However, there is also lesion evidence supporting the unified MTL view. For instance, a recent study by Stark and Squire (2003), which used a similar paradigm to Kroll *et al.* (1996), found that hippocampal patients were impaired in simple recognition and did not show a greater proportion of conjunction errors.

Positron-emission tomography (PET) and functional MRI (fMRI) studies have also yielded evidence supporting the hippocampal–RM view. In the semantic RM domain, for example, greater hippocampal activity has been found for tasks involving the formation of associations among word pairs or word triplets in comparison with rote rehearsal or single-word learning conditions (Henke *et al.* 1999; Davachi and Wagner 2001). In contrast, the parahippocampal gyrus, perirhinal cortex, and entorhinal cortex have been implicated in memory for single items or simple maintenance of multiple items (Wagner *et al.* 1998; Davachi and Wagner 2001; Davachi *et al.* 2003). Outside the semantic domain, studies investigating the formation of relationships between faces and names, faces and houses, and within complex scenes (Henke *et al.* 1997; Montaldi *et al.* 1998; Sperling *et al.* 2001) have found the hippocampus to be more activated in these conditions than in item-based or non-relational conditions. Additionally, tasks involving spatial navigation have found the hippocampus to be involved in successful memory for routes (Maguire *et al.* 1997; Burgess *et al.* 2001). Although these studies provide support for the hippocampal–RM view, there is also functional neuroimaging evidence supporting the unified MTL view. For instance, studies of recognition memory for item-based pictures and words have also found hippocampal activity (Stark and Squire 2000, 2001).

Effects of ageing on prefrontal cortex and medial temporal lobe contributions to relational memory

It is generally accepted that RM decline is a fundamental aspect of age-related cognitive deterioration (Burke and Light 1981; Johnson *et al.* 1993; Naveh-Benjamin 2000). According to Naveh-Benjamin's (2000) **associative deficit hypothesis**, older adults have a deficit in encoding and retrieving links between units of information, including meaningful units (e.g. word pairs) and items with their contexts. According to Johnson's **source monitoring framework** (Johnson *et al.* 1993; Schacter *et al.* 1998), remembering a complex event requires binding its components during encoding, and evaluating and reconstructing the recovered components during retrieval. Thus age-related RM deficits may reflect weak component processing and binding during encoding (Chalfonte and Johnson 1996; Mitchell *et al.* 2000b) and/or impaired component evaluation and reconstruction during retrieval (Mitchell *et al.* 2000b).

The foregoing theoretical accounts are supported by behavioural evidence that older adults are impaired in featural, spatial, and temporal RM (reviewed by Kausler 1994; Spencer and Raz 1995) Regarding featural RM, older adults are impaired in remembering whether information was presented auditorily or visually (Kausler and Puckett 1981a; McIntyre and Craik 1987), in a male or a female voice (Kausler and Puckett 1981b), in upper or lower case letters (Kausler and Puckett 1980), or in a particular colour (Park and Puglisi 1985; but see Chalfonte and Johnson 1996) or font (Naveh-Benjamin 2000). Regarding spatial RM, older adults are impaired in remembering the location of words (Denney *et al.* 1992) or objects (Park *et al.* 1982, 1983) on the screen, buildings and landmarks in a 'tourist' map (Perlmutter *et al.* 1981; Light and Zelinski 1983), real objects in a real room (Utl and Graf 1993), and a platform in a virtual water maze (Moffat *et al.* 2001; Moffat and Resnick 2002). Finally, regarding temporal RM, older adults are impaired in order recall (Kausler *et al.* 1988; Naveh-Benjamin 1990), recency discrimination (McCormack 1982; but see Perlmutter *et al.* 1981), and list-section discrimination (McCormack 1981). The foregoing RM deficits are most likely a consequence of age-related decline in MTL and PFC functions, but neurobiological evidence of age-related RM deficits is very scarce.

Prefrontal cortex

According to the **frontal ageing hypothesis** (Dempster 1992; Moscovitch and Winocur 1995; West 1996), age-related cognitive deficits are primarily due to PFC dysfunction (but see Greenwood 2000). Consistent with this hypothesis, PFC not only shows the greatest amount of age-related atrophy (reviewed by Raz 2004) but it is also affected by pronounced age-related deficits in dopamine function (reviewed by Bäckman and Farde, in press). Moreover, older adults tend to be more impaired in cognitive tasks sensitive to frontal damage, such as interference, recall, and source memory tasks, than in other tasks (Moscovitch and Winocur 1995; West 1996). Furthermore, PET and fMRI studies have repeatedly found significant age-related differences in PFC activity during cognitive performance (reviewed by Cabeza 2001a,b).

Although empirical support for the frontal ageing hypothesis is quite strong, direct evidence linking age-related deficits in RM to PFC dysfunction is in short supply. Indirect evidence has been provided by studies that found positive correlations between the RM performance of older adults and their scores in 'frontal lobe tasks' (Craik *et al.* 1990; Glisky *et al.* 1995; Parkin *et al.* 1995; Henkel *et al.* 1998). For example, Parkin *et al.* (1995) found that older adults' temporal-order memory performance, but not their item memory performance, was positively correlated with performance in a word fluency task. However, these correlations are ambiguous because the so-called 'frontal lobe tasks' depend on the activity of other brain regions in addition to PFC (Esposito *et al.* 1999). To date, the only direct evidence linking older adults' RM deficits with PFC dysfunction has been provided by PET/fMRI studies showing age-related decreases in PFC activity during RM encoding and retrieval.

During RM encoding, age-related decreased in PFC activity have been found for semantic RM (Cabeza *et al.* 1997c), spatial RM (Mitchell *et al.* 2000a), and semantic–featural RM (Iidaka *et al.* 2001). In a semantic RM study (Cabeza *et al.* 1997c), participants were scanned during intentional learning of word pairs. Compared with young adults, older adults showed weaker activity in the left ventrolateral PFC (Fig. 24.2), a region which has been strongly associated with semantic processing and verbal encoding (reviewed by Gabrieli *et al.* 1998; Cabeza and Nyberg 2000). Thus this finding suggests a deficit in older adults' ability to form new semantic associations. In a spatial RM study (Mitchell *et al.* 2000a), object drawings were presented in a 3×3 matrix, and participants were asked to hold in working memory the identity of the object, its location, or both (combination trials). During combination trials, older adults showed weaker medial PFC activity than young adults, possibly reflecting a deficit in binding objects with their screen locations. Finally, in a study by Iidaka *et al.* (2001),

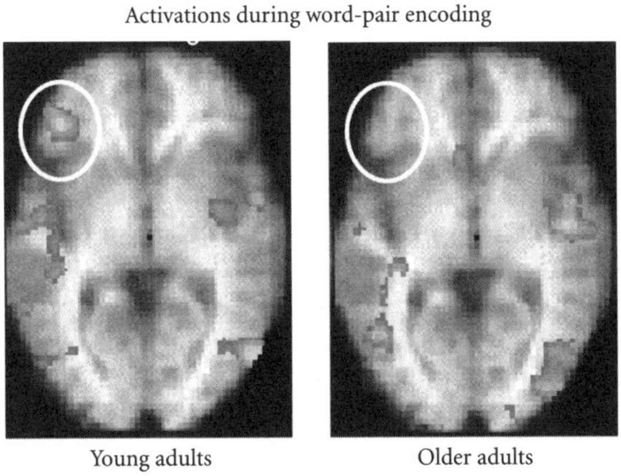

Figure 24.2 During word-pair learning, left ventrolateral PFC was significantly activated in young adults but not in older adults, possibly reflecting age-related deficits in memory encoding processes. See colour plate section. (Based on results originally reported in R. Cabeza, *Psychology and Aging*, **17**, 85–100, 2002.)

participants were scanned while encoding pairs of drawings (related objects, unrelated objects, and abstract designs). Two PFC regions activated by young adults during the encoding of unrelated objects (left ventral and right dorsal) were not activated by older adults, although in a direct comparison the age effect was not significant, possibly because of the small number of subjects.

During RM retrieval, we have found age-related decreases in PFC activity for semantic RM (Cabeza *et al.* 1997c, 2002) and temporal-order RM (Cabeza *et al.* 2000, 2002). In a semantic RM study (Cabeza *et al.* 1997c), we scanned participants while they were recalling word pairs and found an age-related decrease in right PFC activity. At the same time, older adults showed an activation in the left ventrolateral PFC which was not displayed by young adults. As a result, PFC activity was unilateral in young adults but bilateral in older adults. We attributed this change to functional compensation in the ageing brain. In a temporal-order RM study (Cabeza *et al.* 2000), participants studied a list of words and were then scanned while remembering what words were in the list (forced-choice recognition task) and when they occurred within list (recency discrimination task). Compared with the recognition task, the recency task yielded greater right PFC activity in young adults but not in older adults. This finding constituted the first direct evidence linking age-related deficits in context memory with changes in PFC function. Interestingly, as in the foregoing recall study, an age-related increase in activity was found in the PFC hemisphere that was less activated in young adults (left PFC), again suggesting a compensatory mechanism. Thus, during RM retrieval, older adults tend to show less activity in the PFC hemisphere that is most activated by young adults but more activity in the contralateral PFC hemisphere. This pattern has been found for both semantic and temporal-order

RM (Cabeza *et al.* 1997c, 2000). A recent study comparing the effects of ageing on these two forms of RM (Cabeza *et al.* 2002) is described at the end of this chapter.

Medial temporal lobe

The anatomical and functional integrity of MTL declines with ageing, and this decline is associated with deficits in memory performance. Even if milder than PFC decline, MTL decline in healthy ageing is usually reliable (reviewed by Raz 2000). The hippocampus shows significant reductions in neurons (reviewed by West 1993), synapses (Geinisman *et al.* 1995), and overall volume (reviewed by Raz 2000), and the volumes of entorhinal, perirhinal, and parahippocampal cortices are also reduced (Insausti *et al.* 1998). Importantly, age-related MTL atrophy correlates with measures of memory performance (reviewed by Raz 2000). For example, several studies have found that in older adults a larger hippocampal volume is associated with better verbal memory (Jack *et al.* 1999; Petersen *et al.* 2000; Tisserand *et al.* 2000; Hackert *et al.* 2002). The link between age-related RM deficits and MTL decline is also supported by functional neuroimaging studies. Early PET studies suggested that these reductions occurred during encoding (Grady *et al.* 1995) but not during retrieval (Schacter *et al.* 1996; Bäckman *et al.* 1997; Cabeza *et al.* 2000). However, event-related fMRI studies have found them during both encoding (Mitchell *et al.* 2000a; Iidaka *et al.* 2001; Daselaar *et al.* 2003b) and retrieval (Cabeza *et al.* 2004).

In two recent event-related fMRI studies, age-related changes in MTL activity were directly linked to differences between RM and IM (Mitchell *et al.* 2000a; Cabeza *et al.* 2004). In the aforementioned study by Mitchell *et al.* (2000a), in which participants had to maintain in working memory information about objects, locations, or both (combination trials), young adults showed greater left anterior hippocampal activity for combination than for object and location trials (Fig. 24.3), suggesting that this region is involved in binding objects with their locations (i.e. spatial RM encoding). Older adults, in contrast, did not show greater activity for combination trials (Fig. 24.3), possibly because of an age-related deficit in hippocampal binding during spatial RM.

The study by Cabeza *et al.* (2004) investigated, among other issues, the effects of ageing on recollection and familiarity using the remember—know paradigm. Young and older participants were scanned while recognizing words studied before scanning. As illustrated in Figure 24.4, older adults made fewer 'remember' responses but more 'know' responses than young adults. This finding is consistent with evidence that older adults tend to be impaired in recollection but not in familiarity (Parkin and Walter 1992; Jennings and Jacoby 1993; Mantyla 1993;

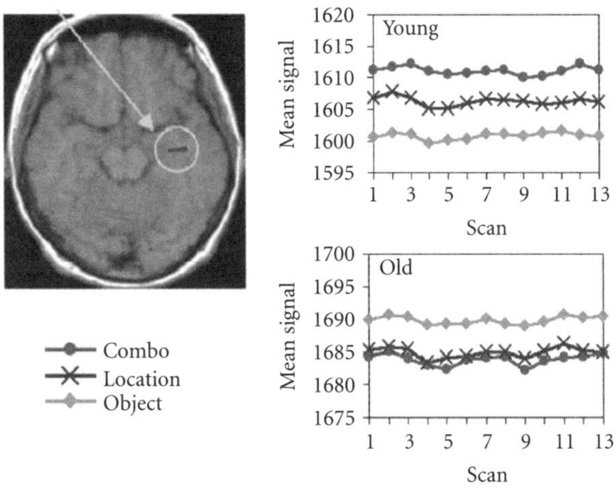

Figure 24.3 During a working memory task, young adults showed greater hippocampal activity when maintaining information about objects in different screen locations (combo trials), than when maintaining the objects or the locations alone (object and location trials). In contrast, older adults did not show greater hippocampal activity for combo trials. (Reproduced from K.J. Mitchell *et al., Cognitive Brain Research*, **10**, 197–206, 2000.) See also colour plate section.

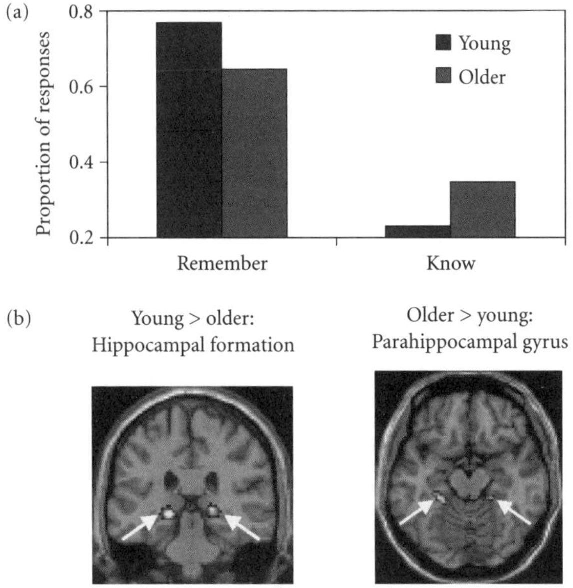

Figure 24.4 (a) During episodic retrieval, older adults produced fewer 'remember' responses (recollection), but more 'know' responses (familiarity), than young adults. (b) During the same episodic retrieval task, the hippocampus was more activated in young adults than in older adults, whereas the parahippocampal gyrus was more activated in older adults than in young adults. The parahippocampal activation in older adults was significantly correlated with the number of 'know' responses in this group, suggesting that this activation reflected an age-related increase in familiarity-based responding. (Reproduced from R. Cabeza *et al., Cerebral Cortex*, **14**, 364–375, 2004.) See also colour plate section.

Java 1996; Searcy *et al.* 1999), and with evidence of a differential effect of ageing on 'remember' and 'know' responses (Parkin and Walter 1992). Analyses of MTL activity during word recognition yielded a dissociation between two MTL regions; whereas a hippocampal region was more activated in young than in older adults, a parahippocampal region was more activated in older than in young adults. Given evidence linking the hippocampus to recollection and cortical MTL regions to familiarity (reviewed by Aggleton and Brown 1999; Yonelinas 2002), this dissociation suggest an age-related reduction in hippocampal-based recollection coupled with an accerelated increase in parahippocampal-based familiarity. Consistent with the latter, the correlation between the parahippocampal activation and the number of 'know' responses in older adults was positive and significant. Although further research is obviously required, this is probably the first evidence linking age-related differences in MTL activity with differential age effects on recollection and familiarity.

Open issues

Despite the great progress made towards clarifying the involvement of PFC and MTL regions in RM and how it changes as a function of ageing, several important issues remain unsolved. These open issues include the following: similarities and differences between RM encoding and retrieval; similarities and differences between various forms of RM; the role of pre-existing associations in the formation and retrieval of new associations; the role of PFC–MTL interactions during RM; and the role of compensation on age-related changes in RM. These five issues are considered in separate sections below

Relational memory encoding versus relational memory retrieval

Very little is known regarding similarities and differences between the neural correlates of RM encoding and RM retrieval. In general, lesion evidence cannot address this issue because memory decrements following brain damage may reflect encoding deficits, retrieval deficits, or both. Some information may be gained by manipulating variables that differentially affect encoding versus retrieval phases (Mangels 1997b), but this evidence is still indirect. In contrast, functional neuroimaging can independently measure neural activity during encoding and during retrieval, and compare them directly with each other. Cross-study comparisons have identified differences in the distributions of encoding and retrieval activations within the PFC (e.g. the HERA model (Tulving *et al.* 1994; Nyberg *et al.* 1996)) and within the MTL (e.g. the HIPER model (Lepage *et al.* 1998; but see Schacter and Wagner 1999)). Only a handful of functional neuroimaging studies have compared RM encoding and retrieval directly within subjects (Mottaghy *et al.* 1999; Iidaka *et al.* 2000; Schmidt *et al.* 2002), and they have all used blocked designs that cannot distinguish successful versus unsuccessful activity.

To address this issue, we recently conducted an event-related fMRI study that measured activity associated with semantic and featural RM during both encoding and retrieval. In the semantic RM condition, participants encoded word pairs, and at test they distinguished between old (identical) and new (recombined) pairs. In the perceptual RM condition, they associated word pairs with different fonts, and at test they distinguished between pairs presented in the same font (identical) or in the font previously seen on a different pair (recombined). Encoding success activity was identified by comparing pairs that were subsequently remembered (hits: identical pairs classified as identical) versus forgotten (misses: identical pairs classified as recombined). This method is known as the subsequent memory paradigm (reviewed by Paller and Wagner 2002). Retrieval success activity was identified by comparing activity for hits and misses during retrieval. One of the main findings of this study was the identification of brain regions that were generally involved in RM regardless of phase (encoding versus retrieval) and information type (semantic versus perceptual). Two of these regions were the left ventrolateral PFC region and the left hippocampus, consistent with the idea that PFC and MTL play a fundamental role in RM.

Directly comparing brain activity during RM encoding and retrieval is also critical for understanding the neural bases of age-related memory deficits because these deficits may reflect difficulties in any of these two phases. Moreover, deficits during one phase may be partly counteracted by compensatory changes during the other phase. For example, weak binding during encoding may be compensated by more careful evaluation during retrieval. In functional neuroimaging studies of ageing, age-related reductions in activity tend to be more pronounced during encoding, whereas age-related increases in activity tend to be more pronounced during retrieval (Cabeza 2001a). One possible interpretation is that older adults attempt to compensate encoding deficits by deploying greater processing resources during retrieval (Schiavetto *et al.* 2002). To investigate this idea, it is critical to compare age-related changes in brain activity during encoding and retrieval within participants, and to use event-related designs that distinguish between successful and unsuccessful activity. The few functional neuroimaging studies of ageing that investigated both encoding and retrieval (Grady *et al.* 1995; Cabeza *et al.* 1997c; Anderson *et al.* 2000; Daselaar *et al.* 2003a) did not investigate RM and did not isolate successful encoding and retrieval activity. Thus this is an important gap in the available data concerning RM and ageing.

Different forms of relational memory

Direct evidence regarding the role of various PFC and MTL subregions in different forms of RM is very scarce. Within PFC, featural RM has been associated with the ventrolateral cortex, and spatial RM with the dorsolateral cortex (Goldman-Rakic *et al.* 1999). However, an alternative view proposes that these regions differ in terms of processes rather than in terms of information kind (Petrides 1994; Owen *et al.* 1999). Within MTL, spatial RM has been associated with the hippocampus and the parahippocampal cortex (reviewed by Burgess *et al.* 2002), featural RM has been associated with the perirhinal cortex (reviewed by Murray 1999; Brown and Aggleton 2001), and temporal RM has been associated with the hippocampus (Dusek and Eichenbaum 1997; Mayes *et al.* 2001). However, most of the foregoing distinctions are based on cross-study comparisons, and very few studies have directly compared different forms of RM within subjects.

There is also little information regarding the effects of ageing on various forms of RM. At the behavioural level, a meta-analysis concluded that RM for spatial and temporal context shows greater age-related decline than RM for stimulus-bound perceptual features, such as colour (Spencer and Raz 1995). One possible explanation is that perceptual features are naturally integrated with the item, and hence are less dependent on self-initiated binding operations. Another explanation is that that featural RM is not true RM because it involves blends rather than representations that preserve the whole as well as the parts (compositionality) (Cohen *et al.* 1997).

It is possible that the critical factor is not the nature of information involved (semantic, spatial, etc.) but whether the items being related are of the same type (intra-type RM, e.g. a word–word pair) or of different type (crosstype RM, e.g. a word–face pair). Intra-type and cross-type RM may differ both within PFC and within MTL. A difference within PFC is suggested by a recent version of Baddeley's working memory model (Baddeley 2000), which postulates not only separate buffers for verbal and visuospatial information (phonological loop and visuospatial sketchpad), but also a third buffer for maintaining and integrating information from different sources (episodic buffer). Baddeley (2000) suggested that the episodic buffer may be mediated by a right anterior/dorsolateral PFC region, which an fMRI study found to be activated during the maintenance of integrated letter/location information (Prabhakaran *et al.* 2000). However, it is unclear how the function of this region differs from that of the medial PFC region which the aforementioned study by Mitchell *et al.* (2000a) found to be activated during combination trials.

Within MTL, although the hippocampal–RM view attributes RM to the hippocampus (Aggleton and Brown 1999; Brown and Aggleton 2001), there is evidence that parahippocampal (reviewed by Burgess *et al.* 2002) and perirhinal (reviewed by Murray 1999) cortices can also support certain kinds of associations. Thus the hippocampal–RM view has been refined by suggesting that the hippocampus is critical not for all kinds of associations, but for associations across different events (Bunsey and Eichenbaum 1996; Dusek and Eichenbaum 1997; Nagode and Pardo 2002) or across different information types (Mayes and Montaldi 1999; Mayes *et al.* 2001). Consistent with this last hypothesis, Vargha-Khadem *et al.* (1997) reported that three patients with selective hippocampal damage were impaired in associative recognition of face–voice and object–location pairs but not in word–word, non-word–non-word, and face–face pairs. Although this finding is very interesting, evidence for the cross-type–intra-type distinction is still very scarce.

Regarding the effects of ageing, there is evidence that older adults are considerably impaired in cross-type RM tasks, such as remembering people's names (Maylor 1990, 1998). In fact, a difficulty in remembering the names of familiar people is one of the most common cognitive complaints in older adults (Martin 1986) and the cognitive skill that they want to improve the most (Cohen and Faulkner 1985). A recent fMRI study found an age-related decrease in left PFC activity during encoding of novel face–name associations (Sperling *et al.* 2003). Although this finding may suggest an age-related deficit in cross-type RM, it is important to note that age-related decreases in left PFC activity during encoding have also been found for intra-type RM (word pairs) (Cabeza *et al.* 1997c). In the case of MTL, the aforementioned finding of age-related decrease in hippocampal activity during maintenance of integrated object/location information (Mitchell *et al.* 2000a) could be interpreted as a deficit in cross-type RM. However, the effects of ageing on intra-type versus cross-type RM have not been directly investigated.

Role of pre-existing associations

Another open issue is the effect of pre-existing associations on new RM learning, which may be positive or negative depending on whether pre-existing associations match or mismatch with novel associations. As an example of a positive influence, learning pairs of related words is typically better and faster than learning pairs of unrelated items (Wicklund *et al.* 1964). Regrettably, very little is known about the neural correlates of this relatedness effect, which has been investigated in only a few functional neuroimaging studies (Mayes *et al.* 1998; Fletcher *et al.* 2000; Lepage *et al.* 2000). PFC activations in these studies have been consistent; left ventrolateral PFC tends to be more activated for unrelated than for related pairs, possibly reflecting greater demands in forming new associations (Fletcher *et al.* 2000; Lepage *et al.* 2000). In contrast, MTL activations have been inconsistent; whereas one study found greater MTL activity for related than for unrelated words (Lepage *et al.* 2000), another study found greater MTL activity for related than for unrelated words (Mayes *et al.* 1998). A speculative account of this difference is that the former finding reflects semantic retrieval for pre-existing associations, whereas the latter finding reflects episodic encoding of novel associations. Clearly, the neural basis of the relatedness effect is an important issue and deserves further investigation.

As for the effects of ageing, there is evidence that pre-experimental associative strength can attenuate and even eliminate age-related deficits in paired-associate learning (but see Verhaeghen *et al.* 1993; reviewed by Kausler 1994). For example, in one study (Zaretsky and Halberstam 1968b) age-related deficits in pair associate learning were large for high-strength pairs, modest for medium-strength pairs, and negligible for high-strength pairs (see also Kausler and Lair 1966; Zaretsky and Halberstam 1968a). These findings are consistent with the resources theory of cognitive ageing (e.g. Craik 1986), which postulates that older adults have reduced processing resources (e.g. attention, working memory) and hence are less impaired in conditions involving greater environmental support. These findings are also consistent with the notion that semantic memory is relatively preserved in older adults (Craik and Jennings 1992; Bäckman *et al.* 2000; Nyberg *et al.* 2003). Thus, older adults' relatively good performance with pairs composed of related words may reflect the recruitment of semantic memory operations to compensate for episodic RM decline. Unfortunately, no functional neuroimaging evidence is available about this issue.

In contrast with the foregoing results, when pre-existing associations are inconsistent with novel associations they tend to impair RM (reviewed by Anderson and Neely 1996) and augment age-related RM deficits (reviewed by Kausler 1994). In the AB–AC paradigm, for example, studying a list of word pairs AB (e.g. apple–piano) followed by a list of partially overlapping pairs AC (e.g. apple–stove) impairs memory for both the first list (retroactive interference) and the second list (proactive interference). The ability to overcome interference depends on the roles of PFC and MTL in establishing strong associations during encoding, and in accessing specific targets and monitoring recovered information during retrieval. Consistent with this idea, PFC and MTL damage tends to increase interference effects (Shimamura *et al.* 1995; Kroll *et al.* 1996). Only two functional neuroimaging studies have investigated the interference effect in episodic memory. In Fletcher *et al.*'s (2000) PET study, participants studied a list of word pairs repeatedly and then studied a list of recombined pairs. Left ventrolateral PFC activity decreased with repetitions but became very active for recombined pairs, suggesting that this region mediates binding operations which are critical for overcoming interference. In Henson *et al.*'s (2002) fMRI study, a multiple interference condition (AB, AC, AD) was compared with a repetition condition (AD, AD, AD). At test, participants recalled the most recent associate (e.g. A→D). During encoding, activity in the left ventrolateral PFC decreased with repetition and increased with interference, consistent with Fletcher *et al.*'s results. During retrieval, activity in the left ventrolateral PFC activity decreased with repetition, possibly reflecting diminished generation demands, whereas activity in the right dorsolateral PFC increased with interference, possibly reflecting augmented monitoring demands.

Turning to ageing, there is evidence that older adults are more sensitive to RM interference than young adults (reviewed by Kausler 1994). This evidence is consistent with the view that ageing is associated with deficits in inhibitory control (Hasher and Zacks 1988; Hasher *et al.* 1999). Among other paradigms, greater interference in older adults has been found during word-pair learning (Lair *et al.* 1969; Winocur and Moscovitch 1983; Kliegl and Lindenberger 1993). For example, enhanced sensitivity to interference in the AB–AC paradigm was found in older adults, particularly among those living in institutions (Winocur and Moscovitch 1983). Although functional neuroimaging studies of cognitive ageing have not investigated interference during RM, they have investigated interference in other paradigms (Jonides *et al.* 2000; Nielson *et al.* 2002). For example, in a verbal working memory task in which interference yielded left ventrolateral PFC activity in young adults, older adults showed reduced interference-related activity in the same region (Jonides *et al.* 2000). It is possible that similar age-related differences in activation will also be found for RM.

PFC–MTL interactions in relational memory

Although in previous sections we have considered the roles of PFC and MTL in RM independently of each other, it is obvious that RM depends not only on the function of these two regions but also on their interaction during encoding and retrieval. Functional interactions between brain regions are very difficult to investigate. Lesions are informative only if they are very selective, affecting a specific white matter bundle but not the neighbouring grey matter. In the case of RM, a critical white matter bundle is the uncinate fasciculus, which directly links the PFC and MTL regions. A few years ago, we reported a case study of a traumatic brain injury patient with a very small lesion that apparently transected the right uncinate fasciculus (Levine *et al.* 1998). In addition to severe retrograde amnesia, this patient showed impaired recollection but preserved familiarity, consistent with the idea that PFC–MTL interactions are particularly critical for RM.

In functional neuroimaging studies, interactions among brain regions have been investigated using network and correlational analyses (reviewed by Nyberg and McIntosh 2001). For example, McIntosh *et al.* (1997) found that during IM retrieval the correlation between left hippocampal and right ventrolateral PFC activations changed as a function of retrieval success. Given that PFC is more critical for RM than for IM, PFC–MTL activity correlations are likely to be greater for RM than for IM. Moreover, they are likely to be greater for successful than for unsuccessful RM.

Investigating PFC–MTL interactions during RM is also important for understanding the effects of ageing on RM because there is evidence that ageing alters functional connectivity, possibly leading to a disconnection among components of neurocognitive networks (age-related disconnection hypothesis). In fact, in a study in which we applied structural equation modelling to PET data, we found significant age-related changes in functional connectivity between PFC and other brain regions during RM encoding and retrieval (Cabeza *et al.* 1997a). In another PET study (Esposito *et al.* 1999), the correlation between activity in the left dorsolateral PFC and the right MTL during performance of the Wisconsin Card Sorting Test was significant in young but not in older adults. This result is consistent with the age-related disconnection hypothesis.

This hypothesis is also supported by evidence that ageing significantly impairs white matter integrity, and that this impairment is correlated with age-related deficits in cognitive performance. *In vivo* measures of white matter integrity are provided by qualitative analyses of white matter hyperintensity (WMH) in MRI images or by quantitative analyses of diffusion tensor imaging (DTI). DTI assesses the integrity of directionally organized white matter pathways by measuring the diffusivity of water molecules. Several studies have found significant correlations between WMH and age-related cognitive deficits (reviewed by Raz 2000). Using DTI, one study found a significant correlation between age-related white matter decline, particularly in anterior brain regions, and age-related executive deficits (O'Sullivan *et al.* 2001) Likewise, we have found significant correlations between age-related white matter deficits and age-related slowing (Madden *et al.* 2003).

Age-related compensation during RM

As mentioned before, several functional neuroimaging studies of RM have found that ageing is associated not only with decreases but also with increases in activation (Cabeza *et al.* 1997c, 2000, 2002). Age-related increases in activation have often been found in PFC regions contralateral to the ones most activated in young adults, thereby leading to a more bilateral pattern of PFC activity in older adults (Cabeza *et al.* 1997c, 2002). Age-related bilateral PFC recruitment is not exclusive to RM, and has been observed for IM and several other cognitive functions, including perception, language, semantic retrieval, working memory, and inhibitory control. These findings have been conceptualized within a model called hemispheric asymmetry reductions in old adults (HAROLD) (Cabeza 2002), which states that, under similar circumstances, PFC activity tends to be less asymmetric in older adults than in young adults. According to a compensation hypothesis, age-related bilateral recruitment reflects an attempt of the ageing brain to counteract neural decline (Cabeza *et al.* 1997c, 2002; Reuter-Lorenz *et al.* 2000), whereas according to a dedifferentiation hypothesis, it reflect an age-related difficulty in recruiting specialized neural mechanisms (Li and Lindenberger 1999; Li 2004).

We investigated these two hypotheses by measuring brain activity during two RM tasks: word-pair cued recall and context recognition (Cabeza *et al.* 1997c, 2002; Reuter-Lorenz *et al.* 2000). As mentioned before, in young adults we had found that the left PFC was more activated for cued recall than for context recognition, possibly reflecting greater production demands, whereas the right PFC was more activated for context recognition than for cued recall, possibly reflecting greater monitoring demands (Cabeza *et al.* 2003). Based on the HAROLD model, we predicted that this hemispheric asymmetry in PFC activity would be reduced in older adults. Moreover, we tested the compensation and dedifferentiation hypotheses by selecting, before the imaging study and on the basis of a memory battery, two different groups of older participants, one group whose memory performance was similar to that of our young participants (Old–High), and another whose memory performance was significantly below that of young participants (Old–Low). Whereas the compensation hypothesis predicts that the HAROLD pattern should be more pronounced in Old–High than in Old–Low participants, the dedifferentiation hypothesis predicts the converse pattern or no differences between elderly groups. As illustrated in Figure 24.5, compared with recall, context recognition was associated with greater right PFC activations in young and Old–Low participants but with bilateral PFC activations in Old–High participants. The finding of HAROLD for high-performing rather than for low-performing elderly has been replicated (Rosen *et al.* 2002) and provides strong support for the compensation hypothesis.

Regarding RM, it is interesting to note that in this study bilateral PFC recruitment in older adults was found during context recognition but not during word-pair recall. During cued recall, both Old–High and Old–Low participants showed left PFC activations, similar to those displayed by young adults (Cabeza *et al.* 2003). Prima facie, this result suggests that compensatory bilateral

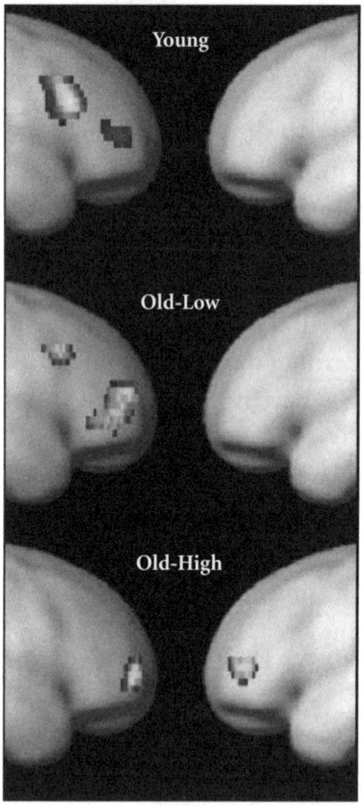

Figure 24.5 Consistent with the compensatory interpretation of bilateral PFC recruitment in older adults, high-performing but not low-performing older adults showed bilateral PFC activation during context memory (Reproduced from R. Cabeza *et al.*, *NeuroImage*, **17**, 1394–1402, 2002). See colour plate section.

recruitment in older adults occurs for some forms of RM (e.g. context memory) but not others (e.g. word-pair recall). However, as noted before, we found bilateral PFC recruitment in older adults in a previous study investigating word-pair cued recall (Cabeza *et al.* 1997c). One possible explanation is that the probability of finding age-related bilateral recruitment increases with task demands (Nolde *et al.* 1998a). Consistent with this idea, in the study in which we found age-related bilateral recruitment during cued recall (Cabeza *et al.* 1997c) we did not find it during a less demanding recognition task, and in the study in which we found bilateral activity during context memory (Cabeza *et al.* 2002) we did not find it during a less demanding cued recall task. As for the function of the PFC regions recruited by older adults, given the production—monitoring hypothesis (Cabeza *et al.* 2003), one may speculate that older adults compensate for deficits in monitoring processes by recruiting additional production processes and vice versa.

Conclusions

In summary, there is a considerable amount of evidence that RM depends on MTL and PFC functions, and that age-related RM deficits are related to the dysfunction of these regions. PFC is assumed to control encoding and retrieval strategies, which tend to be more critical for RM than for IM. Consistently, the effects of PFC lesions are usually greater for RM than for IM tasks, and for recollection than for familiarity. Also, PFC activity tends to be greater for RM than for IM during both encoding and retrieval. The lateralization of these activations seems to depend on both the type of information retrieved (conceptual versus perceptual) and the proportion of retrieval processes involved (production versus monitoring). PFC is the brain region most affected by ageing, both structurally and functionally, and hence PFC dysfunction is assumed to play a major role in age-related cognitive deficits, including RM decline. The link between age-related RM decline and PFC dysfunction is supported by evidence of age-related decreases in PFC activity during RM encoding and retrieval. These decreases are sometimes accompanied by increases in the contralateral PFC region, which have been attributed to functional compensation.

Regarding the contributions of MTL to RM, the hippocampal–RM view attributes them specifically to the hippocampus, whereas the unified MTL view postulates that this region is similarly involved in RM and IM. Although the theoretical debate is still ongoing, the former view is becoming very popular. Consistent with the hippocampal–RM view, hippocampal lesions in animals and humans have been found to produce larger effects on RM than on IM, and several PET/fMRI studies have found greater hippocampal activity for RM than for IM. The anatomical and functional integrity of MTL declines with age, and some of these changes are significantly correlated with measures of memory performance. In two functional neuroimaging studies, age-related deficits in RM were directly linked to differences in MTL activity.

Notwithstanding all these findings, there are several unsolved issues, including the following. First, it is unclear how the neural correlates of RM differ for encoding and retrieval. This gap in the data is problematic not only for understanding general RM mechanisms, but also for understanding age-related changes in RM. Secondly, there is very little evidence regarding the neural correlates of various forms of RM, even though they are likely to involve distinct PFC and MTL subregions and to be differentially affected by ageing. Thirdly, pre-existing associations are known to modulate the formation of new RM and age-related RM decline, but evidence about the neural basis of these effects is very scarce. Fourthly, RM is assumed to depend not only on PFC and MTL functions but on the interactions between these two regions, but evidence about these interactions is virtually non-existent. Finally, even though there is evidence of compensatory brain activity in older adults during RM, it is unclear how this differs for various RM tasks and how it is affected by task demands.

Thus the functional neuroanatomy of RM in young and older adults is a very exciting and challenging research domain. It is exciting because of the great empirical progress made during the last couple of decades and the rich background of theories and ideas about RM. It is challenging because of the complexity of the problem and the considerable number of unsolved issues. Despite these difficulties, the rapid convergence of findings and ideas predicts important breakthroughs in the near future.

References

Aggleton, J.P. and Brown, M.W. (1999). Episodic memory, amnesia, and the hippocampal–anterior thalamic axis. *Behavioral and Brain Sciences*, **22**, 425–444.

Anderson, M.C. and Neely, J.H. (1996). Interference and inhibition in memory retrieval. In *Handbook of Perception and Cognition: Memory* (2nd edn). (ed E.L. Bjork and R.A. Bjork). San Diego, CA: Academic Press, pp 237–313.

Anderson, N.D., Iidaka, T., McIntosh, A.R., Kapur, S., Cabeza, R. and Craik, F.I.M. (2000). The effects of divided attention on encoding- and retrieval-related brain activity: a PET study of younger and older adults. *Journal of Cognitive Neuroscience*, **12**, 775–792.

Bachevalier, J. and Mishkin, M. (1986). Visual recognition impairment follows ventromedial but not dorsolateral prefrontal lesions in monkeys. *Behavioral Brain Research*, **20**, 249–261.

Bäckman, L. and Farde, L. (2004). The role of dopamine systems in cognitive aging. In *Cognitive Neuroscience of Aging: Linking Cognitive and Cerebral Aging* (ed R. Cabeza, L. Nyberg, and D.C. Park). New York: Oxford University Press, pp. 58–84.

Bäckman, L., Almkvist, O., Andersson, J., *et al.* (1997). Brain activation in young and older adults during implicit and explicit retrieval. *Journal of Cognitive Neuroscience*, **9**, 378–391.

Bäckman, L., Small, B.J., and Wahlin, A. (2000). Cognitive functioning in very old age. In *Handbook of Aging and Cognition II* (ed F.I.M. Craik and T.A. Salthouse). Mahwah, NJ: Erlbaum.

Baddeley, A. (2000). The episodic buffer: a new component of working memory? *Trends in Cognitive Sciences*, **4**, 417–423.

Badgaiyan, R.D., Schacter, D.L., and Alpert, N.M. (2002). Retrieval of relational information: a role for the left inferior prefrontal cortex. *NeuroImage*, **17**, 393–400.

Broadbent, N.J., Clark, R.M., Zola, S.M., and Squire, L.R. (2002). The medial temporal lobe and memory. In *The Neuropsychology of Memory* (3rd edn) (ed L.R. Squire and D.L. Schacter). New York: Guilford Press, pp 3–23.

Brown, M.W. and Aggleton, J.P. (2001). Recognition memory. What are the roles of the perirhinal cortex and hippocampus? *Nature Reviews Neuroscience*, **2**, 51–61.

Bunsey, M. and Eichenbaum, H. (1996). Conservation of hippocampal memory function in rats and humans. *Nature*, **379**, 255–257.

Burgess, N., Maguire, E.A., Spiers, H.J., and O'Keefe, J. (2001). A temporoparietal and prefrontal network for retrieving the spatial context of lifelike events. *NeuroImage*, **14**, 439–453.

Burgess, N., Maguire, E.A., and O'Keefe, J. (2002). The human hippocampus and spatial and episodic memory. *Neuron*, **35**, 625–641.

Burke, D.M. and Light, L.L. (1981). Memory and aging: the role of retrieval processes. *Psychological Bulletin*, **90**, 513–514.

Butters, M.A., Kaszniak, A.W., Glisky, E.L., Eslinger, P.J., and Schacter, D.L. (1994). Recency discrimination deficits in frontal lobe patients. *Neuropsychology*, **8**, 343–353.

Cabeza, R. (2001a). Functional neuroimaging of cognitive aging. In *Handbook of Functional Neuroimaging of Cognition* (ed R. Cabeza and A. Kingstone). Cambridge, MA: MIT Press, pp 331–377.

Cabeza, R. (2001b). Cognitive neuroscience of aging: contributions of functional neuroimaging. *Scandinavian Journal of Psychology*, **42**, 277–286.

Cabeza, R. (2002). Hemispheric asymmetry reduction in older adults: the HAROLD model. *Psychology and Aging*, **17**, 85–100.

Cabeza, R. and Nyberg, L. (2000). Imaging cognition II: an empirical review of 275 PET and fMRI studies. *Journal of Cognitive Neuroscience*, **12**, 1–47.

Cabeza, R., McIntosh, A.R., Tulving E., Nyberg, L., and Grady, C.L. (1997a). Age-related differences in effective neural connectivity during encoding and recall. *Neuroreport*, **8**, 3479–3483.

Cabeza, R., Mangels, J., and Nyberg, L., *et al.* (1997b). Brain regions differentially involved in remembering what and when: a PET study. *Neuron*, **19**, 863–870.

Cabeza, R., Grady, C.L., Nyberg, L., *et al.* (1997c). Age-related differences in neural activity during memory encoding and retrieval: a positron emission tomography study. *Journal of Neuroscience* 17, 391–400.

Cabeza, R., Anderson, N.D., Houle, S., Mangels, J.A., and Nyberg, L. (2000). Age-related differences in neural activity during item and temporal-order memory retrieval: a positron emission tomography study. *Journal of Cognitive Neuroscience*, **12**, 1–10.

Cabeza, R., Anderson, N.D., Locantore, J.K., and McIntosh, A.R. (2002). Aging gracefully: compensatory brain activity in high-performing older adults. *NeuroImage*, **17**, 1394–1402.

Cabeza, R., Locantore, J.K., and Anderson, N.D. (2003). Lateralization of prefrontal cortex activity during episodic memory retrieval: evidence for the production-monitoring hypothesis. *Journal of Cognitive Neuroscience*, **15**, 249–259.

Cabeza, R., Daselaar, S.M., Dolcos, F., Prince, S., Budde, M., and Nyberg, L. (2004). Task-independent and task-specific age effects on brain activity during working memory, visual attention and episodic retrieval. *Cerebral Cortex*, **14**, 364–375.

Chalfonte, B.L. and Johnson, M.K. (1996). Feature memory and binding in young and older adults. *Memory and Cognition*, **24**, 403–416.

Cohen, G. and Faulkner, D. (1985). Memory for proper names: age differences in retrieval. *British Journal of Developmental Psychology*, **4**, 187–197.

Cohen, N.J., Poldrack, R.A., and Eichenbaum, H. (1997). Memory for items and memory for relations in the procedural/declarative memory framework. *Memory*, **5**, 131–178.

Craik, F.I.M. (1986). A functional account of age differences in memory. In *Human Memory and Cognitive Capabilities, Mechanisms, and Performances* (ed F. Lix and H. Hagendorf). Amsterdam: North-Holland, pp 499–422.

Craik, F.I.M. and Jennings, J.M. (1992). Human memory. In *The Handbook of Aging and Cognition* (ed F.I.M. Craik and T.A. Salthouse). Hillsdale, NJ: Erlbaum.

Craik, F.I.M., Morris, L.W., Morris, R.G., and Loewen, E.R. (1990). Relations between source amnesia and frontal lobe functioning in older adults. *Psychology and Aging*, **5**, 148–151.

Daselaar, S.M., Veltman, D.J., Rombouts, S.A., Lazeron, R.H., Raaijmakers, J.G., and Jonker, C. (2003a). Neuroanatomical correlates of episodic encoding and retrieval in young and elderly subjects. *Brain*, **126**, 43–56.

Daselaar, S.M., Veltman, D.J., Rombouts, S.A., Raaijmakers, J.G., and Jonker, C. (2003b). Deep processing activates the medial temporal lobe in young but not in old adults. *Neurobiology of Aging*, **24**, 1005–1011.

Davachi, L. and Wagner, A.D. (2001). Hippocampal contributions to episodic encoding: Insights from relational and item-based learning. *Journal of Neurophysiology*, **88**, 982–990.

Davachi, L., Mitchell, J.P., and Wagner, A.D. (2003). Multiple routes to memory: distinct medial temporal lobe processes build item and source memories. *Proceedings of the National Academy of Sciences of the United States of America*, **100**, 2157–2162.

Dempster, F.N. (1992). The rise and fall of the inhibitory mechanism: toward a unified theory of cognitive development and aging. *Developmental Review*, **12**, 45–75.

Denney, N.W., Dew, J.R., and Kihlstrom J.F. (1992). An adult developmental study of the encoding of spatial location. *Experimental Aging Research*, **18**, 25–32.

Dobbins, I.G. and Wagner, A.D. (2005). Recollecting events and detecting novelty: domain-general and domain-sensitive prefrontal retrieval mechanisms. *Cerebral Cortex*, **15**, 1768–1778.

Dobbins, I.G., Rice, H.J., Wagner, A.D., and Schacter, D.L. (2003). Memory orientation and success: separable neurocognitive components underlying episodic recognition. *Neuropsychologia*, **41**, 318–333.

Dusek, J.A. and Eichenbaum, H. (1997). The hippocampus and memory for orderly stimulus relations. *Proceedings of the National Academy of Sciences of the United States of America*, **94**, 7109–7114.

Eichenbaum, H., Otto, T., and Cohen, N.J. (1994). Two component functions of the hippocampal memory system. *Behavioral and Brain Sciences*, **17**, 449–517.

Eldridge, L.L., Knowlton, B.J., Furmanski, C.S., Bookheimer, S.Y., and Engle, S.A. (2000). Remembering episodes: a selective role for the hippocampus during retrieval. *Nature Neuroscience*, **3**, 1149–1152.

Esposito, G., Kirby, G.S., Van Horn, J.D., Ellmore, T.M., and Faith Berman, K. (1999). Context-dependent, neural system-specific neurophysiological concomitants of ageing: mapping PET correlates during cognitive activation. *Brain*, **122**, 963–979.

Fletcher, P.C., Shallice, T., and Dolan, R.J. (2000). 'Sculpting the response space'—an account of left prefrontal activation at encoding. *NeuroImage*, **12**, 404–417.

Gabrieli, J.D., Poldrack, R.A., and Desmond, J.E. (1998). The role of left prefrontal cortex in language and memory. *Proceedings of the National Academy of Sciences of the United States of America*, **95**, 906–913.

Gardiner, J.M. (2001). Episodic memory and autonoetic consciousness: a first-person approach. *Philosophical Transactions of the Royal Society of London, Series B, Biological Sciences*, **356**, 1351–1361.

Geinisman, Y., deToledo-Morell, L., Morell, F., and Heller, R.E. (1995). Hippocampal markers of age-related memory dysfunction: behavioural, electrophysiological and morphological perspectives. *Progress in Neurobiology*, **45**, 223–252.

Giovanello, K.S., Verfaellie, M., and Keane, M.M. (2003). Familiarity-based associative recognition memory in amnesia. *Journal of Cognitive Neuroscience, Supplement*, **C179**, 107.

Glisky, E.L., Polster, M.R., and Routhieaux, B.C. (1995). Double dissociation between item and source memory. *Neuropsychology*, **9**, 229–235.

Goldman-Rakic, P.S., O'Scalaidhe, S.P., and Chafee, M.V. (1999). Domain specificity in cognitive systems. In *The Cognitive Neurosciences* (2nd edn) (ed M.S. Gazzaniga). Cambridge, MA: MIT Press.

Grady, C.L., McIntosh, A.R., Horwitz, B., *et al.* (1995). Age-related reductions in human recognition memory due to impaired encoding. *Science*, **269**, 218–221.

Greenwood, P.M. (2000). The frontal aging hypothesis evaluated. *Journal of the International Neuropsychological Society*, **6**, 705–726.

Hackert, V.H., den Heijer, T., Oudkerk, M., Koudstaal, P.J., Hofman, A., and Breteler, M.M. (2002). Hippocampal head size associated with verbal memory performance in nondemented elderly. *NeuroImage*, **17**, 1365–1372.

Hasher, L. and Zacks, R.T. (1988). Working memory, comprehension and aging: a review and a new view. *Psychology of Learning and Motivation*, **22**, 193–225.

Hasher, L., Zacks, R.T., and Rahhal, T.A. (1999). Timing, instructions, and inhibitory control: some missing factors in the age and memory debate. *Gerontology*, **45**, 355–357.

Henke, K., Buck, A., Weber, B., and Wieser, H.G. (1997). Human hippocampus establishes associations in memory. *Hippocampus*, **7**, 249–256.

Henke, K., Weber, B., Kneifel, S., Wieser, H.G., and Buck, A. (1999). Human hippocampus associates information in memory. *Proceedings of the National Academy of Sciences of the United States of America*, **96**, 5884–5889.

Henkel, L.A., Johnson, M.K., and De Leonardis, D.M. (1998). Aging and source monitoring: cognitive processes and neuropsychological correlates. *Journal of Experimental Psychology: General*, **127**, 251–268.

Henson, R.N.A., Shallice, T., and Dolan, R.J. (1999a). Right prefrontal cortex and episodic memory retrieval: a functional MRI test of the monitoring hypothesis. *Brain*, **122**, 1367–1381.

Henson, R.N.A., Rugg, M.D., Shallice, T., Josephs, O., and Dolan, R.J. (1999b). Recollection and familiarity in recognition memory: an event-related functional magnetic resonance imaging study. *Journal of Neuroscience*, **19**, 3962–3972.

Henson, R.N., Shallice, T., Josephs, O., and Dolan, R.J. (2002). Functional magnetic resonance imaging of proactive interference during spoken cued recall. *NeuroImage*, **17**, 543–558.

Hockley, W.E. (1992). Item versus associative information: further comparisons of forgetting rates. *Journal of Experimental Psychology: Learning, Memory, and Cognition*, **18**, 1321–1330.

Iidaka, T., Anderson, N.D., Kapur, S., Cabeza, R., and Craik, F.I. (2000). The effect of divided attention on encoding and retrieval in episodic memory revealed by positron emission tomography. *Journal of Cognitive Neuroscience*, **12**, 267–280.

Iidaka, T., Sadato, N., Yamada, H., Murata, T., Omori, M., and Yonekura, Y. (2001). An fMRI study of the functional neuroanatomy of picture encoding in younger and older adults. *Cognitive Brain Research*, **11**, 1–11.

Insausti, R., Insausti, A.M., Sobreviela, M.T., Salinas, S., and Martinez-Penuela, J.M. (1998). Human medial temporal lobe in aging: anatomical basis of memory preservation. *Microscopy Research and Technique*, **43**, 8–15.

Jack, C.R., Jr, Petersen, R.C., Xu, Y.C., *et al.* (1999). Prediction of AD with MRI-based hippocampal volume in mild cognitive impairment. *Neurology*, **52**, 1397–1403.

Java, R.I. (1996). Effects of age on state of awareness following implicit and explicit word-association tasks. *Psychology and Aging*, **11**, 108–111.

Jennings, J.M. and Jacoby, L.L. (1993). Automatic versus intentional uses of memory: Aging, attention, and control. *Psychology and Aging*, **8**, 283–293.

Johnson, M.K., Hashtroudi, S., and Lindsay, D.S. (1993). Source monitoring. *Psychological Bulletin*, **114**, 3–28.

Jonides, J., Marshuetz, C., Smith, E.E., Reuter-Lorenz, P.A., Koeppe, R.A., and Hartley, A. (2000). Brain activation reveals changes with age in resolving interference in verbal working memory. *Journal of Cognitive Neuroscience*, **12**, 188–196.

Kausler, D.H. (1994). *Learning and Memory in Normal Aging*. San Diego, CA: Academic Press.

Kausler, D.H. and Lair, C.V. (1966). Associative strength and paired-associate learning in elderly subjects. *Journal of Gerontology*, **21**, 278–280.

Kausler, D.H. and Puckett, J.M. (1980). Adult age differences in recognition memory for a nonsemantic attribute. *Experimental Aging Research*, **6**, 349–355.

Kausler, D.H. and Puckett, J.M. (1981a). Adult age differences in memory for modality attributes. *Experimental Aging Research*, **7**, 117–125.

Kausler, D.H. and Puckett, J.M. (1981b). Adult age differences in memory for sex of voice. *Journal of Gerontology*, **36**, 44–50.

Kausler, D.H., Salthouse, T.A., and Saults, J.S. (1988). Temporal memory over the adult lifespan. *American Journal of Psychology*, **101**, 207–215.

Kesner, R.P., Hopkins, R.O., and Fineman, B. (1994). Item and order dissociation in humans with prefrontal cortex damage. *Neuropsychologia*, **32**, 881–891.

Kliegl, R. and Lindenberger, U. (1993). Modeling intrusions and correct recall in episodic memory: adult age differences in encoding of list context. *Journal of Experimental Psychology: Learning, Memory, and Cognition*, **19**, 617–637.

Kostopoulos, P. and Petrides, M. (2003). The mid-ventrolateral prefrontal cortex: insights into its role in memory retrieval. *European Journal of Neuroscience*, **17**, 1489–1497.

Kroll, N.E.A., Knight, R.T., Metcalfe, J., Wolf, E.S., and Tulving, E. (1996). Cohesion failure as a source of memory illusions. *Journal of Memory and Language*, **35**, 176–196.

Lair, C.V., Moon, W.H., and Kausler, D.H. (1969). Associative interference in the paired-associate learning of middle-aged and old subjects. *Developmental Psychology*, **1**, 548–552.

Lepage, M., Habib, R., and Tulving, R. (1998). Hippocampal PET activations of memory encoding and retrieval: the HIPER model. *Hippocampus*, **8**, 313–322.

Lepage, M., Habib, R., Cormier, H., Houle, S., and McIntosh, A.R. (2000). Neural correlates of semantic associative encoding in episodic memory. *Cognitive Brain Research*, **9**, 271–280.

Levine, B., Black, S.E., Cabeza, R., *et al.* (1998). Episodic memory and the self in a case of isolated retrograde amnesia. *Brain*, **121**, 1951–1973.

Li, S.-C. (2004). Neurocomputational perspectives linking neuromodulation, processing noise, representational distinctiveness, and cognitive aging. In *Cognitive Neuroscience of Aging: Linking Cognitive and Cerebral Aging* (ed R. Cabeza, L. Nyberg, and D.C. Park). New York: Oxford University Press.

Li, S.-C. and Lindenberger, U. (1999). Cross-level unification: a computational exploration of the link between deterioration of neurotransmitter systems dedifferentiation of cognitive abilities in old age. In *Cognitive Neuroscience of Memory* (ed L.-G. Nilsson and H.J. Markowitsch). Seattle, WA: Hogrefe and Huber, pp. 103–146.

Light, L.L. and Zelinski, E.M. (1983). Memory for spatial information in young and old adults. *Developmental Psychology*, **19**, 901–906.

McAndrews, M.P. and Milner, B. (1991). The frontal cortex and memory for temporal order. *Neuropsychologia*, **29**, 849–859.

McCormack, P.D. (1981). Temporal coding by young and elderly adults: a test of the Hasher–Zacks model. *Developmental Psychology*, **17**, 509–515.

McCormack, P.D. (1982). Temporal coding and study-phase retrieval in young and elderly adults. *Bulletin of the Psychonomic Society*, **20**, 242–244.

McIntosh, A.R., Nyberg, L., Bookstein, F.L., and Tulving, E. (1997). Differential functional connectivity of prefrontal and medial temporal cortices during episodic memory retrieval. *Human Brain Mapping*, **5**, 323–327.

McIntyre, J.S. and Craik, F.I.M. (1987). Age differences in memory for item and source information. *Canadian Journal of Psychology*, **41**, 175–192.

Madden, D.J., Whiting, W.L., Huettel, S.A., *et al.* (2003). Age-related change in functional integrity of white matter pathways obtained from diffusion-weighted imaging. *Journal of Cognitive Neuroscience Supplement*, 22.

Maguire, E.A., Frackowiak, R.S.J., and Frith CD (1997). Recalling routes around London: Activation of the right hippocampus in taxi drivers. *Journal of Neuroscience*, **17**, 7103–7110.

Mangels, J.A. (1997a). Relationship between strategic processing and memory for temporal order in patients with frontal lobe lesions. *Neuropsychology*, **11**, 1–15.

Mangels, J.A. (1997b). Strategic processing and memory for temporal order in patients with frontal lobe lesions. *Neuropsychology*, **11**, 1–15.

Mantyla, T. (1993). Knowing but not remembering: adult age differences in recollective experience. *Memory and Cognition*, **21**, 379–388.

Martin, M. (1986). Ageing and patterns of change in everyday memory and cognition. *Human Learning*, **5**, 63–74.

Mayes, A.R. and Montaldi, D. (1999). The neuroimaging of long-term memory encoding processes. *Memory*, **7**, 613–659.

Mayes, A.R., Gooding, P.A., Hunkin, N.M., *et al.* (1998). Storage of verbal associations is sufficient to activate the left medial temporal lobe. *Behavioral Neurology*, **11**, 163–172.

Mayes, A.R., Isaac, C.L., Holdstock, J.S., *et al.* (2001). Memory for single items, word pairs, and temporal order of different kinds in a patient with selective hippocampal lesions. *Cognitive Neuropsychology*, **18**, 97–123.

Maylor, E.A. (1990). Recognizing and naming faces: aging, memory retrieval, and the tip of the tongue state. *Journal of Gerontology*, **45**, 215.

Maylor, E.A. (1998). Retrieving names in old age: short- and (very) long-term effects of repetition. *Memory and Cognition*, **26**, 309–319.

Miller, E.K. and Cohen, J.D. (2001). An integrative theory of prefrontal cortex function. *Annual Review of Neuroscience*, **24**, 167–202.

Milner, B. (1971). Interhemispheric differences in the localization of psychological processes in man. *British Medical Bulletin*, **27**, 272–277.

Milner, B., Petrides, M., and Smith, M.L. (1985). Frontal lobes and the temporal organization of memory. *Human Neurobiology*, **4**, 137–142.

Milner, B., Corsi, P., and Leonard, G. (1991). Frontal-lobe contribution to recency judgments. *Neuropsychologia*, **29**, 601–618.

Mishkin, M., Vargha-Khadem, F., and Gadian, D.G. (1998). Amnesia and the organization of the hippocampal system. *Hippocampus*, **8**, 212–216.

Mitchell, K.J., Johnson, M.K., Raye, C.L., and D'Esposito, M. (2000a). fMRI evidence of age-related hippocampal dysfunction in feature binding in working memory. *Cognitive Brain Research*, **10**, 197–206.

Mitchell, K.J., Johnson, M.K., Raye, C.L., Mather, M., and D'Esposito, M. (2000b). Aging and reflective processes of working memory: binding and test load deficits. *Psychology and Aging*, **15**, 527–541.

Moffat, S.D. and Resnick, S.M. (2002). Effects of age on virtual environment place navigation and allocentric cognitive mapping. *Behavioral Neuroscience*, **116**, 851–859.

Moffat, S.D., Zonderman, A.B., and Resnick, S.M. (2001). Age differences in spatial memory in a virtual environment navigation task. *Neurobiology of Aging*, **22**, 787–796.

Montaldi, D., Mayes, A.R., Barnes, A., *et al.* (1998). Associative encoding of pictures activates the medial temporal lobes. *Human Brain Mapping* **6**, 85–104.

Moscovitch, M. (1992). Memory and working-with-memory: a component process model based on modules and central systems. *Journal of Cognitive Neuroscience*, **4**, 257–267.

Moscovitch, M., and Winocur, G. (1995). Frontal lobes, memory, and aging. *Annals of the New York Academy of Sciences*, **769**, 119–150.

Mottaghy, F.M., Shah, N.J., Krause, B.J., *et al.* (1999). Neuronal correlates of encoding and retrieval in episodic memory during a paired-word association learning task: a functional magnetic resonance imaging study. *Experimental Brain Research*, **128**, 332–342.

Murray, E. (1999). Memory for objects in nonhuman animals. In *The Cognitive Neurosciences* (2nd edn) (ed M.S. Gazzaniga). Cambridge, MA: MIT Press.

Nagode, J.C. and Pardo, J.V. (2002). Human hippocampal activation during transitive inference. *Neuroreport*, **13**, 933–944.

Naveh-Benjamin, M. (1990). Coding of temporal order information: an automatic process? *Journal of Experimental Psychology: Learning, Memory, and Cognition* **16**, 117–126.

Naveh-Benjamin, M. (2000). Adult age differences in memory performance: tests of an associative deficit hypothesis. *Journal of Experimental Psychology: Learning, Memory, and Cognition* **26**, 1170–1187.

Nielson, K.A., Langenecker, S.A., and Garavan H.P. (2002). Differences in the functional neuroanatomy of inhibitory control across the adult lifespan. *Psychology and Aging* **17**, 56–71.

Nolde, S.F., Johnson, M.K., Raye, C.L. (1998a). The role of prefrontal cortex during tests of episodic memory. *Trends in Cognitive Sciences*, **2**, 399–406.

Nolde, S.F., Johnson, M.K., and D'Esposito, M. (1998b). Left prefrontal activation during episodic remembering: an event-related fMRI study. *Neuroreport*, **9**, 3509–3514.

Norman, D.A. and Shallice, T. (1986). Attention to action: willed and automatic control of behavior. In *Consciousness and Self-Regulation: Advances in Research and Theory* (ed R.J. Davidson; G.E. Schawartz, and D. Shapiro D). New York: Plenum, pp 1–18.

Nyberg, L. and McIntosh, A.R. (2001). Functional neuroimaging: network analyses. In *Handbook of Functional Neuroimaging of Cognition* (ed R. Cabeza and A. Kingstone). Cambridge, MA: MIT Press, pp 49–72.

Nyberg, L., Cabeza, R., and Tulving, E. (1996). PET studies of encoding and retrieval: the HERA model. *Psychonomic Bulletin and Review*, **3**, 135–148.

Nyberg, L., Maitland, S.B., Ronnlund, M., *et al.* (2003). Selective adult age differences in an age-invariant multifactor model of declarative memory. *Psychology and Aging*, **18**, 149–160.

O'Sullivan, M., Jones, D.K., Summers, P.E., Morris, R.G., Williams, S.C.R., and Markus, H.S. (2001). Evidence for cortical 'disconnection' as a mechanism of age-related cognitive decline. *Neurology*, **57**, 632–638.

Owen, A.M., Herrod, N.J., Menon, D.K., *et al.* (1999). Redefining the functional organization of working memory processes within human lateral prefrontal cortex. *European Journal of Neuroscience*, **11**, 567–574.

Paller, K.A. and Wagner, A.D. (2002). Observing the transformation of experience into memory. *Trends in Cognitive Sciences*, **6**, 93–102.

Park, D.C. and Puglisi, J.T. (1985). Older adults' memory for the color of pictures and words. *Journal of Gerontology*, **40**, 198–204.

Park, D.C., Puglisi, J.T., and Lutz R. (1982). Spatial memory in older adults: effects of intentionality. *Journal of Gerontology*, **38**, 582–588.

Park, D.C., Puglisi, J.T., and Sovacool, M. (1983). Memory for pictures, words, and spatial locations in older adults: evidence for pictorial superiority. *Journal of Gerontology*, **38**, 582–588.

Parkin, A.J. and Walter, B.M. (1992). Recollective experience, normal aging, and frontal dysfunction. *Psychology and Aging*, **7**, 290–298.

Parkin, A.J., Walter, B.M., and Hunkin, M. (1995). Relationships between normal aging, frontal lobe function, and memory for temporal and spatial information. *Neuropsychology* **9**, 304–312.

Perfect, T.J., Mayes, A.R., Downes, J.J., and Van Eijk, R. (1996). Does context discriminate recollection from familiarity in recognition memory? *Quarterly Journal of Experimental Psychology A*, **49**, 797–813.

Perlmutter, M., Metzger, R., Nezworski, T., and Miller, K. (1981). Spatial and temporal memory in 20 and 60 year olds. *Journal of Gerontology*, **36**, 59–65.

Petersen, R.C., Jack, C.R., Jr, Xu, Y.C., *et al.* (2000). Memory and MRI-based hippocampal volumes in aging and AD. *Neurology*, **54**, 581–587.

Petrides, M. (1994). Frontal lobes and working memory: evidence from investigations of the effects of cortical excisions in nonhumans primates. In *Handbook of Neuropsychology* (ed F. Boller and J. Grafman). Amsterdam: Elsevier, pp. 59–82.

Prabhakaran, V., Narayanan, K., Zhao, Z., and Gabrieli, J.D.E. (2000). Integration of diverse information in working memory within the frontal lobe. *Nature Neuroscience*, **3**, 85–89.

Ranganath, C., Johnson, M.K., and D'Esposito, M. (2000). Left anterior prefrontal activation increases with demands to recall specific perceptual information. *Journal of Neuroscience*, **20: RC108**, 1–5.

Raz, N. (2000). Aging of the brain and its impact on cognitive performance: integration of structural and functional findings. In In *Handbook of Aging and Cognition II* (ed F.I.M. Craik and T.A. Salthouse). Mahwah, NJ: Erlbaum, pp. 1–90.

Raz, N. (2004). The aging brain observed *in vivo*: differential changes and their modifiers. In *Cognitive Neuroscience of Aging: Linking Cognitive and Cerebral Aging* (ed R. Cabeza, L. Nyberg, and D.C. Park). New York: Oxford University Press, pp.19–57

Reed, J.M. and Squire, L.R. (1994). Impaired recognition memory in patients with lesions limited to the hippocampal formation. *Behavioral Neuroscience*, **113**, 3–9.

Reuter-Lorenz, P., Jonides, J., Smith, E.S., *et al.* (2000). Age differences in the frontal lateralization of verbal and spatial working memory revealed by PET. *Journal of Cognitive Neuroscience*, **12**, 174–187.

Rosen, A.C., Prull, M.W., O'Hara, R., *et al.* (2002). Variable effects of aging on frontal lobe contributions to memory. *Neuroreport*, **13**, 2425–2428.

Rugg, M.D., Fletcher, P.C., Chua, P.M., and Dolan, R.J. (1999). The role of the prefrontal cortex in recognition memory and memory for source: an fMRI study. *NeuroImage*, **10**, 520–529.

Ryan, J.D., Althoff, R.R., Whitlow, S., and Cohen, N.J. (2000). Amnesia is a deficit in relational memory. *Psychological Science*, **11**, 454–461.

Schacter, D.L. (1987). Memory, amnesia, and frontal lobe dysfunction. *Psychobiology*, **15**, 21–36.

Schacter, D.L. and Wagner, A.D. (1999). Medial temporal lobe activations in fMRI and PET studies of episodic encoding and retrieval. *Hippocampus*, **9**, 7–24.

Schacter, D.L., Savage, C.R., Alpert, N.M., Rauch, S.L., and Albert, M.S. (1996). The role of hippocampus and frontal cortex in age-related memory changes: a PET study. *Neuroreport* **7**, 1165–1169.

Schacter, D.L., Norman, K.A., and Koutstaal, W. (1998). The cognitive neuroscience of constructive memory. *Annual Review of Psychology*, **49**, 289–3 18.

Schiavetto, A., Kohler, S., Grady, C.L., Winocur, G., and Moscovitch, M. (2002). Neural correlates of memory for object identity and object location: effects of aging. *Neuropsychologia*, **40**, 1428–1442.

Schmidt, D., Krause, B.J., Mottaghy, F.M., *et al.* (2002). Brain systems engaged in encoding and retrieval of word-pair associates independent of their imagery content or presentation modalities. *Neuropsychologia* **40**, 457–470.

Searcy, J.H., Bartlett, J.C., and Memon, A. (1999). Age differences in accuracy and choosing in eyewitness identification and face recognition. *Memory and Cognition*, **27**, 538–552.

Shimamura, A.P. (2002). Memory retrieval and executive control processses. In *Principles of Frontal Lobe Function*. (ed D.T. Stuss and R.T. Knight). New York: Oxford University Press, pp. 210–220.

Shimamura, A.P., Janowsky, J.S., and Squire, L.R. (1990). Memory for the temporal order of events in patients with frontal lobe lesions and amnesic patients. *Neuropsychologia*, **28**, 803–813.

Shimamura, A.P., Jurica, P.J., Mangels, J.A., *et al.* (1995). Susceptibility to memory interference effects following frontal lobe damage: findings from tests of paired-associate learning. *Journal of Cognitive Neuroscience*, **7**, 144–152.

Spencer, W.D. and Raz, N. (1995). Differential effects of aging on memory for content and context: a meta-analysis. *Psychology and Aging*, **10**, 527–539.

Sperling, R.A., Bates, J.F., Cochchiarella, A.J., Schacter, D.L., Rosen, B.R., and Albert, M.S. (2001). Encoding novel face-name associations: a functional MRI study. *Human Brain Mapping*, **14**, 129–139.

Sperling, R.A., Bates, J.F., Chua, E.F., *et al.* (2003). fMRI studies of associative encoding in young and elderly controls and mild Alzheimer's disease. *Journal of Neurology, Neurosurgery, and Psychiatry*, **74**, 44–50.

Squire, L.R. and Knowlton, B.J. (1995). Memory, hippocampus, and brain systems. In *The Cognitive Neurosciences* (ed M.S. Gazzaniga). Cambridge, MA: MIT Press, pp. 825–837.

Squire, L.R. and Zola-Morgan, S. (1991). The medial temporal lobe memory system. *Science*, **253**, 1380–1386.

Stark, C.E.L. and Squire, L.R. (2000). Functional magnetic resonance imaging (fMRI) activity in the hippocampal region during recognition memory. *Journal of Neuroscience*, **20**, 7776–7781.

Stark, C.E. and Squire, L.R. (2001). Simple and associative recognition memory in the hippocampal region. *Learning and Memory*, **8**, 190–197.

Stark, C.E. and Squire, L.R. (2003). Hippocampal damage equally impairs memory for single items and memory for conjunctions. *Hippocampus*, **13**, 281–292.

Stark, C.E., Bayley, P.J., and Squire, L.R. (2002). Recognition memory for single items and for associations is similarly impaired following damage to the hippocampal region. *Learning and Memory*, **9**, 238–242.

Stuss, D.T., Eskes, G.A., and Foster, J.K. (1994). Experimental neuropsychological studies of frontal lobe functions. In *Handbook of Neuropsychology* (ed F. Boller and J. Grafman) Amsterdam: Elsevier, pp. 149–185.

Tisserand, D.J., Visser, P.J., van Boxtel, M.P., and Jolles, J. (2000). The relation between global and limbic brain volumes on MRI and cognitive performance in healthy individuals across the age range. *Neurobiology of Aging*, **21**, 569–576.

Tulving, E. (1985). Memory and consciousness. *Canadian Psychology*, **25**, 1–12.

Tulving, E., Kapur, S., Craik, F.I.M., Moscovitch, M., and Houle, S. (1994). Hemispheric encoding/retrieval asymmetry in episodic memory: positron emission tomography findings. *Proceedings of the National Academy of Sciences of the Unied States of America*, **91**, 2016–2020.

Utl, B. and Graf, P. (1993). Episodic spatial memory in adulthood. *Psychology and Aging*, **8**, 257–253.

Vargha-Khadem, F., Gadian, D.G., Watkins, K.E., Connelly, A., Van Paesschen, W., and Mishkin, M. (1997). Differential effects of early hippocampal pathology on episodic and semantic memory. *Science*, **277**, 376–380.

Verhaeghen, P., Marcoen, A., and Goossens, L. (1993). Facts and fiction about memory aging: A quantitative integration of research findings. *Journal of Gerontology*, **48**, 157–171.

Wagner, A.D., Schacter, D.L., Rotte, M., *et al.* (1998). Building memories: remembering and forgetting of verbal experiences as predicted by brain activity. *Science*, **281**, 1188–1191.

West, M.J. (1993). Regionally specific loss of neurons in the aging human hippocampus. *Neurobiology of Aging*, **14**, 287–293.

West, R.L. (1996). An application of prefrontal cortex function theory to cognitive aging. *Psychological Bulletin*, **120**, 272–292.

Wheeler, M.A. and Stuss, D.T. (2003). Remembering and knowing in patients with frontal lobe tests. *Cortex*, **39**, 827–846.

Wheeler, M.A., Stuss, D.T., and Tulving, E. (1995). Frontal lobe damage produces episodic memory impairment. *Journal of the International Neuropsychological Society*, **1**, 525–536.

Wicklund, D.A., Palermo, D.S., and Jenkins, J.J. (1964). The effects of associative strength and response hierarchy on paired-associate learning. *Journal of Verbal Learning and Verbal Behavior*, **3**, 413–420.

Winocur, G. and Moscovitch, M. (1983). Paired-associate learning in institutionalized and noninstitutionalized old people: an analysis of interference and context effects. *Journal of Gerontology*, **38**, 455–464.

Yonelinas, A.P. (2002). The nature of recollection and familiarity: a review of 30 years of research. *Memory and Language*, **46**, 441–517.

Zaretsky, H.H. and Halberstam, J.L. (1968a). Age differences in paired-associate learning. *Journal of Gerontology*, **23**, 165–168.

Zaretsky, H.H. and Halberstam, J.L. (1968b). Effects of aging, brain damage, and associative strength on paired-associate learning and relearning. *Journal of Genetic Psychology*, **112**, 165–168.

Chapter 25

Binding of memories: adult-age differences and the effects of divided attention in young adults on episodic memory

Moshe Naveh-Benjamin

Introduction

In this chapter we attempt to determine whether there is a common mechanism underlying the adverse effects on episodic memory of ageing and of attention withdrawal in young people. To do so, we compare and contrast the effects of age and of divided attention in younger adults on episodic memory performance. One hypothesis suggested in previous research (the common mechanism hypothesis, discussed below), is that both effects are mediated, at least partially, by a reduction in attentional resources. According to the common mechanism view (Craik 1982, 1986; Craik and Byrd 1982; Rabinowitz *et al.* 1982), a major cause of deficient episodic memory in older adults is their characteristic reduction in attentional resources. These depleted resources prevent older adults from adequately encoding and retrieving information. According to this hypothesis, such a reduction in attentional resources in younger adults (e.g. when their attention is divided among several simultaneous tasks) would result in a similar reduction in memory performance relative to a case where the information is encoded under full attention.

In the first part of the chapter we briefly review the major findings and theories offered to explain the results in each domain (ageing and divided attention in the young) and specify the assumptions and predictions of the common mechanism hypothesis. In the second part we discuss a series of experiments that test an associative deficit (binding) hypothesis (ADH) as one instantiation of the common mechanism hypothesis underlying the poorer episodic memory performance of older adults and of younger adults under divided attention. Finally, in the third part of the chapter we discuss the theoretical implications of the empirical evidence provided in this series of experiments. On the whole, the empirical evidence supports an associative deficit mechanism mediating age-related changes in episodic memory performance, but not younger adults' performance under divided attention. These findings seem consistent with a modified weaker version of the common mechanism hypothesis. The results are taken to support the view that, whereas some aspects of memory performance are affected in a similar way by age and by divided attention in young adults, other aspects of performance may reflect different mechanisms underlying these detrimental effects on episodic memory.

Memory, divided attention, and ageing

Research concerning the effects on episodic memory of divided attention in young adults and of age in older adults has for the most part been carried out independently. Different researchers and different questions, as well as different research paradigms, were used in each of these areas of research. A short review of the major findings and theories suggested in each domain is given below.

Memory and ageing

The ability to learn new information and retrieve previously learned information is essential for successful ageing. Memory researchers interested in lifespan development have attempted to explain adult age differences in memory performance with the aim of both enhancing our understanding the behaviour of older adults and establishing a knowledge base which would constrain memory theories in general. Several hypotheses have been advanced to explain the relatively poor memory performance of the old, including a deficit in semantic processing (Cohen 1979; Craik and Byrd 1982), a failure of metamemory (Perlmutter 1978), a failure of deliberate recollection (Craik 1983, 1986; Jennings and Jacoby 1993; Hay and Jacoby 1999), a reduction in contextual encoding (McIntyre and Craik 1987; Light 1991), a reduction in processing resources (reviewed by Light 1991), a reduction in processing speed (Salthouse 1996), and a failure of inhibitory processes (Hasher and Zacks 1988). Although all the above are related to memory deficits in older adults, especially those deficits which characterize episodic memory, none of them provide an explanation for the full range of phenomena associated with episodic memory deficits in older adults. More recently, following work by Chalfonte and Johnson (1996), an ADH was suggested (Naveh-Benjamin 2000; Naveh-Benjamin *et al.* 2003b, 2004a,b) (see discussion below).

Memory and divided attention in young adults

Studies using the divided attention (DA) paradigm have shown marked effects on memory performance. However, the effects of DA on memory were found to differ depending on the stage of processing, encoding or retrieval, at which the DA was manipulated. Dividing participants' attention between the encoding of the information presented and performing a secondary task had a clear detrimental effect on free recall, cued recall, and recognition memory performance relative to conditions where full attention (FA) is paid to encoding the items (Murdock 1965; Baddeley *et al.* 1984; Craik *et al.* 1996; Naveh-Benjamin *et al.* 1998, 2000a,b). DA at encoding was shown to have a similar effect on a variety of memory features, including memory for frequency of occurrence (Naveh-Benjamin and Jonides 1986), memory for spatial location (Naveh-Benjamin 1987, 1988), and memory for temporal order information (Naveh-Benjamin 1990). Interestingly, DA at retrieval showed only small reductions in free recall, cued recall, and recognition performance (Baddeley *et al.* 1984, Craik *et al.* 1996, Naveh-Benjamin *et al.* 1998, 2000b; Naveh-Benjamin *et al.*, in press; Naveh-Benjamin and Guez 2000).

Manipulations emphasizing the memory or the secondary task also seem to affect the encoding of information. For example, Craik *et al.* (1996) showed that manipulating emphasis at encoding by instructing participants to stress the memory task, the secondary task, or both tasks equally has complementary effects on the two tasks; as attention is switched to the secondary task and away from the memory task, memory performance declines and secondary task performance improves. These results indicate that encoding processes require attention and that the allocation of attention to encoding processes is under the conscious control of the participant.

Several possible mediator mechanisms have been suggested for the effects of DA at encoding (reviewed by Naveh-Benjamin 2002). The reduced processing time hypothesis claims that the decrease in memory performance under DA at encoding occurs because the subjects spend some of their time performing the secondary task, leaving less time for processing the relevant information. However, using a shared time model analysis, Craik *et al.* (1996) showed that the decrease in processing time could explain only part of the memory deficit resulting from DA effects at encoding.

Another possible mediator in the effects of DA at encoding on later memory performance is the level of processing employed by the participants. It makes sense that DA at encoding qualitatively causes encoding to become shallower and less semantically elaborative. This notion was supported behaviourally, for example, in a series of studies during the 1980s (Craik 1982; Craik and Byrd

1982; Rabinowitz *et al.* 1982) which indicated that DA at encoding changes the qualitative nature of encoding such that it becomes less semantic. More recently, neuroimaging studies (Fletcher *et al.* 1995; Anderson *et al.* 2000) have shown that DA at encoding reduces encoding-related brain activity in the left inferior prefrontal cortex, an area shown in other studies to be associated with deep strategic semantic processing (Kapur *et al.* 1994). However, several recent studies reported in the literature complicate this picture. For example, Craik and Kester (2000) provide some counter-results. In a typical study in this series, participants were presented with word pairs and asked to rate the elaboration of the connection which they created for each word pair. This was done under either FA or DA. Results indicated that cued recall performance improved as the rated degree of elaboration increased, and that this happened for both FA and DA conditions. However, in contrast to what is expected by the elaboration of processing hypothesis, memory performance for the DA condition proved substantially lower than under the FA condition at every level of elaboration. This implies that a mechanism other than the amount of strategic elaboration underlies the effects of DA at encoding on later memory performance. In addition, Naveh-Benjamin (2002) showed similar effects of DA at encoding when learning was incidental (no deep-level strategic processing was used) to those under intentional learning when some deep elaborative strategies are used. Such results indicate that DA most likely affects other types of processing in addition to deep effortful strategies.

Therefore it appears that we are still in need of theoretical explanations regarding the effects of age and of DA in the young on episodic memory. As outlined below, the aim of the research reported in this chapter was to determine whether both effects can be explained by a common underlying mechanism, and, in particular, whether an ADH can explain the episodic memory decline associated with old age and with dividing the attention of younger adults at encoding.

Common mechanism

The principle of parsimony, stating that understanding and explaining phenomena should involve as few variables as possible, intends to unify seemingly unrelated phenomena under the same descriptive or explanatory scheme. The recent history of cognitive psychology is characterized by many specific models and theories, each dealing with a particular set of phenomena; therefore a unified approach is lacking in many areas of research.

One such unified approach was suggested by Craik and his collaborators (Craik 1982, 1983; 1986; Craik and Byrd 1982), to explain adult age changes in cognition in general, and in memory in particular. Using the assertion by Birren *et al.* (1983) that 'it would seem that the principal function of psychological research on ageing is to reduce the great variety of changes in behavior associated with age to a smaller number of concepts', Craik (1982) and his colleagues suggested that an age-related reduction in attentional or processing resources may underlie the older person's episodic memory deficiency. Moreover, they related these age-related changes to those occurring in younger adults who are operating under conditions of reduced attentional capacity (e.g. DA). The suggestion is that effortful cognitive operations, such as elaboration at encoding and reconstructive operations at retrieval, require substantial attentional resources and that elderly people have fewer of these resources. According to this suggestion, younger adults under DA conditions presumably invest some of their limited attentional resources in performing the secondary task; therefore, operating with reduced attentional resources devoted to the memory task, they would show patterns of memory performance similar to older adults.

Several studies have supported this common mechanism hypothesis. For example, there is some evidence that older adults encode information in a more stereotyped manner (Rabinowitz *et al.* 1982; Hess *et al.* 1989; Hashtroudi *et al.* 1990). That is, recurring aspects of objects and items can be encoded in a relatively automatic fashion, whereas the changing contextual aspects of a situation require more controlled and attentionally demanding memory operations. In cases when attentional resources are low, there will be a tendency to encode items in terms of their general stereotyped features, resulting in memory for the event being poor since it is not differentiated from other similar encodings. For example, Craik and Byrd (1982) and Craik and Simon (1980) have shown that general retrieval cues are relatively more effective for older subjects, whereas contextual cues are relatively more effective for young subjects. Similar results were reported by Rabinowitz *et al.* (1982) for younger adults under DA conditions, providing support for a common mechanism underlying the effects of age and of attention in the young on episodic memory.

Similar patterns were reported for retrieval. For example, Craik and McDowd (1987) showed that older adults' performance was poorer on cued recall than on recognition tasks compared with younger adults. Such results can be interpreted in terms of the amount of attentional resources required by each; cued recall requires substantial resources to search for the target word, whereas recognition, where subjects are provided with a copy of the original target, requires fewer attentional resources. Younger subjects under DA showed the same pattern of performance: DA at retrieval affected cued recall more than it affected recognition performance.

However, some results reported in the literature are not consistent with such a common mechanism hypothesis underlying the effects of age and of DA in the young on memory performance. One result, recently reported by Craik and Kester (2000) (see details above), showed that DA, unlike age, is not affected by the degree of elaboration of processing carried out during encoding. Similarly, Rabinowitz *et al.* (1982) have shown that, under DA conditions, memory performance for unrelated pairs did not suffer a greater decrease than performance for related pairs relative to an FA condition. This contrasts with the effects of age where older adults show a greater decline in memory for unrelated than for related pairs.

The current work was intended to explore further the feasibility of a common mechanism underlying the effects of age and of DA in young adults on memory. This was done by evaluating whether a deficit in an associative mechanism can mediate both the effect of ageing and that of DA in the young on memory performance.

Associative deficit hypothesis

The ADH is based on the notion that complex events consist of multiple kinds of information sources that are related together. A dominant view in cognitive psychology (e.g. Underwood 1969), assumes that an episode is composed of several attributes (e.g. semantic, acoustic, contextual) which are connected together to create a coherent distinctive unit. An event can include the semantic content, information about the time and place in which it occurred, the acting agents, their characteristics, etc. All these aspects integrated with the internal cognitive state of the person are encoded as an episode. Remembering such an episode requires that at least some of the components are retained, as well as their relationships to each other.

Several suggestions in the literature support a separation within memory of information about single units from information about associative relationships among these units (Anderson and Bower 1973; Humphreys 1976; Murdock 1982; 1993; Gillund and Shiffrin 1984; Johnson 1992; Johnson and Chalfonte 1994; Chalfonte and Johnson 1996). This distinction between item and associative information has been shown by several experiments which yielded different patterns of results for the two types of information (B.A. Dosher 1988, unpublished results; Gronlund and Ratcliff 1989; Hockley 1991, 1992, 1994; Hockley and Cristi 1996).

Associative deficit hypothesis and episodic memory in older adults and in younger adults under divided attention

Chalfonte and Johnson (1996), Bayen *et al.* (2000), and Mitchell *et al.* (2000) have suggested that part of the deficient memory performance in older adults stems from their difficulty in binding the information into complex memories. Naveh-Benjamin and colleagues (Naveh-Benjamin 2000; 2002; Naveh-Benjamin *et al.* 2003b, 2004a,b) proposed and provided support for an associative deficit hypothesis which suggests that an important cause of older adults' episodic memory deficit is their inability to associate together different components of the episode. The hypothesis attributes a substantial part of older adults' deficient memory performance to their difficulty in merging unrelated attributes–units of an episode into a cohesive unit. While each of the components can be memorized to a reasonable degree, the associations which tie the attributes–units to each other grow weaker in old age.

Naveh-Benjamin and colleagues (Naveh-Benjamin 2000; Naveh-Benjamin *et al.* 2003b, 2004a,b) provided converging validity to the hypothesis by demonstrating an associative deficit in older adults for both inter-item relationships and intra-item relationships, and discriminant validity by contrasting and testing competing predictions made by the ADH and by alternative hypotheses (see details below). They did this by employing a procedure suggested by Humphreys (1976), where participants study a list of pairs of items (e.g. word–word, word–font, or face–name pairs) and then receive tests on the items (components) and a test on their association with each other. For item information, participants receive at test some of the original items (words, names, fonts, or faces) with some new items and their task is to recognize the old items. For associative information, participants receive some originally intact pairs, which appeared as pairs at the study phase, and some recombined pairs, which include items that were presented but now the A item is taken from one pair and the B item from a different pair. Participants have to recognize which of the pairs are in their original form.

The common mechanism hypothesis regarding the effects of age and of DA at encoding in the young on memory performance suggests that if the ADH adequately accounts for older adults' deficient episodic memory performance (Naveh-Benjamin 2000; Naveh-Benjamin *et al* 2003b; and see below), then it can also plausibly be assumed to mediate the effects of DA at encoding in the young. In particular, in the present context we would expect DA at encoding to prove more disruptive to the activity of the associative mechanism, which binds together the components of the episode, than to the activity of the mechanism which encodes each component separately. Using task analysis, it appears that the cohesiveness of the episode created is disrupted during DA at encoding, i.e. since participants have to alternate between processing the primary encoding task and the concurrent task, they are unable to engage in uninterrupted merging together and binding of the different components of the episode. This results in the creation of a fragmented encoding unit.

Experiments

We now discuss five experiments which examined the effects of age, on the one hand, and the effects of DA at encoding in young adults, on the other hand, on item and associative information. To assess the effects of age, we used groups of young and old adults (Naveh-Benjamin 2000), while to assess the effects of DA, we used additional groups of younger adults under FA and DA (Naveh-Benjamin *et al.* 2003a). In these experiments we have used several different types of associations, as well as different memory tasks and learning instructions. The younger adult groups consisted of undergraduate students, aged 18–30 years, who participated in the experiment as part of their course requirements. The older adult groups were composed of individuals living independently in the community, aged 65–85, and matched the younger adult groups in education level and in the proportion of males to females. The common mechanism hypothesis predicts that both older adults and younger adults under DA at encoding will exhibit a similar associative deficit.

General methods

We have used a variety of associations in order to increase the external validity of the studies. In the first two experiments, we used the episodic relationships established between two unrelated items which appeared together (inter-unit associations) (Mandler 1979): Experiment 1 used word–non-word pairs, while Experiment 2 used word–word pairs. In Experiment 3 we used the episodic relationships established between different memory attributes (memory for word–font pairs; intra-unit associations) (Mandler 1979). In Experiments 4 and 5, we contrasted predictions made by an ADH with those made by a hypothesis which posits poorer general encoding in older adults and in younger adults under DA. This was done in Experiment 4 by assessing the effects of age and DA at encoding on different memory tasks, and in Experiment 5 by providing pre-experimental semantic support for the creation of associations.

In all the experiments, the younger adults under the DA condition were set a dual-task paradigm with the following features. First, we used well-understood memory paradigms, in which encoding and retrieval phases could be clearly separated. We presented the memory lists either auditorily or visually, depending on the experiment. To avoid modality-specific interference, we presented the memory and the concurrent tasks in different modalities. The concurrent task was either a visual or an auditory continuous choice reaction time (CRT) task, reported in previous studies (Craik *et al.* 1996; Naveh-Benjamin *et al.* 1998, 2000a), in which the participant's response immediately caused the next stimulus to appear. Participants, who were tested individually, were told in all the experiments to pay equal attention to learning the relevant materials and to performing on the secondary task. They had gone through a practice session on all tasks before the experimental trials began.

At the end of the study phase for each experiment, participants had to count backwards by threes for 90 s as an interpolated activity. In all the experiments reported in this article, participants were told to provide a response for each test item once they reached a decision. They had as much time as they needed to make their responses. A response triggered the appearance of the next test item. Moreover, in all experiments, a given stimulus appeared in only one of the tests in order to avoid across-test item re-exposure effects.

Experiment 1

In the first experiment we assessed the degree to which age and DA at encoding in the young differentially affect memory for associative and item information. The type of association used in this experiment was the episodic relationships established between two unrelated items which appeared together (inter-unit associations). Unrelated word–non-word pairs were presented visually for study to younger adults under FA or DA at encoding and to older adults under FA, with instructions to learn for upcoming memory tests. In the DA condition, the secondary task was a continuous 3-CRT task that involved a sequential presentation of auditory tones by the computer, one at a time, and a manual response on a computer keyboard to each tone. One of three tones, which differed from each other in frequency, was presented at random, and the participant's task was to press a pre-designated corresponding key on the keyboard. A response caused the immediate presentation of one of the other two tones at random.

At the end of the interpolated activity, three memory tests (one for words, one for non-words, and one for their associations) were administered to all participants. The order of the tests was counterbalanced across all participants. Item memory was tested by word and non-word recognition tests in which half the items (either the words or the non-words) were studied (targets) and half (words and non-words) were not (distractors). Associative memory was tested by presenting participants with target items only, either as intact pairs (a word and a non-word that were presented together at study) or as recombined pairs (a word and a non-word presented in different pairs at study), and asking them to recognize the intact pairs.

The ADH predicts an interaction between age and type of test where the greatest age effects are expected in the word–non-word associative test. In addition, the ADH predicts an interaction between attention condition in the young and the type of test. Specifically, the differences between FA and DA at encoding conditions are expected to be greatest in the word–non-word association test.

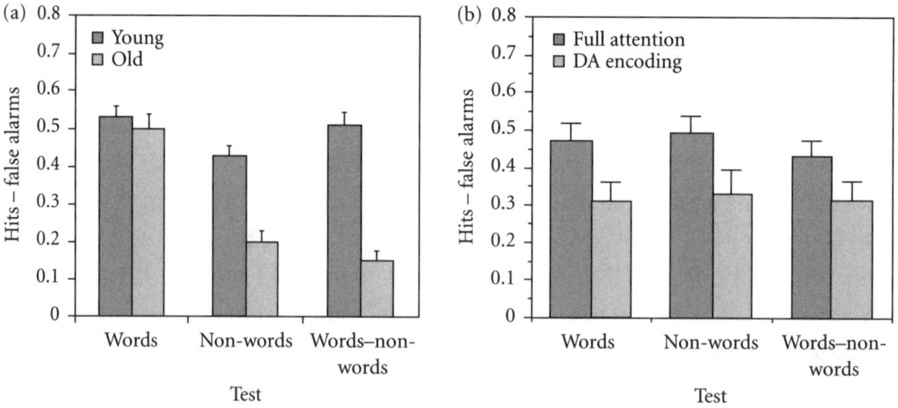

Figure 25.1 (a) Proportion of hits minus proportion of false alarms (± SE) in the item (word and non-word) and the associative (word–non-word) recognition tests for younger and older participants in Experiment 1 (Reproduced from M. Naveh-Benjamin, *Journal of Experimental Psychology: Learning, Memory, and Cognition*, **26**, 1170–1187, 2000.) (b) Proportion of hits minus proportion of false alarms (± SE) in the item (word–non-word) and the associative (word and non-word) recognition tests for each attention condition in Experiment 1 (Reproduced from M. Naveh-Benjamin *et al.*, *Memory and Cognition*, **31**, 1021–1035, 2003.)

Figure 25.1(a) presents results for the proportion of hits minus false-alarm measure (with standard errors) in the different conditions for the younger and older adults. As can be seen, older adults showed overall poorer performance than the young adults under FA. More importantly, older adults appear to be particularly deficient in the word–non-word pair recognition test, which requires associative information. They also exhibit some disadvantage in the non-word recognition test, which was, nevertheless, still smaller than their disadvantage in the word–non-word association test (the interaction of age and test for these conditions was statistically significant). This disadvantage could be accommodated by an ADH, as older participants may not have been able to assimilate these non-words in any obvious way into pre-existing knowledge; apparently they attempted, and failed, to create new associations among the letters of each non-word.

Figure 25.1(b) presents the results for young adults under FA and DA conditions. In contrast with older adults, younger adults under DA did not show any special disadvantage in the word–non-word pair association test. Instead, they showed an overall poorer memory on all three memory tests. Similar patterns of results are obtained when relative-scaled scores are used (Salthouse 1991).

These results indicate that older adults and younger adults under DA exhibit different patterns of performance. Older adults showed a differentially poorer performance in recognition of associative information compared with younger adults under FA. In contrast, younger participants under DA at encoding did not show such a differentially poorer performance in recognition of associative information compared with their performance under FA. Apparently, DA at encoding affects component processing (either word or non-word) to the same degree as it affects the processing of associations among the components. These results support an ADH as the locus of the effects of age on memory performance, but they do not support an ADH as the locus of the effects of DA at encoding on memory performance.

The results of the secondary task in this experiment (and in all other reported experiments) showed that the performance of the participants was poorer under DA than in the baseline conditions. Such results validate the different secondary tasks employed here, showing that the encoding of the relevant materials diverted attentional resources from the secondary task.

Experiment 2

In the second experiment, we wanted to extend the results of Experiment 1 to other types of associations and used different components from those used in Experiment 1. The type of association used in this experiment was the episodic relationships established between two unrelated words which appeared together (inter-unit associations). A second aim of this experiment was to explore whether an associative deficit that older adults showed in Experiment 1 is related to their intention to learn the associative information. In particular, the question was whether older adults' memory for associative information is deficient under both incidental and intentional learning of the associations. In addition, although the results of Experiment 1 do not support an ADH as the locus of the effects of DA at encoding in young, this may be because these participants learned the associations intentionally. It is still possible that DA at encoding may differentially affect the registration of associative information when participants concentrate on the encoding of the components and not of their associations.

Word pairs were presented auditorily to participants for study under instructions to expect either an item recognition test or an associative recognition test. Older adults studied the information under FA conditions, whereas younger adults studied the information under either FA or DA conditions. In the DA condition, younger participants learned the information simultaneously with a secondary visual 4-CRT task (DA). The task involved a visual display on a computer screen and a manual response on a computer keyboard (Craik *et al.* 1996; Naveh-Benjamin *et al.* 1998). The display consisted of four boxes arranged horizontally. An asterisk appeared at random in one of the boxes and the participant's task was to press the corresponding key on the keyboard. A correct response caused the asterisk to move immediately to one of the other boxes at random

As in Experiment 1, item memory was tested by a recognition test in which half the items (words) had been studied (targets) and half had not (distractors). Associative memory was tested by presenting participants with target items only, as either intact pairs (words that were presented together at study) or recombined pairs (words presented in different pairs at study), and asking them to recognize the intact pairs.

Figure 25.2(a) presents the results for the proportion of hits minus the proportion of false alarms for younger and older adults under FA. The figure indicates that older adults showed a differentially poorer performance in recognition of associative information than in item information compared with younger adults, as reflected by the interaction of age and test. It appears that older adults do not encode and store associative information as well as younger adults. In addition, as reflected by the triple interaction of age, study instructions, and test, older adults showed this associative deficit when the information was encoded incidentally under study instructions to pay attention to the single items. Furthermore, this deficit became more pronounced under intentional instructions to learn the pairs. These results differ from those obtained when younger adults were compared under FA and DA conditions (Fig. 25.2(b)). Despite the powerful effects of DA on both item and associative recognition, DA at encoding did not result in a differentially poorer performance in the recognition of associative information than in item information when compared with FA. The absence of both a significant interaction effect of attention and instructions and a significant triple interaction indicates that whatever is disrupted under DA conditions in young adults is not related to whether participants pay attention to the components or to their association with each other.

Experiment 3

Associations are required not only for relating single units together (inter-item connections), as discussed and demonstrated in Experiments 1 and 2, but also for connecting together different attributes within a unit. In order to allow us to evaluate the effects of age and DA in the young on memory for single attributes and their associations, we devised three memory tasks, each of which is supposed to test a different facet of the information. We used the form (font) in which words were presented as the perceptual–contextual attribute. Words were presented for study in one of 18 fonts. We compared memory for the words, for the fonts in

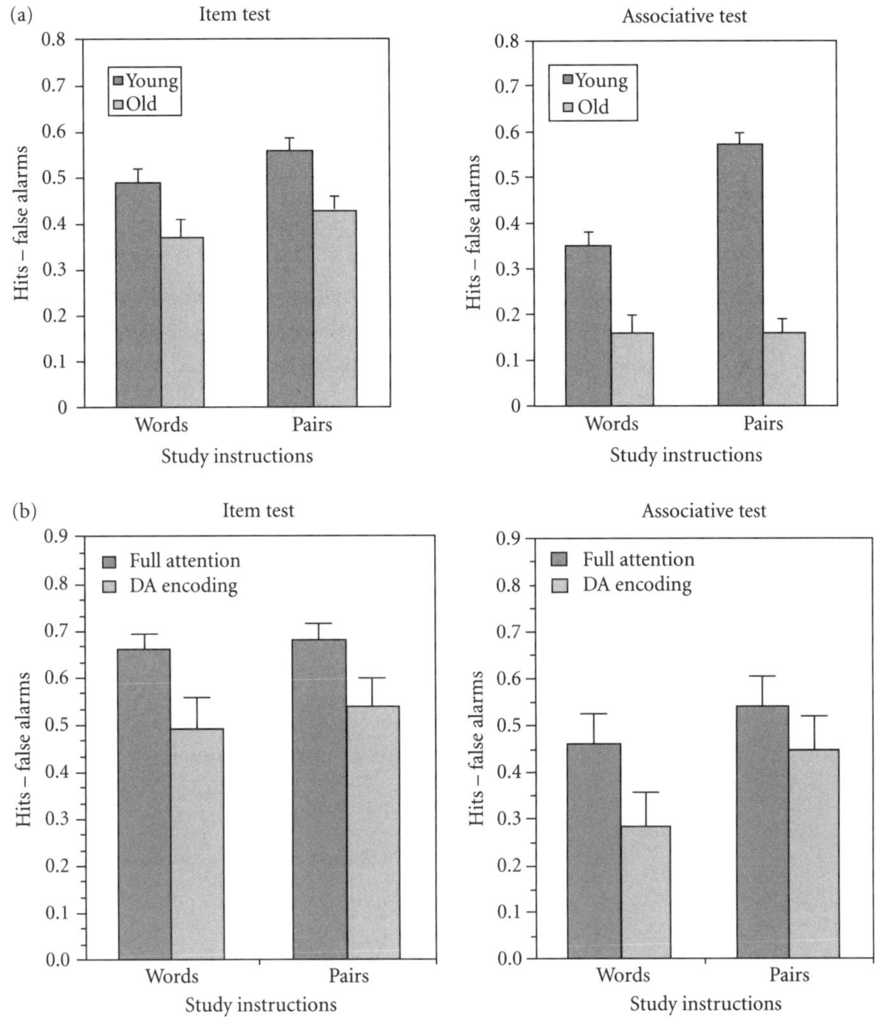

Figure 25.2 (a) Proportion of hits minus proportion of false alarms (± SE) in the item (words) and the associative (word–word) recognition tests for younger and older participants in the different study instruction conditions of Experiment 2. (Reproduced from M. Naveh-Benjamin, *Journal of Experimental Psychology: Learning, Memory, and Cognition*, **26**, 1170–1187, 2000.) (b) Proportion of hits minus proportion of false alarms (± SE) in the item (words) and the associative (word–word) recognition tests for each attention condition in the different study instruction conditions of Experiment 2. (Reproduced from M. Naveh-Benjamin *et al.*, *Memory and Cognition*, **31**, 1021–1035, 2003.)

which the words were presented, and for the relationships (conjunctures) between specific words and specific fonts in older adults and in younger adults under FA and DA conditions. The secondary task was the continuous auditory 3-CRT task employed in Experiment 1.

At the test phase participants received the following.

1. A pure recognition test on the words which in some of the original words (targets) appeared with new words (distractors). All the words at test appeared in a neutral font (which had not been presented at study).
2. A pure recognition test on the fonts in which the original fonts (targets) were mixed with other new fonts (distractors) and were presented without the words (using XXXX) for a recognition test.
3. A recognition test on the conjunctures–associations of words and fonts. In this test only original (target) words and fonts were presented. In half of the cases, the word was presented in the original font (intact events), and in the other half the word was presented in a different font from the one in which it appeared at the study phase, but which had appeared with another word at study (recombined events). Such a test requires participants to possess information about the relationships between the words and the fonts, and it is similar in nature to the recognition test for inter-item associations employed in Experiments 1 and 2.

Figure 25.3(a) presents the results for the proportion of hits minus the proportion of false alarms for younger and older adults under FA conditions. The figure shows an interaction between age and test, indicating that older adults, compared with younger adults, show a differentially poorer performance in recognition of

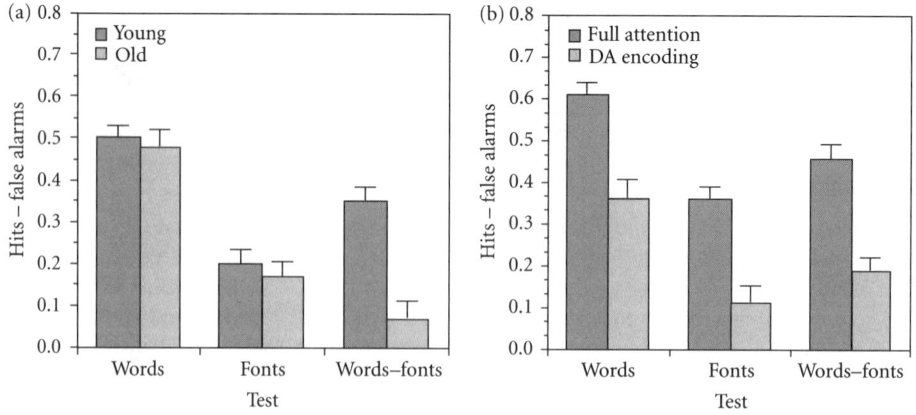

Figure 25.3 (a) Proportion of hits minus proportion of false alarms (± SE) in the word, font, and word–font recognition tests for younger and older participants in Experiment 3. (Reproduced from M. Naveh-Benjamin, *Journal of Experimental Psychology: Learning, Memory, and Cognition*, **26**, 1170–1187, 2000.) (b) Proportion of hits minus proportion of false alarms (± SE) in the word, font, and word–font recognition tests for each attention condition in Experiment 3. (Reproduced from M. Naveh-Benjamin *et al.*, *Memory and Cognition*, **31**, 1021–1035, 2003.)

associative information relating words and fonts, than in component information (either the words or the fonts). It appears that older adults do not encode and store associative information as well as younger adults under FA. In contrast, Figure 25.3(b) shows that, despite the strong effect of DA on both the components (words and fonts) and their links with each other, DA at encoding, compared with the FA condition in the young, does not result in a differentially poorer performance in recognition of associative information than in recognition of item information.

Overall, the results of this experiment indicate an associative deficit in older adults, who appear to have problems in encoding and retrieving information about the associations of contextual and focal elements of episodes. In contrast, younger adults under DA show a similar deficit in a task requiring the association of contextual elements together as in tasks requiring memory for each of the contextual elements separately.

Experiment 4

In this experiment we compared the effects of age and DA at encoding in the young on different memory retrieval tasks. Two hypotheses were contrasted: one that attributes the memory deficiency in old age and in younger adults under DA at encoding to a generally poorer encoding of the information, and the other, an ADH, which attributes this deficit to a selective impairment of the associative mechanism. According to the first hypothesis, the overall poorer encoding in old age and under DA at encoding conditions in the young will result in a weaker memory trace. This will lead to performance in these two groups, relative to FA encoding in younger adults, to be depressed to the same degree in all the retrieval tasks. Another version of this hypothesis would predict that this weaker trace in old age and under DA at encoding could be helped the most at retrieval when supporting conditions exist (e.g. when a recognition test is employed) which could help induce the appropriate mental operations necessary for retrieval (environmental support view) (Craik 1983, 1986). However, in a cued recall test, and even more in a free recall test, where participants do not have much support at retrieval and where they have to initiate the mental operations (search etc.) necessary for recall performance, poor encoding in older adults and in younger ones under DA conditions will significantly affect memory performance. Such a view would predict large effects of age and DA in the young at encoding when a free recall task is used, smaller effects when cued recall is used, and still smaller effects when a recognition task is employed where the poorer encoding in older adults and under DA can be compensated by the supporting conditions at retrieval.

In contrast, an ADH makes different predictions: a cued recall task, which involves the direct encoding and retrieval of specific associations among items, is predicted to be the most sensitive to the effects of age and of DA at encoding in the young. This is because both older participants and young participants under DA conditions will encounter problems in creating and retrieving associations between unrelated pairs of items. Free recall, which also involves, at least indirectly, creating relationships between items (Mandler 1979), is predicted to be somewhat less sensitive to the effects of age and of DA at encoding in the young, as it involves other operations not directly related to the retrieval of specific associations (e.g. initiation of a memory search and generation of cues (Atkinson and Shiffrin 1968)). Finally, item recognition, which is the least dependent on associative information, will be the least sensitive to the effects of age and of DA in the young. A major difference between the general poor encoding hypothesis and the ADH is in their differential predictions regarding the effects of age and of DA at encoding conditions in the young on free recall and cued recall performance; whereas the former predicts either no differential effects of age and DA on the two tasks, or larger effects in free recall, the latter predicts the opposite—larger age and DA effects in cued recall.

To test the contrasting hypotheses discussed above, we compared the effects of age and of DA at encoding in the young on memory performance in three tasks: free recall, cued recall, and recognition. Older participants and younger participants under FA and DA conditions received six lists of unrelated word pairs to study, and after each list they performed one of the three memory tasks. The learning was intentional, and the nature of the tests was known in advance. For the free recall task, participants were told that at the test phase they would have to memorize and write down as many of the targets as possible. For the cued recall task, they were told that at the test phase the first cue word of each pair would be provided, and that their task was to come up with its paired word. Lastly, for the recognition task, they were told that during the test phase they would be given the 12 targets plus 24 distractors, and that their task would be to circle the 12 targets out of the 36 candidate words. The secondary task used was the same continuous auditory 3-CRT task that was employed in Experiments 1 and 3.

In order to compare performance on the three memory tasks directly, we used the proportion of correctly recalled targets in the free recall test, the proportion of correctly recalled targets in the cued recall test, and the proportion of hits minus the proportion of false alarms in the recognition test (see Craik and McDowd (1987) for a similar procedure). Since there were only a few false alarms in the free recall and cued recall tasks, this equated the three tasks in terms of the chance level which was 0.0.

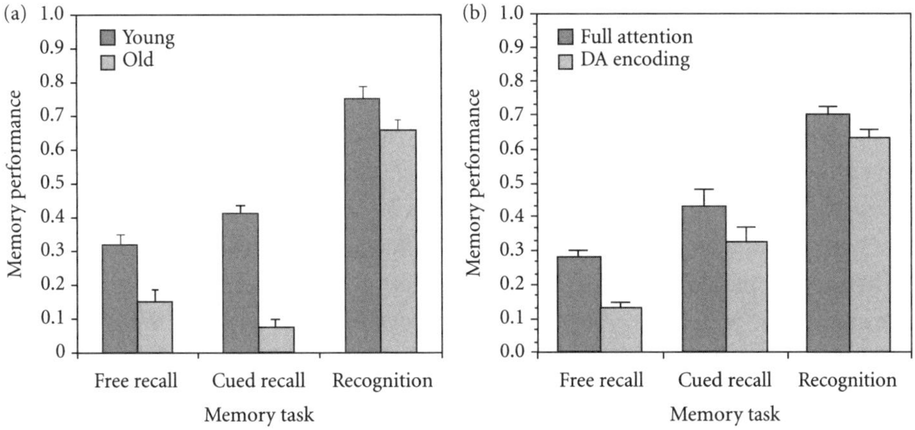

Figure 25.4 (a) Proportion of hit rates (± SE) in the free recall and cued recall tests and the proportion of hit minus false-alarm rates in the recognition test for younger and older participants in Experiment 4. (Reproduced from M. Naveh-Benjamin, *Journal of Experimental Psychology: Learning, Memory, and Cognition*, **26**, 1170–1187, 2000.) (b) Proportion of hit rates (± SE) in the free recall and cued recall tests and the proportion of hit minus false-alarm rates in the recognition test for each attention condition in Experiment 4. (Reproduced from M. Naveh-Benjamin *et al.*, *Memory and Cognition*, **31**, 1021–1035, 2003.)

Figure 25.4(a) presents the means for the above measures for the younger and older adults under FA conditions. As this figure indicates, the interaction of age and test was significant, reflecting the fact that the largest difference between young and older adults was obtained in the cued recall task. Such a pattern is consistent with an ADH, which claims that the cued recall task of unrelated pairs (involving the direct encoding and retrieval of associations) is the most age-sensitive task, even more so than free recall.

In contrast, Figure 25.4(b), which compares the performances of younger adults under FA and DA conditions, indicated a different pattern. The figure reveals that unlike older adults, younger adults under DA at encoding conditions do not show an associative deficit. The young adults under the DA condition do not seem to be differentially disrupted in the encoding and storage of associative information. Rather, they are at a general disadvantage when trying to remember unrelated pairs, since DA at encoding seems to affect performance on the different memory tests to the same degree. These results, coupled with the trend showing that the largest difference between the FA and the DA conditions emerged in the free recall task, with a decreasing effect in the cued recall task and even more so in the recognition task, are all inconsistent with an ADH.

Experiment 5

In this experiment we tested another prediction of an ADH regarding the underlying mechanism that is disrupted in older adults and in younger ones under DA at encoding. Specifically, we contrasted a case where unrelated pairs are employed and new temporospatial episodic relationships have to be created (as in Experiment 4), with a situation in which the creation and retrieval of these associations can be supported by pre-existing semantic associations (e.g. when semantically related pairs are used). In the latter case, where much less episodic distinctiveness is necessary and previous knowledge can support the creation of associations, we would expect much smaller differences, if any, between older and younger adults, as well as between younger adults under FA and DA conditions. In particular, according to an ADH hypothesis, older adults and younger adults under DA conditions should benefit more than younger adults under FA conditions when semantically related rather than unrelated pairs are used in the cued recall task. This is because the use of pre-existing associations will be the most beneficial in encoding associative information in older adults and under DA conditions in the young. Participants under full attention at encoding might also benefit from the semantically related pairs, but to a lesser degree, since, according to an ADH, they encode associative information quite well even when this information is not supported by pre-existing associations.

Participants listened to four lists of word pairs, two with semantically unrelated and two with semantically related pairs, and received a cued recall test after each. They were told to try to learn the pairs, paying special attention to the second word in each pair (the target word). They were also told to pay attention to the first cue word, since it could help them memorize and retrieve the target word. The secondary task was the visual CRT task used in Experiment 2.

Figure 25.5(a) shows the means of proportions correct for younger and older participants under FA for the different pair types. The results indicate that the largest difference between younger and older adults was obtained in the cued recall of unrelated pairs. Such a pattern is consistent with an ADH in older adults, which claims that the cued recall task of unrelated pairs (requiring extensive encoding and retrieval of associations) will show particular sensitivity to age. However, when the cued recall task demands less reliance on the creation of new associations and a greater use of previously learned associations (the semantically related pairs condition), the differences between younger and older adults disappear completely.

In contrast, Figure 25.5(b) indicates that young participants under DA at encoding conditions do not show a differential disadvantage in memory for unrelated pairs. In particular, the deficit for these pairs in the DA condition,

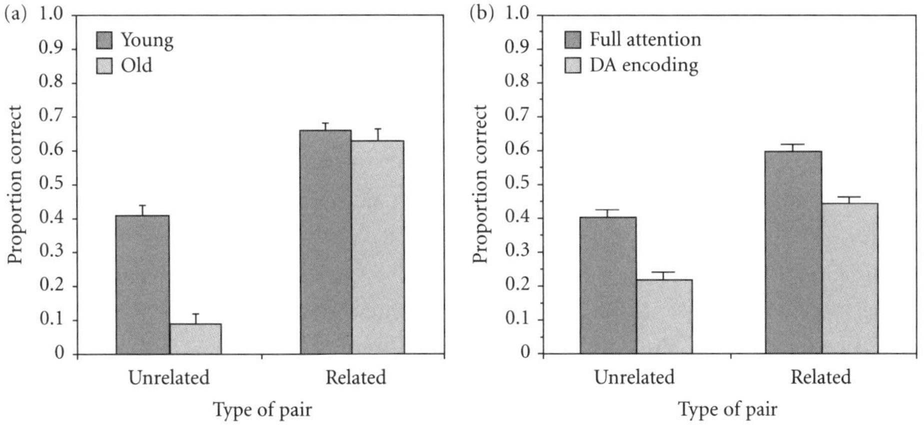

Figure 25.5 (a) Proportion correct (± SE) in the unrelated and related pairs conditions for younger and older adults in Experiment 5. (Reproduced from M. Naveh-Benjamin, *Journal of Experimental Psychology: Learning, Memory, and Cognition*, **26**, 1170–1187, 2000.) (b) Proportion correct (± SE) for each attention condition in the unrelated and related pairs conditions of Experiment 5. (Reproduced from M. Naveh-Benjamin *et al.*, *Memory and Cognition*, **31**, 1021–1035, 2003.)

compared with encoding under FA, is the same as when related pairs are used. Young participants under DA conditions clearly take advantage of the related pairs, but they do so to the same degree under FA conditions. Such results do not support an ADH as the locus of the effects of DA at encoding. If associative processes were particularly interrupted under DA at encoding, as an ADH presumes, we would have expected this to prove particularly detrimental to the encoding of unrelated pairs.

Summary of results

The results of the five experiments are consistent with an ADH which attributes at least part of older adults' deficient explicit episodic memory performance to their decreased ability to encode and retrieve associations among units of information or attributes within events. However, these results are not consistent with an ADH that attributes at least part of the deficient explicit episodic memory performance of younger adults under DA at encoding conditions to their decreased ability to encode associations among units of information or attributes within events.

The reported results do not appear to depend on the scale used because the same patterns emerged regardless of whether we used absolute or scaled scores. In addition, the lack of interaction effect of attention and type of test in the younger adults cannot be attributed to a lack of statistical power of the test: the trends obtained in all five experiments do not show any differential effects of DA on the component and the association tests. In fact, in most of the experiments the effects of DA were somewhat weaker for the associative test than for the component test. In addition, the memory performance results in the younger adults under FA and DA conditions indicate similar patterns, despite the use of different secondary tasks in the different experiments. Finally, performance on the secondary task showed similar patterns in all the experiments, being poorer under DA than in the baseline condition. Such results validate the different secondary tasks employed here, showing that the encoding of the relevant materials diverted attentional resources from the secondary task.

Taken as a whole, the results of the experiments suggest that a deficit in the processing of relationships–associations between single units (an episode's components) probably plays a role in older adults' deficits in episodic memory, but does not play an important role in explaining the poor memory performance of young participants who encoded the information under DA conditions.

Interpretation of the results

In this section we discuss the implications of the reported results for a common mechanism hypothesis, for theoretical perspectives on age-related changes in memory, and for understanding the effects of DA at encoding on memory in the young.

Common mechanism hypothesis

It appears that, despite previous support for the suggestion that reduced attentional resources might be a common mechanism underlying the effects of age and those of DA in young adults on episodic memory, the current results place certain constraints on such an explanation. Although both age and DA in young adults are negatively associated with episodic memory performance, the locus of their effects seems to be somewhat different. Whereas ageing seems to have a particularly disruptive effect on the associative mechanism, reduced attention at encoding in younger adults does not do so but is, instead, related to a general decrease in memory performance. One possibility is that in order to be as disruptive as age, attention may have to be withdrawn both at encoding and at retrieval instead of just at encoding, as was done in the current studies. However, there are several reasons for suspecting that this was not why DA did not have a differentially larger effect on the associative mechanism. First, previous results have shown depleted attentional resources at retrieval to have little or no effect on memory performance (Craik *et al.* 1996; Naveh-Benjamin *et al.* 1998, 2000a,b). Furthermore, these results showed no further decrease in memory performance when attention was divided at both encoding and retrieval compared with a case when attention was divided only at encoding (Craik *et al.* 1996; Anderson *et al.* 1998).

One plausible explanation for the conflict between the results which support the common mechanism hypothesis for age and DA effects in young adults (e.g. Craik 1983; 1986) and those reported here is that age-related changes in memory performance have multiple causes. One important cause is related to depleted attentional resources, which leads to information being encoded less distinctively and more schematically, resulting in poorer memory for item information. Such a mechanism might be operating in both older adults and in younger adults under DA at encoding conditions. The results reported here, in the work of Naveh-Benjamin and colleagues (Naveh-Benjamin 2000; Naveh-Benjamin *et al.* 2003a,b; 2004a,b), and in other previous studies (e.g. Craik 1983, 1986) support such a view by showing clear detrimental effects of both age and DA in the young on memory for item information. The associative deficit, which appears to be unique to older adults, further degrades their memory performance whenever explicit episodic memory is involved. However, it does not appear to affect younger adults further under DA conditions.

Such a suggestion is consistent with evidence and models emerging from the literature on neuropsychology and neuroscience. For example, one noteworthy model is that suggested by Moscovitch (1992), which proposes that episodic memory performance is mediated by two principal components: a modular medial temporal–hippocampal (MTLH) component, whose operations are essentially automatic, and a frontal-lobe component, whose operations are strategic, organizational, and accessible to consciousness and voluntary control. Recent neuroimaging studies indicate that DA at encoding results mostly in decreased brain activation in the left prefrontal region but not in the MTLH regions (Fletcher *et al.* 1995; Anderson *et al.* 2000). Such studies are in line with the results reported in this chapter, showing no differential effects of DA on associative information; they are also consistent with the notion that the MTLH region, which is believed to mediate the merging of different components of an episode into a cohesive unit (Cohen and Eichenbaum 1993), is not differentially affected by DA at encoding. The results of the experiments presented here agree with such a suggestion.

Interestingly, neuroimaging studies (Mitchell *et al.* 2000a) show that age may have some effect not only on the prefrontal regions, but also on the MTLH activity, in line with the results reported by Naveh-Benjamin and colleagues (Naveh-Benjamin 2000; Naveh-Benjamin *et al.* 2003a,b; 2004a,b) showing an associative deficit in older adults.

If the effects of age and DA in the young on memory performance are mediated, at least partially, by different mechanisms, one interesting question is whether there is a way of simulating older adults' associative deficit in younger adults. One possibility arising from the current results is that in order to simulate such a deficit, we need to create conditions which will not allow younger adults to use their associative processing apparatus effectively. One way of doing this is to provide young participants with a secondary task at encoding which requires the processing of associative information, and comparing its effects with those obtained with a secondary task of equal difficulty but where no associative processing is required. We have recently obtained preliminary evidence that supports such a suggestion (Naveh-Benjamin *et al.*, in preparation). Young participants have learnt pairs of words while simultaneously performing a secondary task. This secondary task involved a continuous presentation of pairs of single digits. Participants in one condition had to treat each digit separately, having to judge whether each of the digits was an odd or even number, while participants in the other condition had to evaluate the relationship between the digits, specifically whether one digit was numerically larger or smaller than the other. Results indicated that only the latter task, requiring the consideration of the relations between the digits, affected differentially associative and item recognition performance. In particular, whereas a secondary task requiring the processing of each digit alone affected memory for item and for associative information to the same degree, a secondary task involving associative secondary task affected younger participants' memory for associative information more than that for item information, rendering them similar to older adults. These results seem to indicate that young adults may also show an associative deficit under conditions when the associative mechanism is occupied by other processing and cannot be enlisted to encode the relevant information.

It should be noted that a recent study by Castel and Craik (2003), using the odd-digit secondary task in a word-pair study paradigm and with a somewhat different testing paradigm than the one reported in the current experiments, demonstrated that younger adults under DA at encoding showed poorer performance in associative than in item memory. However, since there were varying types of targets and lures in their study, it was possible to calculate item memory performance in a number of ways, whereas the current experiments offer a more straightforward measure. In addition, the differential decline in associative memory in younger adults under DA at encoding, reported by Castel and Craik (2003), was smaller than the one shown by older adults.

It should be noted that the experiments reported here do not address the issue of perceptual binding (Treisman and Gelade 1980). These researchers claimed that attention is necessary in order to bind together different attributes. However, their methodologies use extremely brief presentations that are very different from those used in the current experiments. In terms of the temporal dimension, it is reasonable to conceptualize the experiments reported in this chapter as dealing with the processing done after initial perceptual processing has taken place.

Relevance to perspectives on age-related changes in memory

Despite the support for an associative deficit underlying some of the older adults' deficit in episodic memory, there are still some issues and questions left open regarding different aspects of an ADH. One question is whether such a deficit shown by older adults stems mostly from problems in creating new associations during encoding or from problems in retrieving such associations at test. There are some indications that the deficit is related to both. The results reported in this chapter can be taken to support such a view in showing a differential associative deficit in older adults which was affected by manipulations at both encoding (instructions, Experiment 2) and retrieval (test types, Experiment 4). These results seem to support the conclusion that older adults' deficient memory for associations is due to problems at both at encoding and in explicit retrieval. However, there is a need for further research on this issue. Glisky *et al.* (2001), using a source memory task, reported results supporting this view.

A second question concerns the distinction between memory for associative versus item information. Item recognition is known to rely, at least partially, on the association created between an item and the experimental context (Tulving and Thomson 1973). If a notable characteristic of older adults is their inability to encode and retrieve associations, as suggested by the ADH, then why is item recognition not hampered in older adults? Such a claim is not incompatible with the view presented here. First, the association between the item and the experimental context may be one of the mediators in the rather moderate effects of age on item recognition reported in the literature and in the experiments of this chapter. The claim advanced by the ADH is that pair recognition more distinctly taps associative information because it is sensitive not only to the relationships between the pairs and the experimental context (as in item recognition), but even more to the specific relationships between the components of each pair. In addition, is appears that the associative deficit is particularly relevant when the task involves explicit retrieval of associations, as is the case in the associative recognition task. The item recognition test does not usually involve explicit retrieval of associations between the item and the context. The large deficits that older adults show in source memory (McIntyre and Craik 1987) and context memory (Spencer and Raz 1995) is consistent with this position, for the tasks used to demonstrate these deficits rely on explicit retrieval of associations between the item and the context.

Another important question is whether the associative deficit demonstrated here affects or is mediated by the type of the associative representation created. We do not yet know whether older adults' memory representation of associations is different from that of younger adults. Is the associative deficit of older adults related to episodic components being represented independently in memory, unlike younger adults, who have a new compound representation qualitatively different from the separate components? Future research may shed some light on this issue (see Rizzuto and Kahana 2001, for a related discussion).

Finally, as pointed out in the original formulation (Naveh-Benjamin 2000), while an ADH suggests a reduced ability of older adults to encode and retrieve associations, it is not committed to the exact micro-level mechanisms responsible for such deficits. These mechanisms may involve a reduction in priming transmitted across connections among units due to declined linkage strength (MacKay and Burke 1990), a decreased efficiency of the simultaneity mechanism (Salthouse 1996), an impaired neuromodulation involved in frontal–hippocampal circuitry (Li *et al.*, in press), or an inefficient binding mechanism (Chalfonte and Johnson 1996; Mitchell *et al.* 2000b) (for a more formal connectionist model, see Chapter 9). We believe that any such microlevel mechanism would have to account for the inefficiency in creating new associations, as well as for the decreased ability to retrieve such associations (see Li *et al.* (in press) for supportive results of a simulation study based on a connectionist network).

Alternative mechanisms involved in the effects of DA at encoding on memory performance in the young

Encoding processes were shown in previous research (Craik *et al.* 1996; Naveh-Benjamin *et al.* 1998; 2000a,b) to be consciously controlled and attention demanding. This was reflected in the findings that division of attention at encoding is associated with a reduction in memory performance and also with a slowing of concurrent RT task. Moreover, changes in task emphasis result in systematic and complementary changes in performance in both tasks. There could be several information processing stages where the detrimental effects of DA occur (Naveh-Benjamin 2002). One is during the initial registration-perception of the information. Another is during the encoding of the event's components. Others are during binding of the components together, and during the elaboration of the whole episode. The final one might be during the consolidation of the episode. The results of the current study appear to suggest that the effects of DA do not interrupt the binding stage but stages that are either upstream or downstream of it.

Other recent results of studies in our laboratory may shed light on the locus of the effects of DA at encoding. For example, we have recently shown (Naveh-Benjamin 2002) that DA at encoding affects memory performance similarly regardless of whether the original encoding was performed with the intention to learn. Two groups of subjects learned words either intentionally (in preparation for an upcoming memory test) or incidentally. For the latter group the cover story used was that we would be measuring the physiological activity associated with paying attention to the words, as reflected by GSR recordings from an electrode attached to a finger. Nothing was mentioned to the participants about the upcoming memory test. Participants encoded the words either under FA or DA and were later asked to free recall the words. The results indicated a general effect of instructions where those participants in the intentional learning condition performed significantly better than their incidental counterparts. There was also a considerable effect of DA. Most interestingly, however, there was no interaction between the two, i.e. the effects of DA were the same under incidental and intentional learning instructions. Since subjects under incidental instructions presumably did not use any encoding strategies (including elaboration), such a pattern of results is consistent with the view that the effects of DA are upstream at an early stage of processing before elaborative strategic processing takes place, possibly related to the initial registration of the information (Naveh-Benjamin *et al.*, submitted).

However, other studies are consistent with the position that the effects of DA are downstream. For example, we have recently conducted a study (Naveh-Benjamin 2002) where subjects were instructed to process the items at either a shallow level (pay attention and make a judgement on the font in which each word appears) or a deeper level (pay attention to the words and provide a pleasantness rating for each). Results indicated that the effects of DA at encoding were much smaller in the latter condition, indicating that the employment of deep-level elaborative processing may provide immunity to the effects of DA on later memory performance. These elaborations must have been done after the initial encoding was completed; this may imply that DA affects the elaboration of the episode. Thus it seems that the effects of DA at encoding may interrupt processing both early on, when it is more automatic, and later, when it is more controlled. This provides a less parsimonious and more complex picture according to which DA during encoding does not affect only one specific type of processes, but instead seems to interfere with a multitude of encoding processes. However, the effects of DA at encoding do not seem to influence the processes involved in associating together the different components of the episodes, as the studies reported in this chapter have shown.

Summary

Overall, the results of the experiments reported in this paper support the ADH suggested recently by Naveh-Benjamin and colleagues (Naveh-Benjamin 2000; Naveh-Benjamin *et al.* (2003b, 2004a,b) because they demonstrate the differentially poorer performance of older adults on memory tasks which require the effective processing of associative information. At the same time, younger adults under DA at encoding do not seem to show this deficit. Such patterns constrain the generality of a common depleted attentional resources mechanism as underlying the decline in episodic memory seen in younger adults under DA conditions and in older adults. The reported results suggest that depleted attentional resources may result in generally poorer encoding of episodes in the case of both young adults under conditions of DA at encoding and older adults. The further differentially poorer performance in tests requiring associative information seems to be uniquely related to the effects of age, but not to the effects of DA.

Acknowledgements

This research was supported in part by grants from the Ben-Gurion University Faculty of Humanities and Social Sciences and the Zlotowski Center for the Neurosciences. I am grateful to members of the memory research group at Ben-Gurion University of the Negev for their help in conducting the research, and to Fergus Craik for his helpful comments on earlier version of this chapter. Part of this chapter was written while I was a visiting scientist at the Rotman Research Institute, Baycrest Centre for Geriatric Care, Toronto, Canada.

References

Anderson, J.R. and and Bower G.H. (1973). *Human Associative Memory*. Washington, DC.: V.H. Winston.

Anderson, N.D., Craik, F.I.M., and Naveh-Benjamin, M. (1998). The attentional demands of encoding and retrieval in younger and older adults. I: Evidence from divided attention costs. *Psychology and Aging*, **13**, 405–423.

Anderson, N.D., Iidaka, T., Cabeza, R., Kapur, S., McIntosh, A.R., and Craik, F.I.M. (2000). The effects of divided attention on encoding- and retrieval-related brain activity: a PET study of younger and older adults. *Journal of Cognitive Neuroscience*, **12**, 775–792.

Atkinson, R.C. and Shiffrin, R.M. (1968). Human memory: a proposed system and its control processes. In The *Psychology of Learning and Motivation: Advances in Research and Theory*, Vol. 2 (ed K.W. Spence and J.T. Spence). New York: Academic Press.

Baddeley, A.D., Lewis, V., Eldridge, M., and Thomson, N. (1984). Attention and retrieval from long-term memory. *Journal of Experimental Psychology: General*, **13**, 518–540.

Bayen, U.J., Phelps, M.P., and Spaniol, J. (2000). Age-related differences in the use of contextual information in recognition memory: a global matching approach. *Journal of Gerontology, Series B, Psychological Sciences and Social Sciences*, **55**, 131–141.

Birren, J.E., Cunningham, W.R., and Yamamoto, K. (1983). Psychology of adult development and aging. *Annual Review of Psychology*, **34**, 543–575.

Castel, A. and Craik, F.I.M. (2003). The effects of aging and divided attention on memory for item and associative information. *Psychology and Aging*, **18**, 873–885.

Chalfonte, B.L. and Johnson, M.K. (1996). Feature memory and binding in young and older adults. *Memory and Cognition*, **24**, 403–416.

Cohen, G. (1979). Language comprehension in old age. *Cognitive Psychology*, **11**, 412–429.

Cohen, N.J. and Eichenbaum, H. (1993). *Memory, Amnesia, and the Hippocampal System.* Cambridge, MA: MIT Press.

Craik, F.I.M. (1982). Selective changes in encoding as a function of reduced processing capacity. In *Cognitive Research in Psychology* (ed F. Klix, J. Hoffman, and E. Van der Meer). Berlin: DVW, pp. 152–161.

Craik, F.I.M. (1983). On the transfer of information from temporary to permanent memory. *Philosophical Transaction of the Royal Society of London, Series B, Biological Sciences*, **302**, 341–359.

Craik, F.I.M. (1986). A functional account of age differences in memory. In *Human Memory and Cognitive Capabilities, Mechanisms and Performance* (ed F. Klix and H. Hagendorf). Amsterdam: North-Holland, pp. 409–422.

Craik, F.I.M. and Byrd, M. (1982). Aging and cognitive deficits: the role of attentional resources. In *Aging and Cognitive Processes* (ed F.I.M. Craik and S.E. Trehub). New York: Plenum Press, pp. 191–211.

Craik F.I.M. and Kester, J.D. (2000). Divided attention and memory: impairment of processing or consolidation? In *Memory, Consciousness, and Brain* (ed E. Tulving). Philadelphia, PA: Psychology Press.

Craik, F.I.M. and McDowd, J. M. (1987). Age differences in recall and recognition. *Journal of Experimental Psychology: Learning, Memory, and Cognition*, **13**, 474–479.

Craik, F.I.M. and Simon, E. (1980). Age differences in memory: the roles of attention and depth of processing. In *New Directions in Memory and Aging* (ed L.W. Poon, J.L. Fozard, L.S. Cermak, D. Arenberg, and L.W. Thomson), pp. 95–112. Hillsdale, NJ: Erlbaum.

Craik, F.I.M., Govoni, R., Naveh-Benjamin, M., and Anderson, N.D. (1996). The effects of divided attention on encoding and retrieval processes in human memory. *Journal of Experimental Psychology: General*, **125**, 159–180.

Fletcher, P.C., Frith, C.D., Grasby, P.M., Shallice, T., Frackowiak, R.S., and Dulan, R.J. (1995). Brain systems for encoding and retrieval of auditory–verbal memory: an *in vivo* study in humans. *Brain*, **118**, 401–416.

Gillund, G. and Shiffrin, R.M. (1984). A retrieval model for both recognition and recall. *Psychological Review*, **91**, 1–67.

Glisky, E.L., Rubin, S.R., and Davidson, P.S.R. (2001). Source memory in older adults: an encoding or retrieval problem? *Journal of Experimental Psychology: Learning, Memory, and Cognition*, **27**, 1131–1146.

Gronlund, S.D. and Ratcliff, R. (1989). Time course of item and associative information: implications for global memory models. *Journal of Experimental Psychology: Learning, Memory, and Cognition*, **15**, 846–858.

Hasher, L. and Zacks, R.T. (1988). Working memory, comprehension, and aging: a review and a new view. In *The Psychology of Learning and Motivation: Advances in Research and Theory*, Vol. 22 (ed G.H. Bower). San Diego, CA: Academic Press.

Hashtroudi, S., Johnson, M.K., and Chrosniak, L.D. (1990). Aging and qualitative characteristics of memories for perceived and imagined complex events. *Psychology and Aging*, **5**, 119–126.

Hay, J.F. and Jacoby, L.L. (1999). Separating habit and recollection in young and older adults: effects of elaborative processing and distinctiveness. *Psychology and Aging*, **14**, 122–134.

Hess, T.M., Donley, J., and Vandermaas, M.O. (1989). Aging-related changes in the processing and retention of script information. *Experimental Aging Research*, **15**, 89–96.

Hockley, W.E. (1991). Recognition memory for item and associative information: a comparison of forgetting rates. In *Relating Theory and Data: Essays on Human Memory in Honor of Bennet B. Murdock* (ed W.E. Hockley and S. Lewandowsky). Hillsdale, NJ: Erlbaum, pp. 227–248.

Hockley, W.E. (1992). Item versus associative information: further comparisons of forgetting rates. *Journal of Experimental Psychology: Learning, Memory, and Cognition*, **18**, 1321–1330.

Hockley, W.E. (1994). Reflections of the mirror effect for item and associative recognition. *Memory and Cognition*, **22**, 713–722.

Hockley, W.E. and Crisi, C. (1996). Tests of encoding tradeoffs between item and associative information. *Memory and Cognition*, **24**, 202–216.

Humphreys, M.S. (1976). Relational information and the context effect in recognition memory. *Memory and Cognition*, **4**, 221–232.

Jennings, J.M. and Jacoby, L.L. (1993). Automatic versus intentional use of memory: Aging, attention, and control. *Psychology and Aging*, **8**, 283–293.

Johnson, M.K. (1992). MEM: mechanisms of recollection. *Journal of Cognitive Neuroscience*, **4**, 268–280.

Johnson, M.K. and Chalfonte, B.L. (1994). Binding complex memories: the role of reactivation and the hippocampus. In *Memory Systems 1994* (ed D.L. Schacter and E. Tulving). Cambridge, MA: MIT Press, pp. 311–350.

Kapur, S., Craik, F.I.M., Tulving, E., Wilson, A.A., Houle, S., and Brown, G.M. (1994). Neuroanatomical correlates of encoding in episodic memory: levels of processing effect. *Proceedings of the National Academy of Sciences of the United States of America*, **91**, 2008–2011.

Li, S-C, Naveh-Benjamin, M., and Lindenberger, U. (2005). Modeling aging deficits of associative binding. *Psychological Science*, **16**, 445–450.

Light, L.L. (1991). Memory and aging: four hypotheses in search of data. *Annual Review of Psychology*, **43**, 333–376.

MacKay, D.G. and Burke, D.M. (1990). Cognition and aging: a theory of new learning and the use of old connections. In *Aging and Cognition: New Knowledge Organization and Utilization* (ed T.M. Hess). Amsterdam: Elsevier, pp. 213–263.

McIntyre, J.S. and Craik, F.I.M. (1987). Age differences in memory for item and source information. *Canadian Journal of Psychology*, **41**, 175–192.

Mandler, G.D. (1979). Organization and repetition: an extension of organization principles with special reference to rote learning. In *Perspectives on memory research* (ed L.G. Nilsson). Hillsdale, NJ: Erlbaum, pp. 293–327.

Mitchell, K.J., Johnson, M.K., Raye, C.L., and D'Esposito, M. (2000a). FMRI evidence of age related hippocampal dysfunction in feature binding in working memory. *Cognitive Brain Research*, **10**, 197–206.

Mitchell, K.J., Johnson, M.K., Raye, C.L., Mather, M., and D'Esposito, M. (2000b). Aging and reflective processes of working memory: binding and test load deficits. *Psychology and Aging*, **15**, 527–541.

Moscovitch, M. (1992). Memory and working-with-memory: a component process model based on modules and central systems. *Journal of Cognitive Neuroscience*, **4**, 257–267.

Murdock, B.B., Jr (1965). Effects of a subsidiary task on short-term memory. *British Journal of Psychology*, **56**, 413–419.

Murdock, B.B., Jr (1982). A theory of storage and retrieval of item and associative information. *Psychological Review*, **89**, 609–626.

Murdock, B.B. (1993). TODAM2: A model for the storage and retrieval of item, associative, and serial-order information. *Psychological Review*, **100**, 183–203.

Naveh-Benjamin, M. (1987). Coding of spatial location information: an automatic process? *Journal of Experimental Psychology: Learning, Memory, and Cognition*, **13**, 595–605.

Naveh-Benjamin, M. (1988). Recognition of spatial location information: another failure to support automaticity. *Memory and Cognition*, **16**, 437–445.

Naveh-Benjamin, M. (1990). Coding of temporal order information: an automatic process? *Journal of Experimental Psychology: Learning, Memory, and Cognition*, **16**, 117–126.

Naveh-Benjamin, M. (2000). Adult-age differences in memory performance: tests of an associative deficit hypothesis. *Journal of Experimental Psychology: Learning, Memory, and Cognition*, **26**, 1170–1187.

Naveh-Benjamin, M. (2002). The effects of divided attention on encoding processes: underlying mechanisms. In *Perspectives on Human Memory and Cognitive Aging* (ed M. Naveh-Benjamin, M. Moscovitch, and H.L. Roediger III). Philadelphia, PA: Psychology Press.

Naveh-Benjamin, M. and Guez, J. (2000). Effects of divided attention on encoding and retrieval processes: assessment of attentional costs and a componential analysis. *Journal of Experimental Psychology: Learning, Memory, and Cognition*, **26**, 1461–1482.

Naveh-Benjamin, M. and Jonides, J. (1986). On the automaticity of frequency coding: effects of competing task load, encoding strategy, and intention. *Journal of Experimental Psychology: Learning, Memory, and Cognition*, **12**, 378–386.

Naveh-Benjamin, M., Craik, F.I.M., Guez, J,. and Dori, H. (1998). Effects of divided attention on encoding and retrieval processes in human memory: further support for an asymmetry. *Journal of Experimental Psychology: Learning, Memory, and Cognition*, **24**, 1091–1104.

Naveh-Benjamin, M., Craik, F.I.M, Gavrilescu, D., and Anderson, N. (2000a). Asymmetry between encoding and retrieval processes: evidence from a divided attention paradigm and a calibration analysis. *Memory and Cognition*, **28**, 965–976.

Naveh-Benjamin, M., Craik, F.I.M., Perratta, J., and Tonev, S. (2000b). The effects of divided attention on encoding and retrieval processes: the resiliency of retrieval processes. *Quarterly Journal of Experimental Psychology*, **53**, 609–626.

Naveh-Benjamin, M., Guez, J., and Marom, M. (2003a). The effects of divided attention on item and associative memory. *Memory and Cognition*, **31**, 1021–1035.

Naveh-Benjamin, M., Hussain, Z., Guez, J., and Bar-On, M. (2003b). Adult-age differences in episodic memory: further support for an associative deficit hypothesis. *Journal of Experimental Psychology: Learning, Memory, and Cognition*, **29**, 826–837.

Naveh-Benjamin, M., Guez, J., Kilb, A., and Reedy, S. (2004a). The associative deficit of older adults: further support using face–name associations. *Psychology and Aging*, **19**, 541–546.

Naveh-Benjamin, M., Guez, J., and Shulman, S. (2004b). Older adults' associative deficit in episodic memory: assessing the role of decline in attentional resources. *Psychonomic Bulletin and Review*, **11**, 1067–1073.

Naveh-Benjamin, M., Kilb, A., and and Fisher, T. Concurrent task effects on memory encoding and retrieval: further support for an asymmetry. *Memory and Cognition*, in press.

Naveh-Benjamin, M., Guez, J., and Sorek, S. The effects of divided attention on encoding processes in memory: mapping the locus of interference, submitted.

Naveh-Benjamin, M., Guez, J., and Drizen. *The effects of type of secondary task on memory for items and associations*, in preparation.

Perlmutter, M. (1978). What is memory the aging of? *Developmental Psychology*, **14**, 330–345.

Rabinowitz, J.C., Craik, F.I.M., and Ackerman, B.P. (1982). A processing resource account of age differences in recall. *Canadian Journal of Psychology*, **36**, 325–344.

Rizzuto, D.S. and Kahana, M.F. (2001). An autoassociative neural network of paired-associative learning. *Neural Computation*, **13**, 2075–2092.

Salthouse, T.A. (1991). *Theoretical Perspective on Cognitive Aging*. Hillsdale, NJ: Erlbaum.

Salthouse, T.A. (1996). The processing-speed theory of adult age differences in cognition. *Psychological Review*, **103**, 403–428.

Spencer, W.O. and Raz, N. (1995). Differential effects of aging on memory for content and context: a meta-analysis. *Psychology and Aging*, **10**, 527–539.

Treisman, A. and Gelade, A. (1980). A feature intergration theory of attention. *Cognitive Psychology*, **12**, 97–136.

Tulving, E. and Thomson, D.M. (1973). Encoding specificity and retrieval processes in episodic memory. *Psychological Review*, **80**, 352–373.

Underwood, B.J. (1969). Attributes of memory. *Psychological Review*, **76**, 559–573.

Chapter 26

Binding of source and content: new directions revealed by neuropsychological and age-related effects

Mark A. McDaniel, Karin M. Butler, and Courtney C. Dornburg

Introduction

The experimental study of memory has for the most part focused on remembering the occurrence of an event. In much research these events typically are the words presented in a list (Craik and Tulving 1975; McDaniel and Masson 1977; Roediger 1980), short prose passages (Einstein *et al.* 1984; Roediger and Wheeler 1993; McDaniel *et al.* 1994), or pictures (Madigan 1983). However, many researchers have begun to consider memory for the source of an event—the 'when', 'where', and 'how' of an event. For instance, studies have examined memory for the temporal differentiation of items ('when') (Underwood and Malmi 1978) and the particular list in which a word appeared (Winograd 1968; Hintzman *et al.* 1973). Others have examined the spatial location in which an item was presented ('where') (Chalfonte and Johnson 1996; Naveh-Benjamin 1987; Glisky *et al.* 2001, Experiment 2; Ellis 1990; Macklin and McDaniel 2005). Finally, some studies have looked at the 'how'—memory for perceptual modality (Durso and Johnson 1980; Belli *et al.* 1994), memory for type font (Naveh-Benjamin and Craik 1995), and memory for the particular speakers who presented the items (Jurica and Shimamura 1999; Dodson and Shimamura 2000; Glisky *et al.* 2001).

The distinction between occurrence information and source information underlies the observation that complete and accurate episodic memory depends not only on memory for an event's occurrence but also on memory for its source, i.e. memory failures can be described in which events are well remembered but their source is not. In one kind of failure, misleading information that is presented subsequent to the original event is falsely remembered as the original event (Loftus 1992). In this memory illusion the original event is not necessarily forgotten, but the sources of the misleading information and the original event become confused (Lindsay and Johnson 1989). In another paradigm, subjects are given lists of associatively related words (bed, rest, awake, dream) that are derived from a common associate (sleep) which is omitted from the list (Deese 1959; Roediger and McDermott 1995). Subjects show robust false recall and false recognition of the non-presented but associatively related word, at least partly because subjects fail to remember that the source of the non-presented item was an internal associative response to the presented items (McEvoy *et al.* 1999; Roediger *et al.* 2001).

In a third kind of memory illusion, people fail to distinguish accurately between actions that they performed and actions that they thought about or imagined. Here again, the occurrence of the event is remembered, but the source of the event is forgotten or confused so that people are said to fail at reality monitoring (Johnson *et al.* 1993). It is this type of memory illusion on which we focus in the present chapter, primarily from the perspective of age-related changes and neuropsychological correlates. We use these aspects as leverage points to begin to explore and illuminate the factors that influence binding of these two major aspects of memory content: event occurrence and event source. The basic and non-controversial idea here is that completely accurate episodic memory requires some binding of occurrence and source features so that the source of the event's occurrence can be accurately identified (Chalfonte and Johnson 1996; Naveh-Benjamin 2000; Glisky *et al.* 2001). However, the factors and processes that support binding remain an entirely open question. After presenting some findings on ageing and source memory for actions, including a new experiment that incorporates a neuropsychological approach, we end the chapter by proposing a new dual-level framework of source memory and binding. First, however, we briefly describe the action memory paradigm (Engelkamp and Krumnacker 1980; Cohen 1981; Saltz and Donnenwerth-Nolan 1981), which has provided the foundation for our work on memory illusions in which imagined actions are believed to have been performed.

A basic characteristic of the action memory paradigm is that the target materials are short descriptions of mini-tasks, which are typically verb–object phrases. Examples are 'smoke the pipe', 'open the book', and 'lift the hat'. The set of mini-task descriptions are unrelated and are presented in lists that participants listen to, usually with the intent of learning the list of phrases. Another essential characteristic is that one encoding condition requires participants to perform the stated action. In our work, paralleling others, this enactment is performed with real objects. A variety of other encoding conditions can be implemented as comparisons with the self-performed condition (for details see Engelkamp 1998). For our purposes, the other encoding condition of interest instructs participants to imagine another actor performing the tasks (Engelkamp *et al.* 1989; Denis *et al.* 1991). Finally, when these two encoding activities are varied within-subjects, participants can be required to make two kinds of recognition judgments during testing. Participants can judge whether a phrase occurred in the study list, and also judge whether it was originally enacted or only imagined (Ecker and Engelkamp 1995). It is this kind of recognition task within the action memory paradigm that we further develop and investigate in order to explore factors that are involved in the binding of an event with its source.

Source memory for actions

Several studies have examined memory for whether actions were enacted or only imagined and found that, much like recall measures, memory for performing an action is better than memory for imagining an action and that this difference between memory for encoding condition is larger for older than for younger adults (Guttentag and Hunt 1988; Cohen and Faulkner 1989; Lee 2000). Of particular concern is whether imagining an action can lead someone to later misremember performing the action (Garry *et al.* 1996; Goff and Roediger 1998). After performing, imagining, or listening to simple action statements, Goff and Roediger (1998) asked participants to indicate how many times they had performed the actions. They found a memory illusion such that imagined actions were identified as performed. In addition, this illusion increased with repeated imagining of the action, i.e. an imagination inflation effect.

In the remainder of this chapter we focus on age-related changes in source memory for actions and possible neuropsychological correlates of these changes. Our focus is prompted by both theoretical and practical concerns. From a theoretical perspective, by examining neuropsychological correlates of source memory performance, we hope to gain a better understanding of the systems that subserve binding and source monitoring. This theme will be developed below in the context of a new experiment that we report.

From a practical perspective, older adults face critical memory demands in health-related activities that require accurate source memory for whether an event was enacted or thought about (imagined). As one salient example, a third of older adults take three or more medications daily (Park and Kidder 1996). It seems plausible that, throughout the day, one could think about taking one medication, have taken another medication, and perhaps both thought about and taken a third medication. This situation seems ripe for producing two kinds of source errors: remembering that an imagined action was performed, and remembering that a performed action was merely thought about. Either kind of source error could lead to medication adherence problems. Misremembering taking a medication that one only thought about taking could lead to undermedication, whereas misremembering that one only thought about taking a medication that was actually taken could lead to overmedication (see McDaniel and Einstein (in press) for experimental demonstrations of such behaviours in habitual prospective memory paradigms). Accordingly, it is important to understand the influence of ageing on source memory in this kind of context.

Lee (2000) examined whether older adults are more susceptible to both of these types of source memory errors than young adults. In a variation of Goff and Roediger's (1998) paradigm, Lee (Experiment 1) found that older adults were more likely to misremember that a simple imagined action had been performed than younger adults, but the effect of repeated imaginings was no greater for old adults than for young adults. Related to the real-world scenario above, these types of source errors might lead to undermedication, especially for older adults. In Experiment 2, Lee addressed whether performing an action might lead to judgements of imagining the action. When given the opportunity, young and older adults indicated incorrectly that actions that had only been performed were imagined. As with the source errors for imagined actions, repeatedly performing an action statement increased this memory error as well. This suggests that source errors leading to overmedication could also occur. However, the likelihood of source errors for performed actions did not differ between the age groups, i.e. the source judgements of older adults were more error prone than the source judgements of younger adults only for action phrases that were imagined, and not for actions that were performed. One initial explanation of these data is that the older adults in Lee's sample were relatively high in frontal functioning, thereby attenuating robust age-related decline in source memory.

Frontal functioning and source memory

Reports of age-related declines in accuracy of source memory for a variety of source information are common in the literature (Glisky *et al.* 1995, 2001; Naveh-Benjamin and Craik 1995; Spencer and Raz 1995; Henkel *et al.* 1998). From a theoretical perspective, these age-related deficits are consistent with the general view that source encoding and binding are dependent on prefrontal systems, as prefrontal decline seems to be a hallmark of normal ageing (West 1996; Raz 2000). Supporting this frontal theory of source memory, in a series of experiments Glisky and her colleagues found that older adults with high frontal functioning scores (based on the neuropsychological tests described below) showed significantly higher source memory performance (for speakers' voices, location of pictured objects) than older adults with low frontal functioning scores. To extend these findings and directly test the frontal theory of source memory in the context of imagination inflation, in conjunction with Amanda Price we conducted a new experiment that distinguished between older adults with relatively high frontal functioning and those with relatively low frontal functioning. Because this new study has not been reported elsewhere, we describe it here in some detail.

A new experiment

Following the work just mentioned, we assessed the frontal functioning of older adults using a composite measure based on five neuropsychological tests that individually have been assumed to tap some aspect of frontal functioning (Glisky *et al.* 1995, 2001; McDaniel *et al.* 1999): modified Wisconsin Card Sort Test (number of categories), verbal fluency, arithmetic from the Wechsler Adult Intelligence Scale Revised (WAIS-R), digit span backwards from the Wechsler Memory Scale III (WMS-III), and mental control from the WMS-III. In factor analyses, Glisky *et al.* (1995) confirmed that these five tests loaded together on a single factor and, further, that they did not load on another factor comprised of tests presumably tapping medial temporal processes. Moreover, Butler *et al.* (2004) reported that this composite measure of frontal functioning, but not each individual measure (except for arithmetic), was reliably sensitive to differences in the performance of older adults on word list recall. From the pool of older adults for whom we collected the neuropsychological assessments, we identified 16 low frontal function (FF) older adults (low FF, $M = -0.825$) with below-average composite scores (according to the normative baseline established in Glisky's laboratory) and 18 high frontal function older adults (high FF, $M = 0.357$) with above-average composite scores. We also included 17 young adults aged between 18 and 31 years in the study.

The experimental procedure was patterned after Lee's (2000) work. A set of action statements was assembled for which most of the actions were performed on one object, the action was typical for that object, and the objects were small and familiar (e.g. 'roll the car across the table'). This set was divided into four subsets of action statements, of which three were presented at study and one was used as new statements for the testing phase. At study, some actions were performed once, twice, or four times, some actions were imagined once, twice, or four times, and some actions were both imagined and performed (either once imagined and once performed or twice imagined and twice performed). (Note that the four subsets of action statements were counterbalanced across these different conditions.) Two weeks later, participants returned for a test on the action statements. The entire set of action statements was presented and participants had to indicate how many times they 'did' the action and how many times they 'imagined' the action, using a response range of 0–8.

Based on the theory that frontal processes subserve encoding and/or binding of source features to event occurrence, we expected that high FF older adults would show more accurate memory for the source of the action statements than low FF older adults. Alternatively, a number of researchers propose that the medial temporal system plays a key role in binding features into complex memories, with these features including inter-item associations as well as context (source) information (Henkel *et al.* 1998; Isaac and Mayes 1999; Naveh-Benjamin 2000) (see also O'Reilly and Rudy (2001) for work supporting medial temporal involvement in context binding for non-human animals). From this perspective, there should be little variation in the performance of older adults across high and low FF groups (assuming that the quality of the information provided to the medial temporal system is not affected by frontal functioning).

The data allowed a rich set of analyses for comprehensively testing these predictions, including source errors for imagined and performed actions and item memory. We report each measure of performance in turn by first comparing the younger and older adults and then examining whether the low and high FF groups differed. In all cases the α level for determining statistical significance was set at $P < 0.05$.

Source memory errors for imagined actions

We first examined source memory errors for the imagined actions. For the imagined actions, a source memory error occurred whenever participants provided a non-zero value (i.e. any response within the 1–8 range) for how many times they 'did' the action. These responses were analysed in two ways: all non-zero responses were simply tabulated as a 'did' response, and each frequency judgement was retained and tabulated. Figure 26.1 shows the mean proportion of 'did' responses to action statements that were only imagined as a function of group (young, high

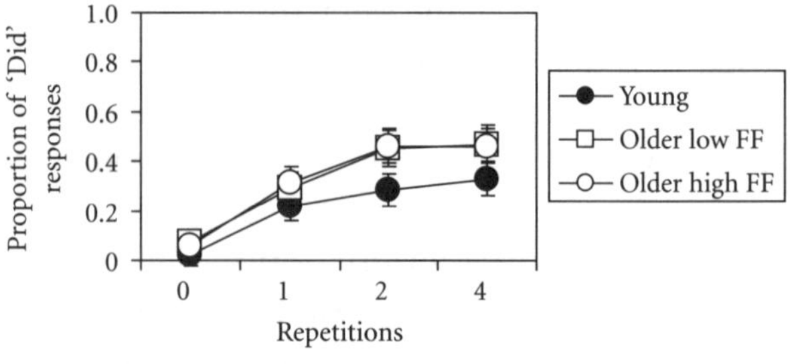

Figure 26.1 Mean proportion of 'did' responses to imagined items.

FF old, low FF old). Older adults incorrectly indicated that an imagined action had been performed 41 per cent of the time, whereas younger adults made this error only 28 per cent of the time ($F(1, 49) = 4.56$, MSE $= 0.13$). The likelihood of incorrectly indicating that an action had been done increased with the number of repetitions (26 per cent, 37 per cent, and 40 per cent errors for actions imagined once, twice, and four times, respectively) ($F(2, 98) = 5.67$, MSE $= 0.04$), but the number of repetitions did not interact with age group ($F < 1$). There was no difference in the likelihood of this type of error between the low and high FF groups ($F < 1$). Correlational analyses similarly revealed that FF scores were not predictive of these incorrect 'did' responses (r-values of -0.05, 0.09, and -0.04 for actions imagined once, twice, and four times, respectively).

The second analysis of source errors to imagined items focused on the judgements for the number of times performed for the actions that had only been imagined. The outcome of this analysis directly paralleled the error analyses above. Young adults gave lower frequency judgements for actions that were only imagined (0.51) compared with older adults (0.85) ($F(1, 49) = 3.40$, MSE $= 1.10$, $P = 0.07$). These frequency judgements became larger as the number of times the item was imagined increased (0.38, 0.73, and 0.93 times performed for actions imagined once, twice, and four times, respectively) ($F(2, 98) = 12.59$, MSE $= 0.28$). Age group did not interact with the number of repetitions ($F < 1$). Again, there was no difference in the frequency judgements given by the low and high FF groups ($F < 1$).

Source memory errors for performed actions

Source memory errors were also made when individuals incorrectly indicated that an action had been imagined when, in fact, it had only been performed. These responses were analysed in two ways as above: all non-zero responses for the number of times imagined were tabulated as an 'imagined' response, and each frequency judgement was retained and tabulated. Figure 26.2 shows the mean proportion of imagined responses to action statements that were only

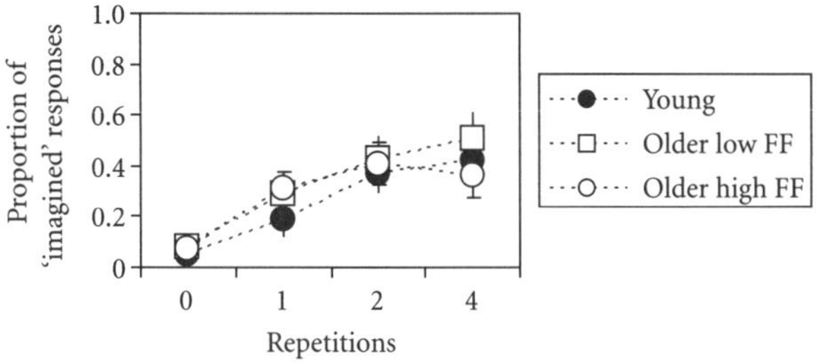

Figure 26.2 Mean proportion of 'imagined' responses to performed items.

performed as a function of group (young, high FF old, low FF old). Unlike source errors for imagined actions, the difference between the younger adults (33 per cent) and the older adults (38 per cent) in the likelihood of erroneously judging performed actions to have been imagined was not significant ($F < 1$). As the number of repetitions of these performed items increased, the items were more likely to be judged incorrectly as imagined (25 per cent, 40 per cent, and 43 per cent errors for items performed once, twice, and four times, respectively) ($F(2, 98) = 14.14$, MSE = 0.03). Age group did not interact with repetitions ($F < 1$). These patterns replicate Lee's (2000) findings. Importantly, the FF groups did not differ in the likelihood of making this kind of source memory error for performed actions ($F < 2.2$). Correlational analyses similarly revealed that FF scores were not predictive of incorrect imagined responses (r-values of −0.01, −0.07, and −0.17 for actions performed once, twice, and four times, respectively). Thus this finding refutes our preliminary idea that the finding in Lee's Experiment 2 of no age differences on incorrect imagined responses to performed actions reflected a sample of older adults with relatively high frontal functioning.

The judgements of the number of times imagined for actions that had only been performed also indicated no age difference in source memory errors for performed actions. Younger adults (0.43) and older adults (0.60) did not significantly differ in their frequency judgements ($F < 1.6$). Increasing repetitions of performed actions increased the frequency of imaging judgements for the actions (0.36, 0.59, and 0.60 times imagined for items performed once, twice, and four times, respectively) ($F(2, 98) = 7.55$, MSE = 0.10). Age group did not interact with repetitions ($F < 1$).

When only the two older adult groups were compared on the frequency of imagining judgements given to performed actions, the low (0.62) and high (0.59) FF groups did not differ in their frequency judgements ($F < 1$). However, unlike the error analysis, FF group did interact with repetitions ($F(2, 64) = 4.54$, MSE = 0.11). Whereas the frequency of imagining judgements of the low FF group increased as the number of repetitions increased (0.38, 0.66, and 0.82 times imagined for items performed once, twice, and four times, respectively), the frequency judgements of the high FF group declined from the two- to the four-repetition condition (0.55, 0.69, and 0.52 times imagined for items performed once, twice, and four times, respectively).

Item memory

Memory for the action statements was examined by ignoring whether the source attribution was correct or not. Younger adults remembered more of the statements (86 per cent) than did the older adults (74 per cent) ($F(1, 49) = 12.60$, MSE $= 0.08$) and performed actions were remembered better (85 per cent) than imagined actions (75 per cent) ($F(1, 49) = 24.73$, MSE $= 0.02$). These two variables did not interact ($F < 1$). When the two groups of older adults (high FF and low FF) were compared there was no effect of FF and no interaction with study condition or number of repetitions ($F < 1.6$).

Discussion

Item memory

Dovetailing with Engelkamp's fundamental work (e.g. Engelkamp 1998), performed actions were remembered better than imagined actions. Our findings reinforce the mnemonic potency of enactment encoding, showing that the self-performance effect emerged even after a delay of 2 weeks between study and test. In addition, we found that although older adults had a worse memory for performed and imagined actions than younger adults, the enactment effect was the same for both age groups (see also Lichty *et al.* 1986). On a recognition test following a 2-week delay, older adults benefited just as much as younger adults from performing an action.

Source memory

The results are interesting from both practical and theoretical perspectives. In everyday life, older adults encounter challenging source demands not unlike those presented here. As previously described, at least a third of older adults juggle complex prescription schedules involving memory for three or more daily medications. During the course of these medication regimes, medication-taking actions could be imagined, enacted, or both. If our results were to translate to medication behaviours, source memory problems for older adults could significantly interfere with their medication regime. For approximately 40 per cent of actions only performed, older adults incorrectly indicated that the action had been imagined, and the same level of confusion was found for actions only imagined. This confusion would be expected to play a role in increasing failure to maintain proper medication.

Although the example of daily medication behaviour involves shorter-term memory demands than explored in our research, health-related memory challenges might occur over longer retention intervals as well. For example, weeks after a doctor's appointment older adults may confuse information that they had thought about sharing with their physician (e.g. episodes involving shortness of breath, dizziness, chronic pain, etc.) with information that they did share during the doctor's visit. If so, this could lead to false assumptions about the maladies that are or are not being treated by the physician. More benign instances of everyday source challenges that may parallel our experiment include remembering whether thank-you notes for some event (some of which are thought about, some sent, and some thought about and sent) were sent or not. Our results suggest that, for both older adults and younger adults, reality-monitoring errors will not be uncommon in this instance.

We now turn to the theoretical implications of our results. The present task, requiring participants to make a judgement about whether an action phrase was enacted or imagined, is similar to other memory tasks commonly classified as source memory tests in which participants must judge whether an event was perceived or imagined. Our task also parallels a broader conceptualization of source as information involved in many-to-one mappings (Glisky *et al.* 2001). In typical studies of source memory, many items are mapped to a few (usually two) sources. The same held here; many action phrases were either enacted or imagined.

However, the current results diverge from previous findings in investigations of frontal processes in the source memory of healthy older adults. Other researchers have reported that the performance of older adults on source memory tasks is related to frontal functioning, with those adults with higher FF showing better source memory than those with lower FF (Craik *et al.* 1990; Glisky *et al.* 1995; Parkin *et al.* 1995). Somewhat unexpectedly, high FF older adults showed memory patterns remarkably similar to that of low FF older adults. For imagination inflation, high FF older adults had significant deficits relative to younger adults and a magnitude of decline equivalent to that shown by low FF older adults. In only one instance did high FF older adults appear to show more accurate source memory than low FF older adults; when an action was performed four times, high FF older adults judged that they had *imagined* the action fewer times than low FF older adults. Further, there were no significant age-related declines in the likelihood that performed actions would be incorrectly judged as imagined, even for low FF older adults (as indexed by the neuropsychological tests). If frontal lobes are involved in source memory (Glisky *et al.* 2001), how might we account for our results?

One potential factor that could contribute to discrepant outcomes regarding frontal contributions to source memory performance is the manner in which frontal functioning is assessed. One or two individual tests have often been used to assess 'frontal' functioning, with the instability of any individual test or restricted variability possibly producing different patterns (Spencer and Raz 1994; Henkel *et al.* 1998; Glisky *et al.* 2001). This was not the case here. We used the composite assessment of frontal functioning based on five tests developed and used by Glisky *et al.* (1995), as well as by Henkel *et al.* (1998), in reporting associations between frontal functioning and the source memory of older adults. Further, we used the same normative group of older adults used by Glisky to determine the composite scores.

However, it might be argued that the differentiation between our low and high FF groups (i.e. the cut-offs separating low from high FF groups) was not great enough to reveal frontally mediated differences in performance. This possibility can also be ruled out. We tested the same sample of younger adults, high FF older adults, and low FF older adults used in the present experiment in another false-memory experiment using the Deese–Roediger–McDermott (DRM) paradigm. In the DRM experiment we found patterns that converged nicely with the usual findings outlined above. The recall performance of high FF older adults was equivalent to that of younger adults and significantly better than low FF older adults (higher veridical recall and lower false recall) (Butler *et al.*, 2004). Thus, in terms of free recall, our findings were in line with the expected relation between frontal functioning and performance (Shimamura 1995).

Perhaps the virtual absence of a relation between frontal functioning and source memory in older adults rests on the increased demands of our source judgement task. Unlike other paradigms, a proportion of the items was presented with both sources (imagined and performed), thus complicating the source decision with the possibility that a target item could have been both imagined and performed, instead of the usual source judgement restricted to one or the other. The idea here is that even high FF older adults do not have the capability to remember source under such demands. However, task difficulty *per se* does not seem to be the critical factor articulating with the relation between frontal functioning and performance. In a clever experiment, Glisky *et al.* (2001, Experiment 1) made the more difficult voice judgement task the item test and the sentence content task the source test. When sentence content (believed to be somewhat easier to encode) was the source test, low FF older adults showed impairment relative to high FF older adults, and performed no better than chance. These same low FF older adults improved to the levels of the high FF older adults when the task was the item memory test, even though that test now involved memory for voice—information ostensibly difficult to encode.

Thus our results are puzzling in light of the 'consensus that the FL's [frontal lobes] are in some way involved in source memory' (Glisky *et al.* 2001, p. 1132; Chalfonte and Johnson 1996). Our results may instead point towards the general perspective that source memory processes, including binding of source to content, are more complicated than can be accommodated by either a frontal explanation (Spencer and Raz 1994) or, more generally, by an explanation based on any single system dedicated to source (Henkel *et al.* 1998; Naveh-Benjamin 2000).

One possibility is that both medial temporal and frontal systems play critical roles in source memory. Henkel *et al.* (1998) suggest that medial temporal regions are important for binding features into complex memories. Assuming that age-related decline in the hippocampal (medial temporal structures) system is not as prominent in normal ageing as is frontal decline (West 1996; Raz 2000), our findings of no age-related deficits in source memory in some cases (no significant age-related deficits in confusing performed items as imagined) dovetail with this idea of medial temporal involvement in binding and source memory.

Henkel *et al.* (1998) also proposed that the frontal regions are important in source memory for more effortful or strategic retrieval and for more complex evaluative processes regarding the source-related features that are retrieved. In support of this idea, they report that for immediate source memory tests (15-min delay), frontal scores (the same as those used in our experiment) did not correlate with older adults' source memory but medial temporal scores did. However, when tested after a 2-day delay, older adults' source memory was correlated with frontal scores (as well as medial temporal scores). Presumably reactivation of the source information would be less effortful on the immediate test and thus would only require medial temporal structures, whereas on the delayed test more strategic and evaluative processes would be required—processes subserved by frontal regions.

Our results cannot be completely accounted for even within this more complex source-monitoring framework. Because our source judgements were collected at a delay considerably longer than the 2-day delay used by Henkel *et al.* (1998), and given the high potential for source confusion in our paradigm (source testing for actions that could be imagined, enacted, or both), this source monitoring account would expect a significant role for frontal regions. Similarly, in our false recall experiment (Butler *et al.* 2004), performance was tested immediately after study, and thus frontal involvement might have been minimized in the source monitoring involved in that illusion. As described above and in Butler *et al.* (2004), our results were the opposite of these expectations. Thus there may be an even more complex set of parameters that are involved in determining the contribution of the medial temporal and frontal systems to source memory. In the next section we amplify this idea, focusing on refining the notion of source, and then we apply our conceptualization to account for the apparent discrepancy between the previous work implicating frontal processes in source memory with the patterns reported here.

A dual-level framework of source memory and binding

In nearly all instances in the experimental literature, source information is incidental, irrelevant, or peripheral to the target content and the significance of the content in the experimental context (for an exception see Rahhal *et al.* 2002). For instance, in the study by Glisky *et al.* (2001), the voice of the speaker presenting sentences that are to be rated on semantic dimensions is irrelevant to the task in hand. Similarly, the room in which a chair appears (in photographs) is peripheral to the task of rating how comfortable the chair is likely to be. We suggest that constraining source (context) information to that which is irrelevant or peripheral (or unimportant, Rahhal *et al.* 2002) is probably overly restrictive and not entirely reflective of the range of possibilities found in everyday experience. For instance, the voice of a speaker (its gender, timbre, prosody, and so on) may be relevant to the content of a message that carries emotional or romantic overtones. Similarly, when assessing the comfort level of a chair in real-world settings, the location of the chair (its source) and other contextual features may not be peripheral.

Building on the above notion, we further suggest that the neuropsychological systems involved in source memory will depend, at least in part, on the degree to which the target source information is relevant or pertinent to the target content information. In line with the modal findings in the literature, our working framework is that memory for source information that is non-focal or peripheral to the content will depend on frontal processes. In contrast, memory for source information that is relevant or pertinent to the content will depend on medial temporal processes. This assumption that the medial temporal structures are involved in source–content binding dovetails with both animal and human work. In the animal literature, researchers have demonstrated that rats can acquire conditioned fear of a particular cage (sources or contexts) by being exposed to shock in that cage. A series of clever studies involving lesion and drug techniques has established that the binding of the animal's representation of the context with the experience of shock is mediated by the hippocampal (medial temporal) structures (O'Reilly and Rudy 2001; Rudy *et al.* 2004). In human work with neuropsychological patients with medial temporal damage, associative binding of various features seems to be impaired (Isaac and Mayes 1999) and many models of human memory assume that medial temporal structures subserve associative binding of information (Moscovitch 1992), including source with content (Chalfonte and Johnson 1996; Henkel *et al.* 1998; Isaac and Mayes 1999).

Our idea is that memory for source information that is pertinent to the focal task will be mediated primarily by medial temporal binding functions, whereas source information that is peripheral or irrelevant to the focal task will require frontal involvement at least for encoding the source (Glisky *et al.* 2001), if not also for binding that source with content (cf. Naveh-Benjamin 2000). This idea has the general flavour of previous conceptualizations that posit different domains of source information and/or that both medial temporal and frontal structures are involved in associative binding of information. However, the present formulation is different from previous conceptualizations on some dimensions.

Spencer and Raz (1995) proposed a distinction between stimulus-bound source features like auditory qualities, shape, or size and extra-stimulus source features like spatial location or temporal order. They suggest that age-related differences in stimulus-bound source features will not be amplified relative to age-related differences in content. In contrast, memory for extra-stimulus source features will pose special challenges for older adults. In its favour, this formulation is consistent with subsequent findings of Naveh-Benjamin and Craik (1995), investigating memory for speaker's voice and type font, and of Glisky *et al.* (2001), investigating memory for speaker's voice and spatial location. Our view takes this idea one step further by emphasizing that even stimulus-bound source features such as speaker's voice, type font, and so on are typically peripheral to the focal processing of content. Therefore memory for this kind of source information may rely on frontal processes that are at risk with age.

Naveh-Benjamin's (2000) basic dichotomy is that the medial temporal systems are responsible for relatively automatic encoding under incidental conditions, whereas the frontal lobes involve more effortful intentional processing of information. This analysis would not seem to capture the findings of Glisky *et al.* (2001, Experiments 3 and 4) which showed that instructions to attend to the source–content relation eliminated the source memory deficits of low FF older adults. Here, intentional processing of the information was not impaired by low frontal functioning.

Rather, the previous results and the new experiment reported in this chapter appear consistent with the idea that when the source is peripheral because of the orienting task or the ecological dynamics between the source and the content (i.e. the normal task of extracting semantic content from language may not ordinarily depend on the speaker's voice, type font, and other perceptual aspects of the source), frontal processes may be involved and required for the spontaneous noticing and incidental encoding of the relation of the source to the content. In these cases, there will be correlations between frontal functioning and source memory (Glisky *et al.* 2001, Experiments 1 and 2).

When the source is not peripheral, because of either the orienting task (e.g. intentional learning of source) or the nature of the source information in relation to the content, frontal processes will not be correlated with source memory.

In the new experiment reported in this chapter, the source of enacting or imaging modifies the content—it is part and parcel of the content. The action event when performed takes on additional features including motor programs involved in enactment, body postures, and kinaesthetic feedback. Indeed, it is the inclusion of these features in the encoding that provides the basis for explaining why subject-performed phrases are better remembered than phrases encoded in any other way (Engelkamp 2001). Thus we suggest that in this case medial temporal structures, not frontal structures, are more prominent in subserving source memory. The observations that medial temporal structures are believed to decline with age, but not as prominently as frontal structures (West 1996; Raz 2000), are compatible with our findings. After the 2-week delay, older adults showed some source memory impairment, as evidenced by more frequent source errors for imagined events, but this impairment was not consistent. Older adults were not significantly more likely than young adults to judge an enacted action as being imagined. These findings appear to be stable, as Lee (2000) reported an identical pattern.

The formulation outlined above might also help to account for the interaction in source memory between age and type of source reported by Rahhal *et al.* (2002). When the source was peripheral (speaker's voice) older adults' source memory was consistently worse than that of younger adults. Our idea is that significant age-related decline in frontal processes would be involved in this age-related source deficit. In contrast, when the source was important (character of the speaker), older and younger adults did not display significantly different levels of source memory. We assume that, for this more pertinent source information, medial temporal structures support source memory and that these structures are sufficiently intact in older adults to support the good performance reported by Rahhal *et al.*

Clearly, the framework just outlined is speculative and awaits further work. As a start, we are conducting an experiment that focuses on source information that is more peripheral (speaker's voice) and less peripheral (performing or imaging action events) within the same experiment and with the same target items. Also, we are assessing both frontal and medial temporal functioning scores. More generally, we have presented our new findings and theoretical ideas in the spirit of stimulating existing frameworks of memory and contributing ideas towards a more complete and fruitful understanding of the processes and systems that serve memory encoding and binding.

Acknowledgments

The preparation of this chapter and the experiment reported were supported by National Institute on Aging Grant AG17481 to Mark McDaniel and Roddy Roediger. We are grateful to the older adults from the New Mexico Aging Processes Study (funded by NIA Grant AG02049) who graciously volunteered their time to participate in the experiment reported. We also thank Roddy Roediger for helpful discussions in formulating this chapter. We especially acknowledge Johannes Engelkamp for his elegant and programmatic work on memory for actions throughout his distinguished scientific career.

References

Belli, R.F., Lindsay, D.S., Gales, M.S., and McCarthy, T.T. (1994). Memory impairment and source misattribution in postevent misinformation experiments with short retention intervals. *Memory and Cognition*, **22**, 40–54.

Butler, K.M., McDaniel, M.A., Dornburg, C.C., Price, A.L., and Roediger, H.L., III (2004). Age differences in veridical and false recall are not inevitable: the role of frontal lobe function. *Psychonomic Bulletin and Review*, **11**, 921–925.

Chalfonte, B.L. and Johnson, M.K. (1996). Feature memory and binding in young and older adults. *Memory and Cognition*, **24**, 403–416.

Cohen, G. and Faulkner, D. (1989). Age differences in source forgetting: effects on reality monitoring and on eyewitness testimony. *Psychology and Aging*, **4**, 10–17.

Cohen, R.L. (1981). On the generality of some memory laws. *Scandinavian Journal of Psychology*, **22**, 267–281.

Craik, F.I. and Tulving, E. (1975). Depth of processing and the retention of words in episodic memory. *Journal of Experimental Psychology: General*, **104**, 268–294.

Craik, F.I.M., Morris, L.W., Morris, R.G., and Loewen, E.R. (1990). Relations between source amnesia and frontal lobe functioning in older adults. *Psychology and Aging*, **5**, 148–151.

Deese, J. (1959). On the prediction of occurrence of particular verbal intrusions in immediate recall. *Journal of Experimental Psychology*, **58**, 17–22.

Denis, M., Engelkamp, J., and Mohr, G. (1991). Memory for imagined actions: Imagining oneself or another person. *Psychological Research*, **53**, 246–250.

Dodson, C.S. and Shimamura, A.P. (2000). Differential effects of cue dependency on item and source memory. *Journal of Experimental Psychology: Learning, Memory, and Cognition*, **26**, 1023–1044.

Durso, F.T. and Johnson, M.K. (1980). The effects of orienting tasks on recognition, recall, and modality confusion of pictures and words. *Journal of Verbal Learning and Verbal Behavior*, **19**, 416–429.

Ecker, W. and Engelkamp, J. (1995). Memory for actions in obsessive-compulsive disorder. *Behavioural and Cognitive Psychotherapy*, **23**, 349–371.

Einstein, G.O., McDaniel, M.A., Bowers, C.A., and Stevens, D.T. (1984). Memory for prose: the influence of relational and proposition-specific processing. *Journal of Experimental Psychology*, **10**, 133–143.

Ellis, N.R. (1990). Is memory for spatial location automatically encoded? *Memory and Cognition*, **18**, 584–592.

Engelkamp, J. (1998). *Memory for Actions*. Hove, UK: Psychology Press.

Engelkamp, J. (2001). Action memory: a system-oriented approach. In *Memory for Actions: A Distinct Form of Memory?* (ed H.D. Zimmer, R.L. Cohen, M.J. Guynn, J. Engelkamp, R. Kormi-Nouri, and M.A. Foley). New York: Oxford University Press, pp. 49–96.

Engelkamp, J. and Krumnacker, H. (1980). Imaginale und motorische Prozesse beim behalten verbalen Materials [Image- and motor-processes in the retention of verbal materials]. *Zeitschrift fuer Experimentelle und Angewandte Psychologie*, **27**, 511–533.

Engelkamp, J., Zimmer, H.D., and Denis, M. (1989). Paired associate learning of action verbs with visual or motor-imaginal encoding instructions. *Psychological Research*, **50**, 257–263.

Garry, M., Manning, C.G., Loftus, E.F., and Sherman, S.J. (1996). Imagination inflation: Imagining a childhood event inflates confidence that it occurred. *Psychonomic Bulletin and Review*, **3**, 208–214.

Glisky, E.L., Polster, M.R., and Routhieaux, B.C. (1995). Double dissociation between item and source memory. *Neuropsychology*, **9**, 229–235.

Glisky, E.L., Rubin, S.R., and Davidson, P.S.R. (2001). Source memory in older adults: an encoding or retrieval problem? *Journal of Experimental Psychology: Learning, Memory, and Cognition*, **27**, 1131–1146.

Goff, L.M., and Roediger, H.L., III. (1998). Imagination inflation for action events: repeated imaginings lead to illusory recollections. *Memory and Cognition*, **26**, 20–33.

Guttentag, R.E. and Hunt, R.R. (1988). Adult age differences in memory for imagined and performed actions. *Journal of Gerontology*, **43**, P107–P108.

Henkel, L.A., Johnson, M.K., and De Leonardis, D.M. (1998). Aging and source monitoring: Cognitive processes and neuropsychological correlates. *Journal of Experimental Psychology: General*, **127**, 251–268.

Hintzman, D.L., Block, R.A., and Summers, J.J. (1973). Contextual associations and memory for serial position. *Journal of Experimental Psychology*, **97**, 220–229.

Isaac, C.L. and Mayes, A.R. (1999). Rate of forgetting in amnesia. II: Recall and recognition of word lists at different levels of organization. *Journal of Experimental Psychology: Learning, Memory, and Cognition*, **25**, 963–977.

Johnson, M.K., Hashtroudi, S., and Lindsay, D.S. (1993). Source monitoring. *Psychological Bulletin*, **114**, 3–28.

Jurica, P.J. and Shimamura, A.P. (1999). Monitoring item and source information: evidence for a negative generation effect in source memory. *Memory and Cognition*, **27**, 648–656.

Lee, S.C. (2000). Imagination inflation for action events: are older adults more susceptible? Unpublished Master's Thesis, Washington University in St. Louis, St Louis, MO.

Lichty, W., Kausler, D.H., and Martinez, D.R. (1986). Adult age differences in memory for motor versus cognitive activities. *Experimental Aging Research*, **12**, 227–230.

Lindsay, D.S. and Johnson, M.K. (1989). The eyewitness suggestibility effect and memory for source. *Memory and Cognition*, **17**, 349–358.

Loftus, E.F. (1992). When a lie becomes memory's truth: memory distortion after exposure to misinformation. *Current Directions in Psychological Science*, **1**, 121–123.

McDaniel, M.A., and Einstein, G.O. (in press). Components of prospective memory most at risk for older adults and implications for medical adherence. In *Social and Cognitive Perspectives on Medical Adherence* (ed D.C. Park and L. Liu). Washington, DC: American Psychological Association, in press.

McDaniel, M.A., Glisky, E.L., Rubin, S.R., Guynn, M.J., and Routhieaux, B.C. (1999). Prospective memory: A neuropsychological study. *Neuropsychology*, **13**, 103–110.

McDaniel, M.A., Hines, R.J., Waddill, P.J., and Einstein, G.O. (1994). What makes folk tales unique: content familiarity, causal structure, scripts, or superstructures? *Journal of Experimental Psychology: Learning, Memory, and Cognition*, **20**, 169–184.

McDaniel, M.A. and Masson, M.E. (1977). Long-term retention: when incidental semantic processing fails. *Journal of Experimental Psychology: Human Learning and Memory*, **3**, 270–281.

McEvoy, C.L., Nelson, D.L., and Komatsu, T. (1999). What is the connection between true and false memories? The differential roles of interitem associations in recall and recognition. *Journal of Experimental Psychology: Learning, Memory, and Cognition*, **25**, 1177–1194.

Macklin, C.B. and McDaniel, M.A. (2005). The bizarreness effect: dissociation between item and source memory. *Memory*, **13**, 682–689.

Madigan, S. (1983). Picture memory. In *Imagery, Memory and Cognition: Essays in Honor of Allan Paivio* (ed J.C. Yuille). Hillsdale, NJ: Erlbaum, pp. 65–89.

Moscovitch, M. (1992). Memory and working-in-memory: a component process model based on modules and central systems. *Journal of Cognitive Neuroscience*, **4**, 257–267.

Naveh-Benjamin, M. (1987). Coding of spatial location information: an automatic process? *Journal of Experimental Psychology: Learning, Memory, and Cognition*, **13**, 595–605.

Naveh-Benjamin, M. (2000). Adult age differences in memory performance: tests of an associative deficit hypothesis. *Journal of Experimental Psychology: Learning, Memory, and Cognition*, **26**, 1170–1187.

Naveh-Benjamin, M. and Craik, F.I.M. (1995). Memory for context and its use in item memory: comparisons of younger and older persons. *Psychology and Aging*, **10**, 284–293.

O'Reilly, R.C. and Rudy, J. W. (2001). Conjunctive representations in learning and memory: principles of cortical and hippocampal function. *Psychological Review*, **108**, 311–345.

Park, D.C. and Kidder, D.P. (1996). Prospective memory and medication adherence. In *Prospective Memory: Theory and Applications* (ed M. Brandimonte, G.O. Einstein, and M.A. McDaniel). Mahwah, NJ: Erlbaum, pp. 369–390.

Parkin, A.J., Walter, B.M., and Hunkin, N.M. (1995). Relationships between normal aging, frontal lobe function, and memory for temporal and spatial information. *Neuropsychology*, **9**, 304–312.

Rahhal, T.A., May, C.P., and Hasher, L. (2002). Truth and character: sources that older adults can remember. *Psychological Sciences*, **13**, 101–105.

Raz, N. (2000). Aging of the brain and its impact on cognitive performance: integration of structural and functional findings. In *Handbook of Aging and Cognition* (ed F.I.M. Craik and T.A. Salthouse). Mahwah, NJ: Erlbaum, pp. 1–90.

Roediger, H.L. (1980). The effectiveness of four mnemonics in ordering recall. *Journal of Experimental Psychology: Human Learning and Memory*, **6**, 558–567.

Roediger, H.L. and McDermott, K.B. (1995). Creating false memories: remembering words not presented in lists. *Journal of Experimental Psychology: Learning, Memory, and Cognition*, **21**, 803–814.

Roediger, H.L. and Wheeler, M.A. (1993). Hypermnesia in episodic and semantic memory. *Psychological Science*, **4**, 207–208.

Roediger, H.L., Watson, J.M., McDermott, K.B., and Gallo, D.A. (2001). Factors that determine false recall: a multiple regression analysis. *Psychonomic Bulletin and Review*, **8**, 385–407.

Rudy, J.W., Huff, N., and Matus-Amat, P. (2004). Understanding contextual fear conditioning: Insights from a two process model. *Neuroscience and Biobehavioral Reviews*, **28**, 675–685.

Saltz, E. and Donnenwerth-Nolan, S. (1981). Does motoric imagery facilitate memory for sentences? A selective interference test. *Journal of Verbal Learning and Verbal Behavior*, **20**, 322–332.

Shimamura, A.P. (1995). Memory and frontal lobe function. In *The Cognitive Neurosciences* (ed M.S. Gazzaniga). Cambridge, MA: MIT Press, pp. 803–813.

Spencer, W.D. and Raz, N. (1994). Memory for facts, source, and context: can frontal lobe dysfunction explain age-related differences? *Psychology and Aging*, **9**, 149–159.

Spencer, W.D. and Raz, N. (1995). Differential effects of aging on memory for content and context: a meta-analysis. *Psychology and Aging*, **10**, 527–539.

Underwood, B.J. and Malmi, R.A. (1978). An evaluation of measures used in studying temporal codes for words within a list. *Journal of Verbal Learning and Verbal Behavior*, **17**, 279–293.

West, R.L. (1996). An application of prefrontal cortex function theory to cognitive aging. *Psychological Bulletin*, **120**, 272–292.

Winograd, E. (1968). List differentiation, recall, and category similarity. *Journal of Experimental Psychology*, **78**, 510–515.

Chapter 27

Age-associated changes in episodic memory: event-related potential investigations of recollection and familiarity

David Friedman

Behavioural studies of age-related changes in episodic memory

Forming new associations between the distinct features of an experience (e.g. time of occurrence, place of occurrence, etc.) is essential for the creation of episodic memories. For example, the common occurrence of recognizing the face of a familiar person as someone you have met before without being able to retrieve the details surrounding that episode (e.g. the person's name, occupation, time, and place of the previous encounter) is an example of a content or item memory devoid of contextual features. A complete memory of that experience requires integrating the content with the context. This latter type of memory is labelled source memory. As attested to by a large experimental literature (Spencer and Raz 1995), normally ageing humans appear to experience greater difficulty in this kind of integration than their young adult counterparts. That is, older adults perform as well as younger subjects on most tests of simple old–new recognition, which only require the identification of an item as old or new, without the necessity to retrieve the contextual details of the initial learning episode (Craik and McDowd 1987). However, older adults are at a considerable disadvantage compared with younger adults when retrieval of source information is required (Spencer and Raz 1995; Fabiani and Friedman 1997; Glisky *et al.* 2001).

Age-related deficits in source memory performance have been observed for a wide variety of contextual information, suggesting a generalized difficulty in encoding and/or retrieving contextual detail. These include, but are not limited to, gender of voice (Senkfor and Petten 1996; Mark and Rugg 1998; Glisky *et al.* 2001), temporal order or recency memory (Fabiani and Friedman 1997), list membership (Trott *et al.* 1999), and whether an item was imagined or perceived (Henkel *et al.* 1998). However, certain types of contextual information, such as temporal order and location, place older adults at an even greater disadvantage (Perlmutter *et al.* 1981; Spencer and Raz 1995; Chalfonte and Johnson 1996; Fabiani and Friedman 1997).

Another consistent finding in the behavioural literature on memory and ageing is that the elderly appear to rely more on familiarity than recollection to make judgements about previously experienced episodes (Gardiner and Java 1990; Grady and Craik 2000) (see Light *et al.* (2000) for a review and caveats. Familiarity, which has been hypothesized to be a global matching process between the item to be retrieved and its previously studied counterpart (Curran 2000), has been linked with the retrieval of the content of a memory. Familiarity is believed to be a relatively automatic process with its products not necessarily available to consciousness. On the other hand, the hallmark of a recollection-based recognition response is the retrieval of the contextual attributes with which the original episode was associated. In contrast with familiarity, recollection is believed to be an effortful process requiring strategic control for its implementation (reviewed by Yonelinas 2002).

The fact that older adults rely more on familiarity than recollection is believed to account for the finding that these participants are not always impaired on item recognition tasks, i.e. old–new recognition memory (Craik *et al.* 1987). This can occur because above-chance performance on these types of recognition memory paradigms can be achieved by relying solely on the familiarity component of recognition memory. However, when source retrieval is required, above-chance performance can typically be supported only by recollection. Hence the age-related deficit in recollection can be masked in traditional old–new recognition memory tasks by familiarity-based performance (Jennings and Jacoby 1997; D. Friedman and H. Gaeta 2002, unpublished results).

This phenomenon has been particularly apparent when familiarity is placed in opposition to recollection using the process dissociation procedures developed by Jacoby (1991). For example, Jennings and Jacoby (1997) (see also D. Friedman and H. Gaeta 2002, unpublished results) asked young and elderly adults to study a list of words and were then given a recognition test in which old and new words were presented with each new word repeated once after a certain number of intervening items (e.g. lags of 4, 12, 24, and 48 intervening items). Subjects had to identify old words only; they responded 'old' to words studied earlier and 'new' to new words regardless of whether the new item was presented for the first or second time in the test list. Recollection of the previous presentation of an item in the test list should have led to its rejection as a target, whereas familiarity gained from the prior presentation of the 'new' test item should have had the opposite effect, leading to mistaken recognition of the repeated test word as having been previously studied. When this occurred it was referred to as a 'repetition error'. In line with expectation, repetition errors increased for the elderly as the interval between the first presentation of a new test item and its repetition was lengthened. Moreover, the estimates of familiarity derived from Jacoby's (1991) equations were equivalent in the young and elderly, whereas the estimates of recollection were reliably lower in the older age group.

In addition to Jacoby's (1991) inclusion–exclusion paradigm described above, the remember–know (R–K) paradigm (Tulving 1985) has also been used to provide support for the distinction between familiarity and recollection (reviewed by Gardiner 2001; Yonelinas 2002). In this paradigm, following a study phase, participants are asked to make old–new recognition judgements. For any item judged old, the participant is asked to make an additional R or K judgement. They are to state R if they know that the item was on the study list and, in addition, can retrieve contextual details (whether idiosyncratic, inherent in the studied item, or experimentally induced); they are to state K if they are certain that the item was on the study list, but cannot retrieve specific details associated with its initial occurrence. On the basis of a number of dissociations between experimental manipulations such as levels of processing (Craik and Lockhart 1972) and the frequency with which old items attract R or K responses, several authors have argued that R and K are surrogates for recollection and familiarity, respectively (but see Gardiner *et al.* 1999). Consistent with an age-related deficit in recollection and preservation of familiarity-based processing, normally ageing older adults tested using the R–K paradigm have generally produced fewer R responses than their young adult counterparts, while producing the same or a greater number of K responses (Bastin and Van der Linden 2003; Clarys *et al.* 2002). These data based on the R–K distinction are consistent with the estimates of familiarity and recollection derived from the process dissociation procedure discussed earlier (Jennings and Jacoby 1997; D. Friedman and H. Gaeta 2002, unpublished results).

One potential explanation for the age-related deficit in source memory is that older adults have difficulty in binding the different aspects of experience into a cohesive integrated whole. There is evidence from behavioural investigations (Chalfonte and Johnson 1996; Henkel *et al.* 1998; Mitchell *et al.* 2000a) and neuroimaging investigations (Mitchell *et al.* 2000b) in support of this hypothesis. The behavioural investigations demonstrate that older adults are at a greater disadvantage when retrieval depends upon the requirement to encode and store a representation of an item in which two or more features (e.g. colour and location) must be integrated or 'bound' compared with the case when only a single feature must be retrieved (e.g. either location or colour). For example, in a working memory task, Mitchell *et al.* (2000a) presented common objects in locations within a 3 × 3 grid. In different conditions, subjects had to encode the object, the location, or both the object and its location for a subsequent test trial probe. Older adults performed as well as young adults when a single feature had to be retrieved, but performed significantly worse when retrieval requirements were such that two previously studied features had to be recognized as a 'unit' (i.e. both the object and the location had to be identical to the studied object and location). In further conditions, these investigators ruled out the possibility that the binding deficit was due to the greater amount of information that had to be maintained when retrieval of bound information was required.

In similar fashion to the study of working memory by Mitchell *et al.* (2000a), Chalfonte and Johnson (1996) described a specific age-related deficit in binding information in episodic memory. In separate study phases, participants were asked to study the distinct features of the item itself, the item's location, the item's colour, the combination of item and location, and the combination of item and colour. In separate test phases, which immediately followed each study phase, subjects were instructed as to which of the features had to be recognized. Although older adults showed a deficit in the recognition of location, there was age equivalence in the recognition of colour and item. On the other hand, when bound information had to be recognized, there was an age-related decline in item–location and item–colour performance accuracy, i.e. older adults appeared to show a deficit in binding information to form richly detailed memories. In a more stringent test of whether the older adults tested by Mitchell *et al.* (2000a) had a disproportionate deficit in binding, the authors constructed a recognition test in which distractors were mispaired old (i.e. previously studied) item features. In this situation, employing an old item feature to distinguish between distractor and target (which could have been done in the initial experiment) would not suffice; only recognition of bound information would lead to good performance. The results indicated that, as in the first experiment, older adults showed a decline in their ability to recognize bound information.

To summarize, the elderly appear to show small or non-existent deficits in item memory when retrieval is tested via yes–no recognition. However, when subjects must retrieve the contextual details of a memory, older adults show reliably worse performance than their young adult counterparts. These generalizations appear to apply to at least three different paradigms for assessing the contribution of recollection and familiarity to age-related changes in episodic memory: the process dissociation, remember–know, and source memory procedures. In the very few extant age-related studies of 'binding', the major finding is that older adults show a greater deficit in encoding/retrieving bound information relative to encoding/retrieving a single feature. We turn now to a consideration of the physiological literature to determine whether it can provide any insight into age-related changes in episodic memory.

Neuroimaging evidence for age-related alterations in episodic memory

Event-related brain potentials (ERPs), as well as positron-emission tomography (PET) and functional MRI (fMRI) data, have contributed to the cognitive ageing database. We first review the ERP studies from the general literature and then present detailed results of two studies conducted in our laboratory. This will be followed by a discussion of results from fMRI investigations.

ERP data

Both ERP (Paller *et al.* 1987) and event-related functional MRI (efMRI) techniques (Wagner *et al.* 1998) provide informative measures of encoding-related activity (reviewed by Paller and Wagner 2002). These are known as subsequent memory effects (SMEs) or the difference in subsequent memory (Dm) effect (Paller *et al.* 1987) because brain activity elicited by a given study item is averaged on the basis of how that item fared during the subsequent test phase, i.e. was it correctly recognized (a hit) or unrecognized (a miss). Unlike studies which assess age-related changes in encoding without respect to subsequent memory performance, the computation of SMEs allows one to infer the psychophysiological correlates of successful performance. Currently, only one ERP study has assessed age-related changes in SMEs. To briefly preview the results which will be described in detail below, Friedman and Trott (2000) demonstrated that younger, but not older, adults showed larger SMEs to study items subsequently associated with R judgements (i.e. recollected with contextual details) than with K judgements (i.e. familiarity-based) made at test. The older adults showed equal magnitude SMEs in subsequent association with R and K judgements. Moreover, younger, but not older, adults showed evidence of activity at scalp regions overlying the left inferior prefrontal cortex (LIPC). Hence these data suggest that, at encoding, older subjects did not differentially encode those items that would be subsequently associated with retrieval of contextual details (remember) from those that would not (know). This, in turn, suggests a difference in encoding between the young and the elderly. These results implicate age-related encoding deficits, perhaps due to a failure to activate LIPC (see the discussion of fMRI studies below), as contributing to the poorer episodic memory performance often observed in the elderly. Apart from ERP studies in our laboratory (Friedman *et al.* 1996), there are (to our knowledge) no other published age-related studies of encoding using the ERP technique.

In the retrieval phase of study–test paradigms, correctly recognized old items typically elicit greater positive amplitude than correctly rejected new items. This has been termed the old–new or episodic memory (EM) effect (Friedman and Johnson 2000). Several subcomponents of the EM effect have been identified in young adults (reviewed by Johnson 1995; Friedman and Johnson 2000; Rugg and Allan 2000; Paller 2001). There are three consistently observed EM effects, all of which are more positive to old than new items. The first, between about 300 and 500 ms, shows a topographic distribution that is maximal over the medial prefrontal scalp and has been referred to as the medial prefrontal EM effect. A subsequent EM effect, active between about 500 and 900 ms, is typically left-sided with verbal material and shows its maximum amplitude over temporo-parietal scalp regions. It has been labelled the left parietal EM effect. A longer-lasting EM effect, a right-lateralized prefrontally oriented electrical activity labelled the right prefrontal EM effect (about 800–2000 ms), occurs later in the ERP sequence and is also larger to old than to new items. The medial prefrontal EM effect has been found not to differ in the ERPs associated with old items given either a K or an R judgement, whereas the left parietal EM effect is larger in association with old items endorsed with an R judgement (Smith 1993; Trott *et al.* 1999). On these bases, as well as a variety of other evidence (e.g. Johnson *et al.* 1998; Rugg *et al.* 1998; Curran 2000), a general consensus is that the medial prefrontal EM effect reflects the familiarity component (but see Tsivilis *et al.* 2001; Yovel and Paller 2004), whereas the left parietal EM effect reflects the recollective component hypothesized to account for memory performance by two-process theories of recognition memory (Mandler 1980).

The functional significance of the right prefrontal EM effect is less certain, but some tentative agreement as to its likely functional role has appeared (Wilding 1999). Findings in the ERP–memory literature suggest that, like LIPC scalp activity during encoding, it is likely to reflect a cognitive control function, perhaps related to evaluating the products of retrieval dependent upon the requirements of the memory task (e.g. for guiding the search for and/or retrieval of episodic information). Although speculative, it could also reflect the temporary storage of the attributes of previous experience (e.g. item and context information) that have been unitized or bound in a working memory buffer.

With respect to ageing, the medial prefrontal EM effect has been reported to be similar in young and old adults (Swick and Knight 1997) (see retrieval-related data below), which is in keeping with the putative age invariance of familiarity-based processing. On the other hand, some investigators have shown the left parietal EM effect to be reduced in older relative to younger subjects (Swick and Knight 1997; Rugg *et al.* 1997; Joyce *et al.* 1998), consistent with the hypothesized age-related deficit in recollection-based retrieval. With the exception of Mark and Rugg (1998), investigators have shown the right prefrontal EM effect to be reduced or absent in the waveforms of the elderly (Senkfor and Van Petten 1996; Trott *et al.* 1999; Wegesin *et al.* 2002). Hence, although the number of studies is limited, the results are generally concordant with the notion that familiarity-based response is preserved in the elderly, whereas recollective responding undergoes some age-related change; see the example from D. Friedman and H. Gaeta (2002, unpublished results) given below. In contrast, the severely limited ERP encoding data that exist suggest that the putative deficit in recollection during retrieval may be due to encoding-related deficiencies. The lack of the right prefrontal EM effect in the majority of ageing studies suggests that some of the age-related deficit in recollection may be due to a failure to monitor the products of retrieval and/or to effectively retrieve bound information as unitized episodes (Mitchell *et al.* 2000b) and implicates deficiencies in prefrontal cortical control in the episodic memory decrements observed in elderly samples.

ERP data from an inclusion–exclusion paradigm

An example of an age-related decrement in the parietal EM effect in a condition in which familiarity is pitted against recollection is shown in Figure 27.1 (D. Friedman and H. Gaeta 2002, unpublished results). The data were recorded in an inclusion–exclusion paradigm modelled after the experiment of Jennings and Jacoby (1997) described earlier. The participants were 12 young and 12 older healthy adults. During all test phases new words were repeated at either a lag of either 0 or 4. In addition to the exclusion condition employed by Jennings and Jacoby (1997), in which new and repeated items during the test phase had to be excluded (only items from the study phase were to be endorsed as targets), Friedman and Gaeta added a second exclusion condition in which the subject's task was to detect the presence of lag 0 or lag 4 words (i.e. all repeated items during the test phase) and exclude previously studied old or unstudied new words. In Figure 27.1, the difference mean data (i.e. old minus new) from the inclusion (simple old–new recognition of repeated items) and the second exclusion condition are illustrated at a midline posterior parietal scalp site. Table 27.1 presents the amplitudes for these conditions together with the recollection and familiarity values computed according to Jacoby (1991). Importantly, the only condition in which a reliable EM effect is not elicited is for the elderly for a lag 4 item that should have been endorsed as a target. Note also that, in this condition,

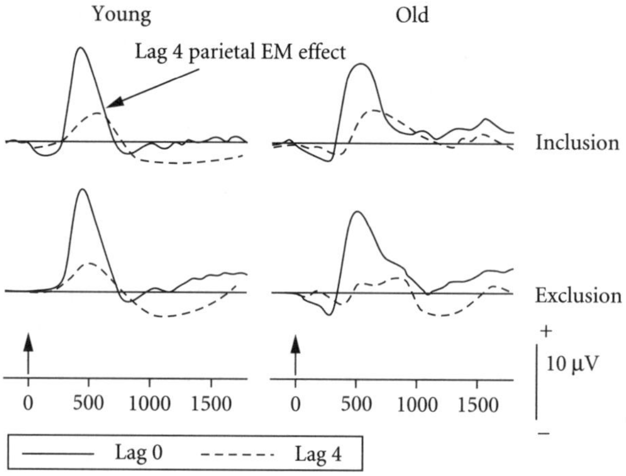

Figure 27.1 Grand mean difference waveforms at a posterior midline electrode location averaged across subjects within each age group to items repeated at lag 0 or lag 4 during the test phase. Waveforms from the inclusion task are depicted in the first row, with waveforms from the exclusion condition illustrated in the bottom row. Arrows mark stimulus onset with time lines every 500 ms. (Reproduced from D. Friedman and H. Gaeta 2002, unpublished results.)

Table 27.1 Grand average (± SD) ERP difference mean amplitudes for the young and elderly at a posterior midline scalp site (roughly equivalent to Pz in the 10/20 system) together with values of recollection *R* and familiarity *F* computed according to Jacoby (1991).

	ERP difference mean amplitude (μV)		***R***	***F*[a]**
	Inclusion	**Exclusion**		
Young ($N = 12$)				
Lag 0	11.9 (3.3)*	13.5 (4.9)*	0.96 (0.04)	–
Lag 4	3.6 (2.9)*	3.7 (5.0)*	0.82 (0.11)	0.75 (0.25)
Elderly ($N = 12$)				
Lag 0	10.9 (6.0)*	9.9 (6.9)*	0.88 (0.10)	–
Lag 4	4.0 (3.6)*	1.3 (3.9)	0.53 (0.23)	0.79 (0.16)

[a] Familiarity values were not computed at lag 0 because the majority of young and old subjects showed a probability of 1 for correctly responding 'yes' during inclusion and a probability of zero for erroneously responding 'yes' in the exclusion condition.

* Significantly different from zero at $P < 0.03$.

the values of recollection produced by the elderly are dramatically reduced relative to the young, whereas the values of familiarity do not differ between age groups. One interpretation of this reduction is that the elderly had difficulty in endorsing the item as a target because, at a lag of 4, it could not be discriminated reliably from a studied old item. In other words, in this condition the older adult's tendency to respond on the basis of familiarity overwhelmed any benefit that could have arisen from a recollection-based process. This age-related difference could have been due to a faulty (prefrontal?) control process in the elderly which failed to monitor the source of previous experiences or failed to bind the item's content with its context, leading the older adult to incorrectly attribute the lag 4 item to the study episode. However, based on these data alone, this is a purely speculative interpretation. Some support for a faulty control process comes from the study by Trott *et al.* (1999) described below.

ERP data from a source memory paradigm with remember–know judgements

A study in which the ERP data indicate that the older adult may have difficulty in encoding item–context associations and/or monitoring the source of previous experience is provided by Trott *et al.* (1999). Most investigators of age-related ERP phenomena have concentrated on the retrieval phases of recognition memory paradigms. To our knowledge, there have been no studies of encoding-related activity with elderly participants other than that by Trott *et al.* (1999). One of the reasons for initiating this study was to determine whether encoding difficulties, retrieval difficulties, or some combination of both might be responsible for age-related change in episodic memory function.

Complete details of this study can be found in Trott *et al.* (1999), and only brief methodological details will be provided here. Sixteen healthy young and 16 healthy older women viewed simple sentences of the form noun 1—verb—noun 2: for example, 'The **dragon** sniffed the **fudge**'. The two nouns in each sentence were unassociated based on a pilot study performed with 20 individuals who did not participate in the ERP experiment. In each study phase there were two lists of eight sentences. The sentences were presented one word at a time with a 1200 ms inter-stimulus interval (ISI). There were eight study–test phases, with recognition testing following immediately after each study phase. Subjects were not given specific encoding instructions, but were told that their memory for the nouns and the list in which they were presented would be tested following each study series. During each recognition test phase, an equal number of old ($N = 32$) and new ($N = 32$) nouns was presented in two-noun sequences separated by an ISI of 2 s. Subjects first made a speeded and accurate old–new judgement to each noun via reaction time. If either noun was judged old, additional remember–know and list 1–list 2 judgements were solicited. These latter judgements were untimed.

Figure 27.2 shows the grand mean percentage correct and corrected recognition scores. Figure 27.2(a) shows that the percentage accuracy data are consistent with previous investigations; the older participants show a non-significant trend towards a lower hit rate and higher false-alarm rate than the younger subjects,

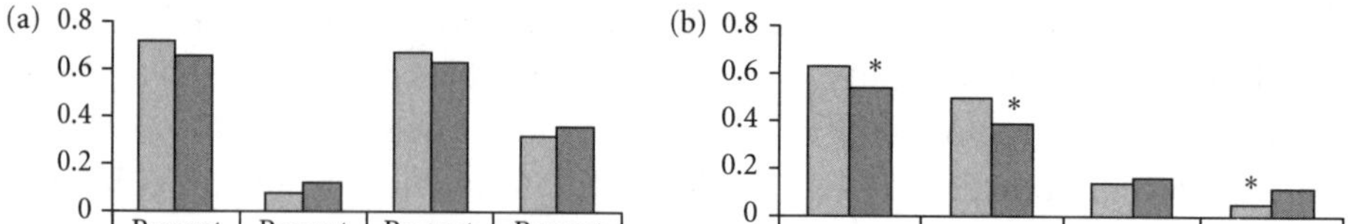

(a)

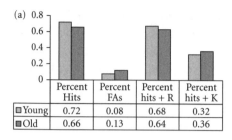

	Percent Hits	Percent FAs	Percent hits + R	Percent hits + K
Young	0.72	0.08	0.68	0.32
Old	0.66	0.13	0.64	0.36

(b)

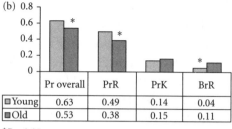

	Pr overall	PrR	PrK	BrR
Young	0.63	0.49	0.14	0.04
Old	0.53	0.38	0.15	0.11

*$P < 0.05$

Figure 27.2 (a) Grand mean percentage of hits and false alarms (FAs), and the percentage of hits attracting R and K judgments in the two age groups. (b) Grand mean corrected recognition scores (Pr) computed according to Snodgrass and Corwin (1988) for overall recognition performance and for hits attracting remember and know judgments. The measure of bias (Br) is also shown for hits attracting R judgments. *Reliable difference between young and old.

with a smaller percentage of hits attracting R judgements and a greater percentage of hits associated with K judgements. However, the picture changes when the corrected recognition scores (hits minus false alarms) are considered (Snodgrass and Corwin 1988) (Figure 27.2(b)). Here, the old differ from the young in the accuracy of discriminating old from new items, and this is primarily driven by their remember responses, as the corrected recognition memory scores do not differ for know responses. Moreover, the old show a less conservative bias than the young when applying R judgements to old items. Note that, based on these behavioural data alone, it is difficult to determine whether encoding difficulties impacted the age-related memory differences observed in Figure 27.2.

Encoding phase data

The ERP data can shed light on these issues, as can be seen in Figure 27.3. As mentioned earlier, because the ERPs at study were averaged as a function of subsequent memory performance at test, the ERP data can provide some insight into whether age-related encoding differences had some impact on the behavioural differences observed in Figure 27.2. Grand mean study phase data (collapsed across nouns 1 and 2 and the eight study phases) averaged as a function of subsequent performance during the test phases are shown for the young and elderly samples in Figure 27.3. Note that there are large SMEs for both age groups, i.e. there is a positive-going modulation of the subsequently correct (hit) waveforms relative to the subsequently incorrect (miss) waveforms. In the young, the ERPs to study nouns that are subsequently correctly recognized and associated with an R judgement are significantly larger than those that are subsequently correctly recognized and associated with a K judgement. Moreover, only those ERPs to study trials subsequently associated with an R judgement are

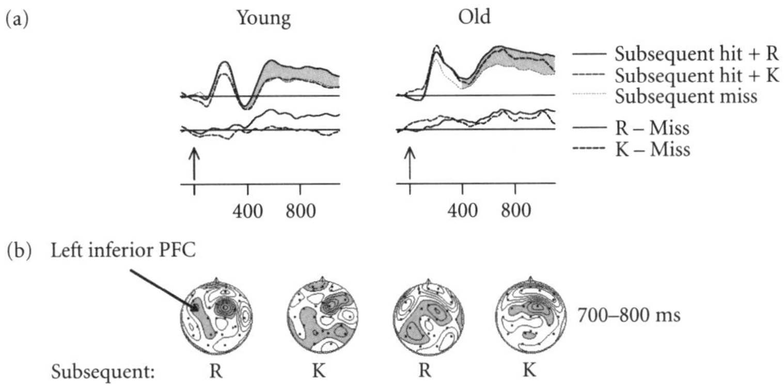

Figure 27.3 (a) Grand mean study phase ERPs averaged across subjects within each age group. The data are averaged as a function of subsequent memory performance according to whether the item was correctly recognized and received an R or K judgment, and whether the item was subsequently unrecognized or missed. The ERP data of the young are illustrated in the first column, and those of the old are shown in the second column. Arrows mark stimulus onset with time lines at 600 ms. Shaded areas in the waveforms indicate the subsequent memory effect. (b) CSD maps computed on the subsequently remember minus missed and know minus missed difference waveforms between 700 and 800 ms, separately for the young and older adults (depicted below their respective waveforms). The separation between isopotential lines is 0.02 μV/cm^2. Shaded regions, negativity; unshaded regions, positivity.

reliably larger than study trials that would later be missed; this is not the case with the ERPs to study trials later attracting a K judgement. This is clearly seen in the second row of waveforms in Figure 27.3(a), where the subsequently correct minus subsequently incorrect difference waveforms are shown. The pattern for the older adults is quite different. ERPs to study nouns subsequently associated with hits attracting either R or K judgements do not differ in magnitude from one another, and both are reliably larger than the ERPs to study nouns that were subsequently missed. This can also be observed in the second row of older adult waveforms. These data suggest that, for the young, some nouns were distinctively encoded, i.e. those that would later attract R judgements, whereas such differential encoding did not appear to take place for the older adults. Hence, consistent with this interpretation, older adults may have encoded the majority of items without using an elaborative strategy, thereby failing to ensure that some items would be distinctively encoded. On this view, in contrast with the young adults, the subsequent distinction between R and K judgements would be blurred for the elderly, most likely because of impoverished encoding activity during the study phase.

We now turn to a consideration of the scalp topography data to determine whether they can shed light on the age-related encoding differences that are apparent in the pattern of waveform differences described above. Scalp current source density (CSD) topographies, which primarily reflect cortical activity (Nunez and Pilgreen 1991), are shown in Figure 27.3(b). Note that, for the young, there is negative activity over the inferior prefrontal scalp that appears larger for trials associated with a subsequent R judgement compared with those subsequently attracting K judgements. There is also evidence of right-sided positive activity for trials associated with subsequent R judgements only. Further, the topographies associated with the two conditions show little similarity.

In contrast, the older participants show bilateral areas of positive activity and little evidence of negative activity over the left inferior prefrontal scalp. Moreover, the distribution for study trials associated with subsequent R and K judgements looks remarkably similar. This suggests that the processing reflected by the ERP SMEs in the young and the elderly are different. As described in more detail in the discussion of fMRI data below, these topographic data may be consistent with the notion that a contributing factor to the older adult's deficient encoding might be a failure to recruit the LIPC.

Retrieval phase data

Figure 27.4 shows the grand mean retrieval phase data for young and elderly participants. The ERP waveforms are depicted at the top and the corresponding CSD topographic maps are illustrated at the bottom of the figure. The data depict the same conditions as shown in Figure 27.3, that is, hits associated with remember and K judgements, as well as the ERPs elicited by nouns that were correctly rejected as new or foil items. For the young adults, there is again a clear distinction between the ERPs associated with hits that attracted remember and those that attracted K judgements. The ERPs elicited by hits associated with a K judgement show the early EM effect active between about 300 and 500 ms, i.e. this aspect of the ERP waveform is more positive than that elicited by a new noun. The same relation holds for the ERPs elicited by hits associated with an R judgement. On this basis, the 300–500 ms region of the waveform may reflect familiarity-based recognition, as both types of old items should have been equally familiar. In contrast, only the ERPs associated with R judgements show a subsequent positive-going modulation of the waveforms that appears active between about 500 and 800 ms. This latter phenomenon suggests that the parietal EM effect is associated with recognition based on recollection, as presumably more information of a contextual nature would have been retrieved in association with a R judgement than with a K judgement.

The pattern for the old at the frontal and parietal scalp sites appears similar to that for the young, although the waveforms of the three conditions are not as

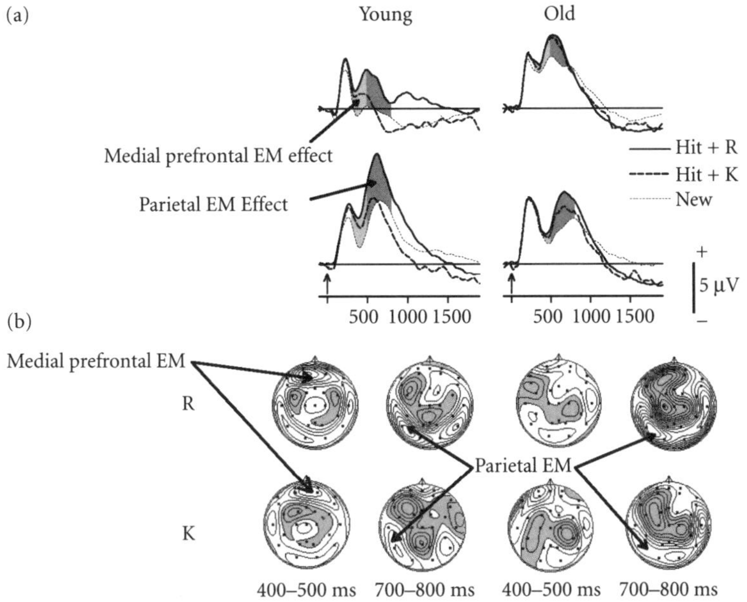

Figure 27.4 (a) Grand mean ERPs averaged across subjects within each age group at midline frontal and parietal electrode sites. Light grey shading indicates the region of the medial prefrontal EM effect and dark grey shading indicates the region of the left parietal EM effect. Arrows mark stimulus onset with time lines every 500 ms. (b) CSD maps of the medial prefrontal (400–500 ms) and left parietal (700–800 ms) EM effects shown below the respective waveforms for the young and old groups. The separation between isopotential lines is 0.02 $\mu V/cm^2$. Shaded regions, negativity; unshaded regions, positivity.

clearly demarcated as those observed in the data for the young. Note that, at the frontal scalp site, the ERPs associated with R and K judgements do not differ in magnitude, whereas both differ from the ERP elicited by correctly identified new items. This effect, like that in the young, occurs earlier in time than that observed at the parietal scalp site. Based on the assumption that the early EM effect reflects familiarity, this result would argue for an intact familiarity mechanism in the data of the elderly. In contrast with the data at the frontal scalp electrode, at the parietal site the ERPs associated with R judgements differ in magnitude from those associated with K judgements in highly similar fashion to the data of the young. However, although the parietal EM effect associated with R and K judgements appears to differ in magnitude from the ERPs elicited by new items, only the difference between the ERPs associated with R judgements and those associated with new items was actually reliable for this later region of the waveform.

In addition to the medial prefrontal and left parietal EM effects, Trott *et al.* (1999) also observed the right prefrontal EM effect described earlier.

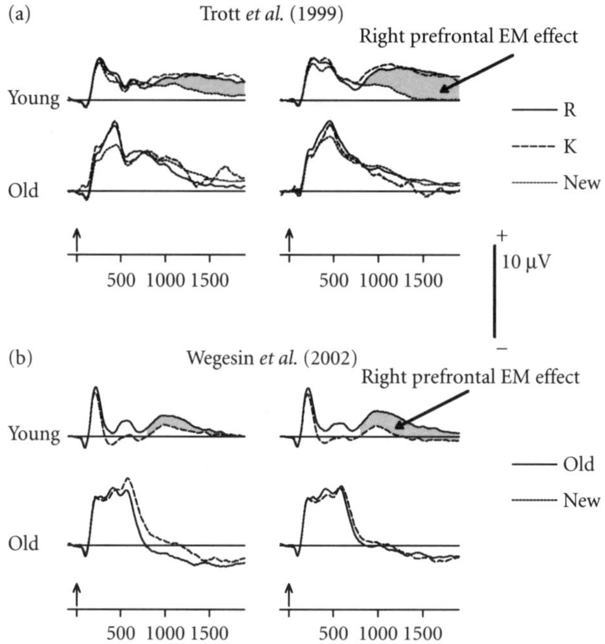

Figure 27.5 Grand mean ERPs averaged across subjects within each age group at left and right prefrontal scalp sites. Data are from the source memory studies by (a) Trott *et al.* (1999) and (b) Wegesin *et al.* (2002). The Trott *et al.* data are shown at prefrontal electrode sites over left and right eye locations for the same conditions as illustrated in Figure 27.4. Wegesin *et al.* (2002) did not employ R–K judgments, but used the same list judgment procedure as Trott *et al.* (1999). They did not use the same prefrontal locations as Trott *et al.* Hence, the data are illustrated at FP1 and FP2. Arrows mark stimulus onset with timelines every 500 ms. The shaded regions of the waveforms indicate the right prefrontal EM effect.

Figure 27.5(a) shows this activity at the left and right prefrontal regions of the scalp. Only the young adults show the right prefrontal EM effect (indicated by grey shading), which is clearly larger over the right than the left hemiscalp. It is of equal magnitude in association with correctly recognized old items that attracted either R or K judgements.

A similar phenomenon can be observed in the replication data of Wegesin *et al.* (2002) shown in Figure 27.5(b). The figure depicts the ERPs associated with correctly rejected new items and those associated with old items whose source (i.e. list 1 or list 2) was correctly attributed. Wegesin *et al.* (2002) modified the design used by Trott *et al.* (1999) to make the source judgement task easier, as one hypothesis for the lack of right prefrontal activity in the ERPs of the elderly subjects studied by Trott *et al.* was that their source memory performance was at chance levels. However, despite the improved and above-chance source memory performance of the elderly participants in the study by Wegesin *et al.* (2002), the right prefrontal EM effect was still not observed.[1]

Right prefrontal activity follows mean reaction time to correctly recognized old items, which averaged about 920 ms for the young and about 1070 ms for the elderly in the study by Trott *et al.*, and about 800 ms for the young and about 965 ms for the elderly in the study by Wegesin *et al.* Therefore it does not appear to reflect either familiarity- or recollection-based processes, which most likely would have preceded the behavioural response. Rather, this activity appears to be associated with some kind of post-retrieval processing (Wilding 1999). The exact nature of these post-retrieval processes is currently unclear (Friedman and Johnson 2000; Rugg and Wilding 2000; Wilding and Sharpe 2002). A possibility in the current experimental situation is that the presence of the right prefrontal EM effect in the data of the young indicates that the products of retrieval have been stored in working memory. Because the R and K (and list) judgements are delayed relative to the old–new decision, the information stored in working memory (presumably representations of the content and context of the current item) would have been consulted in order to make the appropriate R or K judgement. This would account for the equal-magnitude right prefrontal EM effects in association with R and K judgements in the data for the young. Although it is difficult to infer intracranial sources simply based on the pattern of electrical activity on the scalp, the prefrontal scalp activity in the data of the young is consistent with several fMRI studies of working memory in which prefrontal activations have been observed when information must be maintained in a short-term working memory buffer (Fletcher and Henson 2001).

The lack of right prefrontal activity in the ERP data of the older subjects suggests that these maintenance operations may not have been performed by the majority of participants in this age group. An alternative, but not necessarily exclusive, interpretation is that the products of retrieval were 'fuzzy' because of the possibility that the older adults encoded fewer items 'deeply' compared with the young (based upon the encoding phase data presented earlier). This may have resulted in the older adults employing a more liberal criterion in judging items as remembered (Fig. 27.2). Hence, as mentioned earlier, the distinction between R and K judgements would have been blurred for the elderly, possibly because the majority of items were shallowly encoded (Fig. 27.3), i.e. the lack of distinction at encoding in the ERPs associated with items subsequently given R and K judgements. On this view, the lack of the right prefrontal EM effect in the data of the elderly could have resulted from a failure to maintain coordinated representations of context and content information that would have enabled well-informed distinctions between R and K judgements.

To summarize at this juncture, in contrast with the study phase data, both young and old participants appear to show highly similar patterns of ERP response during the retrieval phase in both the magnitudes and scalp distributions of the medial prefrontal and parietal EM effects, albeit with the elderly lagging the young by approximately 100 ms and showing somewhat reduced amplitude of the left parietal EM effect. To the extent that the medial prefrontal EM effect can be associated with familiarity, and the left parietal EM effect with recollection, the data suggest that the elderly may not be deficient in employing both these behavioural processes to support episodic memory retrieval. However, the lack of the right prefrontal EM effect in the data of the elderly suggests impairment in post-retrieval processing, possibly in maintaining the products of retrieval in working memory.

Functional MRI and positron-emission tomography data

Although the ERP has exquisite temporal resolution, it cannot match the functional neuroimaging techniques, such as PET and fMRI, in degree of spatial resolution. Therefore it is useful to determine whether the results of the age-related functional imaging studies that do exist show convergence with the ERP studies reviewed above. With the caveat that the proposed pairing of ERP and fMRI/PET results remains speculative, the attempt to combine the data provided by the ERP with those available from fMRI/PET can nevertheless be informative.

The physiological correlates of the encoding and retrieval of bound information from long-term memory have not been assessed extensively, especially with respect to ageing. In the only study of this phenomenon that currently exists, (Mitchell *et al.* 2000b) showed that young, but not older, adults had an activation pattern consistent with a right prefrontal–medial temporal lobe (MTL) circuit during a working memory paradigm. This network was activated to a greater extent when bound information had to be retrieved. In another neuroimaging study of working memory with young adult participants, Prabhakaran *et al.* (2000) demonstrated that the extent of right prefrontal activation was related directly to the extent to which an integrated representation had to be retrieved. Together, these limited findings suggest that, at least in working memory, feature binding requires the right prefrontal cortex to maintain the integrated information and/or influence MTL activity. Based on these studies, the lack of right prefrontal scalp activity in the ERP data of the elderly in the investigation by Trott *et al.* (1999)may be consistent, as stated above, with a failure on the part of the older subjects to maintain the representations of previous experience in working memory.

To our knowledge, there are no other age-related ERP, PET, or fMRI data that deal with the issue of binding in either working or episodic memory. However, there are a number of fMRI/PET studies whose focus has been either encoding or retrieval (and, more rarely, both) of episodic memories. Hence the results of these studies might aid in the interpretations of the ERP data described above.

Encoding

Morcom *et al.* (2003) used event-related fMRI (efMRI) to assess encoding-related activity in the only age-related haemodynamic study of SMEs that currently exists. Participants made semantic animate–inanimate decisions to a series of words during which scanning occurred. Subjects were not imaged during recognition memory testing, which followed the study phase by either a short (10–15 min) or long (30 min) delay. There were two major results, which did not differ as a function of memory test delay: (1) a number of regions, which included, but were not limited to, the LIPC (Brodmann area 47) and the left hippocampus, showed age-invariant correlations with subsequent memory performance (i.e. showed greater activation to remembered than to forgotten items); (2) in the prefrontal cortex, the SMEs were more bilateral in the data of the old compared with those of the young, consistent with recent age-related haemodynamic studies of memory (Cabeza 2002).

The data of Morcom *et al.* (2003) suggest a possible explanation for the lack of scalp activity over LIPC in the ERPs[2] of the elderly in the data shown in Figure 27.3. Trott *et al.* (1999) did not give any specific encoding instructions. A well-established phenomenon evinced in the behavioural literature is that older adults typically fail to spontaneously encode items to semantic or 'deep' levels (Hashtroudi *et al.* 1989), which typically engenders low levels of subsequent memory performance. The results of haemodynamic studies of young adults generally indicate that the LIPC is activated to a greater extent for items that are subsequently remembered, possibly because this brain region is usually activated when items are retrieved from semantic memory, whether during semantic retrieval tasks *per se* or during encoding phases for subsequent recognition memory testing. Hence the failure to demonstrate scalp activity over the LIPC may be consistent with older adults failing to 'deeply' encode the study items spontaneously. Thus one possible interpretation of these data is that a failure to elaborate the stimuli semantically led to contextually impoverished memory traces which, when a retrieval attempt was made, failed to reconstitute the item and its context as a unitized episode.

A compelling demonstration of the role of the LIPC in elaborative encoding has been provided by Anderson *et al.* (2000) using PET scanning. These investigators used full- and divided-attention conditions with young and older adults during both encoding and retrieval phases. Subjects had to memorize word pairs and, to facilitate subsequent memory performance, were instructed to construct an image linking the two words. Dividing attention primarily affected the encoding and not the retrieval phases for both age groups. During full attention, older adults produced less haemodynamic activity in the LIPC and poorer memory performance than the young adults. However, during divided attention conditions, LIPC activity during encoding and subsequent memory performance was decreased for both age groups. These data suggest that dividing attention and ageing have a similar effect on LIPC activity, which serves to reduce the amount of elaborative processing that can be engaged. Hence these PET data concur with the ERP subsequent memory data described earlier in suggesting that one reason for age-related episodic memory deficits is a failure to semantically elaborate to-be-memorized material.

Other neuroimaging evidence also points to age-related deficits in brain regions that appear to support semantic elaboration, although some contradictory findings are also apparent. Using efMRI, Logan *et al.* 2002) found that older adults under-recruited left inferior frontal regions implicated in meaning elaboration during intentional encoding, which was accompanied by poorer recognition memory performance relative to the young. In contrast, when older subjects were given an elaborative task (abstract/concrete), this under-recruitment was reversed, although there was still a (non-significant) trend for the older subjects to perform at a lower level than the young. On the other hand, using the same abstract/concrete encoding task as Logan *et al.* (2002), Stebbins *et al.* (2002) found that LIPC activity during encoding was significantly weaker in their older subjects (they did not include a recognition test phase). During face encoding, Grady *et al.* (2002) reported an increase in activations during deep semantic encoding (pleasantness judgement) relative to shallow encoding in both young and old age groups in bilateral Brodman areas 10 and 47. Like the data of Logan *et al.* (2002), the Grady *et al.* data indicate that older adults can recruit these regions in the service of semantic encoding when given a task that constrains encoding activity. However, although the older adults were able to improve their performance via deep encoding, the magnitude of their left prefrontal activation was smaller, consistent with their poorer performance, relative to the young, during the subsequent recognition of items from the pleasantness task.

Hence, the majority of age-related haemodynamic studies of encoding appear to demonstrate weaker left inferior prefrontal activations for elderly relative to young subjects. These reduced activations are typically accompanied by lower recognition performance for the older subjects. However, the picture has recently become somewhat more complicated. Although the results of some investigations show reduced activity in the elderly relative to the young in left-hemisphere brain regions implicated in semantic retrieval and elaboration, these have sometimes been accompanied by contralateral activations that are larger than those observed for the young, leading to a more bilateral pattern of activation in the elderly (for reviews and experimental demonstrations, see Cabeza 2002; Cabeza *et al.* 2002; Logan *et al.* 2002; Morcom *et al.* 2003). This has led some authors to propose that these contralateral activations are 'compensatory', and may only characterize the haemodynamic data of a subset of elderly individuals who are better performers than their peers (Cabeza *et al* 2002; Logan *et al.* 2002; Daselaar *et al.* 2003). To date, this more bilateral pattern, relative to the data of the young, has not been observed in ERP studies, although interpretations of ERP data as consistent with a 'compensation' hypothesis have been published (Friedman 2003). Hence the generalizability of this phenomenon to other techniques is unknown. Interestingly, in the one age-related study of working memory and binding that does exist (Mitchell *et al.* 2000b), there appears to be no evidence of this type of bilateral pattern in the haemodynamic data of the older sample. Thus the haemodynamic data on compensation appear to be silent with respect to item–context binding. Another complication is the fact that, with the exception of the study by Morcom *et al.* (2003), none of the other efMRI age-related studies of encoding have computed SMEs. Hence, with the exception of limited ERP data (Friedman and Trott 2000), the results of the vast majority of haemodynamic investigations are based on activity that reflects both successful and unsuccessful encoding.

Retrieval

The ERP retrieval data described above suggest a deficit in a right prefrontal mechanism, which might reflect a working memory component active during episodic retrieval. Can the age-related neuroimaging investigations of retrieval add to this very preliminary hypothesis? In general, haemodynamic data based on young adults indicate that retrieval of previous episodes engages a network of brain regions, with prominent activation in the left and right prefrontal cortex. Some investigators have suggested that the magnitude of prefrontal activity (and whether it is asymmetrical in the left or right prefrontal cortex) reflects the extent to which retrieval requires executive control (Nolde *et al.* 1998a,b; Mayes and Montaldi 2001; but see Habib *et al.* 2003). Specific posterior neocortical regions, where the multimodal representations of past events are presumably stored, are also involved. Hence it is likely that the prefrontal cortex serves to control processes that guide access to and retrieval of these representations (Henson *et al.* 1999), although it is also possible that specialized mnemonic functions are carried out by different regions of the prefrontal cortex. There have been several haemodynamic studies of memory retrieval and ageing (reviewed by Cabeza 2001; Grady 2000). Unlike young adults, elderly adults exhibit a more bilateral pattern of prefrontal activation (Schacter *et al.* 1996; Cabeza *et al.* 1997; Madden *et al.* 1999), which typically results in right-sided activations of similar magnitude when compared to the young.

One difficulty limiting unequivocal interpretation of the extant age-related haemodynamic studies of memory retrieval is that the experiments have not typically been designed to test the veracity of dual-process theories of recognition memory. This appears to be the case, for example, for the right prefrontal activation that has been observed consistently in studies of retrieval in the data of young adults. Whereas several studies have attempted to determine whether this activity reflects 'monitoring' of the products of retrieval in young adults (reviewed by Fletcher and Henson 2001), to our knowledge this has not been attempted in studies of older adults. Similarly, with few exceptions (Cabeza *et al.* 2000), age-related haemodynamic studies of recollection versus familiarity and source versus item memory do not exist. This hinders attempts to use the age-related haemodynamic data concerning retrieval to aid in interpreting the lack of the right prefrontal EM effect observed in the study by Trott *et al.* (1999) described above, or to assist in interpreting age-related changes in recollection and familiarity.

However, a recent efMRI study by Cabeza *et al.* (2004) suggests an intriguing possibility with respect to age-related changes in recollection and familiarity. In this study, young and elderly participants studied a list of 40 words while making living–non-living judgements. Subjects were scanned during the test phase, which included three types of trials: working memory, visual attention, and episodic recognition (for the 40 previously presented words). The three trial types were cued randomly on a trial-by-trial basis. During episodic recognition trials subjects had to judge whether their recognition of old items was accompanied by specific contextual details (an R response) or not (a K response), or whether the item was new (i.e. not previously studied). R and K judgements were included only to encourage participants to use recollection to retrieve items, as the small number of old trials precluded categorizing the fMRI data into those associated with R and K judgements.

Young adults ($M = 77$ per cent) produced reliably more R responses than the old ($M = 65$ per cent), while older adults ($M = 35$ per cent) produced more K responses than the young ($M = 23$ per cent), again suggesting that older adults rely more on familiarity than the young. A highly interesting, but unpredicted, age-related finding was observed for the medial temporal lobes. Young adults activated the hippocampus more than older adults, whereas older adults activated the parahippocampal region more than young adults. Because some theorists have hypothesized that the hippocampus is essential for recollection-based retrieval, but not familiarity-based recognition, while the parahippocampal region subserves familiarity-based responding, but not recollection (Aggleton and Brown 1999; Eichenbaum 2003), this tantalizing result could be taken to mean that the elderly relied more on familiarity than recollection, which would be consistent with the behavioural research reviewed earlier and the R and K findings from the investigation by Cabeza *et al.* (2004) investigation. However, a great deal of caution must be exercised as the result was not predicted and, to our knowledge, has not been reported previously. Thus it requires replication.

Conclusions

Based on a variety of evidence from different imaging techniques as well as behavioural procedures, older adults appear to be more impaired when conscious recollection of previous experience is required compared with when automatic familiarity-based responding will suffice. Whether assessed using the process dissociation, remember–know, or source memory paradigms, the weight of the evidence suggests that older adults are always at a disadvantage when contextual details must be retrieved in addition to item content. However, the majority of these investigations were performed during the retrieval phases of memory tasks and few data exist that speak to the issue of whether the deficit in recollection-based processing has its origin during the encoding phases of recognition memory paradigms. One of the ERP studies described here (Friedman and Trott 2000) suggests that encoding has a critical influence which may be more important than that of retrieval. However, this conclusion is premature until more studies directly compare the encoding and retrieval phases of recognition memory paradigms. Nevertheless, regardless of the locus of the episodic memory deficit, it is likely that older adults have greater difficulty in forming unitized representations that are comprised of associations between unrelated items, a problem that has recently been formalized as the associative deficit hypothesis (ADH) (Naveh-Benjamin *et al.* 2003; see also Chapter 25). The ADH has been advanced on the basis of age-related difficulties in forming new associations between two unrelated words or pictures and therefore appears to be a more specific case of a general age-related binding problem. Hence these associations could be, for example, between items and their spatial locations (Chalfonte and Johnson 1996), between items and their list membership (Trott *et al.* 1999), or between items and the gender of the voice in which they were presented (Senkfor and Petten 1996; Mark and Rugg 1998). Future behavioural, ERP, and haemodynamic investigations will undoubtedly shed greater light on the age-related nature of the processes and brain regions that are altered when binding of separate features is required for good episodic memory performance.

Notes

1. Mark and Rugg (1998) reported intact right prefrontal EM effects in the data of their elderly subjects. The reasons for this discrepancy are not known, but some possibilities have been considered by Mark and Rugg (1998), Trott *et al.* (1999), and Rugg and Morcom (2004).
2. The relations between a given ERP component and fMRI activation in a specific region of the brain are currently unknown. Nonetheless, it is highly unlikely that ERP and fMRI data will converge completely, as ERPs can only be observed for those intracranial fields that have the correct orientation with respect to the scalp, which is not a limitation of the fMRI technique. Similarly, for example, the fMRI signal may be reduced or absent for regions of the brain that are associated with susceptibility artefacts, a restriction that does not apply to the ERP technique. Currently, a series of converging operations has typically been employed to determine correspondences between the two types of data. For example, if SMEs show similar relations to the experimental variables in both the ERP and fMRI laboratories, this would be good evidence that the mechanisms underlying the SMEs in the two datasets might be similar (for expanded discussions of these issues, see Luck (1998) and Rugg (1998)).

Acknowledgements

The author thanks Mr C.L. Brown III for computer programming and technical assistance, and Mr J. Cheng for technical assistance. Sincere thanks are due to Dr Y. Cycowicz, Dr M. Fabiani, Dr H. Gaeta, Dr D. Nessler, Dr W. Ritter, Dr J.G. Snodgrass, Dr C. Trott, and Dr D. Wegesin for their contributions to the research reported here and for discussions concerning these data. Preparation of this paper was supported in part by grants AG05213 and AG09988 from the National Institute on Aging, grant HD14959 from the National Institute of Child Health and Human Development, and the New York State Department of Mental Hygiene.

References

Aggleton, J.P. and Brown, M.W. (1999). Episodic memory, amnesia, and the hippocampal-anterior thalamic axis. *Behavioral and Brain Sciences*, **22**, 425–489.

Anderson, N.D., Iidaka, T., Cabeza, R., Kapur, S., McIntosh, A.R., and Craik, F.I. (2000). The effects of divided attention on encoding- and retrieval-related brain activity: a PET study of younger and older adults. *Journal of Cognitive Neuroscience*, **12**, 775–792.

Bastin, C. and Van der Linden, M. (2003). The contribution of recollection and familiarity to recognition memory: a study of the effects of test format and aging. *Neuropsychology*, **17**, 14–24.

Cabeza, R. (2001). Cognitive neuroscience of aging: contributions of functional neuroimaging. *Scandinavian Journal of Psychology*, **42**, 277–286.

Cabeza, R. (2002). Hemispheric asymmetry reduction in older adults: the HAROLD model. *Psychology and Aging*, **17**, 85–100.

Cabeza, R., Grady, C.L., Nyberg, L., ***et al.*** (1997). Age-related differences in neural activity during memory encoding and retrieval: a positron emission tomography study. *Journal of Neuroscience*, **17**, 391–400.

Cabeza, R., Anderson, N.D., Houle, S., Mangels, J.A., and Nyberg, L. (2000). Age-related differences in neural activity during item and temporal- order memory retrieval: a positron emission tomography study. *Journal of Cognitive Neuroscience*, **12**, 197–206.

Cabeza, R., Anderson, N.D., Locantore, J.K., and McIntosh, A.R. (2002). Aging gracefully: compensatory brain activity in high-performing older adults. *NeuroImage*, **17**, 1394–1402.

Cabeza, R., Daselaar, S.M., Dolcos, F., Prince, S.E., Budde, M., and Nyberg, L. (2004). Task-independent and task-specific age effects on brain activity during working memory, visual attention and episodic retrieval. *Cerebral Cortex*, **14**, 364–375.

Chalfonte, B.L. and Johnson, M.K. (1996). Feature memory and binding in young and older adults. *Memory and Cognition*, **24**, 403–416.

Clarys, D., Isingrini, M., and Gana, K. (2002). Mediators of age-related differences in recollective experience in recognition memory. *Acta Psychologica*, **109**, 315–329.

Craik, F.I.M., Byrd, M., and Swanson, J.M. (1987). Patterns of memory loss in three elderly samples. *Psychology and Aging*, **2**, 79–86.

Craik, F.I.M. and Lockhart, S. (1972). Levels of processing: a framework for memory research. *Journal of Verbal Learning and Verbal Behavior*, **11**, 671–684.

Craik, F.I.M. and McDowd, J.M. (1987). Age differences in recall and recognition. *Journal of Experimental Psychology: Learning, Memory, and Cognition*, **13**, 474–479.

Curran, T. (2000). Brain potentials of recollection and familiarity. *Memory and Cognition*, **28**, 923–938.

Daselaar, S.M., Veltman, D.J., Rombouts, S.A., Raaijmakers, J.G., and Jonker, C. (2003). Neuroanatomical correlates of episodic encoding and retrieval in young and elderly subjects. *Brain*, **126**, 43–56.

Eichenbaum, H. (2003). How does the hippocampus contribute to memory? *Trends in Cognitive Science*, **7**, 427–429.

Fabiani, M. and Friedman, D. (1997). Dissociations between memory for temporal order and recognition memory in aging. *Neuropsychologia*, **35**, 129–141.

Fletcher, P.C. and Henson, R.N. (2001). Frontal lobes and human memory: insights from functional neuroimaging. *Brain*, **124**, 849–881.

Friedman, D. (2003). Cognition and aging: a highly selective overview of event-related potential (ERP) data. *Journal of Clinical and Experimental Neuropsychology*, **25**, 702–720.

Friedman, D. and Johnson, R. (2000). Event-related potential (ERP) studies of memory encoding and retrieval: a selective review. *Microscopy Research and Technique*, **51**, 6–28.

Friedman, D. and Trott, C. (2000). An event-related potential study of encoding in young and older adults. *Neuropsychologia*, **38**, 542–557.

Friedman, D., Ritter, W., and Snodgrass, J.G. (1996). ERPs during study as a function of subsequent direct and indirect memory testing in young and old adults. *Brain Research: Cognitive Brain Research*, **4**, 1–13.

Gardiner, J.M. (2001). Episodic memory and autonoetic consciousness: a first-person approach. *Philosophical Transactions of the Royal Society of London, Series B: Biological Sciences*, **356**, 1351–1361.

Gardiner, J.M. and Java, R.I. (1990). Recollective experience in word and nonword recognition. *Memory and Cognition*, **18**, 23–30.

Gardiner, J.M., Ramponi, C., and Richardson-Klavehn, A. (1999). Response deadline and subjective awareness in recognition memory. *Consciousness and Cognition*, **8**, 484–496.

Glisky, E.L., Rubin, S.R., and Davidson, P.S.R. (2001). Source memory in older adults: an encoding or retrieval problem? *Journal of Experimental Psychology: Learning, Memory, and Cognition*, **27**, 1131–1146.

Grady, C.L. (2000). Functional brain imaging and age-related changes in cognition. *Biological Psychology*, **54**, 259–281.

Grady, C.L. and Craik, F.I. (2000). Changes in memory processing with age. *Current Opinion in Neurobiology*, **10**, 224–231.

Grady, C.L., Bernstein, L.J., Beig, S., and Siegenthaler, A.L. (2002). The effects of encoding task on age-related differences in the functional neuroanatomy of face memory. *Psychology and Aging*, **17**, 7–23.

Habib, R., Nyberg, L., and Tulving, E. (2003). Hemispheric asymmetries of memory: the HERA model revisited. *Trends in Cognitive Sciences*, **7**, 241–245.

Hashtroudi, S., Parker, E.S., Luis, J.D., and Reisen, C.A. (1989). Generation and elaboration in older adults. *Experimental Aging Research*, **15**, 73–78.

Henkel, L.A., Johnson, M.K., and De Leonardis, D.M. (1998). Aging and source monitoring: cognitive processes and neuropsychological correlates. *Journal of Experimental Psychology: General*, **127**, 251–268.

Henson, R., Shallice, T., and Dolan, R.J. (1999). Right prefrontal cortex and episodic memory retrieval: a functional MRI test of the monitoring hypothesis. *Brain*, **122**, 1367–1381.

Jacoby, L.L. (1991). A process dissociation framework: separating automatic from intentional uses of memory. *Journal of Memory and Language*, **30**, 513–541.

Jennings, J.M. and Jacoby, L.L. (1997). An opposition procedure for detecting age-related deficits in recollection: telling effects of repetition. *Psychology and Aging*, **12**, 352–361.

Johnson, R. (1995). Event-related potential insights into the neurobiology of memory systems. In *Handbook of Neuropsychology*, Vol. 10 (ed F. Boller and J. Grafman). Amsterdam: Elsevier, pp. 135–163.

Johnson, R., Jr, Kreiter, K., Russo, B., and Zhu, J. (1998). A spatio-temporal analysis of recognition-related event-related brain potentials. *International Journal of Psychophysiology*, **29**, 83–104.

Joyce, C.A., Paller, K.A., McIsaac, H.K., and Kutas, M. (1998). Memory changes with normal aging: behavioral and electrophysiological measures. *Psychophysiology*, **35**, 669–678.

Light, L.L., Prull, M.W., Voie, D.J.L., and Healy, M.R. (2000). Dual process theories of memory in old age. In *Models of Cognitive Aging* (ed T.J. Perfect and E.A. Maylor). Oxford: Oxford University Press, pp. 238–300.

Logan, J.M., Sanders, A.L., Snyder, A.Z., Morris, J.C., and Buckner, R.L. (2002). Under-recruitment and non-selective recruitment: dissociable neural mechanisms associated with aging. *Neuron*, **33**, 827–840.

Luck, S.J. (1999). Direct and indirect integration of event-related potentials, functional magnetic resonance images, and single-unit recordings. *Human Brain Mapping*, **8**, 115–120.

Madden, D.J., Gottlob, L.R., Denny, L.L., *et al.* (1999). Aging and recognition memory: changes in regional cerebral blood flow associated with components of reaction time distributions. *Journal of Cognitive Neuroscience*, **11**, 511–520.

Mandler, G. (1980). Recognizing: the judgement of previous occurrence. *Psychological Review*, **87**, 252–271.

Mark, R.E. and Rugg, M.D. (1998). Age effects on brain activity associated with episodic memory retrieval: an electrophysiological study. *Brain*, **121**, 861–873.

Mayes, A.R. and Montaldi, D. (2001). Exploring the neural bases of episodic and semantic memory: the role of structural and functional imaging. *Neuroscience and Biobehavioral Reviews*, **25**, 555–573.

Mitchell, K.J., Johnson, M.K., Raye, C.L., Mather, M., and D'Esposito, M. (2000a). Aging and reflective processes of working memory: binding and test load deficits. *Psychology and Aging*, **15**, 527–541.

Mitchell, K.J., Johnson, M.K., Raye, C.L., and D'Esposito, M. (2000b). fMRI evidence of age-related hippocampal dysfunction in feature binding in working memory. *Cognitive Brain Research*, **10**, 197–206.

Morcom, A.M., Good, C.D., Frackowiak, R.S.J., and Rugg, M.D. (2003). Age effects on the neural correlates of successful memory encoding. *Brain*, **126**, 213–229.

Naveh-Benjamin, M., Hussain, Z., Guez, J., and Bar-On, M. (2003). Adult age differences in episodic memory: Further support for an associative-deficit hypothesis. *Journal of Experimental Psychology: Learning, Memory, and Cognition*, **29**, 826–837.

Nolde, S.F., Johnson, M.K., and D'Esposito, M. (1998a). Left prefrontal activation during episodic remembering. *Neuroreport*, **9**, 3509–3514.

Nolde, S.F., Johnson, M.K., and Raye, C.L. (1998b). The role of prefrontal cortex during tests of episodic memory. *Trends in Cognitive Sciences*, **2**, 399–406.

Nunez, P.L. and Pilgreen, K.L. (1991). The spline-Laplacian in clinical neurophysiology: a method to improve EEG spatial resolution. *Journal of Clinical Neurophysiology*, **8**, 397–413.

Paller, K.A. (2001). Neurocognitive foundations of human memory. In *The Psychology of Learning and Motivation*, Vol. 40 (ed D.L. Medin). San Diego, CA: Academic Press, pp. 121–145.

Paller, K.A. and Wagner, A.D. (2002). Transforming experience into memory: observations of mind and brain. *Trends in Cognitive Sciences*, **6**, 93–102.

Paller, K.A., Kutas, M., and Mayes, A.R. (1987). Neural correlates of encoding in an incidental learning paradigm. *Electroencephalography and Clinical Neurophysiology*, **67**, 360–371.

Perlmutter, M., Metzger, R., Nezworski, T., and Miller, K. (1981). Spatial and temporal memory in 20 to 60 year olds. *Journal of Gerontology*, **36**, 59–65.

Prabhakaran, V., Narayanan, K., Zhao, Z., and Gabrieli, J.D. (2000). Integration of diverse information in working memory within the frontal lobe. *Nature Neuroscience*, **3**, 85–90.

Rugg, M.D. (1998). Convergent approaches to electrophysiological and hemodynamic investigations of memory. *Human Brain Mapping*, **6**, 394–398.

Rugg, M.D. and Allan, K. (2000). Memory retrieval: an electrophysiological perspective. In *The Cognitive Neurosciences*, Vol. 2 (ed M. Gazzaniga). Cambridge, MA: MIT Press.

Rugg, M.D. and Morcom, A.M. (2004). The relationship between brain activity, cognitive performance and aging: the case of memory. In *Cognitive Neuroscience of Aging: Linking Cognitive and Cerebral Aging* (ed R. Cabeza, L. Nyberg, and D.C. Park). New York: Oxford University Press.

Rugg, M.D. and Wilding, E.L. (2000). Retrieval processing and episodic memory. *Trends in Cognitive Sciences*, **4**, 108–115.

Rugg, M.D., Mark, R.E., Gilchrist, J., and Roberts, R.C. (1997). ERP repetition effects in indirect and direct tasks: effects of age and interitem lag. *Psychophysiology*, **34**, 572–86.

Rugg, M.D., Schloerscheidt, A.M., and Mark, R.E. (1998). An electrophysiological comparison of two indices of recollection. *Journal of Memory and Language*, **39**, 47–69.

Schacter, D.L., Savage, C.R., Alpert, N.M., Rauch, S.L., and Albert, M.S. (1996). The role of hippocampus and frontal cortex in age-related memory changes: a PET study. *Neuroreport*, **7**, 1165–1169.

Senkfor, A.J. and Petten, C.V. (1996). ERP measures of source and item memory in young and elderly subjects. Paper presented at the Society for Psychophysiological Research, Vancouver, BC.

Smith, M.E. (1993). Neurophysiological manifestations of recollective experience during recognition memory judgements. *Journal of Cognitive Neuroscience*, **5**, 1–13.

Snodgrass, J.G. and Corwin, J. (1988). Pragmatics of measuring recognition memory: applications to dementia and amnesia. *Journal of Experimental Psychology: General*, **117**, 34–50.

Spencer, W.D. and Raz, N. (1995). Differential effects of aging on memory for content and context: a meta-analysis. *Psychology and Aging*, **10**, 527–539.

Stebbins, G.T., Carrillo, M.C., Dorfman, J., *et al.* (2002). Aging effects on memory encoding in the frontal lobes. *Psychology and Aging*, **17**, 44–55.

Swick, D. and Knight, R.T. (1997). Event-related potentials differentiate the effects of aging on word and nonword repetition in explicit and implicit memory tasks. *Journal of Experimental Psychology: Learning, Memory, and Cognition*, **23**, 123–142.

Trott, C.T., Friedman, D., Ritter, W., Fabiani, M., and Snodgrass, J.G. (1999). Episodic priming and memory for temporal source: event-related potentials reveal age-related differences in prefrontal functioning. *Psychology and Aging*, **14**, 390–413.

Tsivilis, D., Otten, L.J., and Rugg, M.D. (2001). Context effects on the neural correlates of recognition memory. an electrophysiological study. *Neuron*, **31**, 497–505.

Tulving, E. (1985). Memory and consciousness. *Canadian Psychologist*, **26**, 1–12.

Wagner, A.D., Schacter, D.L., Koutstaal, M.R.W., *et al.* (1998). Building memories: remembering and forgetting of verbal experiences as predicted by brain activity. *Science*, **281**, 1188–1191.

Wegesin, D.J., Friedman, D., Varughese, N., and Stern, Y. (2002). Age-related changes in source memory retrieval: an ERP replication and extension. *Cognitive Brain Research*, **13**, 323–338.

Wilding, E.L. (1999). Separating retrieval strategies from retrieval success: an event-related potential study of source memory. *Neuropsychologia*, **37**, 441–454.

Wilding, E.L. and Sharpe, H. (2002). Episodic memory encoding and retrieval: recent insights from event-related postentials. In *The Cognitive Electrophysiology of Mind and Brain* (ed A. Zani and A.M. Proverbio). New York: Academic Press, pp. 169–196.

Yonelinas, A.P. (2002). The nature of recollection and familiarity: a review of 30 years of research. *Journal of Memory and Language*, **46**, 441–517.

Yovel, G. and Paller, K.A. (2004). The neural basis of the butcher-on-the-bus phenomenon: when a face seems familiar but is not remembered. *NeuroImage*, **21**, 789–800.

Chapter 28

Episodic memory impairment in preclinical Alzheimer's disease: the role of encoding, consolidation, and retrieval factors

Brent J. Small and Lars Bäckman

Introduction

In recent years, there has been great interest in preclinical Alzheimer's disease (AD). The preclinical phase is believed to represent a period of time prior to the diagnosis of AD where individuals who are at higher risk of developing this disease exhibit differences on a variety of characteristics as compared with those who will remain free of AD over a follow-up period. These differences have been shown to include decreased volume of select brain regions and elevated values on several serum and cerebrospinal fluid indices, as well as poorer performance on a variety of tests of cognitive performance (reviewed by DeKosky and Marek 2003). The notion of a preclinical period of AD suggests that individuals who may be at risk of developing AD could be identified and interventions may be attempted. This is a critically important issue, as recent projections suggest that over the next 50 years the number of people diagnosed with clinical AD in Western countries is expected to increase to over four times the current number (Brookmeyer *et al.* 1998; Hebert *et al.* 2003). Additional evidence suggests that early intervention to delay the onset of the disease can result in a significant reduction in the number of cases of AD (Brookmeyer *et al.* 1998). Although the long-term efficacy of pharmacological interventions is limited at the present time (Flicker 1999; Rockwood *et al.* 2003), future medications may be more effective.

In this chapter we focus on the nature of cognitive deficits in preclinical AD, with special emphasis on its impact on episodic memory functioning. Specifically, we are interested in documenting the prevalence and magnitude of cognitive deficits, as well as identifying the potential implications of the results as a means of early detection of future AD patients. We will begin by describing methodological features of studies that have examined preclinical AD. Next, we will describe evidence concerning the generality of cognitive deficits in preclinical AD, with particular emphasis on impairments in tests of episodic memory. Finally, we will describe some work that has attempted to improve understanding of the source of the episodic memory deficit in preclinical AD, with reference to the role of binding processes.

Methodological features of studies of preclinical Alzheimer's disease

An important feature of studies that examine preclinical AD is to assess functioning prior to the diagnosis of AD among individuals, some of whom will eventually receive a dementia diagnosis. This is done by assessing individuals over a longitudinal follow-up interval, even if cognitive performance is obtained from only a single time point. In a typical study, all participants are assessed at a baseline measurement point where cognitive functioning is evaluated and all participants are free of a diagnosis of AD. At a later point, which may range from annual assessments to multiple years between follow-up intervals, individuals return and their diagnostic status (non-demented, AD) is re-evaluated. At this point, some of the individuals will receive a diagnosis of AD. As a result, their initial cognitive performance test scores are believed to represent the time during which individuals are in the preclinical phase of the disease.

Although the general methodological strategy described above is the norm in the study of preclinical AD, there is a great deal of variability in study design that can affect the nature of the results observed. For example, most studies assess the cognitive status of individuals at only a single point in time (e.g. Tierney *et al.* 2000), making inferences with regard to the nature of changes in cognitive performance during preclinical AD impossible to derive (but see Chen *et al.* 2001; Bäckman *et al.* 2001a). Secondly, there can be significant variability in the time between assessment and clinical diagnosis. For example, in some cases relatively short follow-up periods (2–3 years) are used (e.g. Celsis *et al.* 1997), but in some cases the follow-up period can be more than 5 years (e.g. Visser *et al.* 2001). Further, some studies assess subjects annually, but when the data are compared, individuals who convert to AD at any point along the follow-up period, ranging from 1 to 15 years of follow-up in one case (Elias *et al.* 2000), are combined into the preclinical group. This variation has the potential to influence which cognitive ability domains are affected preclinically, as well as the magnitude of the cognitive deficits.

Cognitive deficits in preclinical Alzheimer's disease

From the standpoint of measuring cognitive deficits in preclinical AD, two main classes of studies characterize the literature. In the first, cognitive performance is indexed with single relatively broad measures of cognitive performance using tests such as the Mini-Mental State Examination (MMSE; Folstein *et al.* 1987). Using such measures, a number of studies have reported significantly poorer performance among individuals who will go on to be diagnosed with AD (e.g. Huang *et al.* 2000; Lange *et al.* 2002). Although some studies have decomposed performance on the global measures to evaluate specific subdomains of cognitive functioning (e.g. Small *et al.* 1997b, 2000), the main disadvantage of the global measures of cognitive performance is their relative lack of sensitivity to subtle levels of impairment, as well as their limited ability to comprehensively assess multiple domains of cognitive ability.

In the second class of studies, preclinical cognitive deficits have been assessed using broader neuropsychological test batteries. The advantage of these measures is the greater sensitivity of the instruments, as well as detailed information about the specificity of deficits in terms of whether some abilities are more affected than others. The major disadvantage of the comprehensive batteries is the amount of expertise and administration time that they require.

Research with the broader neuropsychological batteries has demonstrated preclinical cognitive deficits across a variety of tasks, including psychomotor speed (Masur *et al.* 1994), perceptual speed (Fabrigoule *et al.* 1998), executive functioning (Albert *et al.* 2001), verbal ability (Jacobs *et al.* 1995), abstract reasoning (Fabrigoule *et al.* 1996), and visuospatial performance (Howieson *et al.* 1997). The results obtained using measures of global cognitive performance, as well as the detailed assessment of multiple domains of cognitive functioning by the more comprehensive batteries, suggest that the cognitive impairment in preclinical AD is relatively generic.

However, the presence of statistically significant impairments across multiple ability domains does not necessarily inform us about the relative magnitude of cognitive deficits across each domain. To address this issue, we recently conducted a meta-analysis of the literature on cognitive deficits in preclinical AD (Bäckman *et al.* 2005). To be included in the meta-analysis, the studies had to have AD as a diagnostic outcome for some individuals, assess cognitive functioning at a baseline assessment point, and provide sufficient statistical test information to allow effect-size parameters to be calculated. In this case, we computed the effect-size measure d, which represents group differences as a function of standard deviation units. In total, we identified 48 studies which included 1246 preclinical AD cases and 9119 controls.

To evaluate whether deficits of cognitive functioning in preclinical AD are general, in that multiple ability domains are affected, or specific to only some cognitive abilities, we categorized the cognitive tests into eight broad measures. These included (prototypical tests in parentheses) global cognitive ability (MMSE), episodic memory (Wechsler Memory Scale), verbal ability (Controlled Oral Word Association Test), visuospatial skill (Block Design), primary memory (Forward Digit Span), attention (Trailmaking A), perceptual speed (Digit Symbol), and executive functioning (Wisconsin Card Sorting Test).

The results of this meta-analysis are shown in Figure 28.1. The *d*-value and the associated 99 per cent confidence interval (CI) are presented for each cognitive ability domain. In all cases, higher scores indicate greater deficits among the preclinical AD group. It is clear from the figure that cognitive deficits in preclinical AD are rather generic in nature, in as much as statistically significant group differences were observed for all domains except primary memory ($d = 0.00$). Further, in many of the non-memory domains of functioning, the differences were greater than 1 SD, including global cognitive ability ($d = 1.19$), perceptual speed ($d = 1.11$), and executive functioning ($d = 1.07$). Among the remaining ability domains, the effect sizes were moderate to large for verbal ability ($d = 0.79$), visuospatial skill ($d = 0.64$), and attention ($d = 0.62$).

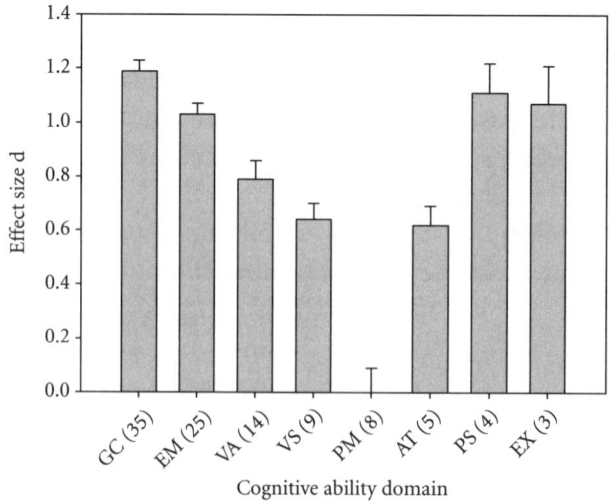

Figure 28.1 Effect size *d* by cognitive ability domain: GC, global cognitive ability; EM, episodic memory; VA, verbal ability; VS, visuospatial skill, PM, primary memory; AT, attention; PS, perceptual speed; EX, executive functioning; Numbers in parentheses refer to the number of studies contributing to the calculation of the effect size.

Episodic memory in preclinical Alzheimer's disease

Although it is clear that multiple cognitive abilities may be affected preclinically, as demonstrated by the results of the meta-analysis described above, episodic memory has been the main focus of interest in this domain of research. This probably reflects the fact that persons who eventually become diagnosed as having AD initially present with memory complaints, as well as a wealth of neurological evidence indicating that initial changes in the brains of AD patients occur to limbic structures (Goldman *et al.* 2001; Gao *et al.* 2004), especially the hippocampus which is well known to be important for successful memory performance (Squire 1992).

Indeed, the results of our meta-analysis demonstrate sizeable preclinical deficits in episodic memory performance. Specifically, across the 25 studies that included tests of episodic memory, the average effect size was greater than 1 SD (d = 1.03, 99 per cent CI 0.99–1.08). Further, research has demonstrated that within the domain of episodic memory, persons who will go on to be diagnosed with AD exhibit differences across a variety of task manipulations, i.e. preclinical deficits have been observed for both verbal (Howieson *et al.* 1997; Chen *et al.* 2001) and non-verbal (Albert *et al.* 2001; Fowler *et al.* 2002) tasks. In addition, impairments have been reported for tasks that vary in terms of retention interval (Linn *et al.* 1995; Chen *et al.* 2001) and for all manner of retrieval conditions, including free recall (Fabrigoule *et al.* 1998; Rubin *et al.* 1998), cued recall (Bäckman *et al.* 2001a; Chen *et al.* 2001), and recognition (Small *et al.* 1997a; Bondi *et al.* 1999).

With regard to the nature of the episodic memory deficit in preclinical AD, variability in the manner in which material to be remembered is presented to participants, the length of the retention interval, and the retrieval conditions may provide insight into the source of the deficit. As a start, it is clear from the results of our meta-analysis that the passive holding of information in the mind, as indexed by tests of primary memory, is well preserved in preclinical AD. Rather, the source of episodic memory deficit in preclinical AD stems from processes associated with committing something to memory. Information relevant to this idea comes from studies that have examined the influence of cognitive support on episodic memory performance in preclinical AD. Cognitive support refers to the characteristics of tasks that make successful retrieval of information more or less likely (reviewed by Bäckman *et al.* 1990). In the normal ageing literature, older adults are clearly able to benefit from the provision of cognitive support at encoding or retrieval (reviewed by Bäckman *et al.* 2001b).

In terms of preclinical AD, variability in episodic memory tasks as a function of cognitive support has important implications in terms of whether persons who will go on to develop AD can benefit to the same degree as individuals who will remain free of dementia. In the clinical AD literature, research has demonstrated that persons with AD are less able to benefit from supportive conditions than individuals who are free of dementia. In particular, it appears that in order for benefits to be observed, persons with AD must received support at both encoding and retrieval (Bäckman and Herlitz 1996; Almkvist *et al.* 1999).

Much less is known about the ability of persons with preclinical AD to benefit from supportive conditions. We examined the impact of cognitive support on the episodic memory performance of three groups of participants: cognitively intact elderly, persons with clinical AD, and individuals who were diagnosed with AD after a 3-year follow-up period (Bäckman and Small 1998). Participants were tested on two occasions separated by approximately 3 years. The preclinical AD group is of particular interest. At time 1, these individuals were still considered cognitively normal in terms of the absence of a dementia diagnosis. However, at time 2 they were diagnosed with AD. Thus we were able to examine the overall performance of this group, as well as the ability to benefit from cognitive support, as they underwent the transition from cognitively intact to prevalent AD. The episodic memory tasks varied in terms of time presented for study (fast versus slow presentation rate), organizability of material at encoding (unrelated versus organizable words), and availability of cues at retrieval (free recall versus cued recall).

The results for the three participant groups are shown in Figure 28.2. There are two important characteristics in this figure that are relevant to the nature of episodic memory deficits in preclinical AD. First, the three participant groups are quantitatively different, with the cognitively intact group performing the best, the clinical AD group the worst, and the preclinical AD group occupying an intermediate position. Thus, consistent with the meta-analysis results reported earlier, the preclinical AD group was deficient 3 years before clinical diagnosis. Secondly, the shape of the graphs is functionally similar for the cognitively intact and preclinical AD groups, but not for the clinical AD participants. The clinical AD group obtained no benefit across the first two additions of cognitive support. Improvement is only seen when memory performance is supported at both encoding (organizable words) and retrieval (cued recall). In contrast, the preclinical AD group was able to improve following each provision of cognitive support, similar to the cognitively intact participants. Thus the preclinical group appeared qualitatively similar to, but quantitatively different from, the cognitively intact group during the preclinical phase of the disease, but became more similar to the clinical group, in terms of the nature of the cognitive deficits, after diagnosis.

The performance of the three groups of participants at the second measurement time is also shown in Figure 28.2. This is most relevant for the preclinical

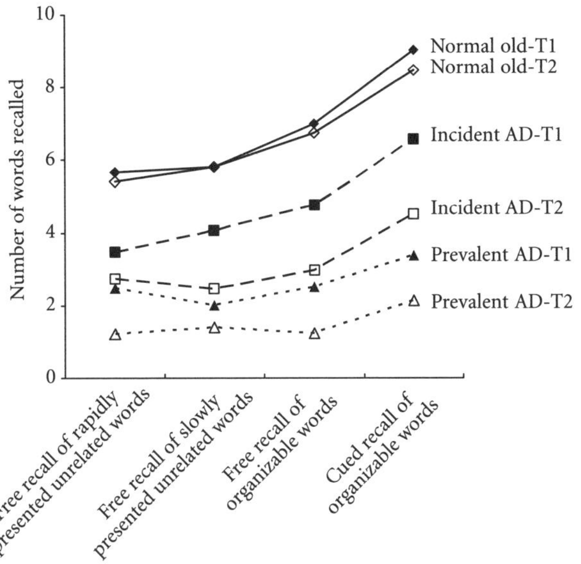

Figure 28.2 Episodic memory performance in normal old adults, incident AD patients, and prevalent AD patients across level of cognitive support at baseline T1 (3 years before diagnosis) and follow-up T2 (diagnosis). (Adapted from L. Bäckman and B.J. Small, *Psychology and Aging*, **13**, 267–276, 1998.)

AD cases, because this is the time at which the clinical diagnosis of AD was made. At this point, unlike their performance 3 years earlier, the now clinical AD participants perform more like the prevalent AD participants from time 1, i.e. significant gains in performance were only seen for cued recall of organizable words, the most supported condition.

The results of the study by Bäckman and Small (1998) provide some information relevant to the encoding and retrieval capabilities of persons with preclinical AD. Their ability to benefit from extra study time suggests that their encoding capabilities are not entirely compromised. However, this group was still at a quantitative disadvantage, in terms of their overall memory performance relative to the cognitively intact group. Additional results from our meta-analysis (Bäckman *et al.* 2005) may provide further information about the encoding and retrieval capabilities of persons in preclinical AD. Figure 28.3 shows the preclinical deficit associated with episodic memory relative to task characteristics, including retention interval (immediate, delayed), retrieval support (recall, recognition), and study materials (verbal, non-verbal).

Several aspects of the data in Figure 28.3 are noteworthy. First, the preclinical deficit associated with AD is sizeable across all task manipulations, i.e. all the episodic memory conditions are impaired preclinically in AD. Secondly, there is variation in the magnitude of the deficit relative to the task variation. Specifically, immediate assessment of performance, testing with recognition, and using non-verbal materials all produced smaller effect sizes. In terms of the relevance of the

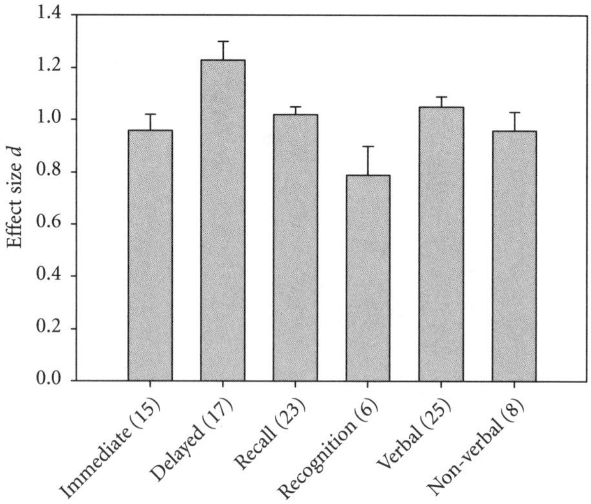

Figure 28.3 Effect size *d* by episodic memory task manipulation. Numbers in parentheses refer to the number of studies contributing to the calculation of the effect size.

current results to the encoding, consolidation, and retrieval abilities in preclinical AD, provided that delayed testing taxes consolidation processes to a greater extent than immediate testing, this is consistent with the view that failure in transferring information from temporary storage to a more permanent memory representation is a characteristic feature of the episodic impairment in preclinical AD (Bäckman and Small 1998). In addition, the greater deficits associated with recall, compared with recognition memory, suggest that retrieval deficits may also underlie the performance decrements seen in preclinical AD. However, it is important to reiterate that, the preclinical deficits were sizable and statistically significant across all episodic memory task conditions.

The results of the individual studies that have examined episodic memory in preclinical AD, as well as the results of the meta-analytis, suggest that impairments in binding of episodic memories are one of the many cognitive deficits associated with preclinical AD. Further evidence for the relevance of episodic memory binding in AD was reported by White and Ruske (2002). They demonstrated that initial discriminability values derived from the forgetting function of a delayed matching to sample test, a measure of encoding ability, was deficient among AD patients relative to controls. These authors argued for the importance of the cholinergic system in mediating these encoding deficits.

Neuroanatomical correlates of preclinical Alzheimer's disease

The importance of the cholinergic neurotransmitter system and associated brain regions in clinical and preclinical AD has been well documented (reviewed by Jagust 2000). For example, research has documented reduced volume of the hippocampus and entorhinal cortex early in the course of AD (Killiany *et al.* 2000; Fox *et al.* 2001). In addition, Gao *et al.* (2004) recently demonstrated that the linear width of the medial temporal lobe accurately discriminated between persons with mild AD and cognitively intact controls. Preclinical changes in the hippocampal complex are entirely consistent with the behavioural manifestations of preclinical AD in terms of the presence of significant episodic memory deficits. Considerable evidence is available from lesion studies (Squire 1992; Vargha-Khadem *et al.* 1997), structural imaging (Laakso *et al.* 1998), and functional imaging (reviewed by Cabeza and Nyberg 2000; Langley and Madden 2001), demonstrating the importance of these brain areas for successful episodic remembering.

Although the brain regions described above are relevant to the episodic memory deficit associated with preclinical AD, the results of our meta-analysis also demonstrated that the cognitive impairment in preclinical AD is more widespread. Thus it is becoming increasingly clear that brain structures other than those in the medial temporal lobe are also impacted preclinically. Specifically, volume reductions have been reported for the anterior cingulate gyrus (Killiany *et al.* 2000), the posterior cingulate gyrus and the neocortical tempororparietal regions (Fox *et al.* 2001), as well as for the frontal regions (van der Flier *et al.* 2002). Further, changes in brain structure and metabolism have been observed on more global measures, such as an increase in white matter hyperintensities (Wolf *et al.* 2000) and a reduction of whole-brain glucose metabolism (Silverman *et al.* 2001). Obviously, the fact that many brain regions and functions are implicated in preclinical AD is consistent with the observation of a global cognitive impairment.

Prognostic value of preclinical cognitive deficits

In this chapter we have clearly demonstrated that persons who go on to receive a diagnosis of AD are different across a variety of cognitive ability measures compared with individuals who remain non-demented. However, in these studies, the evaluation of cognitive performance, with respect to whether preclinical cognitive deficits were present, is retrospective to the point at which the clinical outcome (AD, non-demented) was established. A more interesting issue is the extent to which performance on the cognitive ability measures serves as a prognostic marker of diagnostic outcome. Unfortunately, our ability to identify people at risk of developing AD in the future is not yet exact. For example, in our study of 15 preclinical AD cases and 105 persons who remained free of dementia, the sensitivity of the diagnosis based upon performance on tests of episodic memory was rather poor, with only four of the 15 AD cases identified correctly for a sensitivity value of 27 per cent, although the specificity of the tests in correctly identifying dementia-free participants was quite good at 98.1 per cent (103/105)

Thus a relevant question concerns how we might improve our ability to identify persons prognostically. Many perspectives of episodic memory binding have been discussed in this book. We argue that adopting a multifaceted approach to the identification of preclinical AD cases is also very important. By using brain-based information about differences between persons who will or will not go on to develop AD, we may be able to increase our accuracy of classification. Indeed, Marquis *et al.* (2002) reported that a measure of memory performance and an indicator of hippocampal volume discriminated well between persons who would or would not go on to develop AD. Future approaches with respect to the identification of individuals at risk may benefit from the inclusion of multiple risk factors (e.g. genetic predisposition, hypertension, head trauma, low education) and early markers (e.g. depressive symptoms, family reports of cognitive impairment).Such hybrid disease prediction models would also allow the examination of potential interactive effects between different factors in signalling AD development at the earliest possible time (Bäckman *et al.* 2005).

Conclusions

In this chapter we have provided evidence for cognitive impairment across multiple domains of functioning during the preclinical phase of AD. With respect to episodic memory performance, deficits were observed globally as well as across multiple task conditions. In all cases, persons who would go on to develop AD were deficient in tasks that placed demands upon retrieval of materials as well as tasks that varied encoding conditions. The results demonstrate that episodic memory is just one of many preclinical cognitive deficits and this translates to observations of widespread involvement of multiple brain regions preclinically.

Acknowledgements

The preparation of this chapter was supported by grants to Lars Bäckman from the Swedish Research Council and the Swedish Council for Working Life and Social Research.

References

Albert, M.S., Moss, M.B., Tanzi, R., and Jones, K. (2001). Preclinical prediction of AD using neuropsychological tests. *Journal of the International Neuropsychological Society*, **7**, 631–639.

Almkvist, O., Fratiglioni, L, Agüero-Torres, H., Viitanen, M., and Bäckman, L. (1999). Cognitive support at episodic encoding and retrieval: similar patterns of utilization in community-based samples of Alzheimer's disease and vascular dementia patients. *Journal of Clinical and Experimental Neuropsychology*, **21**, 816–830.

Bäckman, L. and Herlitz, A. (1996). Knowledge and memory in Alzheimer's disease: a relationship that exists. In *The Cognitive Neuropsychology of Alzheimer-Type Dementia* (ed R.G. Morris). Oxford: Oxford University Press, pp. 89–104.

Bäckman, L. and Small, B.J. (1998). Influences of cognitive support on episodic remembering: tracing the process of loss from normal aging to Alzheimer's disease. *Psychology and Aging*, **13**, 267–276.

Bäckman, L., Mäntylä, T., and Herlitz, A. (1990). The optimization of episodic remembering in old age. In *Successful Ageing: Perspectives from the Behavioural Sciences* (ed P.B. Baltes and M.M. Baltes). Cambridge: Cambridge University Press, pp. 118–163.

Bäckman, L., Small, B.J., and Fratiglioni, L. (2001a). Stability of the preclinical episodic memory deficit in Alzheimer's disease. *Brain*, **124**, 96–102.

Bäckman, L., Small, B.J., and Wahlin, Å. (2001b). Aging and memory: cognitive and biological perspectives. In *Handbook of the Psychology of Aging* (5th edn) (ed J.E. Birren and K.W. Schaie). San Diego, CA: Academic Press, pp. 349–377.

Bäckman, L., Jones, S., Berger, A.-K, Jonsson Laukka, E., and Small, B.J. (2005). Cognitive impairment in preclinical Alzheimer's disease: a meta-analysis. *Neuropsychology*, **19**, 520–531.

Bondi, M.W., Salmon, D.P., Galasko, D., Thomas, R.-G, and Thal, L.J. (1999). Neuropsychological function and apolipoprotein E genotype in the preclinical detection of Alzheimer's disease. *Psychology and Aging*, **14**, 295–303.

Brookmeyer, R., Gray, S., and Kawas, C. (1998). Projections of Alzheimer's disease in the United States and the public health impact of delaying disease onset. *American Journal of Public Health*, **88**, 1337–1342.

Cabeza, R. and Nyberg, L. (2000). Imaging cognition. II: An empirical review of 275 PET and fMRI studies. *Journal of Cognitive Neuroscience*, **12**, 1–47.

Celsis, P., Agniel, A., Cardebat, D., Demonet, J.F., Ousset, P.J., and Puel, M. (1997). Age-related cognitive decline: a clinical entity? A longitudinal study of cerebral blood flow and memory performance. *Journal of Neurology, Neurosurgery, and Psychiatry*, **62**, 601–608.

Chen, P., Ratcliff, G., Belle, S.H., Cauley, J.A., DeKosky, S.T., and Ganguli, M. (2001). Patterns of cognitive decline in pre-symptomatic Alzheimer's disease: a prospective community study. *Archives of General Psychiatry*, **58**, 853–858.

DeKosky, S.T. and Marek, K. (2003). Looking backward to move forward: early detection of neurodegenerative disorders. *Science*, **302**, 830–834.

Elias, M.F., Beiser, A., Wolf, P.A., Au, R., White, R.F., and D¥Agostino, R.B. (2000). The preclinical phase of Alzheimer's disease: a 22-year prospective study of the Framingham cohort. *Archives of Neurology*, **57**, 808–813.

Fabrigoule, C., Lafont, S., Letenneur, L., Rouch, I., and Dartigues, J. F. (1996). WAIS similarities subtest performances as predictors of dementia in elderly community residents. *Brain and Cognition*, **30**, 323–326.

Fabrigoule, C., Rouch, I., Taberly, A., *et al.* (1998). Cognitive processes in preclinical phase of dementia. *Brain*, **121**, 135–141.

Flicker, L. (1999). Acetylcholinesterase inhibitors for Alzheimer's disease. *British Medical Journal*, **318**, 615–616.

Folstein, M.F., Folstein, S.E., and McHugh, P.R. (1975). 'Mini-Mental State': a practical method for grading the cognitive state of patients for the clinician. *Journal of Psychiatric Research*, **12**, 189–198.

Fowler, K S., Saling, M.M., Conway, E.L., Semple, J.M., and Louis, W.J. (2002). Paired-associate performance in the early detection of DAT. *Journal of the International Neuropsychological Society*, **8**, 58–71.

Fox, N.C., Crum, W.R., Scahill, R.I., Stevens, J.M., Janssen, J.C., and Rossor, M.N. (2001). Imaging of onset and progression of Alzheimer's disease with voxel-compression mapping of serial magnetic resonance images. *Lancet*, **358**, 201–205.

Gao, F.Q., Black, S.E., Leibovitch, F.S., Callen, D.J., Rockel, C.P., and Szalai, J.P. (2004). Linear width of the medial temporal lobe can discriminate Alzheimer's disease from normal aging: the Sunnybrook Dementia Study. *Neurobiology of Aging*, **25**, 441–448.

Goldman, W.P., Price, J.L., Storandt, M., *et al.* (2001) Absence of cognitive impairment or decline in preclinical Alzheimer's disease. *Neurology*, **56**, 361–367.

Hebert, L.E., Scherr, P.A., Bienias, J.L., Bennett, D.A., and Evans, D.A. (2003). Alzheimer disease in the US population: prevalence estimates using the 2000 census. *Archives of Neurology*, **60**, 1119–1122.

Howieson, D.B., Dame, A., Camicioli, R., Sexton, G., Payami, H., and Kaye, J.A. (1997). Cognitive markers preceding Alzheimer's dementia in the healthy oldest old. *Journal of the American Geriatrics Society*, **45**, 584–589.

Huang, C., Wahlund, L., and Dierks, T. (2000). Discrimination of Alzheimer's disease and mild cognitive impairment by equivalent EEG sources: a cross-sectional and longitudinal study. *Clinical Neurophysiology*, **11**, 1961–1967.

Jacobs, D.M., Sano, M., Dooneief, G., Marder, K., Bell, K.L., and Stern, Y. (1995). Neuropsychological detection and characterization of preclinical Alzheimer's disease. *Neurology*, **45**, 317–324.

Jagust, W.J. (2000). Neuroimaging in dementia. *Neurologic Clinics*, **18**, 885–897.

Killiany, R.J., Gomez-Isla, T., Moss, M., *et al.* (2000). Imaging to predict who will get Alzheimer's disease. *Annals of Neurology*, **47**, 430–439.

Laakso, M.P., Soininen, H., Partanen, K., *et al.* (1997). MRI of the hippocampus in Alzheimer's disease: Sensitivity, specificity, and analysis of the incorrectly classified subjects. *Neurobiology of Aging*, **19**, 23–31.

Lange, K.L., Bondi, M.W., Salmon, D.P., *et al.* (2002). Decline in verbal memory during preclinical Alzheimer's disease: examination of the effect of APOE genotype. *Journal of the International Neuropsychological Society*, **8**, 943–955.

Langley, L.K. and Madden, D.J. (2000). Functional neuroimaging of memory: Implications for cognitive aging. *Microscopy Research and Technique*, **51**, 75–84.

Linn, R.T., Wolf, P.A., Bachman, D.L., *et al.* (1995). The 'preclinical phase' of probable Alzheimer's disease. *Archives of Neurology*, **52**, 485–490.

Marquis, S., Moore, M.M., Howieson, D.B., *et al.* (2002). Independent predictors of cognitive decline in healthy elderly persons. *Archives of Neurology*, **59**, 601–606.

Masur, D.M., Sliwinski, M., Lipton, R.B, Blau, A.D., and Crystal, H.A. (1994). Neuropsychological prediction of dementia and the absence of dementia in healthy elderly persons. *Neurology*, **44**, 1427–1432.

Rockwood, K., Wallack, M., and Tallis, R. (2003). The treatment of Alzheimer's disease: success short of cure. *Lancet Neurology*, **2**, 630–633.

Rubin, E.H., Storandt, M., Miller, J.P., *et al.* (1998). A prospective study of cognitive function and onset of dementia in cognitively healthy elders. *Archives of Neurology*, **55**, 395–401.

Silverman, D.H.S., Small, G.W., Chang, C.Y., *et al.* (2001). Positron emission tomography in evaluation of dementia: Regional brain metabolism and long-term outcome. *Journal of the American Medical Association*, **286**, 2120–2127.

Small, B.J., Herlitz, A., Fratiglioni, L., Almkvist, O., and Bäckman, L. (1997a). Cognitive predictors of incident Alzheimer's disease: a prospective longitudinal study. *Neuropsychology*, **11**, 413–420.

Small, B.J., Viitanen, M., and Bäckman, L. (1997b). Mini-Mental State Examination item scores as predictors of Alzheimer's disease: incidence data from the Kungsholmen project, Stockholm. *Journal of Gerontology: Medical Sciences*, **52**, 299–304.

Small, B.J., Fratiglioni, L., Viitanen, M., Winblad, B., and Bäckman, L. (2000). The course of cognitive impairment in preclinical Alzheimer's disease: 3- and 6-year follow-up of a population-based sample. *Archives of Neurology*, **57**, 839–844.

Squire, L.R. (1992). Memory and the hippocampus: a synthesis from findings with rats, monkeys, and humans. *Psychological Review*, **99**, 195–231.

Tierney, M.C., Szalai, J.P., Dunn, E., Geslani, D., and McDowell, I. (2000). Prediction of probable Alzheimer disease in patients with symptoms suggestive of memory impairment. *Archives of Family Medicine*, **9**, 527–532.

van der Flier, W.M., van den Heuvel, D.M.J., Weverling-Rijnsburger, A.W.E., *et al.* (2002). Cognitive decline in AD and mild cognitive impairment is associated with global brain damage. *Neurology*, **59**, 874–879.

Vargha-Khadem, F., Gadian, D.G., Watkins, K.E., Connelly, A., Van Paesschen, W., and Mishkin, M. (1997). Differential effects of early hippocampal lesions on episodic and semantic memory. *Science*, **277**, 376–380.

Visser, P.J., Verhey, F.R., Ponds, R.W., and Jolles, J. (2001). Diagnosis of preclinical Alzheimer's disease in a clinical setting. *International Psychogeriatrics*, **13**, 411–423.

White, K.G. and Ruske, A.C. (2002). Memory deficits in Alzheimer's disease: the encoding hypothesis and cholinergic function. *Psychonomic Bulletin and Review*, **9**, 426–437.

Wolf, H., Ecke, G.M., Bettin, S., Dietrich, J., and Gertz, H.J. (2000). Do white matter changes contribute to the subsequent development of dementia in patients with mild cognitive impairment? A longitudinal study. *International Journal of Geriatric Psychiatry*, **15**, 803–812.

Index